2025
全国医学博士英语统考
词汇巧战通关 第16版

环球卓越医学考博命题研究中心 / 组编
梁莉娟　张秀峰 / 主编

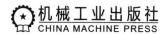

机械工业出版社
CHINA MACHINE PRESS

本书是全国医学博士英语统一考试辅导丛书之一。

本书充分考虑了医学考博考生时间紧张、战线长、攻克考试难度大等特点,为考生提供的词汇备考方案突出一个"巧"字。我们将医学考博词汇按难易程度和考查范畴分为六大部分,前五部分是词汇单元,第六部分是词组搭配。五个词汇单元为:基础词汇、核心意义词汇(A-K)、核心意义词汇(L-Z)、低频词汇和医学专用词汇。可以说,这是一本不可多得的高效且人性化的医学词汇书,不仅可用作备考复习的资料,而且在平时的工作中也是很实用的工具书。

图书在版编目(CIP)数据

全国医学博士英语统考词汇巧战通关 / 环球卓越医学考博命题研究中心组编;梁莉娟,张秀峰主编. 16版. -- 北京:机械工业出版社, 2024.8. --(卓越医学考博英语应试教材). -- ISBN 978-7-111-76636-0

Ⅰ. R

中国国家版本馆CIP数据核字第2024E06M78号

机械工业出版社(北京市百万庄大街22号 邮政编码100037)
策划编辑:孙铁军　　责任编辑:孙铁军　苏筛琴
责任校对:夏晓琳　　责任印制:单爱军
保定市中画美凯印刷有限公司印刷
2024年9月第16版第1次印刷
148mm×210mm・16.5印张・2插页・1078千字
标准书号:ISBN 978-7-111-76636-0
定价:60.00元

电话服务	网络服务
客服电话:010-88361066	机 工 官 网:www.cmpbook.com
010-88379833	机 工 官 博:weibo.com/cmp1952
010-68326294	金　书　网:www.golden-book.com
封底无防伪标均为盗版	机工教育服务网:www.cmpedu.com

丛书序
PREFACE

这是一套由全国知名医学博士英语统考培训机构"环球卓越"（优路教育旗下品牌）策划，联手医学博士英语资深辅导专家，为众多志在考取医学博士的考生量身定制的应试辅导用书。国家医学考试中心于2019年底修订了考试大纲，对全国医学博士外语统一考试的题型及各部分分值进行了局部调整。新大纲仍然设置了听力对话、听力短文、词语用法、完形填空、阅读理解和书面表达6种题型，但调整了具体命题形式，其中听力部分变化最大。"15个短对话+1个长对话+2个短文"的经典组合成为历史，从2020年开始，"5个短对话+5个小短文"的搭配将在很长一段时间内成为考生要面对的题型。考试时间为3个小时（含播放录音及收发卷时间）。

考纲的变化并未改变对考生能力的考查方向，因此为了帮助广大考生在较短的时间内系统备考，在听、说、读、写4个方面得到强化训练，全面提高英语应用和交际能力，顺利通过考试，本套"卓越医学考博英语应试教材"仍然是广大考生朋友们很好的选择。本丛书紧密结合最近几年卫生部组织的医学博士英语统一考试命题情况，针对最新考试大纲进行了修订，并针对新题型编写了大量针对性练习。本丛书包含《全国医学博士英语统考词汇巧战通关》《全国医学博士英语统考综合应试教程》《全国医学博士英语统考实战演练》三本传统综合分册，《医学考博阅读理解高分全解》《医学考博英语听力28天训练计划》两本专项分册，以及《18天攻克医学考博英语核心词》的单词小分册。传统分册从基础到综合再到真题实战，从模块详解到全套试题，高屋建瓴，逐步推进。阅读专项分册对分值较高的阅读理解进行字、词、句、语篇的详解和训练，从技术（语言知识）到技巧（做题方法），精讲多练。听力专项分册则根据听力训练的规律和考试考查目标，按天设置训练内容，分解目标，逐步达成最终目标。

本丛书的特点如下：

一、紧贴考试，实用性强

策划编写本丛书的作者常年在教学一线授课，从基础英语到医博考前辅导，积累了大量的应试辅导实战经验。丛书内容是他们多年辅导经验的提炼和结晶，实用性非常强，专为医学考博考生定制，是目前市面上较全面、系统的医学考博英语应试教材。

二、紧扣大纲，直击真题

本丛书紧扣最新大纲，体例设置与大纲保持一致；各部分考点紧密结合最新历年真题，还原真实考场环境，命题思路分析透彻，重点突出，讲解精确；各部分内容严格控制在大纲规定的范围之内，让考生准确把握考试的重点、难点及命题趋势。

三、内容精练，讲练结合

传统分册《全国医学博士英语统考词汇巧战通关》《全国医学博士英语统考综合应试教程》和《全国医学博士英语统考实战演练》简单精练，通过突破词汇基础关、学习各种题型应试方法以及在高质量实战中历练，考生可在有限的时间内进行全面复习，把握重点，比较系统地完成考前准备。阅读分册《医学考博阅读理解高分全解》则是根据考生的具体情况，分模块予以详解，提升基础，总结技巧，各个击破。听力专项《医学考博英语听力28天训练计划》则专练听力，循序渐进，按天分配学习任务，力争高分。核心词汇专项《18天攻克医学考博英语核心词》在使用词频软件完整统计近十年全套真题的基础上，将该统计结果和大纲词汇进行比较，最后确定出记忆任务的内容和安排。按天设置，不断重复。

四、超值服务，锦上添花

本丛书附带赠送精品服务，由优路教育为每位购书读者提供专业的服务和强大的技术支持。具体为：

1. 《医学考博英语听力28天训练计划》附赠内容：优路教育"2025年医学考博（统考）《英语听力28天训练计划》图书赠课英语（20节）"网络视频课程。使用方法：刮开书籍封底的兑换码，扫描书籍封底二维码关注【优路医学考试】微信公众账号后，点击【兑换课程】–【点击这里兑换课程】的链接，输入兑换码，输入姓名手机号，将自动跳转至您的课程页，开始观看课程。后续看课路径：关注【优路医学考试】服务号，在底部菜单栏【我要学习】–【我的课程】查看课程。（可通过扫描文末二维码，关注后兑换课程）

2. 《18天攻克医学考博英语核心词》附赠内容：优路教育"2025年医学考博（统考）《18天攻克医学考博英语核心词》图书赠课英语（20节）"网络视频课程。使用方法：刮开书籍封底的兑换码，扫描书籍封底二维码关注【优路医学考试】微信公众账号后，点击【兑换课程】–【点击这里兑换课程】的链接，输入兑换码，输入姓名手机号，将自动跳转至您的课程页，开始观看课程。后续看课路径：关注【优路医学考试】服务号，在底部菜单栏【我要学习】–【我的课程】查看课程。（可通过扫描文末二维码，关注后兑换课程）

3. 《全国医学博士英语统考实战演练》附赠内容：优路教育"2025年医学考博（统考）《实战演练》图书赠课英语（10节）"网络视频课程。使用方法：刮开书籍封底的兑换码，扫描书籍封底二维码关注【优路医学考试】微信公众账号后，点击【兑换课程】–【点击这里兑换课程】的链接，输入兑换码，输入姓名手机号，将自动跳转至您的课程页，开始观看课程。后续看课路径：关注【优路医学考试】服务号，在底部菜单栏【我要学习】–【我的课程】查看课程。（可通过扫描文末二维码，关注后兑换课程）

4. 《全国医学博士英语统考综合应试教程》附赠内容：优路教育"2025年医学考博（统考）《综合应试教程》图书赠课英语（10节）"网络视频课程。使用方法：刮开书籍封底的兑换码，扫描书籍封底二维码关注【优路医学考试】微信公众账号后，点击【兑换课程】–【点击这里兑换课程】的链接，输入兑换码，输入姓名手机号，将自动跳转至您的课程页，开始观看课程。后续看课路径：关注【优路医学考试】服务号，在底部菜单栏【我要学习】-【我的课程】查看课程。（可通过扫描文末二维码，关注后兑换课程）

5.《全国医学博士英语统考综词汇巧战通关》附赠内容：优路教育"2025年医学考博（统考）《词汇巧战通关》图书赠课【学习卡】英语（10节）"网络视频课程。使用方法：刮开书籍封底的兑换码，扫描书籍封底二维码关注【优路医学考试】微信公众账号后，点击【兑换课程】-【点击这里兑换课程】的链接，输入兑换码，输入姓名手机号，将自动跳转至您的课程页，开始观看课程。后续看课路径：关注【优路医学考试】服务号，在底部菜单栏【我要学习】-【我的课程】查看课程。（可通过扫描文末二维码，关注后兑换课程）

6.《医学考博阅读理解高分全解》附赠内容：优路教育"2025年医学考博（统考）《阅读理解高分全解》图书赠课【学习卡】英语（8节）"网络视频课程。使用方法：刮开书籍封底的兑换码，扫描书籍封底二维码关注【优路医学考试】微信公众账号后，点击【兑换课程】-【点击这里兑换课程】的链接，输入兑换码，输入姓名手机号，将自动跳转至您的课程页，开始观看课程。后续看课路径：关注【优路医学考试】服务号，在底部菜单栏【我要学习】-【我的课程】查看课程。（可通过扫描文末二维码，关注后兑换课程）

优路教育技术支持及服务热线400-8835-981，可以帮您解决兑换及观看课程中的技术问题。您也可以登录优路教育网站www.youlu.com，在"医学博士英语"栏目下获取更多的学习资料和资讯。

编　者

2024年5月于北京

扫码关注后兑换课程

前言
FOREWORD

　　本书是全国医学博士英语统一考试辅导丛书之一。结合今年考试中词汇的分布情况，本次进行了较大幅度修订。

　　本次修订不仅充分考虑了医学博士考生时间紧张、战线长、攻克考试难度大等特点，同时结合近年考试中词汇考查的重点及难点分布规律，将医学考博词汇按难易程度和考查范畴调整为基础词汇、核心意义词汇、低频词汇和医学专用词汇，便于考生根据自身的英语水平和复习时间选择合适有效的复习策略。英语水平较高的读者可以重点复习高频词汇；医学专用词汇不适合背诵记忆，只是在考试复习时便于术语的查找，同时也可成为工作中的好帮手。

　　本书进行了大幅度的修订。首先，对基础词汇进行了分层，分成"活跃基础词汇"和"普通基础词汇"，前者具有重要的表意功能和结构功能，构成了各类英语考试中最重要的框架，修订时予以详解且配套讲解视频，以帮助考生夯实基础，后者则是用法简单、意义单一的基础词，出现频率较低，修订时用表格形式展示，简单清楚。其次，按照是否具有常见意义的标准对核心意义词汇进行了精简。没有较为重要意义的单词被删除，或被挪至低频词汇部分，供考生学有余力时复习。最后，增加了低频词汇的词条。这样一来，复习重点变得精炼，减少了考生的复习范围，主次更加清晰，难易更加明确，在结构上更有利于考生合理分配复习时间和精力。本次修订中增加视频讲解作为辅助，考生可以得到更为明确的指导，使得本书更具应试性。本次修订后，该书具有以下特点：

1. 基础详解，真正打牢应试基底

本次修订删除了与考试题型较为脱节的测试部分，用大量篇幅来详解搭建考试框架的积极基础词汇。通过对近十年真题词汇词频的统计发现，超高频考试词汇几乎都是考生容易忽略的基础词，但这些词无论从意义上还是结构上，都是测试内容的核心基础。因此本次修订对基础部分全面推翻，重新布局，既保证对此类功能基础词的讲解透彻，同时用表格罗列简单基础词，让考生从基础部分便充满信心。

2. 等级分明，有效把握复习重点

正文划分为三个等级：基础词汇、核心意义词汇、低频词汇。核心意义词汇是考试频率较高且常用的词汇，更需要考生关注其用法。低频词汇收录的是较为生僻复现率低的单词，考生时间不充裕时，可忽略本部分。本书对各部分重点词汇给出了经典例题和经典例句。另外，英语中有许多特殊用法、习惯搭配和重要语法等考点，本书在相关词条下设有【名师导学】栏目，虽寥寥数语，却能一针见血地解开许多考生百思不解的疑惑。【名师导学】栏目中增加了"近义词"内容，不仅便于考生扩大词汇量，而且直击考试中的词汇考题，迅速提分。【经典例句】和【经典例题】用来展示重点词汇的用法及在考试中出现的形式。例句或者例题大多出自历年真题，以帮助考生将词汇复习与考试有机结合起来。考生在分级学习的基础上，还可将本书作为工具书使用，查找会更方便。

通过本书附录中的"考博英语常见同义词一览表"，考生能从容应对词汇考题中的同义词替换部分，同时扩展词汇量。

3. 专业突出，科学掌握医学专用词汇

医学专业词汇在医学考博中至关重要，是考生不容忽视的。本书将医学专业词汇进行了全面完善的整理、归类和扩充，对常见单词的普通含义及医学含义进行了对比归类，便于考生尽快熟悉并掌握专业词汇，也可供考生平时工作中理解医学英语时速查之用。

4. 记忆有方，快速攻克词汇堡垒

本书词汇充分发挥【联想记忆】的功效，运用前后缀、联想记忆等方法，采用以词带词的编排方式，让考生开阔视野，举一反三，成串记忆，横向扩充词汇量。另外，本书还给出了很多【巧记】方法，通俗易懂，生动形象，能够有效地帮助考生快速记忆词汇。同时，全书词汇均有外教朗读的录音作为配套，跟随正确的发音，对于医学专用词汇，尤为重要，恰当利用本书录音，可使记忆事半功倍。

由于编者水平有限，书中错误之处在所难免，敬请同行和广大读者批评指正！

编　者

2024年6月于北京

目 录
CONTENTS

丛书序
前　言

常见词缀	001
第一部分　基础词汇	009
活跃基础词汇	010
普通基础词汇	083
第二部分　核心意义词汇（A-K）	091
第三部分　核心意义词汇（L-Z）	233
第四部分　低频词汇	349
第五部分　医学专用词汇	391
第六部分　词组搭配	423
附　　录	483
考博英语常见同义词一览表	483
高频词复习检测表	507

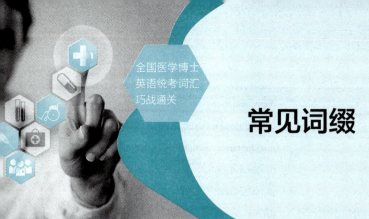

常见词缀

一个英语单词，通过增加前缀、后缀或者另一个单词，便能构成大量新词，这就是我们常常提到的构词法。英语词汇浩瀚无边，如果我们靠死记硬背，恐怕连常用的单词都记不完，记住了含义也没有用，因为单词通过增加前缀和后缀，不仅能改变词义，还能改变词性，而单词的词性在句法中又至关重要。前缀可以增加、改变或加强一个单词的意义，有少数的前缀也可以改变单词的词性，后缀则更多地决定一个单词的词性。因此我们常常将后缀分为名词后缀、动词后缀、形容词后缀和副词后缀。

前缀和后缀数量有限，常用的也就 100 多个，但由这些常用词缀构成的单词数量却是相当庞大的。因此对于复习备考的考生来讲，掌握必要的构词法十分必要。同时，因为篇幅所限，本书（恐怕任何一本词汇书都如此）仅会列出某个单词最常见的词性形式，其他形式则需要读者通过构词法在运用中自行辨认。

下面我们就将常见的词缀分门别类地进行展示。

常见的前缀

1. 表示否定意义的前缀

a-, an-	amoral, anarchy, anonymous, asymmetry（不对称）
dis-	disadvantage, disgrace, dishonest, dislike, distract
in-, il-, im-, ir-	independent, indifferent, indispensable, invalid; illegal, illiterate; impossible, immortal; irregular, irrelevant

001

（续）

non-	nonfiction, nonsense
un-	unable, unemployment
male-, mal-	maladjustment, malfunction, malnutrition
mis-, 表示"错误的"	misfortune, mislead, mistake, mistreat
pseudo-, 表示"假的"	pseudoscience
de-, 表示"反向的"	deform, degenerate, degrade, devalue
dis-, 表示"反向"动作	disable, disapprove, disarm, discharge, discourage, discover, disconnect
anti-, ant-, 表示"对立的"	antiaircraft, antiknock, antiforeign, anticlockwise
contra-, contro-, 表示"对立的"	contradiction, controflow（逆流）
counter-, 表示"对立的"	counteraction, counterattack, countermeasure

2. 表示空间位置、方向关系的前缀

circum-, circu-, 表示"周围, 环绕"	circumlunar, circumpolar, circumstance; circuit
de-, 表示"在下方, 向下"	decapitate, deduce, depress, descend
en-, em, 表示"在内部, 进入"	encage, enclose, endanger; embed（埋入, 嵌入）
ex-, ec-, es-, 表示"外部, 外"	exceed, exclude, exit, expose, export; eclipse
in-, il-, im-, ir-, 表示"向内, 在内"	inborn, include, income, inland, invade, inside; illumine; immigrate, implant, import; irrigate
inter-, intel-, 表示"在……间, 相互"	interchange, interlude, international, interaction, interview, intellectual
intra-, intro-, 表示"向内, 在内部"	intra-school; introduce
medi-, med-, mid-, 表示"中, 中间"	Mediterranean; media; midline, midwife
out-, 表示"在上面, 在外部"	outline, outside, outward
over-, 表示"在上面, 在外部"	overlook, overhead, overboard, overpass
pre-, 表示"在前, 在前面"	prefix, preface（前言）, preposition
pro-, 表示"在前, 向前"	proceed, proclaim, progress, prolong
re-, 表示"向后"	recede
super-, sur-, 表示"在……之上"	superficial, superstructure; surface

3. 表示时间、序列关系的前缀

ante-, anti-, 表示"先前,早于,预先"	antecedent, antemeridian; anticipate
ex-, 表示"先,故,旧"	expresident, ex-husband
fore-, 表示"在前面,先前,前面"	forecast, forefather, foreknowledge, foresee, foresight, foretell, foretime
post-, 表示"在后,后"	postdoctoral, postgraduate, postlude
pre-, pri-, 表示"在前,事先,预先"	preface（前言）, preheat, prelude, prejudice, preview, prewar, prehistory
pro-, 表示"在前,先,前"	prologue（开场白）, prophet（预言家）
re-, 表示"再一次,重新"	recall, reform, retell, review, rewrite

4. 表示比较程度、差别关系的前缀

by-, 表示"副,次要的"	byproduct, by-talk（闲话）, bywork（副业,兼职）
extra-, 表示"超越"	extrajudicial, extraordinary, extrasensory
hyper-, 表示"超过,极度"	hypersonic（超声速的）, hypertension（高血压）
out-, 表示"超过,过分"	outbid（出价高于……）, outlaw, outlive, outnumber
sub-, suc-, sur-, 表示"低,次,副,亚"	subdivide, subordinate, subtropical（亚热带）, subtitle
super-, sur-, 表示"超过"	supernature, superpower; surplus, surpass
under-, 表示"不足"	underdeveloped, underestimate, undergrown
vice-, 表示"副,次"	vice-chairman, vice-minister, vice-president

5. 表示"共同,相等"意思的前缀

com-, col-, cop-, con-, cor-, co-, 表示"共同,一起"	combine, commemorate, compress, colleague, copious, contemporary, correlation, coexist, cooperate
syn-, syl-, sym-, 表示"同,共,和,类"	synonym, sympathy, symphony

6. 表示"分离,离开"意思的前缀

a-, ab-, abs-, 表示"分离,离开"	away, apart; abstract; abstain（弃权）
de-, 表示"离去,除去"	depart, decolour
dis-, di-, dif-, 表示"分离,离开"	disarm（缴械）, distract; divorce
for-, 表示"离开,脱离"	forget, forgive
se-, 表示"分离,隔离"	seduce, select, seclude（隐居）, separate

7. 表示加强意思的前缀

a–, alike, amaze, arouse; ad–, adjoin, adhere（黏附）

8. 表示变换词类作用的前缀

| be-, 动词前缀 | befool, befriend, belittle |
| en-, 动词前缀 | enable, enslave, enrich |

9. 表示数量关系的前缀

mon-, uni-, un-, 表示"单一"	monotone（单调），monopoly, monarch; uniform, unicellular（单细胞），unanimous
ambi-, bi-, di-, twi-, 表示"二，两，双"	ambiguous, amphibian（两栖动物）; bicycle, bilateral, bilingual, bimonthly, biweekly; dioxide, diploma; twin
tri-, 表示"三"	triangle, tricycle, trilateral
quadr(i)-, 表示"四"	quadrennial
penta-, 表示"五"	pentagon
hexa-, 表示"六"	hexagon, hexagram
sept-, 表示"七"	septangle
octa-, octo-, 表示"八"	octopus
deca, deci-, 表示"十，十分之一"	decade, decimals
hecto-, hect-, centi-, 表示"百，百分之一"	hectometer; centimeter
kilo-, centi-, 表示"千，千分之一"	kilometer
myria-, mega-, meg-, 表示"万，万分之一"	megabyte
multi-, 表示"多"	multilingual, multiply, multipurpose
poly-, 表示"许多"	polycentric, polysyllable
hemi-, semi-, pene-, pen-, 表示"半，一半"	hemisphere; semiconductor, semitransparent; peninsula

10. 表示特殊意义的前缀

arch-, 表示"首位的，第一的，主要的"	architect, archbishop
auto-, 表示"自己，独立，自动"	automobile, autobiography
bene-, 表示"善，福"	benefit
eu-, 表示"优，美好"	euphemism
macro-, 表示"大，宏大"	macroscopic（宏观的）
magni-, 表示"大"	magnificent
micro-, 表示"微"	microscope

11. 表示术语的前缀

aud-, 表示"听，声"	audience
bio-, 表示"生命，生物"	biology
ge-, 表示"地球，大地"	geography
phon-, 表示"声，音调"	phonograph
tele-, 表示"远离"	television, telephone

常见的后缀

1. 名词后缀

○ 具有某种职业或动作的人

-an, -ian, 表示"……地方的人，精通……的人"	American, historian
-al, 表示"具有……职务的人"	principal
-ant, -ent, 表示"……者"	merchant, servant; agent
-arian, 表示"……派别的人，……主义的人"	humanitarian, vegetarian
-ate, 表示"具有……职责的人"	candidate, graduate
-crat, 表示"某种政体、主义的支持者"	democrat, bureaucrat
-ee, 表示"动作承受者"	employee, examinee
-eer, 表示"从事……的人"	engineer, volunteer
-er, 表示"从事某种职业的人，某地的人"	banker, observer, Londoner, villager
-ese, 表示"……国人，……地方的人"	Japanese, Cantonese
-ess, 表示阴性人称名词	actress, hostess, manageress
-ian, 表示"……地方的人，信仰……教的人，从事……职业的人"	Christian, physician（内科医生），musician
-icist, 表示"……家，……能手"	physicist
-ist, 表示"从事……研究者，信仰……主义者"	pianist, communist, dentist, artist, chemist
-logist, 表示"……学家，研究者"	biologist, geologist（地质学家）
-or, 表示"……者"	author, doctor, operator

○ 具有抽象含义的名词

-acy, 表示"性质，状态，境遇"	accuracy, diplomacy
-age, 表示"状态，行为，身份及其结果，总称"	courage, storage, marriage
-al, 表示"动作，过程"表示具体的事物	refusal, arrival, survival, denial, approval manual, signal, editorial, journal

（续）

◎具有抽象含义的名词

后缀	例词
-ance, -ence, 表示"性质, 状况, 行为, 过程, 总量, 程度"	endurance, importance; diligence, difference, obedience
-ancy, -ency, 表示"性质, 状态, 行为, 过程"	frequency, urgency, efficiency
-bility, 表示"动作, 性质, 状态"	possibility, feasibility
-craft, 表示"工艺, 技巧"	woodcraft, handicraft
-cracy, 表示"统治, 支配"	bureaucracy, democracy
-cy, 表示"性质, 状态, 职位, 级别"	bankruptcy（破产）, supremacy
-dom, 表示"等级, 领域, 状态"	freedom, kingdom, wisdom
-ery, -ry, 表示"行为, 状态, 习性"	bravery, bribery; rivalry
-ety, 表示"性质, 状态"	variety, dubiety（怀疑）
-faction, -facture, 表示"作成, ……化, 作用"	satisfaction; manufacture
-hood, 表示"资格, 身份, 年纪, 状态"	childhood, manhood, falsehood
-ice, 表示"行为, 性质, 状态"	notice, justice, service
-ine, 表示"带有抽象概念"	medicine, discipline, famine
-ing, 表示"动作的过程, 结果"	building, writing, learning
-ion, -sion, -tion, -ation, -ition, 表示"行为的过程, 结果, 状况"	action, solution, conclusion, destruction, expression, correction
-ism, 表示"制度, 主义, 学说, 信仰, 行为"	socialism, criticism, heroism
-ity, 表示"性质, 状态, 程度"	purity, reality, ability, calamity
-ment, 表示"行为, 状态, 手段及其结果"	treatment, movement, judgment, punishment, argument
-mony, 表示"动作的结果, 状态"	ceremony, testimony
-ness, 表示"性质, 状态, 程度"	kindness, tiredness, friendliness
-ship, 表示"情况, 性质, 技巧, 技能, 身份, 职业"	hardship, membership, friendship
-th, 表示"动作, 性质, 过程, 状态"	depth, wealth, truth, length, growth
-tude, 表示"性质, 状态, 程度"	latitude, altitude（海拔）
-ure, 表示"行为, 结果"	exposure, pressure, failure, procedure

◎具有"学术, 科技"含义

后缀	例词
-graphy, 表示"……学, 写法"	biography, calligraphy, geography
-ic, ics, 表示"……学, ……法"	logic; mechanics, optics, electronics
-ology, 表示"……学, ……论"	biology, zoology, technology
-nomy, 表示"……学, ……术"	astronomy, economy
-ry, 表示"学科, 技术"	chemistry, cookery, machinery

（续）

◎表示"细小"

-cle	particle
-cule	molecule（分子）
-el	parcel
-en	chicken, maiden
-ling	duckling
-let	booklet

2. 形容词后缀

◎具有"属性，倾向，相关"的含义

-able, -ible	movable, comfortable, applicable; visible, responsible
-al	natural, additional, educational
-an, ane	urban, suburban, republican
-ant, -ent	distant, important; excellent
-ar	similar, popular, regular
-ary	military, voluntary
-ic, -atic, ical	politic, historic; systematic; physical
-ine	masculine, feminine, marine
-ing	moving, touching, daring
-ish	foolish, bookish, selfish
-ive	active, impressive, decisive
-ory	satisfactory, compulsory
-il, -ile, -eel	fragile, genteel（文雅的）

◎表示"相像，类似"

-like	manlike, childlike
-ly	manly, fatherly, scholarly, motherly
-some	troublesome, handsome

◎表示"充分的"

-ful	beautiful, wonderful, helpful, truthful
-ous	dangerous, generous, courageous, various

（续）

◎表示方向	
-ern	eastern, western
-ward	downward, forward
◎表示国籍、语种、宗教	
-an	Roman, European
-ese	Chinese
-ish	English, Spanish
◎其他含义	
-less, 表示否定	countless, stainless, wireless

3. 动词后缀

-ize, -ise, 表示"做成，变成，……化"	modernize, organize
-en, 表示"使成为，引起，使有"	quicken, weaken, soften, harden
-fy, 表示"使……化，使成"	beautify, purify, intensify, signify, simplify
-ish, 表示"使，令"	finish, abolish, diminish, establish
-ate, 表示"成为……，处理，作用"	separate, operate, indicate

4. 副词后缀

-ly	possibly, swiftly, simply
-ward, -wards	downward, upward; inwards
-ways	always, sideways

第一部分
基础词汇

全国医学博士英语
统考词汇巧战通关

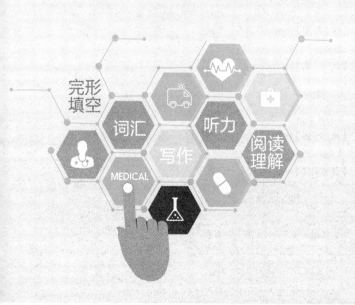

活跃基础词汇

☐ **ability** [əˈbiləti]	*n.* 能力；才能，才干 【同义词】capacity, capability, competence 【反义词】inability, incapacity 【固定搭配】of great/exceptional ability 能力卓越；of high/low/average ability 能力高/低/一般；to the best of one's ability 尽其所能
☐ **able** [ˈeɪbl]	*a.* 有能力的，能干的（比较级/最高级 abler/ablest） 【同义词】capable, competent, talented, efficient, qualified 【反义词】unable, incapable, incompetent, inefficient, unqualified 【固定搭配】be able to do sth. 能做，会做
☐ **about** [əˈbaʊt]	*prep.* 关于，对于；在……周围，在……附近 【同义词】concerning, regarding 【固定搭配】be about to（do）即将（不跟表示将来的时间状语）；go about doing sth.（着手）做某事；see about doing sth. 负责处理某事；What about doing...? ……怎么做？……好吗？（用于提出建议）How about doing...? 做……如何？come about 发生；成为现实；leave...about 到处乱放；turn about 向后转，转身过来；set about 着手处理，开始做
☐ **above** [əˈbʌv]	*prep.* 在……上面；超过 *a.* 上面的；上述的 *ad.* 在上面，以上 【固定搭配】above all 首先，尤其
☐ **accept** [əkˈsept]	*vt.* 同意，认可；接受，领受 【反义词】refuse, deny
☐ **acceptable** [əkˈseptəbl]	*a.* 可接受的；合意的
☐ **acceptance** [əkˈseptəns]	*n.* 接受，接纳；承认；赞同 【反义词】refusal
☐ **achieve** [əˈtʃiːv]	*vt.* 完成，达到；获得 【联想记忆】achievable *a.* 可完成的
☐ **achievement** [əˈtʃiːvmənt]	*n.* 完成，达到；成就，成绩
☐ **across** [əˈkrɒs]	*ad.* 横越，横断 *prep.* 在……对面

☐ **act** [ækt]	*n.* 行为，动作；（一）幕；法令，条例 *v.* 行动；起作用；表演 【固定搭配】act on/upon 按……行动，对……起作用，作用于；act as = serve as 担任，充当；act for 代理
☐ **action** ['ækʃən]	*n.* 行动；作用 【固定搭配】in action 在活动，在运转；out of action 失去作用；有故障；take action 采取行动；into action 实施，实行；actions speak louder than words 行动比言语更响亮，说得好不如做得好
☐ **active** ['æktiv]	*a.* 活动的，活跃的；积极的，主动的
☐ **add** [æd]	*vt.* 加，加上；增加，增进；进一步说/写 *vi.* 增添 【固定搭配】add to 增加，添加，补充；add (up) to = total (up) to 总计，等于；add fuel to the fire/flames 火上浇油
☐ **addition** [ə'diʃən]	*n.* 加，加法；附加部分，增加（物） 【联想记忆】additional *a.* 附加的，另加的，额外的 【固定搭配】in addition 另外；in addition to = apart/aside from 除……之外
☐ **admire** [əd'maiə]	*vt.* 羡慕，赞赏，钦佩 【联想记忆】admiration *n.* 钦佩，赞美，羡慕；admiring *a.* 赞赏的，羡慕的；admiringly *ad.* 羡慕地；admirable *a.* 值得赞赏的，令人羡慕的；admirer *n.* 钦佩者 【固定搭配】admire sb. for sth. 因某事敬佩某人
☐ **advertise/-ize** ['ædvətaiz]	*vt.* 做广告，宣传 【联想记忆】advertiser *n.* 广告商，广告公司；advertising *n.* 广告活动，广告业；advertisement *n.* 广告 【固定搭配】advertise sth. 为……做广告；advertise for... 登广告（公布，征聘）……
☐ **advice** [əd'vais]	*n.* 忠告，意见 【固定搭配】take/give advice 接受/给予建议；a piece of advice 一条建议；follow one's advice 遵从……建议/嘱咐；on one's advice 依照……的建议/嘱咐行事
☐ **advisable** [əd'vaizəbl]	*a.* 明智的，可取的 【固定搭配】It is advisable that... 最好……（从句中谓语动词用原形表示虚拟语气）
☐ **advise** [əd'vaiz]	*v.* 忠告，意见 【固定搭配】advise sb. to do sth. 建议某人做某事，接不定式；advise doing sth. 建议做某事，接动名词；advise sb. (of sth.) 通知，正式告知
☐ **affair** [ə'fɛə]	*n.* 事，事情，事件
☐ **after** ['ɑ:ftə]	*prep./conj.* 在……之后 *ad.* 以后，后来 【固定搭配】after all 毕竟，虽然这样；after a while 过了一会儿；be after = look for 探求，寻找；look after 照管；one after another 一个接一个地；take after 长得像，性格上像
☐ **against** [ə'genst, ə'geinst]	*prep.* 对（着），逆；反对，违反；靠，靠近；和……对比

age
[eidʒ]

n. 年龄；时代　*vi.* 变老

【固定搭配】at the age of 在……岁的时候；for ages 长期；the aged 老年人

ago
[ə'gəu]

ad. 以前；……前

【辨　　析】ago, before:
ago 从此刻起的以前，除 since...ago 短语用于完成时外，一般均用于过去时；
before 从过去某时刻起的以前，常用于过去完成时。

agree
[ə'gri:]

vi. 同意，赞同；（to）一致，适合；商定，约定

【联想记忆】agreement *n.* 同意，一致，协定，协议；disagree *vi.* 不一致，不适宜；disagreeable *a.* 不愉快的，不为人喜的，厌恶的；agreeably *ad.* 愉悦地，令人愉快地；disagreement *n.* 意见不一，分歧，不和，争论

【固定搭配】agree on/upon 同意（用于双方协商同意的事）；agree with 与……意见一致（接"人"或 what 从句）；agree with 适合（接"事物"）；agree to 同意，答应（接受计划、安排、建议等）如 I couldn't agree more. 我完全同意。It was agreed that ... 大家一致同意……；agree to differ 同意保留不同意见

agreement
[ə'gri:mənt]

n. 同意，一致；协议，协定，契约

【反　义　词】disagreement

【固定搭配】in agreement with = in accordance with 同意，与……一致；reach/arrive at/come to an agreement 达成协议

ahead
[ə'hed]

ad. 前头，在前，向前，领先，占优势

【固定搭配】ahead of 在……前，先于；ahead of schedule/time = in advance 提前；look ahead 展望未来；go ahead 前进；去吧

aim
[eim]

vi. 瞄准，对准　*vt.* 旨在；瞄准；针对　*n.* 目标，目的

【派　生　词】aimless *a.* 无方向的；无目的的

【固定搭配】aim at 瞄准，针对；旨在

alarm
[ə'lɑ:m]

n. 惊恐；警报；警报器　*vt.* 惊动，惊吓；向……报警

【派　生　词】alarmed *a.* 担心，害怕；alarming *a.* 使人惊恐的，引起恐慌的，骇人的

【固定搭配】alarm clock 闹钟

alcohol
['ælkəhɔl]

n. 酒精，乙醇

【联想记忆】alcoholic *a.* 含有乙醇的，含有酒精的　*n.* 酒鬼，酗酒者

alike
[ə'laik]

a. 相同的，相似的

【反　义　词】unlike

【辨　　析】like, alike:
like（*a.* 相像的）可做定语和表语，前可加 very。alike 只做表语，前面不可加 very，常加 much。

alive
[ə'laiv]

a. 活着的；活跃的，活泼的

【反　义　词】dead

【辨　　析】alive, living, live, lively:
alive 表示"活着的，在世的"，多指劫后余生，大难不死，并且只做表语或补语。living 表示"活着的，现存的"，多做定语。live 表示"活着的；现场的；现场直播的"。lively 表示"充满生机和活力的；欢快的"。

all
[ɔːl]

a. 全部的，所有的；非常的，极度的 *pron.* 全部，一切 *ad.* 完全，很

【固定搭配】above all 首先，尤其是；all but 几乎，差不多；除……外全部；all out 全力以赴；all over 到处，遍及；all right 行，可以；顺利，良好；at all 完全，根本；in all 总计，共计

allow
[əˈlau]

vt. 允许，准许；给予 *vi.* 考虑到

【联想记忆】allowable *a.* 允许的，正当的，可承认的；allowance *n.* 津贴，补助；宽容；允许

【固定搭配】allow for 考虑到，顾及；allow of 允许；allow doing 允许做；allow sb. to do 允许某人做

almost
[ˈɔːlməust]

ad. 几乎，差不多

【辨　析】almost, nearly:
nearly 在作"几乎，差不多，差一点就……"解释时，后可跟名词、动词、形容词、副词等，可与 almost 通用。但 almost 后面经常可以接否定词 no, none, nothing, never 等，表示"几乎不，差不多都不"，而 nearly 则不可以这样使用，且 nearly 常与数字连用。

alone
[əˈləun]

a. 独自，单独 *ad.* 仅仅，只

【固定搭配】leave sth./sb. alone 不惊动，不变动；let alone sth./doing sth. 更不用说

【辨　析】alone, lonely:
alone 做表语或状语，不能做修饰语，表示"独自一人的"，无感情色彩。lonely 意为"孤独的，寂寞的"，含有感情色彩。

along
[əˈlɔŋ]

prep. 沿着 *ad.* 向前

【联想记忆】alongside *prep.* 在……旁边，沿着……；与……一起，与……同

【固定搭配】all along 始终，一直；along with = together with 与……在一起；get along with 与……相处

although
[ɔːlˈðəu]

conj. 虽然，即使

among(st)
[əˈmʌŋ(st)]

prep. 在……之中，在……之间

【同 义 词】amid, between

【辨　析】among, between, amid:
among 指在三者或三者以上的人/物之间。between 指在两者之间。amid 指在……的过程中，或在……的四周。

ancient
[ˈeinʃənt]

a. 古代的，古老的

【反 义 词】modern *a.* 现代的

announce
[əˈnauns]

v. 宣布，通告

【联想记忆】announcement *n.* 通告，宣告

【辨　析】announce, declare:
announce 指宣布，宣告一个决定，也可指通过广播通知。declare 指郑重地公开某一重大事件，也可指个人向外界声明自己的态度、意见等。

another
[əˈnʌðə]

a. 另一的，不同的；别的 *pron.* 另一个

【固定搭配】one after another 一个接一个；one another = each other 互相

☐ **appear** [əˈpiə]	*vi.* 出现，出场，问世；好像是 【反 义 词】disappear
☐ **appearance** [əˈpiərəns]	*n.* 出现，出场，露面；外表，外观 【反 义 词】disappearance
☐ **area** [ˈɛəriə]	*n.* 面积；地区；范围；领域 【辨 析】area, district, region, zone: area 指界限不分明的地区，一块较大面积的地区，但不是行政上的地理单位。district 指行政单位区域，例如海淀区。region 指较大的行政区域，或具有某种特色的自然地域单位，例如香港特别行政区。zone 指具有特殊性质的地区，以特有的外貌或特点而区别于临近部分的地区或区域，例如 subtropical zone "亚热带"，或 special economic zone "经济特区"。
☐ **arrival** [əˈraivəl]	*n.* 到来，到达；到达者，抵达物 【反 义 词】departure
☐ **arrive** [əˈraiv]	*vi.* 到来，到达；（at）达成，得出 【反 义 词】depart 【派 生 词】arrival *n.* 到来，到达；到达物 【固定搭配】arrive at 到达较小的地方，达到；come to, get to, reach in 到达较大的地方；arrive at conclusion 得出结论
☐ **as** [æs]	*conj.* 在/当……的时候；如……一样；由于，因为 *prep.* 作为，当作 【固定搭配】as...as... 与……一样；as for/to 至于，就……而言；as if/though 好像，仿佛；as long as = so long as 只要，如果，既然；not as/so...as 不如……那样；as a matter of fact 事实上；as a result 结果；as far as...be concerned 就……而言；as follows 如下；as usual 照常；as regards 相当于；with reference to, concerning 关于，至于；as well 也，还；as well as 既……又……
☐ **at** [æt, ət]	*prep.* （表示地点、位置、场合）在，于；（表示时刻、时节、年龄）在，当；（表示目标、方向）对，向；（表示速度、价格等）以
☐ **awake** [əˈweik]	*a.* 醒着的；意识到的 *vt.* 唤醒，唤起 *vi.* 醒来，醒悟，觉悟 【辨 析】awake, awaken, wake, waken: awake 是不及物动词，意思是"醒来"，通常用"觉醒，醒悟"的比喻义。awaken 是及物动词，意为"使……醒，使……醒悟"，常用于被动语态和比喻当中。wake 是普通用词，多做不及物动词，可以与 up 连用，表示真正的"醒来，唤醒"。waken 是及物动词，一般用在被动语态里，意为"唤醒"。
☐ **away** [əˈwei]	*ad.* 离开，远离 【固定搭配】right away 立刻，马上

B

back [bæk]	*ad.* 向后，后退；回复 *n.* 背，背面，后面 *a.* 后面的，背后的 *vt.* 使后退；支持 【辨　析】at the back, behind： behind 指在后面，但不是整体中的部分。at the back 则是整体中的部分。例如：Our room was at the back of the hotel. 我们的房间在旅馆里靠后面的位置。There's a lovely wood just behind our hotel. 就在我们旅馆的后面有一片秀丽的树林。 【固定搭配】back and forth 来回，往返；back down/off 放弃，让步，退却；back up 支持，援助
beat [biːt]	*vt.* 打，敲；打败，取胜 *vi.*（心）跳动 *n.* 敲击；跳动；拍子，节拍；（警察、哨兵）巡逻路线 【固定搭配】beat about the bush 绕弯子说话；beat off 打退；beat time 打拍子；beat up sb. 痛打某人；beat about for 到处寻找；beat back 击退；beat down 杀……价格 【辨　析】beat, defeat, win： win, beat 和 defeat 都可表示"战胜，打败"。win 后面通常接物，defeat 和 beat 后只接人。
because [bɪˈkɔz]	*conj.* 因为 【固定搭配】because of 由于，因为
before [bɪˈfɔː]	*prep./conj.* 在……之前 *prep.* 在……前面 *ad.* 从前，早些时候 【固定搭配】before long 不久以后；long before 很早以前 例如：He began as an actor, before starting to direct films. 他先是当演员，后来才开始执导影片。
begin [bɪˈɡɪn]	*v.* 开始，启动 【反 义 词】end 【派 生 词】beginner *n.* 初学者 【固定搭配】begin with/begin by doing sth. 从……开始；to begin with 首先，第一；begin as sth. 起初是，本来是
beginning [bɪˈɡɪnɪŋ]	*n.* 开始，开端；起因 【反 义 词】end 【固定搭配】at the beginning of 在……之初；in the beginning = at first 开始；from beginning to end 从头至尾
behind [bɪˈhaɪnd]	*prep.* 在……后面，落后于 *ad.* 在后，落后 【固定搭配】fall behind = lag behind 落后；leave behind 留下，忘掉；behind the times 落后于时代；behind schedule 延迟；on schedule 按时
belief [bɪˈliːf]	*n.* 相信；信仰，信条，信念 【辨　析】disbelief, unbelief： disbelief 对某事的不信和怀疑。unbelief 宗教上的怀疑和无信仰。

believe [bi'li:v]	vt. 相信，认为 vi. 相信，信任，信奉 【联想记忆】believable a. 可信的；unbelievable a. 不可相信的；难以置信的 【固定搭配】believe in 信仰，信奉，对……有信心；make believe = pretend/affect 假装；seeing is believing 眼见为实；believe it or not 信不信由你 【辨　析】believe，believe in： believe sb. 相信某人的话。believe in sb. 信赖某人。 例如：I can believe him, but I can't believe in him. 我可以相信其言，但不能信任其人。
belong [bi'lɔŋ]	vi.（to）属，附属；归类于 【联想记忆】belongings n. 动产，财物
below [bi'ləu]	prep. 在……下面，在……以下 ad. 在下面，以下，向下 【反　义　词】above
bend [bend]	n. 弯曲，曲折处 vt. 折弯，使屈曲 【固定搭配】bend the truth 扭曲事实；on bended knees 央求，苦苦哀求
beneath [bi'ni:θ]	prep. 在……（正）下方，在……底下 ad. 在下方
beside [bi'said]	prep. 在……旁边，与……相比
besides [bi'saidz]	ad. 而且，还有，除此之外 prep. 除……之外（尚有……） 【辨　析】besides，except： besides 表示"除……之外"，除去的也包括在整体内，例如：What other sports do you like besides football? 除足球外你还喜欢哪些运动？except 指除此以外，除去的不包含在整体之内，例如：I like all sports except football. 除了足球，什么运动我都喜欢。
between [bi'twi:n]	prep. 在……中间，在……之间 ad. 当中，中间 【固定搭配】between you and me/between ourselves 我们之间的秘密；few and far between 不常有，稀少
beyond [bi'jɔnd]	prep. 在……较远的一边，晚于；超出（能力、范围等）；除……之外 ad. 在那边，在更远处 【固定搭配】be beyond sb. = to be too difficult for someone to understand 对某人来说很难理解；beyond repair/control/belief = impossible to repair, control, believe
bitter ['bitə]	a. 苦味的；痛苦的；严寒的 【反　义　词】sweet 【联想记忆】bitterness n. 苦味，辛酸；bitterly ad. 伤心地，愤怒地
book [buk]	n. 书，书籍 vt. 预订 【联想记忆】bookish a. 书本上的，好学的；书呆子气的；bookmark n. 书签；bookworm n. 书呆子；蛀书虫；bookshelf n. 书架；bookcase n. 书架，书柜 【固定搭配】book in 登记入住旅馆；预订（旅馆房间）；签到，报名；be booked up（车票、住处等）预订一空；by the book 按常规，依照惯例
bottom ['bɔtəm]	n. 底，底部；尽头，末端；（口语）屁股 【反　义　词】top 【联想记忆】bottomless a. 无底的，深不可测的；深奥的，高深莫测的 【固定搭配】from the bottom of one's heart 真诚地；诚挚地；衷心地；at bottom 归根结底，本质上，实质上；bottom up 干杯；bottomless pit 无底洞，无休止的情况

breadth [bredθ]	*n.* 宽度,（布的）幅宽；（船）幅,量度,范围；宽宏大量,宽容
break [breik]	*vt.* 打破,打碎；损坏,破坏；违反；中止 *n.*（课间或工间）休息时间 *vi.* 破,破裂 【联想记忆】breakable *a.* 易碎的；breakage *n.* 易碎物品 【固定搭配】break away (from) 脱离,逃跑；break down 分解,瓦解；（机器）损坏；break in 强行进入,破门而入；打断,插嘴；break into 撬开,闯入；break off 中断,突然停止；break out 突然发生,爆发；break through 突破；break up 打碎,拆散,结束,垮掉；give sb. a break 饶了某人吧 [口语]
bring [briŋ]	*vt.* 拿来,带来；产生,引起；使处于某种状态 【固定搭配】bring about 使发生,致使；bring forward 将……提前；提议；bring out 使出现,使显露；bring up 抚养,教育；提出问题；bring forth 提出；产生；bring down 降低；打倒
build [bild]	*vt.* 修建,建造,建设 【联想记忆】builder *n.* 建造者；building *n.* 建筑物,大楼 【固定搭配】build up 增长；积累；增强；build sth. (of/out of)（用……）构筑,建造（以建造物做直接宾语）；build sth. into 用（某物）建造成……（以材料作为直接宾语）
but [bət, bʌt]	*conj.* 但是,可是,然而 *prep.* 除……之外 *ad.* 只,仅仅 【固定搭配】but for 要不是,如果没有；cannot but = cannot choose/help but（后接动词原形）只得,不得不；nothing but 那不过是,只是；last but one 倒数第二
by [bai]	*prep.* 在……旁,靠近；被,由；在……前,到……为止；经,沿,通过；[表示方法,手段]靠,用,通过；按照,根据 *ad.* 在旁,近旁；经过 【固定搭配】by and by 不久以后,将来；by far... 得多；by hand 用手；by heart 牢记,凭记忆；by oneself 单独地,独自地；by air (railway, sea, plane, bus, etc.) 乘飞机（火车、轮船、飞机、公共汽车等）；by and large 总的来说,大体上,基本上

call [kɔːl]	*vt.* 给……命名,称呼；认为……是；大声呼叫,召唤；给……打电话 *vi.* 拜访,访问；大声呼叫,召唤；打电话 *n.* 打电话；叫声；短暂拜访；要求 【固定搭配】call at a place 访问某地；call for 要求,需求；call forth 激发,使出；call off 取消；call on/upon 访问,拜访；号召,呼吁；call up 召集,动员；打电话；call out 召唤（尤指应付紧急事件）；指示（工人）罢工

☐ **calm** [kɑ:m]	*a.* 安静的，镇静的；（天气）无风的；（海面）平静的 *v.* （使）平静，（使）镇定 *n.* 平静，风平浪静 【固定搭配】calm down（人）平静下来；（自然现象）平息下来；the calm before the storm 暴风雨前的平静
☐ **can** [kæn, kən]	*aux. v.* 能，会；可能；可以 *n.* 罐头，铁罐，易拉罐 【固定搭配】can't help doing 禁不住；can't help but (do) 不能不，不得不；can have done（对过去发生情况的推测）可能做过……
☐ **care** [kɛə]	*n.* 注意，小心；挂念；照顾，照料 *vi.* 关心，计较；在意 【固定搭配】care for 照管，关心；care about 关心，关注，关怀；take care 留心；保重；take care of 照顾，照料；承当，处理，负责；with care 小心，慎重；I couldn't care less 我根本不在乎（不在意）
☐ **career** [kəˈriə]	*n.* 生涯，经历；专业，职业 【固定搭配】career woman 职业女性 【辨　析】career, position, profession: career 意为"职业；专业；生涯"，既可指一般工作，也可指专业性较强的职业。position 意为"职业，职务"，主要指工作岗位。profession "职业"，尤指受过长期专门训练才能从事的工作，如医生、教师、律师等。
☐ **careful** [ˈkɛəful]	*a.* 小心的，注意的，谨慎的；细心的，周密细致的 【联想记忆】carefully *ad.* 小心地，谨慎地；carefulness *n.* 仔细，慎重
☐ **careless** [ˈkɛəlis]	*a.* 粗心的，疏忽的；漫不经心的，不介意的 【联想记忆】carelessly *ad.* 粗心地；carelessness *n.* 粗心
☐ **carry** [ˈkæri]	*vt.* 搬运，运送，携带，佩戴，怀有；传送，传播；支撑，支持 【固定搭配】carry on 继续，坚持下去；从事，经营；carry out 执行，贯彻；carry through 完成；be carried away 很激动，冲昏头脑；carry forward 推进；发扬；carry off 夺去生命；获得（奖），意外成功
☐ **case** [keis]	*n.* 事实，情况；案件；病例；箱子，盒子；[语法]格 【固定搭配】in any case 总之，无论如何；in case 假如，以防；in that case 既然那样，假使那样的话；in case of 假如，万一；in no case 无论如何都不，决不；in the case of 就……而言；as the case may be 根据具体情况，视情况而定
☐ **cash** [kæʃ]	*n.* 现金，现款 *vt.* 把……兑换 【联想记忆】cashier *n.* 出纳员 【固定搭配】pay in cash 以现金支付；cash down 货到付款；ready cash 现款；cash on delivery 货到付款
☐ **cast** [kɑ:st]	*vt.* 投，掷，抛；铸造 *n.* 演员表
☐ **catch** [kætʃ]	*vt.* 捕，捉；赶上；感染，得病；听清楚，领会，理解 【固定搭配】catch up with 追上，赶上；catch on 理解，明白；catch one's eye 引人注目；catch sight of（突然）发现；catch up on 在……方面赶上，补做，补上；catch on to (doing) sth. 理解，了解
☐ **center** [ˈsentə]	*n.* 中心，中央 *v.* 集中

第一部分 基础词汇

central ['sentrəl]
a. 中心的，中央的，中枢的；主要的

chance [tʃɑ:ns]
n. 机会；可能性；偶然性，运气 *v.* 敢于……，冒险
【固定搭配】by chance 偶然，碰巧；take a chance 冒险
【辨　析】chance, fortune, luck, opportunity:
chance 尤指希望发生的事的可能性，含有未知和不可预测的成分。fortune 指命运、际遇、影响人生的机会或运气，也指巨款。luck 指幸运、运气，强调碰巧发生。opportunity 指良机，合适或有利的机会或时间。

change [tʃeindʒ]
v./n. 改变，变化 *vt.* 换，兑换 *n.* 找头，零头
【联想记忆】changeable *a.* 易变的，可改变的；changed *a.* 与以前截然不同的，变化大的
【固定搭配】change one's mind 改变主意；change A for B 用 A 去换 B；change hands 易主，转手

chat [tʃæt]
vi./n. 聊天
【联想记忆】chatter *v.* 喋喋不休
【固定搭配】have a chat with sb. 与某人聊天

cheap [tʃi:p]
a. 便宜的，价钱低的；低劣的，蹩脚的；庸俗可鄙的
【反　义　词】expensive, costly, dear
【联想记忆】cheaply *ad.* 便宜地；cheapness *n.* 廉价

cheat [tʃi:t]
vt. 欺骗，骗取 *vi.* 作弊；对某人不忠 *n.* 欺骗；骗子
【固定搭配】cheat sb. (out) of sth. 骗取某人的某物；cheat sb. into the belief that 哄骗某人相信……

check [tʃek]
vt./n. 检查，核对；制止，控制 *n.* 支票，账单；方格子图案，格子织物
【固定搭配】check in 办理登记手续；check out 结账后离开；check up/(up) on 校对，检验，检查；check sth. out 调查，查证，核实；check over/through 仔细检查，核查；a health check 体检；hold/keep sth. in check 控制，制止

choice [tʃɔis]
n. 选择；选择机会；被选中的东西，入选者，精华；供选择的种类
a. 精选的，上等的
【固定搭配】have no choice but to do 别无他法，只好做……

choose [tʃu:z]
vt. 选择，挑拣；决定，愿意，偏要
【固定搭配】choose to do 愿意做；can't choose but = can't help but 不得不（接动词原形）

clean [kli:n]
a. 清洁的，干净的 *vt.* 弄清洁，擦干净
【反　义　词】dirty
【联想记忆】cleanly *ad.* 干净地；清白地；cleanness *n.* 干净
【固定搭配】clean up 收拾干净，清除；做完，完成；do a clean job 干得很出色；clean out 打扫干净；清除

clear [kliə]
a. 明亮的，清澈的；晴朗的 *ad.* 清楚，清晰 *vt.* 清除；澄清；晴朗起来
【联想记忆】clearance *n.* 清理，清除，空隙
【固定搭配】clear up 解释，澄清；（天气）变晴；clear away 清理
【辨　析】clear, apparent, evident, obvious, plain, distinct:
clear 清晰的，不模糊的；apparent 表面上的，明显的；evident（被证明为）显然的；obvious 一目了然的；plain 简明了的，简朴的；distinct 独特的，不同的

019

close [kləuz] *v.* [kləus] *a.*	*v.* 关，关闭；结束，停止；合拢，合上，包住 *n.* 结束 *a.* 近的；紧密的；齐根的；封闭的；亲密的 *ad.* 接近，紧挨着 【反 义 词】open, far 【固定搭配】close down（广播电台、电视台）停止播音，停播；（工厂等的）关闭，歇业；close up 关闭；停歇；come to a close 结束；bring...to a close 使……结束 【辨　　析】be close to, be closed to: be close to 离……近；be closed to 不向……开放。
colleague [ˈkɔli:g]	*n.* 同事，同僚
come [kʌm]	*vi.* 来，来到；出现，产出 【固定搭配】come about = take place 发生，产生；come across 偶遇，碰到；发生效果；come off 成功，奏效；come on 请，来吧，快点；come out 出版，刊出；传出，显出，长出；结果是，结局是；come round/around = call on/upon 来访；前来；come to = come round/around 苏醒，复原；come through = pull through 经历，脱险；come true 实现，达到；come up 提出；come down with 病倒；come into effect = take effect 生效；come by 偶然得到；come to terms with 接受；come up 出现
comfort [ˈkʌmfət]	*vt./n.* 慰问，安慰 *n.* 安逸，舒适 【反 义 词】discomfort
comfortable [ˈkʌmfətəbl]	*a.* 安慰的，舒适的，轻松自在的 【反 义 词】uncomfortable 【联想记忆】comfortably *ad.* 舒适地
command [kəˈmɑ:nd]	*vt./n.* 命令，指挥 *n.* 掌握，运用能力 【固定搭配】command sb. to do sth. 指挥（命令）某人做某事；do sth. at/by sb.'s command 奉某人之命做某事；be at sb.'s command 愿受某人的指挥；听某人的吩咐
commander [kəˈmɑ:ndə]	*n.* 司令官，指挥官
conference [ˈkɔnfərəns]	*n.* 会议，讨论会 【固定搭配】in conference 商讨 【辨　　析】见 assembly
congratulate [kənˈgrætjuleit]	*vt.* 祝贺，向……贺喜 【固定搭配】congratulate sb. on sth. 向某人道贺
congratulation(s) [kənˌgrætjuˈleiʃən(z)]	*n.* 祝贺，恭喜
connect [kəˈnekt]	*vt.* 连接，联系 【联想记忆】connector *n.* 连接器；connective *a.* 连接的 *n.* 连接词；disconnect *v.* 拆开，分离，断开 【固定搭配】connect...with... 把……与……相连

connection
[kə'nekʃən]

n. 联系，连接，关系；转车，转机
【同 义 词】combination, link, relationship
【反 义 词】disconnection
【固定搭配】in connection with/to 与……有关；in this connection 由于这事，为此

conquer
['kɔŋkə]

vt. 征服，战胜
【联想记忆】conquest *n.* 攻占，征服；战利品　conquerable *a.* 可征服的，可击败的　conqueror *n.* 征服者，胜利者
【反 义 词】surrender

corner
['kɔ:nə]

n. 角，角落　*v.* 使……陷入困境，使……走投无路；控制（买卖活动），垄断
【固定搭配】around/round the corner 来临；在拐角处；in the corner of 在某物里面的角落；at the corner of 在某物外面的角落；cut corners 走捷径；be in tight corner 陷入困境；turn the corner 转危为安，脱离危险，好转，渡过难关，脱离困境

correct
[kə'rekt]

a. 正确的；恰当的，合适的　*vt.* 改正，修改，矫正
【联想记忆】correction *n.* 改正，修正　correctly *ad.* 正确地；恰当地

cost
[kɔst]

n. 成本，费用，代价　*v.* 值，花费
【固定搭配】at all costs = at any cost 无论如何，不惜任何代价；at the cost of 以……为代价；know to one's cost 吃了苦头之后才……，亲身体验到；sth./doing sth. cost sb. sth. 某物／做某事花费某人……，注意该搭配中 cost 不能用人做主语，例如：I bought a bottle of perfume in Paris, which cost me $15. 我在巴黎买了一瓶香水，花了我 15 美元。

costly
['kɔstli]

a. 昂贵的；代价高的；价值高的，豪华的
【辨　　析】costly, dear, expensive, precious, priceless, valuable：
costly 指某物由于稀有、雅致、珍贵或手艺精湛等因素而价格昂贵，也指在时间或精力方面代价过大。dear 指非常受珍视的，宝贵的。expensive 意为"费用大的，豪华的，以高价为标志的"。precious 意为"宝贵的，贵重的"，指无法用钱去衡量人或物的价值，或珍贵的感情。priceless 意为"无价的，昂贵的"，用来描述具有不可估价的东西。valuable 意为"贵重的，有价值的"，修饰商品时指价格高，在修饰商品以外的事物时，指的是其有价值。

couple
['kʌpl]

n. 对，双；夫妇
【辨　　析】couple, pair：
couple 指任何两件东西，如 a couple of cats 两只猫。pair 指两件不可分开的东西，如 a pair of shoes 一双鞋。

courage
['kʌridʒ]

n. 勇气，胆量
【联想记忆】courageous *a.* 勇敢的，有胆量的

course
[kɔ:s]

n. 进程，过程；课程；（一）道（菜）
【固定搭配】of course 自然，当然，无疑；in the course of 在……的过程中，在……期间；in course of 及时地；在适当时候

cover ['kʌvə]	v. 遮盖，覆盖；掩护，掩盖；包括，涉及 n. 覆盖物；套；封面 【联想记忆】coverage n. 新闻报道；覆盖范围 【反 义 词】uncover 【固定搭配】cover up 掩盖；take cover 藏身，躲避，避难；under cover 秘密地，暗中；cover...with 掩盖，用……遮盖
crazy ['kreizi]	a. 疯狂的；愚蠢的；狂热爱好的，着迷 【固定搭配】be crazy to do sth. 干……是荒唐的；be crazy about/on (doing) sth. 对（做）……着迷；be crazy for sth./sb. 渴望某物/迷恋某人
create [kri'eit]	vt. 创造，创作；产生；制造，建立 【联想记忆】creation n. 创造；创作物
creative [kri(:)'eitiv]	a. 有创造力的，创造性的 【联想记忆】creativity n. 创造力
creature ['kri:tʃə]	n. 人；生物；动物
crop [krɔp]	n. 农作物，庄稼；收成，产量 v. 收割，收获；剪短，修剪
cross [krɔs]	v. 越过，穿过；使交叉，使相交 n. 十字形，十字架 a. 交叉的，横穿的 【固定搭配】cross out 删去；取消
crossing ['krɔsiŋ]	n. 横越，横渡；交叉点，渡口
crowd [kraud]	n. 人群，群众 v. 挤满，拥挤
crowded ['kraudid]	a. 拥挤的
crude [kru:d]	a. 天然的，未加工的；简陋的；粗鲁的 【反 义 词】refined 【辨 析】crude, raw: crude 天然的，未提炼的，如 crude oil（原油）；raw 生的，未煮熟的。
cruel ['kru:əl]	a. 残忍的，残酷的；令人痛苦的 【联想记忆】cruelty n. 残忍，残酷
crush [krʌʃ]	n./v. 压碎，榨；压垮
cry [krai]	v./n. 叫，喊，哭泣
curve [kə:v]	v. 弄弯，使成曲线 n. 曲线，弯曲
cut [kʌt]	v./n. 切，剪，割，削；删，缩减 n. 伤口 【固定搭配】cut back 削减，减少；cut down 削减，减少，降低；cut in 插嘴，打断；cut off 切掉，剪去，删去；cut out 切去；删除；cut short 突然停止；简化；cut across 抄近路穿过

danger ['deɪndʒə]	*n.* 危险,威胁 【反 义 词】safety, security 【固定搭配】in danger 在危险中;垂危;out of danger 脱离危险
dangerous ['deɪndʒrəs]	*a.* 危险的,不安全的 【反 义 词】safe, secure
dare [dɛə]	*vt.* 敢于,胆敢;激(某人做某事),问(某人)有没有胆量(做某事) *aux. v.* 敢,胆敢 【固定搭配】做情态动词时的否定式为 daren't,后接动词原形,用于疑问句、否定句和条件句;做及物动词时后接名词或动词不定式。
dark [dɑːk]	*a.* 黑暗的,昏暗的;深色的,近乎黑色的 *n.* 黑暗,暗处;暗色,阴影 【反 义 词】bright 【联想记忆】darken *v.* (使)变暗,(使)变黑,处于暗淡之中 【固定搭配】in the dark 在暗处,秘密地,完全不知道;keep/leave sb. in the dark 不让某人知道
date [deɪt]	*n.* 日期,年代;约会 *v.* 定日期;约 【固定搭配】out of date 过时的,陈旧的;up to date 最新的,最近的,现代的
dawn [dɔːn]	*n.* 黎明,曙光 *vi.* 破晓;开始发展 【反 义 词】dusk *n.* 薄暮,黄昏 【固定搭配】at dawn 拂晓,天一亮
dead [ded]	*a.* 死的,废弃了的 【反 义 词】living, alive
deadline ['dedlaɪn]	*n.* 最后期限,截止日期
death [deθ]	*n.* 死,死亡;消亡,毁灭 【反 义 词】birth
decide [dɪ'saɪd]	*v.* 决定,裁决 【固定搭配】decide on/upon doing sth. 决定干某事;decide against doing sth. = decide not to do sth. 决定不干某事
decision [dɪ'sɪʒən]	*n.* 决定,决心;果断 【联想记忆】decisive *a.* 决定性的
deed [diːd]	*n.* 行为,行动;功绩,事迹
deep [diːp]	*a.* 深的,深刻的;深奥的;深切的 *ad.* 深入地,深刻地 【反 义 词】shallow 【联想记忆】deepen *v.* (使)加深;deeply *ad.* 深深地;deepness *n.* 深刻,深切

delicious [di'liʃəs]	*a.* 美味的，芬芳的
destroy [dis'trɔi]	*vt.* 破坏，摧毁；消灭，扑灭；打破，粉碎 【反 义 词】construct 【联想记忆】destroyer *n.* 破坏者，起破坏作用的东西；驱逐舰；destructive *a.* 破坏（性）的；(in)destructible *a.*（不）可破坏的，（不）易毁坏的
detail ['di:teil, di'teil]	*n.* 细节；详情；枝节，琐事 *vt.* 详述，详谈 【固定搭配】in detail 详细地
detailed ['di:teild]	*a.* 详细的
device [di'vais]	*n.* 设备，装置；炸弹；方法，计谋
die [dai]	*vi.* 死，死亡 【反 义 词】live 【联想记忆】dead *a.* 死亡的，死了的；death *n.* 死亡；deadly *a.* 致命的 *ad.* 极其，非常 【固定搭配】die down 渐渐消失，平息；die out 消失，灭绝；die off（植物）相继枯死，（声音）渐渐消失；die of 死于（疾病、饥饿等）；die from 死于（受伤等）
differ ['difə]	*vi.* 不同，相异 【固定搭配】differ from 不同于，和……意见不一致
difference ['difərəns]	*n.* 差别，差异；分歧，争论 【固定搭配】make a difference 有影响，很重要；make no difference 没有关系；没有影响
different ['difərənt]	*a.* 差异的，不同的 【固定搭配】be different from 不同于 【辨　　析】different, diverse, various： different 意为"不同的"，指事物间的不同或本质上的不同。diverse 意为"不同的，多变的"，指多种多样的，形形色色的。various 意为"各种各样的，不同的"，强调种类的不同或种数的繁多，不强调本质的差别。
difficult ['difikəlt]	*a.* 困难的，艰难的；难应付的，难满足的 【联想记忆】difficultly *ad.* 困难地 【反 义 词】easy
difficulty ['difikəlti]	*n.* 困难，难事；困境 【固定搭配】in difficulty (ies) = in trouble 处境困难；have difficulty (in) doing sth. 在做某事方面有困难；have difficulty with sth. 对某事有困难
digital ['didʒitl]	*a.* 数字的，数码的
direct [di'rekt, dai'rekt]	*a./ad.* 径直的（地），直接的（地）；率直的（地）；正好的（地），恰好的（地）*vt.* 把……对准；指示；管理，指导 【反 义 词】indirect 【固定搭配】direct sb. to do 指挥某人；direct sth. at/to 把……指向，针对

第一部分 基础词汇

direction [diˈrekʃən, daiˈrekʃən]	n. 方向，方位；趋势，动向；指导，指令；[pl.] 用法说明 【固定搭配】in the direction of 朝着……方向
directly [diˈrektli, daiˈrektli]	ad. 直接地，直截了当地；恰好；立即，马上
director [diˈrektə, daiˈrektə]	n. 主任，处长，局长；主管，董事；导演
disappear [ˌdisəˈpiə]	v. 消失，消散，失踪；不复存在，灭绝 【联想记忆】disappearance n. 消失，不见 【反 义 词】appear
disappoint [ˌdisəˈpɔint]	vt. 令人失望，使人扫兴 【联想记忆】disappointment n. 失望；使人失望的人（事情）；disappointed a. 失望的；disappointing a. 使人失望的，令人扫兴的 【固定搭配】be disappointed with/at/about 对……感到失望
discover [disˈkʌvə]	vt. 发现；暴露，显示 【联想记忆】discoverer n. 发现者
discovery [disˈkʌvəri]	n. 发现
discuss [disˈkʌs]	v. 讨论 【联想记忆】discussion n. 讨论；discussible a. 可议论的，可讨论的
disease [diˈzi:z]	n. 疾病
distance [ˈdistəns]	n. 距离，路程；远方，远处 【固定搭配】at a distance 隔开一段距离；in the distance 在远处；keep distance with 与……保持距离；keep sb. at a distance 同……疏远
distant [ˈdistənt]	a. 远的；疏远的，冷漠的
district [ˈdistrikt]	n. 区，地区，行政区
disturb [disˈtə:b]	vt. 扰乱，妨碍；打扰，使不安 【联想记忆】disturbing a. 烦扰的
disturbance [disˈtə:bəns]	n. 动乱；骚扰，干扰；（身心）失调
divide [diˈvaid]	vt. 分开，划分，隔开；分配，分享，分担；除以 【联想记忆】divider n. 分割者，间隔物，分配器；圆规；division n. 分开，分割，区分；除法；公司;（军事）师；分配，分界线；divisional a. 分割的，分区的；部门所有的；divided a. 分开的 【固定搭配】divide into 分为，分成；divide sth. with sb. 与某人一起承担某事
division [diˈviʒən]	n. 分割，分裂；除法

divorce [di'vɔːs]	v./n. 离婚，离异；分离 【反 义 词】marry, marriage
do [duː]	aux.v. （用于实义动词前构成疑问句和否定句的助动词）；（代替动词用于加强语气）vt. 做，干，办；完成，做完；产生 vi. 做，行动，进行；合适 【固定搭配】do away with 消失；丢掉；do one's best 尽力而为；do without 没有……也行，将就；have nothing/something to do with 与……无关 / 有关；do up 扣上；包扎，修理，修葺，整新；dos and don'ts 行为准则，须知
drag [dræg]	v. 拖拉，拖拽 【固定搭配】drag on 拖得太久，持续太久
draw [drɔː]	v. 画，绘制，拔出，抽出，抽（签），抓（阄）vt. 拖（动），拉（动），牵引；获取，领取，提取，引起，吸引 vi. 向……移动，行进 n. 抽奖，抽签；平局，和局 【固定搭配】draw up 写出，画出，草拟；draw in（天）黑了，（日）渐短；（车船等）驶进，到站；draw on 凭借，吸收，利用；接近，靠近
drawing ['drɔːiŋ]	n. 图画，素描；机械图
dream [driːm]	n. 梦；梦想，幻想 v. 做梦，幻想 【固定搭配】dream of/about 梦想；dreams come true 梦想成真 【联想记忆】nightmare n. 噩梦；daydream n. 白日梦
dress [dres]	n. 服装，女装，童装 v. 给……穿衣，打扮；包扎（伤口） 【反 义 词】undress 【联想记忆】dressed a. 穿戴整齐的；dressing n. 调味料；dressing room 更衣室，化妆间 【固定搭配】dress up 穿上盛装，打扮得漂漂亮亮
drift [drift]	n./v. 漂，漂流 【辨　　析】drift, float： drift 指漂流，被气流或水流携带着运动。float 指浮动，保持悬在流体的表层内或表面的状态而不沉下去。
drop [drɔp]	n. 下降；滴，水滴 v. 投下，落下；降低 【固定搭配】drop by/in 顺便来访；drop out 退出，退学；脱离，不参与；drop off 逐渐减少；睡着
drown [draun]	v. 淹死，淹没 【固定搭配】drown oneself in... 埋头于……
drug [drʌg]	n. 药品；[pl.] 麻醉药，毒药 【联想记忆】druggist n. 药商，药剂师，药材商
drum [drʌm]	n. 鼓；鼓状物
drunk [drʌŋk]	a. 酒醉的 【固定搭配】be drunk with 陶醉于……中

dry [draɪ]	a. 干的，干旱的；口干的，口渴的；干巴巴的，枯燥的 vt. 使干燥，晒干 【反 义 词】wet 【固定搭配】dry up 干涸，干旱
dull [dʌl]	a. 钝；愚笨，迟钝；阴暗，沉闷，单调；暗淡，阴郁 【反 义 词】sharp
dumb [dʌm]	a. 哑的，无声的 【联想记忆】deaf a. 聋的
dump [dʌmp]	v./n. 倾卸，倾倒
duty ['dju:ti]	n. 职责；义务，责任；税，关税 【联想记忆】dutyfree a. 免关税的 【固定搭配】off duty 下班；be/go on duty 值班，当班 【辨　　析】duty，tariff，tax： duty（通常作复数）指对各种具体物品所征收的税款。tariff 指政府对进出口货物所征收的关税。tax 泛指普通百姓和营业单位向国家交纳的各种税金。

earn [ə:n]	vt. 赚得，挣得；博得，赢得，获得 【联想记忆】earning n. 收入 【固定搭配】earn one's living = make a living 谋生，挣钱
easy ['i:zi]	a. 容易的；不费力的；舒适的，舒畅的 ad. 小心；慢些；轻点 【反 义 词】difficult; uneasy, careful 【固定搭配】take it easy=take your time 别紧张，慢慢来；沉住气，从容点；easier said than done 说时容易做时难；go easy on sb. 对某人温和（宽容）些
educate ['edju(:)keit]	vt. 教育，培养，训练；教导；教养 【联想记忆】educator n. 教师；教育家
education [,edju(:)'keiʃən]	n. 教育，培养
either ['aɪðə(r)]	pron.(两者中)任何一方，任何一个 ad. [与 not 连用]也(不); [与 or 连用]或……或……，不是……就是…… 【固定搭配】either...or... 或……或……，不是……就是……；注意，either 做代词当主语时，谓语用单数；either...or 做并列主语时，句子的谓语依从后的主语而定。
elect [i'lekt]	v. 选举，推选；选择，抉择 【固定搭配】elect sb. + 职位（不带冠词）选某人做……；elect sb.(to...) 把某人选入机构或组织中

□ **election** [iˈlekʃ(ə)n]	*n.* 选举
□ **electric** [iˈlektrik]	*a.* 电的，带电的，电动的；令人兴奋的，刺激的 【联想记忆】electrify *vt.* 使充电，使通电，使电气化；electrification *n.* 充电，电气化；electronic *a.* 电子的；electronics *n.* 电子学 【辨　析】electric, electrical, electronic： electric 导电的，电动的，发电的。electrical 关于电的。electronic 电子的。
□ **electrical** [iˈlektrik(ə)l]	*a.* 电的，电气科学的
□ **electrician** [ilekˈtriʃ(ə)n]	*n.* 电学家，电工
□ **electricity** [ilekˈtrisiti]	*n.* 电，电学，电气，电流，电力
□ **electron** [iˈlektrɔn]	*n.* 电子
□ **electronic** [ilekˈtrɔnik]	*a.* 电子的，电子仪器的
□ **electronics** [ilekˈtrɔniks]	*n.* 电子学
□ **else** [els]	*ad.* 其他，另外，别的；[与 or 连用]否则 【固定搭配】or else 否则，要不然
□ **energy** [ˈenədʒi]	*n.* 活力，精力；能，能量 【联想记忆】energetic *a.* 精力充沛的；积极的
□ **enjoy** [inˈdʒɔi]	*vt.* 欣赏，喜爱；享受，享有 【联想记忆】enjoyable *a.* 可爱的；令人愉快的，有趣的；enjoyment *n.* 愉快，乐事，享受 【固定搭配】enjoy oneself 过得快乐
□ **enough** [iˈnʌf]	*a.* 足够的，充足的 *ad.* 足够 【固定搭配】enough is enough 够了，行了，适可而止；have had enough of sth./sb. 对……已经厌烦透了，再也忍受不住
□ **enter** [ˈentə]	*v.* 走进，进入；参加，加入；写入，登录 【固定搭配】enter into 进入，参加；开始；成为……的一部分
□ **environment** [inˈvaiərənmənt]	*n.* 环境，四周，外界 【联想记忆】environmental *a.* 环境的，与环境有关的
□ **envy** [ˈenvi]	*vt./n.* 妒忌，羡慕 【联想记忆】envious *a.* 羡慕的 【固定搭配】feel envious at/for 对……嫉妒
□ **equal** [ˈiːkwəl]	*a.* 同等的，相等的；平等的；胜任的 *n.* (地位等)相同的人，匹敌者 *v.* 等于，比得上 【反　义　词】unequal 【联想记忆】equality *n.* 同等，平等，相等；equally *ad.* 平等地 【固定搭配】be equal to = amount to 等于；be equal to (doing) sth. 能胜任（做）某事

equip [i'kwip]	vt. 装备，配备；（在智力上、体力上）使有准备 【固定搭配】be equipped for 准备好，对……有准备；be equipped with 装（配）备；安装
equipment [i'kwipmənt]	n. 装备，设备，器材 【辨析】apparatus, equipment: apparatus 既可指某种具体的由许多不同零件构成的复杂的仪器、装置或器械，又可指它们的总称。 equipment 多指成套的或重型的设备或装备，通常用作不可数名词。
escape [is'keip]	vi. 逃跑；逃避，避免；漏出，渗出 【固定搭配】escape from 逃逸
event [i'vent]	n. 事件，大事，事变；比赛项目 【联想记忆】eventful a. 变故多的，多事的 【固定搭配】in the event of 万一，若；in the event 结果，到头来；at all events/in any event 无论如何
evolution [,i:və'lu:ʃən, ,evə-]	n. 进化，演化；发展，渐进 【联想记忆】evolutionary a. 进化的
evolve [i'vɔlv]	v. （使）进化，（使）演化；（使）发展，（使）演变 【联想记忆】evolvement n. 发展，进化
exact [ig'zækt]	a. 确切的，精确的
examination [ig,zæmi'neiʃən]	n. 考试，测验；检验，检查，审查
examine [ig'zæmin]	vt. 检查，审查，调查；考试
example [ig'zɑ:mpl, ig'zæm-]	n. 例，实例；范例，榜样 【固定搭配】for example 例如
except [ik'sept]	vt. 把……除外；不计；不包括 conj. 除了；只是 prep. 除了……之外，若不是，除非 【固定搭配】except for 除……以外
exception [ik'sepʃən]	n. 例外 【联想记忆】exceptional a. 例外的，异常的 【固定搭配】with the exception of 除……之外
exchange [iks'tʃeindʒ]	vt. 交换，交流；调换，兑换 n. 交换台，交易所 例如：We exchanged our opinions about the event at the meeting. 在会上，我们就此事交换了意见。 【固定搭配】exchange A for B = substitute A for B 用 A 去换 B
excite [ik'sait]	vt. 激动，使兴奋；激发，刺激，唤起
excited [ik'saitid]	a. 兴奋的 【联想记忆】excitedly ad. 兴奋地

□ **excitement** [ik'saitmənt]	*n.* 刺激，兴奋
□ **excuse** [iks'kju:z] *vt.* [iks'kju:s] *n.*	*vt.* 原谅 *n.* 借口，理由 【固定搭配】excuse sb. for doing sth. 原谅某人做某事
□ **exist** [ig'zist]	*vi.* 在，存在
□ **existence** [ig'zistəns]	*n.* 存在，生存 【固定搭配】come into existence 出现，产生，成立；in existence 存在的；bring...into existence 使产生
□ **expand** [iks'pænd]	*v.* 扩大，增加；扩张，发展 *vi.* 详述 【反 义 词】contract
□ **expansion** [iks'pænʃən]	*n.* 扩充，开展；膨胀 【反 义 词】contraction
□ **expect** [iks'pekt]	*vt.* 期待，盼望；料想，预期 【联想记忆】expectation *n.* 期待；预料
□ **expense** [iks'pens]	*n.* 开销，花费；[*pl.*] 费用 【固定搭配】at the expense of 在牺牲……的情况下，以……为代价
□ **expensive** [iks'pensiv]	*a.* 昂贵的，高价的，花钱多的 【反 义 词】inexpensive, cheap
□ **experience** [iks'piəriəns]	*n.* 经验，感受，体验；经历，体验 【联想记忆】experienced *a.* 有经验的 【反 义 词】inexperience
□ **experiment** [iks'perimənt]	*n.* (~ on/with) 试验，实验 【辨　析】experiment, test, trial： experiment 指为研究某事物的发生或为获得新知识而进行仔细试验的过程。 test 指通过试验、检查、使用、比较等就其是否正确、合格等方面做出决定。 trial 指对人或物进行试验以确定其效果或价值等。
□ **explain** [iks'plein]	*vt.* 解释，说明 【固定搭配】explain to sb. that/explain sth. to sb. 向某人解释…… 【辨　析】explain, interpret： explain 作"解释，说明"讲时，指解释不明之事。 interpret 意为"解释，说明"，侧重于用特殊的知识、信念、判断、了解或想象去阐明特别难懂的事物。
□ **explanation** [,eksplə'neiʃən]	*n.* 解释，说明 【联想记忆】explanatory *a.* 说明的
□ **export** [iks'pɔ:t] *v.* ['ekspɔ:t] *n.*	*v.* 输出，出口 *n.* 出口商品 【联想记忆】exporter *n.* 出口商；ex- 朝外……，向外……

face [feis]	*n.* 脸，面，表面 *vt.* 面临，面向 【联想记忆】facial *a.* 面部的 【固定搭配】face to face 面对面地；face up to 大胆面对；in the face of 面对，在……前面；不顾；make faces (a face) 做怪相，做鬼脸
fail [feil]	*vi.* 失败，不及格；衰退，减弱 *vt.* 未能；使失望；没通过 【反义词】succeed 【固定搭配】fail in (doing) sth. 在……失败；fail to do sth. 没有（没能）做
failure ['feiljə]	*n.* 失败，不及格；失败者；没做到；失灵（翻译时，常做"未能，不能"讲） 【反义词】success
faint [feint]	*vi.* 发晕，昏过去 *a.* 微弱的，模糊的
fair [fɛə]	*a.* 公平的，合理的；相当的，中等的，尚好的；晴朗的；美丽的，金发的 *n.* 定期集市，交易会，博览会 【反义词】unfair
fairly ['fɛəli]	*ad.* 公平地，公正地；相当，完全
faith [feiθ]	*n.* 信任，信用；信念，信心；信仰 【固定搭配】in faith 真正地，真实地；in good faith 诚意地，诚实地；have faith in 相信，信任；lose faith in 失去对……的信念；不再信任
faithful ['feiθfl]	*a.* 守信的，忠实的；详确的，可靠的 *n.* 信徒 【固定搭配】be faithful to = be devoted/loyal to 忠实于
fall [fɔ:l]	*vi.* 落下，跌落，降落；跌倒，坠落，陷落 *n.* 秋天 【固定搭配】fall behind 落后；fall back 后退，退却；fall out 争吵，闹翻；fall back on 求助于
false [fɔ:ls]	*a.* 假的；伪造的，人造的；虚伪的
fame [feim]	*n.* 名声，名望
familiar [fə'miljə]	*a.* 熟悉的，通晓的 【固定搭配】be familiar with 通晓……，熟悉……；be familiar to 为……所熟悉
far [fɑ:]	*a.* 远的，遥远的，久远的 *ad.* 很大程度上；远 【固定搭配】as far as/so far as 只要；就……而言；far from 决不，绝非；by far[修饰比较级、最高级]……得多，最；so far 迄今为止（比较级 farther/further；最高级 farthest/furthest.）

fare [fɛə]	*n.* 车费，船费 【辨　析】fare, fee, charge: fare 指交通费用。fee 指法律或组织机构规定的固定费用，如会费、学费、入场费、报名费、手续费等，也指对职业性的服务所支付的报酬，如医生的诊费等。charge 指购买货物或获得服务所付出的价钱。
farewell [fɛə'wel]	*int.* 再会，别了　*n.* 告别
fashion ['fæʃən]	*n.* 样子，方式；流行，风尚，时髦 【固定搭配】in/out of (the) fashion 合时尚 / 不合时尚
fashionable ['fæʃənəbl]	*a.* 流行的，时髦的
fast [fɑːst]	*a./ad.* 快，迅速；紧，牢 【固定搭配】hold fast to 坚持（思想、原则等）
fault [fɔːlt]	*n.* 缺点，缺陷；过失，过错 【固定搭配】at fault 出了毛病；感到困惑；应受责备；find fault with 挑剔，抱怨 【辨　析】fault, error: fault 一般指小并且可宽容的缺点、错误。 error 指思想或行动背离正题轨道或没有得到正确指引而出现的偏差或错误。
faulty ['fɔːlti]	*a.* 有错误的，有缺点的
favo(u)r ['feivə]	*n.* 好感，喜爱；恩惠；帮助，支持　*vt.* 赞成，支持 【固定搭配】in favor of 赞成，支持；有利于
favo(u)rable ['feivərəbl]	*a.* 顺利的，有利的；称赞的，赞成的 【固定搭配】be favo(u)rable for 对某事有利；be favo(u)rable to 赞同；（对某人）有利，有益
favo(u)rite ['feivərit]	*a.* 最喜爱的　*n.* 最喜爱的人或物
feed [fiːd]	*vt.* 喂养，饲养；养活（全家，一群人）；供应，提供；满足 *vi.*（婴儿或动物）吃东西 [过去式和过去分词为 fed] *n.*（婴儿的）一次喂奶；动物的饲料 【固定搭配】feed on 以……为食，以……为能源；be fed up with 厌烦
fetch [fetʃ]	*vt.*（去）拿来；请来，带来
fever ['fiːvə]	*n.* 发热，发烧；热病；狂热，兴奋，激动 【固定搭配】have/run a high/slight fever 发高 / 低烧
few [fjuː]	*a.* 不多，少数，很少，几乎没有几个 *pron.* 很少人（或事物、地方） 【固定搭配】a few 少许，一些；quite a few 不少，有相当数目
fight [fait]	*v./n.* 打架，战斗，斗争 【固定搭配】fight for/against 为 / 向……战斗
fill [fil]	*v.* 装满，充满，填充；占据，担任，补缺 【固定搭配】fill in 填充，填写；fill out 填好，填表；fill up 装满，填满

□ **film** [film]	n. 电影，胶卷；膜，薄层 vt. 把……摄成电影
□ **final** ['fainəl]	a. 最后的，最终的；决定性的
□ **finally** ['fainəli]	ad. 最后，终于
□ **find** [faind]	v. 找，找到；发现，发觉，感到 【固定搭配】find out 发现，查明，找出
□ **finding** ['faindiŋ]	n. 发现；[pl.] 调查结果
□ **fine** [fain]	a. 美好的，优良的，优秀的；晴朗的，明朗的；纤细的；精细的，精致的 n./vt. 罚款
□ **firm** [fə:m]	a. 坚固的，结实的，稳固的；坚定的，坚决的，坚强的 n. 公司，商号 【固定搭配】be firm with sb. 对某人严格
□ **fit** [fit]	a. 适合的，恰当的，合身的；健康的，健壮的 vt. 适合，适应，配合 【固定搭配】fit in (with) 适合，适应；符合；be fit to do 适合于做；be fit for 能胜任，适合于；keep fit 保持健康 【辨　析】fit, match, suit: fit 表示合身，指尺寸和形状合适。match 表示相配、和谐。suit 表示花色、款式、式样等适合、适当，指合乎条件、身份、口味、需要等。
□ **fitness** ['fitnis]	n. 适当，恰当，合理；健康
□ **flow** [fləu]	vi. 流，流动；漂浮，飘扬 n. 流动，流量，流速
□ **fond** [fɔnd]	a. [表语] 喜爱的，爱好的；[定语] 深情的，溺爱的，慈爱的 【固定搭配】be fond of 喜爱，喜好
□ **for** [fɔ:; fə]	prep. 就……而言，对于；代替，代表；[表示对象] 为，为了，对于，给；[表示时间、数量、距离] 达到；[表示目的、方向] 向着；[表示等值关系] 换；[表示身份] 当作，作为；[表示赞成、支持] 拥护 【固定搭配】for all 尽管，虽然
□ **forbid** [fə'bid]	vt. 禁止，不许，不准 【反　义　词】permit, allow 【固定搭配】forbid sb. to do sth. 禁止某人做某事 【辨　析】forbid, prohibit, ban: forbid 指命令不许做（某事）或用（某物），通常为个人行为。prohibit 指由权威禁止，是正式的或法律上的。ban 指由法律或官方命令的强制性禁止。
□ **force** [fɔ:s]	n. 力，力量，力气；暴力，武力；[pl.] 军队，部队 vt. 强迫，迫使；强行，强加；促使 【联想记忆】forceful a. 强有力的；有说服力的；有效的 【固定搭配】in force 大批；生效；come/go/put...into force 施行，实施，实行；force sb. to do sth. = force sb. into doing sth. 强迫某人做某事

forecast ['fɔ:kɑ:st]	vt./n. 预测，预报
foreign ['fɔrin]	a. 外国的，对外的；外国产的，外国来的；外来的，异质的 【反 义 词】home, domestic
forget [fə'get]	v. 忘记，忘记做；不再把……放在心上 【反 义 词】remember 【联想记忆】forgetful a. 健忘的；不经心的，疏忽的；forgettable n. 容易被忘的 【语法考点】forget to do 忘记要做的事；forget doing sth. 忘记已经做过的事；leave sth. somewhere 表示"把某物忘在某处"。
forgive [fə'giv]	n. 原谅，饶恕，宽恕；免除 【固定搭配】forgive sb. for (doing) sth. 原谅某人做某事 【语法考点】forgave（过去式），forgiven（过去分词）
fortunate ['fɔ:tʃənit]	a. 幸运的，走好运的，吉利的 【固定搭配】be fortunate to do sth. 幸运（侥幸）地做某事；be fortunate in 在……方面很幸运
fortunately ['fɔ:tʃənitli]	ad. 幸运地，交好运地 【反 义 词】unfortunately 不幸地
fortune ['fɔ:tʃən]	n. 机会，命运，运气；大笔的钱；财富 【反 义 词】misfortune 不幸 【固定搭配】make a fortune 发财，致富
found [faund]	vt. 成立，建立，创办
foundation [faun'deiʃən]	n. 成立，建立，创办；基础，地基；根据；基金 【联想记忆】foundational a. 基本的，基础的 【固定搭配】lay a solid foundation for 为……打下坚实的基础
frame [freim]	n. 框架，框子；骨架，体格 vt. 装框子
framework ['freimwə:k]	n. 框架，构架；基本结构
frank [fræŋk]	a. 坦白的，直率的
free [fri:]	a. 自由的，无约束的；(~ of) 免费的，免除的；自由开放的，畅通的；空闲的，空余的 vt. 使自由，解放 【固定搭配】for free 免费地，无偿地；set free 释放，解放；free from 无……的，不受……影响的；free of 脱离，无……的
frequency ['fri:kwənsi]	n. 频繁；频率
frequent ['fri:kwənt]	a. 频繁的

☐ **fresh** [freʃ]	*a.* 新的，新鲜的；有生气的；清新的，凉爽的；新颖的，独特的；淡水的
☐ **friction** ['frikʃən]	*n.* 摩擦，摩擦力
☐ **frighten** ['fraitn]	*vt.* 使惊恐，吓唬 【联想记忆】frightened *a.* 受惊吓的；害怕的 【固定搭配】frighten sb. into (out of) doing sth. 使某人吓得做（不做）某事
☐ **from** [frɔm, frəm]	*prep.* [表示起点] 从，自从；[表示离开, 脱离] 离；[表示出来, 来源] 根据，按；[表示原因, 动机] 由于，出于；去除，免除，阻止
☐ **frost** [frɔst, frɔ:st]	*n.* 霜，降霜；严寒
☐ **full** [ful]	*a.* 满的，充满的；完全的，充分的 【固定搭配】in full 全部地；to the full 完全地，充分地，彻底地；be full of 充满
☐ **fun** [fʌn]	*n.* 玩笑，乐趣；有趣的人/事 【固定搭配】for/in fun 开玩笑，不是认真地；make fun of 取笑
☐ **further** ['fə:ðə]	*ad.* (far 的比较级) 更远地，更大程度上，而且，此外；进一步地 *a.* 另外的，更多的；更远的 *vt.* 促进，增进 【辨　析】far 的比较级有两种： far-farther-farthest 指（距离）远；far-further-furthest 指（程度）进一步。
☐ **furthermore** [,fə:ðə'mɔ:(r)]	*ad.* 而且，此外

☐ **gain** [gein]	*v.* 获得，赢得；增加，增进；（钟表）走快 *n.* 赢利；收益，利润；增加，增进，获得 【反　义　词】lose, loss 【固定搭配】gain in 增加，更加；gain on 逼近，赶上；gain by/from (doing) sth. 从某物中获益，得到好处
☐ **gamble** ['gæmbl]	*n./v.* 赌博，投机 【联想记忆】gambler *n.* 赌徒 【固定搭配】gamble at cards 打牌赌博；gamble in 投机买卖；gamble on 把赌注压在……上，做……投机生意
☐ **game** [geim]	*n.* 游戏，玩耍；比赛，[*pl.*] 运动会；猎物，野味 【固定搭配】give the game away 不慎泄露秘密（计谋），露出马脚；play games 闹着玩，不认真对待；play the game 遵守规则；办事公道；做事讲道德

gather ['gæðə]	*vi.* 聚集，集合；收集，采集；逐渐增加 【固定搭配】gather together 集合；聚集
get [get]	*vt.* 获得，得到；使得，使变得，成为；感染（疾病）*vi.* 到达，抵达 【固定搭配】get across 解释清楚，使人了解；get along (with) 相处，有进展，有起色；get away (from) 逃脱，离开；get down to 开始认真考虑，开始着手做；get in 收获；到达，进站；get off 下车，从……下来；离开，动身，开始；get on (with) 继续做；一上车；在……方面取得进展；get out of 逃避，改掉；get over 克服，（从病中）恢复过来；get through 结束，完成；接通电话；get together 集会，聚会；get up 起床，起立；get in the way 成为障碍；get rid of 除去，摆脱
give [giv]	*v.* 给，提供，授予；举行，举办；交给，托付；传授；进行；赠送 【固定搭配】give in 投降，让步，认输；上交；give up 放弃；give back 送还，恢复；give away = get out 泄露，暴露，出卖；give off 发出，放出；give out = hand out 分发，分派；give way(to) 让位于，被……替代；give rise to 引起，造成
glance [glɑːns]	*n.* 一看，一瞥；*vi.* 看一眼，看一看 【固定搭配】at a glance 一看就，一瞥之下；at first glance 乍一看，一看就……；take a glance at 浏览
glow [gləu]	*vi.* 发热，发光，发红的热
go [gəu]	*vi.* 去，离去，走；开动，运行，进行；变为，成为；（时间）过去，（事情）进行；被放置 【固定搭配】go about = set about 着手做；go after = go in for 追逐，追求 【联想记忆】go after, run after, be in pursuit of, be after, chase after, seek after/for 追逐；go ahead 开始；前进；go along with 陪同前行，随行；go around/round 足够分配；go by 经过，放过，过去；遵照或依照；go for 竭力获得；go in for, take up 从事，致力于；go into, look into, inquire into 研究，讨论，调查；go off 爆炸；离去；go on(with) 继续，持续；go out, die out 熄灭；go over, glance over 浏览；go through 完成，检查，审查；go with 陪同前行；与……一致，与……调和；go without, do without 没有，缺乏；无需，没有……也行；go back on/upon/from, run counter to 违背，背叛；go up 上升，增长；go along with, agree with 赞同；go wrong 走入歧途；不对头，出毛病
goal [gəul]	*n.* 终点，球门；目标，目的；进球得分
good [gud]	*a.* 好的，美好的；好心的，善良的；有本事的，擅长的；乖的，恭顺的；*n.* 善，好事；好处，利益 【固定搭配】for good 永久地，一劳永逸地；good for 有效，适用，胜任；as good as 实际上等于，简直是；和……几乎一样；do good to 有益于（反：do harm to）；too good to be true 好得令人难以置信；be good at 擅长于；It's no good/use + doing 干……无用
govern ['gʌvən]	*v.* 统治，治理；支配，影响
government ['gʌvənmənt]	*n.* 政府，内阁；管理，支配；政治，政体

governor [ˈgʌvənə]	n. 地方长官，总督；州长；主管，理事，董事
graceful [ˈgreisfl]	a. 优美的，文雅的 【反 义 词】disgraceful，graceless
grade [greid]	n. 等级，级别，年级；分数，成绩 vt. 分级，记成绩 【固定搭配】make the grade 达到标准，成功
gradual [ˈgrædjuəl]	a. 逐渐的，逐步的 【联想记忆】gradually ad. 逐渐地
graduate [ˈgrædʒuət] n. [ˈgrædʒueit] vi.	n. 毕业生；研究生 vi. 毕业 【联想记忆】graduation n. 毕业；postgraduate n. 研究生
graph [grɑ:f]	n.（曲线）图，图解
grasp [grɑ:sp]	vt. 掌握，理解；抓紧，抓住
grateful [ˈgreitfl]	a. 感激的，感谢的 【反 义 词】ungrateful 【固定搭配】be/feel grateful to sb. for sth. 因某事而感激某人
great [greit]	a. 大，极大；重大的；伟大的；美妙的
greedy [ˈgri:di]	a. 贪吃的，嘴馋的；贪婪的；渴望的 【反 义 词】generous 【固定搭配】be greedy for/of/after 渴望得到
gross [grəus]	a. 总的；毛（重）的；粗鲁的，粗俗的 【反 义 词】net a. 净（重）的
ground [graund]	n. 地面，土地；场地，场所；根据，理由 【固定搭配】gain ground 获得进展，占优势；get off the ground 进行顺利；开始；on the ground of 以……为理由，根据
group [gru:p]	n. 群，小组 vt. 分组聚集
grow [grəu]	vi. 生长，发育；增长，发展，渐渐变得，成为；种植，栽培 vt. 种植，栽种 【固定搭配】grow up 长大，成人，崛起；grow out of 长得太大而穿不上衣服；起因于，来自于（由于成长）抛弃（早年的习惯）
grown-up [ˌgrəunˈʌp] a. [ˈgrəunˌʌp] n.	a. 成长的，成熟的，成人的 n. 成年人
growth [grəuθ]	n. 生长，增长，发展；增长量
guard [gɑ:d]	v./n. 守卫，保卫，提防 n. 哨兵，警卫，看守 【固定搭配】on (one's) guard against 值（当）班，警戒；谨慎；off (one's) guard 疏忽，大意，不提防；不值班

H

☐ **habit** ['hæbit]	n. 习惯，习性，脾性 【联想记忆】habitual a. 日常的，平常的，惯常的，习惯的 【固定搭配】be in the habit of 有……习惯；get/fall into the habit of 养成……习惯；get out of the habit 改掉习惯
☐ **hand** [hænd]	n. 手；人手，职工，雇员；指针 v. 交出，传递 【联想记忆】handful a. 一把；一小撮，少数，少量 【固定搭配】at hand 在手边，在附近；hand down 传下来，传给，往下递；hand in 交上，递交；hand in hand 手拉手；联合，连在一起；hand on 传下来，依次传递；hand out 分发，发给；hand over 交出，移交，让给；on hand 在手边，临近；on the one hand... on the other hand... 一方面……，另一方面……；by hand 用手
☐ **handsome** ['hænsəm]	a.（男子）漂亮的，俊俏的；（女子）端正健美的；慷慨的，可观的 【反 义 词】ugly
☐ **hang** [hæŋ]	vt. 吊，悬挂；吊死，绞死 vi. 悬挂，吊着 【固定搭配】hang about 闲荡，徘徊，逗留；hang on 紧抓不放，（电话）不挂断；hang on to 紧握住；继续保留；hang up 挂断（电话）
☐ **happen** ['hæpən]	vi. 发生；（后接不定式）碰巧 【固定搭配】happen to do 碰巧，恰好
☐ **happy** ['hæpi]	a. 幸福的，快乐的；乐意的；合适的；幸运的 【反 义 词】unhappy, sad, upset 【联想记忆】happiness n. 幸福，快乐；happily ad. 幸福地，愉快地，恰当地，幸亏
☐ **harbo(u)r** ['ha:bə]	n. 港口，海港；避难所，藏身处 vt. 隐匿，窝藏
☐ **hard** [ha:d]	a. 硬的，坚硬的；困难的；冷酷无情的 ad. 努力地，猛烈地；严厉地 【固定搭配】be hard on/upon sb. 对某人严厉，对某人要求苛刻，对某人硬心肠 【联想记忆】be severe on/upon/with，be strict with 对某人厉害，对某人严厉
☐ **harden** ['ha:dn]	vt. 硬化，变硬
☐ **hardly** ['ha:dli]	ad. 几乎不，简直不，仅仅 【固定搭配】barely...when/before；scarcely...when/before；no sooner...than 一……就，注意 hardly 与 scarcely 和 barely 一样，当放在句首时后面的主谓须部分倒装，即 hardly...when 一……就，例如：Hardly had we got home when he knocked on the door. 我们刚到家，他就敲门了。
☐ **harm** [ha:m]	n./vt. 损害，伤害，危害 【联想记忆】harmful a. 有害的，伤害的；harmless a. 无害的 【固定搭配】come to no harm 未受到伤害；do harm to 损害，对……有害

harvest ['hɑːvist]	*n./v.* 收获，收割，收成；结果
	【联想记忆】harvestless *a.* 不生产的，无收获的；harvestman *n.* 收割者
hate [heit]	*n.* 恨，憎恨 *vt.* 不喜欢，不愿
	【固定搭配】hate to do（指做具体事）讨厌做某事；hate doing（指习惯性地）讨厌做某事
hatred ['heitrid]	*n.* 憎恶，憎恨，怨恨
	【反 义 词】love
have [hæv]	*aux.v.* 已经，曾经 *vt.*（后接不定式）必须，不得不；有，具有；从事，进行；体会，经受；使，让；吃，喝，吸（烟）
	【固定搭配】have back 要回，收回；have on 穿着，戴着；have to do with 与……有关；have to/have got to 不得不，必须；have...in mind 牢记……；have sb. do sth./get sb. to do sth. 让某人做某事；have/get sth. done 让别人做某事
	【辨　　析】must, mustn't, have to, not have to：must（主观上）必须。mustn't 禁止。have to（客观上）必须，不得不。not have to 不必。
head [hed]	*n.* 头，头顶；顶部，前部；首脑，首长 *vt.* 领导，主管；居……之首；（朝待定方向）行进
	【固定搭配】head for 朝……走去；above/over one's head 在某人头顶；太深奥，难得不能理解；make head or tail of 弄清楚，了解；off one's head 发疯的；keep one's head 保持镇静；put heads together 集思广益；use one's head 动脑筋
health [helθ]	*n.* 健康，卫生
	【固定搭配】be in good/poor health 身体好 / 不好
healthy ['helθi]	*a.* 健康的，健壮的；有益健康的；正常合理的
hear [hiə]	*vt.* 听见；听说，得知；倾听，听取；审讯，听证
	【联想记忆】hearing *n.* 听力，听觉；解释机会，听证会
	【固定搭配】hear about/of 听说；hear from（通过电话、信件等）得以联络；hear sb. do sth. 听见某人做某事；hear sb. doing sth. 听见某人在做某事
heart [hɑːt]	*n.* 心，心脏；中心，要点；内心，心肠
	【联想记忆】hearty *a.* 衷心的，亲切的；精神饱满的，丰盛的；heartily *ad.* 尽情地，强烈地；极为
	【固定搭配】at heart 在内心，实质上；heart and soul 全心全意；lose heart 丧失勇气，失去信心
heavy ['hevi]	*a.* 重的，沉重的，繁重的；大量的；猛烈的
	【联想记忆】heavily *ad.* 沉重地；猛烈地；大量地
help [help]	*v.* 帮助，救助；改善状况，促进，搀扶，带领，使进食，款待 *n.* 帮助，援助；佣人；助手，帮手
	【固定搭配】can not help doing 禁不住；忍不住；help oneself 自取所需（食物等）

☐ **helpful** ['helpfl]	*a.* 有帮助的；有益的	
☐ **helpless** ['helplis]	*a.* 无助的；无依靠的 【联想记忆】helplessly *ad.* 无能为力地，无望地	
☐ **hide** [haid]	*vt.* 隐藏，躲藏；隐瞒 *vi.*（躲）藏 【固定搭配】hide sth. from sb. 对某人隐瞒某事	
☐ **high** [hai]	*a.* 高的；高度的；高级的，高尚的 *ad.* 在高处 【固定搭配】It is high time that... 该是做……的时候了（谓语动词用过去式）	
☐ **highly** ['haili]	*ad.* 高度地，很，非常 【辨　析】high，highly： high 是指具体的"高"。highly 的意思是抽象的，意为"高度地，极为称颂地"。	
☐ **hint** [hint]	*n./v.* 暗示，示意 *n.*［常 *pl.*］建议，点子；提示，线索，迹象 【固定搭配】give/drop sb. a hint 给人暗示；take a hint 会意	
☐ **hire** ['haiə]	*v./n.* 雇用，租借 【固定搭配】for/on hire 供出租；供雇用	
☐ **history** ['histəri]	*n.* 历史；来历，经历，履历；病历，病史 【联想记忆】historic *a.* 历史上著名的，具有重大历史意义的	
☐ **historical** [his'tɔrikəl]	*a.* 历史的，有关历史的 【辨　析】historical，historic： historical 指历史上存在或发生过的。historic 指历史上有名的，有历史意义的。	
☐ **hit** [hit]	*v./n.* 打击，击中，对（某人、某事物或某地）产生不良的或意外的影响；碰撞 【固定搭配】hit upon/on 忽然想出；无意中发现	
☐ **hold** [həuld]	*vt.* 拿住，握住，持有；掌握（权利），担任（职务）；举行，召开（会议）；认为，相信；吸引；占据，守卫，托住，支撑；包含，容纳 *vi.* 持续，保持；适用 *n.* 船舱；握住；控制，掌握 【固定搭配】get hold of 抓住，掌握；hold back 阻挡，踌躇，退缩不前；hold on 握住不放；hold to（使）坚持，信守，忠于；hold up 举起，支撑，承载；阻挡，使停止	
☐ **household** ['haushəuld]	*n.* 户，家庭 *a.* 家庭的，家常的 【辨　析】household，family，home： household 是抽象的家庭，并含有家事、家务之意。 family 着重强调家庭成员。 home 强调的是"家"的概念。	
☐ **how** [hau]	*ad.* 怎么，怎样；多少，多么 【固定搭配】how about 如何，怎么样；how is it that 为什么，什么原因使得……	
☐ **however** [hau'evə]	*ad.* 无论，不管 *conj.* 然而，可是，不过	

第一部分 基础词汇

if [if]	conj. 如果，假使 【固定搭配】if only 要是……就好了；only if 只要，只有
ill [il]	a. 有病的；坏的，恶意的 ad. 坏，不利 【固定搭配】be ill with 患……病；speak ill of 说……的坏话 【辨　析】ill, sick: ill 和 sick 做表语时都表示"有病的"。而做定语时 ill 通常表示"坏的，邪恶的"，ill will "恶意"，ill treatment "虐待"；sick 表示"令人作呕的，生病的"，a sick smell "令人恶心的气味"，a sick person "病人"。
illegal [iˈli:gəl]	a. 不合法的，非法的
illness [ˈilnis]	n. 病，疾病
image [ˈimidʒ]	n. 像；肖像，形象；影像，图像
imagination [i͵mædʒiˈneiʃən]	n. 想象，想象力；空想，幻想
imagine [iˈmædʒin]	vt. 想象，设想；料想 【辨　析】imaginary, imaginable, imaginative: imaginary 意为"想象的，虚构的，假想的"。 imaginable 意为"可想象的"，往往放在所修饰词后面。 imaginative 意为"想象力丰富的"。
immediate [iˈmi:djət]	a. 立即的，即时的；直接的，最接近的 【联想记忆】immediately ad. 立即，马上；直接地，接近地；（做连接词引导时间状语从句）一……就
import [imˈpɔ:t]	vt. 输入，进口 n. (pl.) 进口商品，进口物质
importance [imˈpɔ:təns]	n. 重要；重要性 【固定搭配】be of (great) importance = be (very) important（非常）重要；be of no importance = be not important 不重要
important [imˈpɔ:tənt]	n. 重要的，重大的；有地位的，显要的 【固定搭配】It is important that... 主语从句表主观判断，从句谓语用"(should) + 动词原形"表虚拟。
impossible [imˈpɔsəbl]	a. 不可能的，做不到的

041

in [in]	prep. [表示地点、场所、位置]在……里，在……中；[表示时间]在……期间，在……以后；[表示工具、方式]以……方式；[表示状态、情况]在……中，处于；[表示范围、领域、方向]在……之内，在……方面 ad. 向里，向内；在家里，屋里 【固定搭配】be in for 肯定会经历（麻烦等）；注定遭受；in that 因为，原因在于；have it in for 跟……过不去 例如：The teacher has always had it in for me. 那位老师总跟我过不去。 Private companies are thought to be beneficial in that they promote competition. 私企的优点在于它能促进相互竞争。
include [in'klu:d]	vt. 包括，包含，计入 【联想记忆】inclusive a. 包含的；范围广的，内容丰富的 【反 义 词】exclude 排除，排斥
income ['inkəm]	n. 收入，所得，进款 【反 义 词】expense 花费 【辨　析】income, revenue: income 个人的收入。revenue 国家、组织的收入。
increase [in'kri:s]	v./n. 增加，增长，增进 【反 义 词】decrease, reduce, diminish，on the decline 【固定搭配】on the increase 正在增加，不断增长；increase by 增加了……；increase to 增加到……
increasingly [in'kri:siŋli]	ad. 日益，越来越多地
indeed [in'di:d]	ad. 的确，确实
independent [,indi'pendənt]	a. 独立的，自治的，有主见的；自立的，自力更生的 【固定搭配】be independent of 独立……之外，不受……
indirect [,indi'rekt]	a. 间接的，迂回的
individual [,indi'vidjuəl]	a. 个别的，单独的；独特的 n. 个人，个体 【辨　析】individual, personal, private: individual 指独立于他人的，意为"单独的，个别的"，与 general（普遍的）和 collective（集体的）相对。personal 意为"个人的，亲自的。"private 意为"私人的，秘密的"，与 public（公共的，共有的）相对。
industrial [in'dʌstriəl]	a. 工业的；产业的 【辨　析】industrial, industrious: industrial 意为"工业的，产业的"，例如：the industrial areas of England 英格兰的工业地区。industrious 意为"勤劳的，勤奋的"，例如：an industrious student 勤勉的学生。
industry ['indəstri]	n. 工业，产业
infect [in'fekt]	vt. 传染，感染；（用快乐的、好的思想感情）感染……；影响 【联想记忆】infection n. [医] 传染，传染病，影响，感染；infectious a. 有传染性的，易传染的，有感染力的 【固定搭配】be infected with 感染上……，沾染上……

inform [in'fɔ:m]	vt. 通知，告诉，报告；告发，告密 【联想记忆】informative a. 情报的，提供情报的，见闻广博的 【固定搭配】inform sb. of sth. 把某事告知某人；inform against/on sb. 告发，检举某人
information [ˌinfə'meiʃən]	n. 消息，资料，情报 【辨　析】information, intelligence: information 强调提供给别人的情报、信息。intelligence 尤指军事情报。
injection [in'dʒekʃən]	n. 注射，注入，喷射
injure ['indʒə]	vt. 伤害，损害，损伤
injury ['indʒəri]	n. 损伤，伤害，毁坏；伤口
inner ['inə]	a. 内部的，里面的；内心的
insert [in'sə:t]	vt. 插入 【联想记忆】insertion n. 插入
inside ['in'said]	prep. 在……里，在……内　a. 内部的，里面的，内幕的　ad. 在内部，在里面　n. 内部，里面，内侧
insist [in'sist]	vi. 坚持，坚持主张，强烈要求；一贯　vt. 坚持，坚决主张，坚决认为 【联想记忆】insistence n. 坚持，坚决主张 【固定搭配】insist on/upon 坚持，坚持认为 【辨　析】insist, persist: insist 着重坚持某种意见、主张或观点，后接介词 on/upon 或 that 从句。persist 指对某种行动坚持不懈或对某种意见固执不改，后接介词 in，当"坚持说，反复说"解时，可与 insist 换用。
inspect [in'spekt]	vt. 检查，调查，视察 【联想记忆】inspection n. 调查，视察；inspector n. 检察官
inspire [in'spaiə]	vt. 使产生灵感；鼓舞，感动 【联想记忆】inspiration n. 鼓舞，鼓励；启发，灵感；inspiring a. 鼓舞的
instrument ['instrumənt]	n.（精密的）器械，仪器，工具 【固定搭配】musical instrument 乐器
insult ['insʌlt]	vt./n. 侮辱，凌辱
insurance [in'ʃuərəns]	n. 保险，保险费
insure [in'ʃuə]	vi. 保险，替……保险；保证 【固定搭配】insure sb./sth. against 给某人或某物保险，以防……
interact [ˌintər'ækt]	vi. 相互作用/影响 【固定搭配】interact with 与……相互作用，相互影响

interaction [ˌɪntərˈækʃn]	n. 交互作用，交感；交互；合作
interest [ˈɪntrɪst]	n. 兴趣，关心，注意；利息，利率；[pl.] 利益 【固定搭配】be interested in 对……感兴趣 in the interest(s) of 为了……的利益 【辨　析】interesting, uninterested, disinterested: interesting 意为"有趣的，引人入胜的"。uninterested 意为"没兴趣的，不关心的"。disinterested 意为"公平的，不偏袒的"。
internal [ɪnˈtɜːnl]	a. 内，内部的；国内的，内政的 【反　义　词】external
international [ˌɪntə(ː)ˈnæʃənəl]	a. 国际的，世界的
into [ˈɪntu, ˈɪntə]	prep. 到……里，进入；成为
introduce [ˌɪntrəˈdjuːs]	vt. 介绍；引进，引导，带领，传入；推行，提出 【固定搭配】introduce...to 把……介绍给（人或物）；introduce...into 把……传入，引入（地方等）。
introduction [ˌɪntrəˈdʌkʃən]	n. 介绍，引进，传入；引论，导言，绪论；入门
invade [ɪnˈveɪd]	vt. 侵入，侵略，侵害
invasion [ɪnˈveɪʒən]	n. 侵入，侵略
invent [ɪnˈvent]	vt. 发明，创造，捏造，虚构
invention [ɪnˈvenʃən]	n. 发明，创造，捏造，虚构
inventive [ɪnˈventɪv]	a. 发明的，有发明才能的
inventor [ɪnˈventə(r)]	n. 发明者，发明家，创造者
invest [ɪnˈvest]	v. 投资，投入 【固定搭配】invest in 对……投资，买进
investment [ɪnˈvestmənt]	n. 投资，投资额
invitation [ˌɪnvɪˈteɪʃən]	n. 邀请，招待；请柬 【固定搭配】at the invitation of sb. 应某人邀请
invite [ɪnˈvaɪt]	vt. 邀请，招待 【联想记忆】inviting a. 诱人的，吸引人的 【固定搭配】invite sb. to somewhere/to do sth. 邀请某人赴／做……
inward(s) [ˈɪnwəd(z)]	a. 内心的，向内的 【反　义　词】outward(s)

□ **iron** ['aiən]	*n.* 铁；烙铁，熨斗 *v.* 烫（衣），熨平 【固定搭配】iron out 熨平；消除（困难）等
□ **irrigate** ['irigeit]	*vt.* 灌溉，修水利 *vi.* 进行灌溉 【联想记忆】irrigation *n.* 灌溉
□ **item** ['aitəm]	*n.* 项目，条款；一条（新闻）

□ **join** [dʒɔin]	*v.* 结合，接合，连接；参加，加入 【固定搭配】join in 参加；join...to... 把……与……连在一起
□ **judge** [dʒʌdʒ]	*n.* 法官，裁判员；评判员，裁判 *vt.* 评价，鉴定；认为，断定，判断；审判，裁判，裁决 【联想记忆】lawyer, attorney *n.* 律师；witness *n.* 证人；sentence *v./n.* 宣判，verdict *n.* 判/裁决；criminal *n.* 罪犯；defendant *n.* 被告；accuser *n.* 原告；suit *v.* 起诉 【固定搭配】judging from/by 由……观察，由……做出判断
□ **judg(e)ment** ['dʒʌdʒmənt]	*n.* 审判，判决；判断力，识别力；意见，看法，判断 【固定搭配】in one's judg(e)ment 依某人来看，按某人的看法

□ **keep** [ki:p]	*vi.* 保持，坚持 *vt.* 保留，保存；保持；保守，遵守；防守，保卫；抑制，防止，扣留，留住；赡养，饲养；经营，管理 【固定搭配】keep back 留意，照看；keep down 阻止，阻挡；隐瞒，保留；keep off 不接近，避开；keep on 继续，保持；keep out of 躲开，置身……之外；keep to 坚持，信守；keep up 继续，坚持；保持，维持；keep up with 跟上，不落后
□ **key** [ki:]	*n.* 钥匙；答案，解答，键，琴键；方法，关键 *a.* 主要的，关键的 【固定搭配】作"解答，回答"含义时要接介词 to。如 key/answer/solution/reply/response/reaction to。

kind [kaind]	n. 种类 a. 仁慈的，和善的，亲切的 【联想记忆】kindness n. 仁慈，亲切，好意；友好行为 kindly a. 仁慈的，宜人的，舒适的 ad. 仁慈地，友好地，令人舒适地 【固定搭配】in kind 以实物（偿付）；以同样的方法；kind of 有点儿，有几分；of a kind 同类的；it's kind of sb. to do sth. 某人做某事真好
knit [nit]	v. 编织；接合，黏合 【联想记忆】knitting n. 编织品，针织
knock [nɔk]	n./v. 敲，敲打；碰撞 【固定搭配】knock about/around 到处游荡；knock down 撞倒，击倒；knock off 击倒，停止工作；从（价格）中减去；knock out 打昏，淘汰
know [nəu]	vt. 知道，了解，懂得；认识，熟悉；识别，认出 vi. 了解，知道 【联想记忆】known a. 已知的，闻名的，普遍认可的 【固定搭配】know better (than) 很懂得，明事理（而不至于）；be known as 被称为，被认为是；be known to 为……所熟知；be known for 因……而出名
knowledge ['nɔlidʒ]	n. 知识，学识；知道，了解 【联想记忆】knowledgeable a. 有知识的，博学的 【固定搭配】to one's knowledge 据……所知；acquire/obtain/get knowledge 获得知识；enlarge/broaden/widen knowledge 扩充知识；a thirst for knowledge 求知欲

labo(u)r ['leibə]	n. 劳动，工作；劳力，劳方 v. 劳动，苦干 【固定搭配】physical labor 体力劳动；mental labor 脑力劳动
lag [læg]	vi./n. 落后，滞后 【固定搭配】lag behind 落后
large [lɑ:dʒ]	a. 大的，广大的；大规模的，众多的 【固定搭配】at large 总体地；详细地；by and large 大体上，总的来说
largely ['lɑ:dʒli]	ad. 大部分，基本上；大规模地
last [lɑ:st]	a. 最后的；最近的；上一个的 ad. 最后，最近 vi. 持续，持久 【反义词】first 【联想记忆】lastly ad. 最后，终于；lasting a. 持久的，耐久的，稳定的 【固定搭配】at last 最终，终于 【辨析】last, terminal: last 指在一系列人、事物，特别是同类中居最后的。terminal 指"到头的，极限的"。

late
[leit]

a./ad. 迟，迟到 *a.* 晚的，晚期的；已故的；后期的，末期的
【反 义 词】early

lately
['leitli]

ad. 最近，近来

later
['leitə]

ad. 后来；过一会儿
【固定搭配】later on 以后，后来
【辨　　析】late 的比较级有两种：
later（最高级为 latest）；latter（最高级为 last）。later 指时间上较迟；latter 指顺序上居后。

latter
['lætə]

a. 后者的；后一半的　*n.* 后者
【固定搭配】the former..., the latter... 前者……，后者……

law
[lɔ:]

n. 法律，法规；法则，定律
【联想记忆】lawful *a.* 合法的，法定的
【辨　　析】law, rule, regulation：
law 意为"法律，法规"，指由立法机关制定的行为准则，也可指自然规律。rule 意为"规则，规定"，指民间组织为指导或控制人们行为或行动而制定的条规，也可指事物发展的规律。regulation 意为"规则，规章"，指由政府或权力机构所制定的规则、法令、章程，要大家共同遵守。

lay
[lei]

vt. 放，搁；下（蛋）；铺设；设置，布置
【固定搭配】lay down 放下；拟订；铺设；lay off（临时）解雇；休息；lay out 安排，布置，设计；摆开，陈列，展示
【辨　　析】lay, lie：
lay—laid—laid—laying 放下，铺设；lie—lay—lain—lying 躺下；lie—lied—lied—lying 说谎。

layer
['leiə]

n. 层

layout
['leiaut]

n. 布局，安排，设计

lead
[li:d]

n. 铅；领先地位　*v.* 领导，率领，领先；引导，带领；导致，通向
【固定搭配】lead to 通向；导致，引起；hold the lead 保持领先地位

leader
['li:də]

n. 领袖，领导者

leadership
['li:dəʃip]

n. 领导
【固定搭配】under the leadership of 在……的领导下

leading
['li:diŋ]

a. 领先的；一流的，最主要的

leak
[li:k]

vi. 漏，渗漏；泄露，走漏　*n.* 漏洞，裂缝；泄露
【联想记忆】leakage *n.* 漏，泄漏；leaky *a.* 渗漏的，易漏的

leap
[li:p]

v. 跳跃，跳过

learn [lə:n]
v. 学习，学会，记住；获悉
【联想记忆】learning n. 知识，学问
【固定搭配】learn...by heart 牢记……，背下来；learn from 向……学习；learn of (about) 听说，获悉

learned ['lə:nid]
a. 有学问的，博学的

least [li:st]
a. 最小的，最少的
【反 义 词】most
【固定搭配】at least 最低限度；least of all 最不，尤其；not in the least 丝毫不，一点也不；to say the least 最起码

leave [li:v]
vi. 离开，出发 vt. 离开留下，剩下，使处于；忘带；交给，托付 n. 许可，同意；休假
【反 义 词】arrive, reach, remain, stay
【固定搭配】leave behind 落后；把……留下；忘带；leave off 停止，中断；leave out 省略，遗漏；take (one's) leave of 向……告辞

lend [lend]
vt. 出借，借给
【固定搭配】lend oneself to 适合于；lend sb. a hand 帮……一把

length [leŋθ]
n. 长，长度
【固定搭配】at length 最后，终于；详细地；go to great lengths 竭尽全力

lengthen ['leŋθən]
vt. 伸长，延长
【反 义 词】shorten
【辨 析】lengthen, extend, prolong, stretch:
lengthen 指在空间或时间上变得更长，不包括宽度的延长；extend 指长度、宽度、期限、意义、影响等方面都超过目前的范围，可指时间、空间方面的扩大或延长；prolong 指时间的延长，超过一般或正常的限度；stretch 指由曲变直、由短变长的伸展。

less [les]
a./ad. 更少，较少，更小
【反 义 词】more
【固定搭配】even (still, much) less 更不用说（用于否定句）；no less than 不少于，多达；none the less 仍然
【辨 析】no less than, not less than:
no less than 意为"不少于"，强调的是数目之大；not less than 意为"至少有……"。

level ['lev(ə)l]
n. 水平；水准，等级 a. 平的 vt. 弄平；夷平
【反 义 词】uneven
【固定搭配】level off/out 做水平运动，呈平稳状态；be level with 与……齐平

lie [lai]
vi. 躺，平放；位于；处于，在于 n. 谎言 v. 说谎
【固定搭配】take lying down 甘受（挫败等）lie in 位于……

life [laif]
n. 生命；寿命，一生；生活，生计
【固定搭配】bring to life 使复活，给……以活力；come to life 苏醒过来，开始有生气；for life 一生，终身

lifestyle ['laifstail]	*n.* 生活方式
lifetime ['laiftaim]	*n.* 一生,终身
lift [lift]	*v.* 提起,举起;消散,(云雾)升起 *n.* 举起;升起;电梯,升降机;搭便车 【反 义 词】lower 【辨 析】lift, raise, elevate: lift 指将笨重物体从地上或较低处提升到较高处。raise 指不费力地将物体提升。elevate 多用于抽象事物,如地位、情操等的提高。
light [lait]	*n.* 光,光线,光亮;灯,灯光 *vt.* 点,点燃;照亮,照耀 *a.* 轻的;轻捷的,轻快的;淡(色)的;明亮的 【联想记忆】lighten *vt.* 照亮,使照亮;减轻(负担),缓和;使轻松;愉快 【固定搭配】bring to light 揭露,将……曝光;come to light 显露,暴露;in (the) light of 鉴于,由于;light up 照亮,点燃;容光焕发;shed/throw/cast light on/upon 使人了解,阐明 【反 义 词】darkness
lighting ['laitiŋ]	*n.* 照明;灯光;点火
lightning ['laitniŋ]	*n.* 闪电 *a.* 闪电般的,快速的
like [laik]	*v.* 喜欢,喜爱;想要 *prep.* 像,同……一样 *a.* 同样的,相像的,类似的 【反 义 词】dislike, unlike 【辨 析】dislike, unlike, liking: dislike 意为"不喜欢,厌恶"。unlike 意为"不像,和……不同",是介词。liking 是名词,意为"爱好"。
likely ['laikli]	*a.* 可能的;似乎适合的 *ad.* 大概,多半 【反 义 词】unlikely 【联想记忆】likelihood *n.* 可能,可能性
limit ['limit]	*n.* 界限,限度;[*pl.*] 范围 *vt.* 限制,限定 【固定搭配】within limit 适度地 【辨 析】limit, confine, restrict: limit 为一般用词,指数量、程度或范围上的限制。confine 为限制某人的活动范围。restrict 多指权威或官方的限制。
limitation [ˌlimi'teiʃən]	*n.* 缺陷,限额,限制 【辨 析】limit, limitation: limit 常用复数,表示"界限,极限",指在一定范围内人或物不得或无法超越的限制、界限或极限。limitation 指外来干涉因素(如法律、环境、风俗习惯等)对人或物所实施的限制或约束,用作复数时,指智力、能力等的局限或缺陷。
limited ['limitid]	*a.* 被限定的,有限的 【联想记忆】unlimited *a.* 无限制的 limitless 无限制的;无限度的

line [lain]	*n.* 线，线条；行，行列；航线，交通线，通信线 *v.* 排队，排列 【固定搭配】in line 排成直线，成一排；in line with ……一致，与……符合；line up 排队，使排成一行；on line 联机的；out of line 不成直线，不一致，出格；line up 排成行；安排
link [liŋk]	*v.* 连接，联系 *n.* 联系
little ['litl]	*a.* 小的，幼小的；矮小的，渺小的；不多的，少到几乎没有的 *ad.* 不多，几乎没有 【固定搭配】a little 一些，少许，稍许，一点儿；little by little 逐渐地；quite a little 相当多，不少
live [liv]	*vi.* 住，居住；生活，过活，生存 *vt.* 过生活 [laiv] *a.* 活的，有生命的；实况播送的 【固定搭配】live on/by 靠……生活，以……为食；live through 度过，经受住；live up to 无愧于，不辜负；live with 与……一起生活，忍受，忍耐；live sth. down 使（往日的难堪、丑闻、罪行等）淡忘 【辨　　析】live on, live by： live on 是指"以……为食"；live by 是指"以某种手段生活"。
livelihood ['laivlihud]	*n.* 生计，谋生之道
lively ['laivli]	*a.* 活泼的，活跃的；令人兴奋的
liver ['livə]	*n.* 肝；肝脏
living ['liviŋ]	*a.* 活的，现存的 *n.* 生活，生计 【固定搭配】make/gain/earn a living 谋生；living standard 生活水平
load [ləud]	*v.* 装，装载，装填 *n.* 负荷，负担 【固定搭配】be loaded with 装满；a load of 大量的；loads of 很多
loan [ləun]	*n.* 贷款；借款；借 *v.* 借 【反　义　词】borrow 【固定搭配】on loan 暂借
local ['ləukəl]	*a.* 地方的，当地的；局部的 【联想记忆】locally *ad.* 在本地，局部地
lock [lɔk]	*n.* 锁 *v.* 上锁，锁住 【固定搭配】lock up 将……封锁；把……监禁起来
logic ['lɔdʒik]	*n.* 逻辑，逻辑学
logical ['lɔdʒikəl]	*a.* 逻辑（上）的，符合逻辑的 【反　义　词】illogical
lonely ['ləunli]	*a.* 孤独的，寂寞的；荒凉的，人迹稀少的 【反　义　词】happy 【联想记忆】loneliness *n.* 孤独，寂寞

☐ **long** [lɔŋ]	*a.* 长的，长远的；长期的 *ad.* 长久地，长期地 *vi.* 渴望 【反 义 词】short, shortly 【联想记忆】be hungry for，be thirsty for 渴望 【固定搭配】no longer 不再，已不；as/so long as 只要；before long 不久以后；long for 渴望……
☐ **look** [luk]	*vi./n.* 看，注视 *v.* 好像，显得 *n.* 脸色，外表 【联想记忆】seek for/after，be in pursuit of，be/go/run after，hunt for 寻求，追求 【固定搭配】look after 照顾，关心，照料；look at 看，注视；look back 回顾，回头看；look down upon 看不起；look for 寻找，寻求；look forward to 盼望，期待；look in 顺便看望，顺便访问；look into 窥视，调查，过问；look on 旁观；look out 注意，警惕；look over 检查，查看，调查；look through 浏览，温习；look up 查找，查阅，寻找，查出；look up to 尊敬，敬仰
☐ **loose** [lu:s]	*a.* 松的，宽的，松散的
☐ **loosen** ['lu:sn]	*vt.* 解开；松开 【反 义 词】tighten
☐ **lose** [lu:z]	*vt.* 丢，失去，丧失；失败，输；失落；迷（路） 【固定搭配】lose oneself 迷路；lose oneself in 专心致志于；lose one's heart 泄气；lose no time 不浪费一点儿时间，立即着手
☐ **loss** [lɔs]	*n.* 丧失，丢失；亏损，损失；失败 【固定搭配】at a loss 困惑，不知所措
☐ **lost** [lɔst]	*a.* 失去的；错过的，浪费掉的；无望的，迷路的 【固定搭配】be lost 迷路；be lost in 陷入……
☐ **lot** [lɔt]	*pronoun.* 许多；大量 *n.* 场地 【固定搭配】a lot/a lot of/lots of 大量；非常，相当
☐ **low** [ləu]	*a.* 低，矮；低级的，下层的，卑贱的；低声的 【反 义 词】high

☐ **mad** [mæd]	*a.* 发疯的；恼火的；愚蠢的，不明智的；痴迷的 【固定搭配】be mad at sb./sth. 对某人（某事）恼火；be mad with sth. 因某事而发狂；be mad about/for/on 特别喜欢，痴迷
☐ **magnificent** [mæg'nifisnt]	*a.* 壮丽的；华丽的；富丽堂皇的，宏伟的，极好的；值得赞扬的 【反 义 词】simple，plain

major [ˈmeidʒə]	*a.* 较大的；重要的 *n.* 专业 【反 义 词】minor 【固定搭配】major in 主修
majority [məˈdʒɔriti]	*n.* 多数，大多数 【反 义 词】minority 【固定搭配】be in the majority 占多数；gain the majority 获得多数票
make [meik]	*vt.* 使，做，制造 【联想记忆】makeup *n.* 化妆品 【固定搭配】make for 走向，冲向；make one's way 前进，行进；make out 开列，书写；看出，辨认出；理解，了解；make up 拼凑，组成，构成；编造（故事、谎言等）；make up for 补偿，弥补 【辨　　析】make, manufacture, produce： make 指用手或机器进行简单生产。manufacture 指机器的大规模生产。produce 既可指物质生产，又可用于描述抽象事物的产生。
manage [ˈmænidʒ]	*vt.* 管理；设法；对付 【联想记忆】manageable *a.* 易支配的，易处理的
management [ˈmænidʒmənt]	*n.* 管理；经营，处理
manager [ˈmænidʒə]	*n.* 经理，管理者
mankind [mænˈkaind]	*n.* 人类
manner [ˈmænə]	*n.* 方式，方法；礼貌；态度，举止 【固定搭配】all manner of 各种各样的，形形色色的；in a manner of speaking 不妨说，在某种意义上
many [ˈmeni]	*a.* 许多的 *n.* 许多（人） 【固定搭配】a great/good many 许多，大量；many a 许多的（many a + 单数名词，做主语时谓语动词用单数；a good/great many + 复数名词，做主语时谓语动词用复数。）
mark [mɑ:k]	*n.* 记号，标记，痕迹；分数 *vt.* 记分，打分；做标记，标志 【固定搭配】mark down 记下；降低……的价格；降低……的分数；mark off 画出，画线分开；mark up 提高……的价格，提高……的分数
master [ˈmɑ:stə]	*n.* 主人，雇主；能手，名家，大师；硕士 *vt.* 掌握，精通 【联想记忆】masterpiece *n.* 名著，杰作 【固定搭配】be master of... 掌握……；控制……；精通……
match [mætʃ]	*n.* 火柴；比赛，竞赛；对手，敌手 *v.* 匹配，相配 【固定搭配】match...for/in... 在……方面与……匹敌；match up to 符合期望，与（预想）一致；make a match 做媒；meet one's match 遇到对手
mate [meit]	*n.* 伙伴，配偶 *v.* 使交配

material
[mə'tiəriəl]

n. 材料，原料；资料 *a.* 物质的，实物的，具体的

【反 义 词】immaterial, spiritual

【联想记忆】materialize *vt./vi.* 使……物质化，使具体化；实现；materialism *n.* 唯物主义；实利主义

【辨　　析】material, matter, substance：
material 指用于造物的原材料，可用于抽象或具体物质。matter 指与精神相对的实体，是构成世界的一切。substance 通常指某个具体的或特殊种类的物质。

matter
['mætə]

n. 物质，物体；事情，情况，事态；毛病，麻烦事 *vi.* 要紧，有关系

【固定搭配】for that matter 就此而言；in the matter of 关于；no matter 无论，不管

mean
[mi:n]

vt. 意指，意味着；意欲，打算 *a.* 低劣的，平庸的；吝啬的；平均的 *n.* 平均值

【固定搭配】be meant to do 打算做，必须做；be meant for 为……而有，注定要属于……；mean to do 打算做……；mean doing 意味着……

meaning
['mi:niŋ]

n. 意义，意思

means
[mi:nz]

n. 方法，手段，工具

【固定搭配】by all means 尽一切办法，务必；by any means 无论如何；by no means 决不；by means of 用，凭借

meanwhile
['mi:nwail]

n. 其时，其间 *ad.* 同时，当时

【固定搭配】in the meanwhile = in the meantime 在此期间，另一方面

measure
['meʒə]

vt. 量，测量；估量 *n.* 度量单位，计量标准；[*pl.*] 措施，方法

【固定搭配】beyond measure 不可估量，极度，过分；for good measure 另外；measure up 合格，符合标准；take measures 采取措施

measurement
['meʒəmənt]

n. 测量，量度；尺寸，宽度，长度

medical
['medikəl]

a. 医学的，医疗的；医药的；内科的

medicine
['medsin]

n. 内服药，医药；医学

mend
[mend]

vt. 修理，修补，缝补

【固定搭配】mend one's ways 改过，改正错误

【辨　　析】mend, patch, repair：
mend 是把坏了的简单物品，如衣服、鞋袜等修好，使其能再用。patch 表示"修补，打补丁"。repair 指把损坏或有故障的复杂大件物品，如机器、车辆、建筑物等，恢复其原来性能、形状、质量等。

mental
['mentl]

a. 思想的，精神的；智力的，脑力的

mention
['menʃən]

vt./n. 提及，说起，讲述

【固定搭配】as mentioned above 如上所述；not to mention = without mentioning 更不必说，除……外，还

☐ **mere** [miə]	*a.* 仅仅的，纯粹的 【辨　析】mere, only： mere 和 only 都是"仅仅"的意思。mere 用于冠词之后名词之前，而 only 用于冠词之前。
☐ **merely** ['miəli]	*ad.* 仅仅，只不过 【固定搭配】not merely...but also 不仅……而且……
☐ **merit** ['merit]	*n.* 优点，价值 【反　义　词】demerit, disadvantage
☐ **merry** ['meri]	*a.* 欢乐的，兴高采烈的 【反　义　词】sad，unhappy
☐ **mess** [mes]	*n.* 混乱，混杂，脏乱 【联想记忆】messy *a.* 肮脏的，凌乱的，杂乱的 【固定搭配】in a mess 乱七八糟；make a mess of 把……弄糟；mess about/around 瞎忙；浪费时间，闲荡；mess up 把……弄糟/弄乱 【辨　析】disorder, mess： mess 着重指脏、乱；而 disorder 则指没条理、没顺序的凌乱。
☐ **method** ['meθəd]	*n.* 方法，办法 【联想记忆】methodical *a.* 秩序井然的，有条不紊的，有条理的
☐ **mild** [maild]	*a.* 温暖的，暖和的；温和的，温柔的；（烟、酒）味淡的 【联想记忆】mildly *ad.* 温和地，适度地，略微地；mildness *n.* 温和，温暖
☐ **mind** [maind]	*n.* 头脑，精神；理智；想法，意见；心情，心思 *v.* 留心，注意；介意，在乎；照料 【固定搭配】keep... in mind 记住……；have in mind 想到，考虑到；make up one's mind 决定，下决心；never mind 不要紧，没关系；to my mind 依我看，我认为 mind 作"介意"讲时，其后跟 if 条件句或动名词，但不能接动词不定式，如：Do/Would you mind if...? 或 Do/Would you mind (one's) doing...?
☐ **minor** ['mainə]	*a.* 较小的，较少的，较次要的 *n.* 辅修科目 *vi.* 辅修 【固定搭配】minor in 兼修，辅修
☐ **minority** [mai'nɔriti]	*n.* 少数，少数派；少数民族
☐ **miracle** ['mirəkl]	*n.* 奇迹，令人惊奇的人/事
☐ **misconduct** [,mis'kɔndʌkt]	*n.* 行为不检
☐ **miserable** ['mizərəbl]	*a.* 痛苦的，悲惨的；低劣的，贫乏的 【联想记忆】misery *n.* 痛苦，苦恼，悲惨，不幸
☐ **mislead** [mis'li:d]	*vt.* 使误入歧途；把……带错路；使误解
☐ **miss** [mis]	*n.* 小姐 *vt.* 未击中，没达到；未看到，未注意到；没赶上；遗漏，省去；怀念 【固定搭配】miss out 不包括；错过机会

mix [miks]	vt. 混合，掺和；混淆，混乱 【固定搭配】mix up 混合，混淆 【辨 析】mix, blend: mix 是把两个以上不同的东西混合起来。blend 是把两个以上近似的东西混合起来，另外调制出新的东西。
mixture ['mikstʃə]	n. 混合，混合物
mobile ['məubail]	a. 运动的，活动的；流动的
mode [məud]	n. 方式，样式 【固定搭配】be in mode 流行；be out of mode 不流行；follow the mode 追随时尚
model ['mɔdl]	n. 样式；模型；模特儿；模范，典型 vt. 做……的模型；模仿，依……仿造 【固定搭配】after/on the model of 以……为模范；model (...) on/after 模仿，仿制
modern ['mɔdən]	a. 现代的，近代的；新式的 【反 义 词】ancient, antique, out-of-date
modernization [ˌmɔdənai'zeiʃən]	n. 现代化
modest ['mɔdist]	a. 端庄的，朴素的；谦虚的，谦逊的；适度的 【反 义 词】immodest, excessive
modesty ['mɔdisti]	n. 谦虚，谦逊
moment ['məumənt]	n. 片刻，瞬间，时刻 【联想记忆】momentary a. 瞬间的，刹那间的 【固定搭配】at the moment 此刻；for the moment 暂时，目前；in a moment 一会儿；the moment（that）一……就……
monitor ['mɔnitə]	n. 班长；监测器，显示器 v. 监听，监测
mood [mu:d]	n. 心情，情绪；语气 【固定搭配】be (not) in the mood for/to do sth. 有/没有情绪做某事；be in good (bad) mood 情绪好/不好
moon [mu:n]	n. 月球，月亮；卫星
more [mɔ:(r)]	a. 更多的，较多的 ad. 更，更多地 【固定搭配】more or less 或多或少，多少有点；more and more 越来越；no more 不再；once more 再一次，又一次
moreover [mɔ:'əuvə]	ad. 此外；而且

☐ **most** [məust]	*a.* 最多的，最大的 *ad.* 最，非常，极 *pron.* 大多数，大部分 【反 义 词】least 【固定搭配】at most/at the most 最多，至多；make the most of 充分利用 【辨　　析】most, most of： most 后可直接跟名词（可数或不可数），同时，也可接由形容词修饰的名词。注意：跟可数名词时，谓语动词要用复数形式。如：Most boys like playing football. 大部分男孩都喜欢踢足球。most 后不能直接跟由定冠词、指示代词或物主代词所修饰的名词，那么，遇到这些情况要用 most of 代替 most。如：I spent most of my time learning to play the piano last year. 去年我把大部分时间都花在学弹钢琴上了。
☐ **mostly** ['məustli]	*ad.* 主要地；一般地；通常地
☐ **motion** ['məuʃən]	*n.* 动，运动；提议，动议 【固定搭配】in motion 在动，运转中
☐ **move** [muːv]	*vt.* 移动，搬动，迁移；感动 *n.* 动，动作，行动 *vi.* 动，走动；搬家，迁移
☐ **must** [mʌst, məst]	*v.* 必须，应当；必定，务必 【语法考点】must + have done 对过去事情的肯定推测。
☐ **mysterious** [mis'tiəriəs]	*a.* 神秘的，可疑的，难以理解的
☐ **mystery** ['mistəri]	*n.* 神秘，神秘的事，悬疑小说
☐ **myth** [miθ]	*n.* 神话

☐ **name** [neim]	*n.* 名字，名称；名声，名望；名义 *vt.* 给……取名；列举；任命，提名 【联想记忆】namely *ad.* 也就是 【固定搭配】in the name of 以……的名义；name after 根据……命名
☐ **narrow** ['nærəu]	*a.* 狭的，狭窄的；狭隘的 【联想记忆】narrowly *ad.* 勉强地，精细地；narrowness *n.* 狭小，小气 【反 义 词】broad, wide
☐ **native** ['neitiv]	*n.* 土著，当地人 *a.* 本国的，本地的，土生的 【反 义 词】foreign 【固定搭配】native land 祖国；native place 故乡；native language 本国语；go native 入乡随俗

natural ['nætʃərəl]	a. 自然界的，天生的；天赋的，固有的 【反 义 词】artificial, unnatural
nature ['neitʃə]	n. 自然，自然界；本性，性质，天性 【固定搭配】by nature 本性上，生性；in nature 性质上，实质上
nearly ['niəli]	ad. 差不多，几乎 【固定搭配】not nearly 远不及，根本没有
neat [ni:t]	a. 整洁的，简洁的；优美的，精致的；利索的 【反 义 词】untidy
necessarily ['nesisərili]	ad. 必然，必定；当然 【固定搭配】not necessarily 未必（表部分否定）
necessary ['nesisəri]	a. 必要的，必需的；必然的 【反 义 词】unnecessary 【固定搭配】if necessary 如有必要
necessity [ni'sesiti]	n. 必要性，必然性；必需品 【固定搭配】of necessity 无法避免地，必定
need [ni:d]	v./n. 必须，必要；缺少 aux. v. 需要，必须 【联想记忆】needy a. 贫困的，贫穷的 【固定搭配】in need of 需要
neither ['naiðə, 'ni:ðə]	a.（两者）没有一个的 pron. 两者都不 ad. 也不 【固定搭配】neither...nor（既）不……也不（neither...nor 连接两个主语时，谓语动词的形式根据 nor 后面的主语形式来确定。如：Neither he nor I agree with this. = Neither I nor he agrees with this.）
never ['nevə]	ad. 永不，从不；绝不
nevertheless [,nevəðə'les]	ad. 仍然，不过
noble [nəubl]	a. 贵族的；高尚的；宏伟的 【反 义 词】humble
nobody ['nəubədi]	pron. 没有人 【反 义 词】everybody
none [nʌn]	pron. 谁也不，哪个都不 ad. 一点也不 【固定搭配】none but 除……之外没有，只有；none other than 正是；none too 一点也不
nor [nɔ:]	conj. 也不
normal ['nɔ:məl]	a. 一般的，正常的，标准的；正规的；精神健全的 n. 常态，通常标准，一般水平 【联想记忆】normality n. 常态；normalizable a. 可规范化的；normalize v. 规范化；normalization n. 正常化，标准化
normally ['nɔ:məli]	ad. 一般地；通常地

not [nɔt]	ad. 不，没
note [nəut]	n. 笔记；（外交）照会；注解，注释；备忘录；票据，纸币；音符 vt. 注意，记录 【联想记忆】notable a. 值得注意的；显著的，著名的 【固定搭配】compare notes 交换意见；of note 显要的，有名望的；take note of 注意，留意 【辨　析】note, notice： note "注意"，指用心观察或仔细注意。notice 多指偶然看到或无意识地注意到，强调注意的结果。
nothing [ˈnʌθiŋ]	n. 微不足道的人或事 pron. 没有东西，什么也没有；毫无趣味的事 【固定搭配】be nothing to 对……无所谓；for nothing 不花钱地，徒劳地；have nothing to do with 与……无关；nothing but 只有，只不过
notice [ˈnəutis]	vt. 注意到，看到 n. 注意，认识；通知，通告，布告 【反 义 词】overlook 【联想记忆】notify vt. 通知，告知，报告 【固定搭配】at short/a moment's notice 提前很短的时间通知；get notice 被解雇；take notice of 注意
noticeable [ˈnəutisəbl]	a. 显而易见的，显著的，值得注意的
novel [ˈnɔvəl]	n. 长篇小说 【联想记忆】novelty n. 新奇，新颖
novelist [ˈnɔvəlist]	n. 小说家 【联想记忆】writer n. 作家；author n. 作者；dramatist n. 剧作家；playwright n. 剧作家；scriptwriter n. 电影剧本作家
nowhere [ˈnəuwɛə]	ad. 哪儿也不，什么地方都没有 【反 义 词】everywhere 【固定搭配】get nowhere 使无进展，使不能成功；nowhere near 远远不，远不及

observation [ˌɔbzəˈveiʃən]	n. 观察，监视；评论，意见 【联想记忆】observatory n. 天文台，气象台 【固定搭配】observation on/upon... 关于……的评论；keep...under (close) observation 对……（密切）监视

observe [əbˈzəːv]

vt. 观察，注意到，看到；遵守；说，评论
【反 义 词】ignore, overlook, violate
【联想记忆】observable *a.* 看得见的，引人注目的；observing *a.* 观察力敏锐的
【固定搭配】observe on/upon 评论

observer [əbˈzəːvə]

n. 观察员，观察家

obtain [əbˈtein]

vt. 获得，得到
【反 义 词】lose
【联想记忆】obtainable *a.* 能得到的，能达到的

obvious [ˈɔbviəs]

a. 明显的，显而易见的
【反 义 词】vague, obscure

obviously [ˈɔbviəsli]

ad. 明显地，显然地

odd [ɔd]

a. 奇数的；奇怪的，古怪的；临时的，不固定的；大约的
【反 义 词】even, normal
【固定搭配】against (all) the odds 尽管有极大的困难，尽管极为不利；at odds (with) 与……不和，与……争吵，与……不一致；odds and ends 零星杂物，琐碎物品
【辨　　析】odd, queer, peculiar, strange：
odd 指一反常态或出乎意料，不寻常。queer 表示"古怪的，怪僻的，神经不正常的"。peculiar 强调与众不同，强调奇异的独特性。strange 所指范围较广泛，泛指一切异乎寻常或较少看到乃至新奇的东西。

of [ɔv, əv]

prep. [表示从属关系]……的；由……制成[或组成]的；含有……的，装有……的；[表示性质，状况]；[表示位置，距离]；关于；[表示同位关系]；[表示数量，种类]；[表示部分或全部]；由于，因为；[表示分离，除去，剥夺][表示行为主体或对象]

off [ɔːf, ɔf]

ad. 离，距，离开；切断，停止；中止；完，光；剪掉，扣掉，消除 *prep.* 从……离开，离……，偏离
【固定搭配】be well off 富有的；off and on 断断续续地，间歇地，有时
【联想记忆】from time to time, off and on 断断续续地；very soon, at once, right away, in no time 立刻；give off 散发；come off 成功

offer [ˈɔfə]

v. 提供，提出；愿意给予；奉献 *n.* 提供，提议；报价，出价
【固定搭配】offer one's hand 握手；offer to do 主动做某事；on offer 削价出售
【联想记忆】give sb. sth., give sth. to sb., provide/supply sb. with sth. 向某人提供

omit [əuˈmit]

vt. 删除，省略，省去；遗漏，忽略
【联想记忆】omission *n.* 省略，疏忽，失职

on [ɔn]

prep. 在……上；靠近，在……旁；关于，有关；在……时候，在……后立即；朝，向，针对；凭，根据；向前，（继续）下去；在从事……中，处于……情况；在……供职，（是）……成员 *ad.* (放/穿/连接)上；向前，（继续）下去
【固定搭配】and so on 等等；off and on 断断续续地，不时地；on and on 不断地；later on 不久，后来；be on 行得通的，认可的

once [wʌns]	ad. 一次，一度，曾经 conj. 一旦……就…… 【固定搭配】all at once 突然；同时，一起；at once 立刻，马上；once for all 一劳永逸地，永远地
only [ˈəunli]	ad. 只，仅仅 a. 唯一的 【固定搭配】not only...but (also) 不但……而且；only if 只有……才；only too 极，非常；an only child 独生子女；only to do 结果是（表示意外的结果，only + 状语放在句首时，句子谓语用倒装结构。not only... but also 连接并列主语时，句子谓语的形式根据 but (also) 后的主语形式来定。）
onto [ˈɔntu]	prep. 到……之上，在……之上
open [ˈəupən]	a. 开着的；开放的；公开的，公共的；诚实的，坦率的；营业的；开阔的，空旷的 v. 打开；开始，开张，开放 【反 义 词】closed 【固定搭配】be open to 易接受……的，暴露于……的；in the open air 在露天；in the open 公开地；open up 开辟，开发；an open secret 公开的秘密；open letter 公开信；open-minded 愿接受新思想的，无偏见的
opening [ˈəupəniŋ]	a. 开始的，开幕的 n. 洞，孔，通道；开，开始，开端；空地；（职务的）空缺 【反 义 词】end, terminal
openly [ˈəupənli]	ad. 公然地，公开地；直率地，坦白地
operate [ˈɔpəreit]	vi. 操作，运转；动手术，开刀 vt. 操作，操纵，进行 【固定搭配】operate on 给……动手术
operation [ˌɔpəˈreiʃən]	n. 操作，工作，运转；手术；运算；有效，起作用，发生影响 【固定搭配】bring/put... into operation 使实施，使执行；come/go into operation 实施，执行；in operation 工作中，运转中；起作用，生效，实施
operational [ˌɔpəˈreiʃənl]	a. 操作的，运作的
opportunity [ˌɔpəˈtjuːniti]	n. 机会 【固定搭配】take the opportunity to do sth./of doing sth. 趁机，借此机会
opposite [ˈɔpəzit]	a. 对面的，对立的；相反的 n. 对立物，对立面 prep. 在……对面 【反 义 词】same 【联想记忆】opposition n. 反对 【固定搭配】be opposite to 与……相对/相反
or [ɔː; ə]	conj. 或，或者；否则，要不然 【固定搭配】or else 否则；or so 大约；or rather 或者更确切地说

□ **order** ['ɔ:də]	*n./v.* 命令 *v.* 定制，订购 *n.* 顺序，次序；等级；秩序，治安；订货，订货单 【反 义 词】disorder 【固定搭配】in order that 以便；in order to 以便，为了；in order 整齐，秩序井然；out of order 发生故障，失调
□ **orderly** ['ɔ:dəli]	*a.* 整齐的，有条理的 【反 义 词】disorderly, orderless
□ **ordinary** ['ɔ:dinəri]	*a.* 平常的，正常的；普通的；平淡的 【反 义 词】extraordinary, unusual 【固定搭配】out of ordinary 不寻常的；非凡的
□ **other** ['ʌðə]	*a.* 另外的，别的；另一个的，其他的 *pron.* 别的东西，别人 【固定搭配】every other 每隔一个的；none other than 不是别人（或他物）而正是；other than[用于否定句] 除……之外
□ **otherwise** ['ʌðəwaiz]	*conj.* 否则，要不然 *ad.* 另外，别样，不同；在其他方面，除此以外
□ **ought** [ɔ:t]	*v./aux.* (~ to + *v.*) 应当，应该
□ **over** ['əuvə]	*prep.* 在……上方；高于，超过；在（做）……时候；越过，横跨；关于，在……方面；到处，遍及 *ad.* 翻过来；以上，超过；越过；在 / 向那边；结束 【反 义 词】under, beneath, below 【固定搭配】all over again 再一次，重新；over and over (again) 一再地，再三地；over and above 另外，此外
□ **overall** ['əuvərɔ:l]	*a.* 全面的，综合的；全部的，总计的
□ **overcome** [,əuvə'kʌm]	*vt.* 战胜，克服 【固定搭配】be overcome by/with 被……压倒
□ **own** [əun]	*a.* 自己的；特有的 *vt.* 拥有 【固定搭配】come to one's own 显示自身的特点（或价值）；on one's own 独自，靠自己；own up 坦白地承认，供认；hold one's own 坚守立场，不被击败；支撑得住
□ **owner** ['əunə]	*n.* 物主，所有权人 【辨 析】owner, possessor： owner 指财产的合法占有人，强调所有权。possessor 则指对事物现在具有使用权、支配权的人。
□ **ownership** ['əunəʃip]	*n.* 所有（权）；所有制

P

pace [peis]	*n.* 步伐，速度；一步，步距 *v.* 踱步（于）；为……定速度，为……的标兵 【固定搭配】keep/lead pace with（与……）并驾齐驱，保持一致；set the pace 起带头作用 【联想记忆】catch up with 赶上；keep up with 与……看齐；赶上 【辨 析】pace, rate, speed, velocity: pace 意为"步速，速度，节奏"，也指运动的速率。rate 意为"速率，比率"，指速度、价值、成本等，作速度讲时强调单位时间内的速度。speed 意为"速率，速度"，指任何事物持续运动时的速度，尤指车辆等无生命事物的运动速度。velocity 意为"速度"，技术用语，指物体沿着一定方向运动时的速率。
pack [pæk]	*n.* 包，包裹；一群，一组，一堆；一副（纸牌）*v.* 包装，把……打包，整理行装；装进，塞进；塞满，充满 【固定搭配】a pack of 一群……，一盒……；pack away 把……收好；pack in 停止，放弃；pack off 把……打发走；pack up 不再做某事；放弃某事物；（指机器、发动机等）不工作或不运转，出毛病，有故障；把……收好
package ['pækidʒ]	*n.* 包装，包裹，箱；一揽子交易（或计划、建议等） 【固定搭配】a package deal/offer 一揽子交易
pain [pein]	*n.* 痛苦，疼痛；[*pl.*] 努力，劳苦 【反 义 词】relief 【联想记忆】painkiller 止痛片 【固定搭配】be in pain 疼痛；苦恼；take pains 努力，尽力，下苦功；bear/endure/stand pain 忍受痛苦
painful ['peinfl]	*a.* 痛苦的，疼痛的；费心的，费力的
panic ['pænik]	*n.* 惊慌，恐慌 *a.* 恐慌的，惊慌的 *v.* 受惊，惊慌 【固定搭配】in panic 处于恐慌中；panic sb. into doing sth. 因惊吓而做某事
parallel ['pærəlel]	*a.* 与……平行的；并列的；类似的 *n.* 平行线；纬线；极其相似的人（或情况、事件等）；相似处 【固定搭配】draw a parallel between 对照，比较；be parallel to/with 与……平行；without (a) parallel 无与伦比的
part [pɑ:t]	*n.* 部分；成分；角色，作用；零件 *v.* (使)分开，分离，分别 【反 义 词】join 【固定搭配】do one's part 尽自己的职责；for one's part 就个人来说；in part 部分地，在某种程度上；on the part of 在……方面，就……而言；part with 放弃，出让；play a part (in) 扮演角色，参与，起作用；take part (in) 参加，参与
particular [pə'tikjulə]	*a.* 特殊的，特别的；特定的；（过分）讲究的，挑剔的 *n.*[*pl.*] 细节，详情 【反 义 词】usual, general 【固定搭配】be particular about 对……挑剔；in particular 特别，尤其；详细地

particularly
[pə'tikjuləli]
ad. 特别地，尤其地

pass
[pɑ:s]
vt. 超过，越过；穿过；终止，消失；传递；（时间）流逝，消磨（时间）；正式通过，批准；通过（考试等），及格 n. 考试及格；通行证，护照；关隘
【固定搭配】pass away 去世，逝世；pass by 经过，走过；pass off 中止，停止；pass over 省略，忽略，回避；pass out 失去知觉，昏倒；pass through 穿过……，经历……

patch
[pætʃ]
n. 小片，小块，补丁 vt. 补，修补
【固定搭配】patch up 解决（争吵、麻烦）等；修补，修理

patent
['peitənt]
n. 专利权，专利品 a. 特许的，专利的 vt. 取得……的专利权，给予……专利权

path
[pɑ:θ]
n. 小路，路线，途径

patience
['peiʃəns]
n. 忍耐，耐心
【固定搭配】run out one's patience 失去耐心；with patience 耐心地；out of patience with 对……失去耐心

patient
['peiʃənt]
a. 能忍耐的，有耐心的 n. 病人，患者
【反 义 词】impatient
【固定搭配】be patient with sb. 对某人有耐心，能容忍的；be patient of sth. 对某事有耐心的，能容忍的

pause
[pɔ:z]
n./v. 中止，暂停
【辨　析】cease, pause, stop: cease 主要指逐渐而缓慢地结束。pause 是"暂停"的含义。stop 指运动、行为、活动进程等突然停止。

pay
[pei]
v. 付款，缴纳；付清；给予，致以（问候），进行（访问）n. 工资，薪饷；报酬
【固定搭配】pay back 偿还，回报；pay off 还清（债务）；付清工资；解雇（某人）；向……行贿；得到好结果，取得成功；pay up 全部付清
【辨　析】pay, salary, wage：
pay 为 salary 和 wage（薪金、工资）普通用语的统称。salary 是按年或月付给白领阶层的薪资，尤指专业人士。wage 指按周、日或小时付给劳动者的工资，尤指体力劳动者。

payment
['peimənt]
n. 支付，付款；报酬，报偿
【固定搭配】in payment for 以偿付，以回报

peculiar
[pi'kju:ljə]
a. 特殊的，独特的；古怪的
【固定搭配】be peculiar to 是……所特有的
【辨　析】见 odd

perfect
['pə:fikt]
a. 完善的，完美的；完全的，十足的 vt. 使完美，改进

perfection
[pə'fekʃən]
n. 完全，完美；完成
【固定搭配】to perfection 完美地，尽善尽美地，完全地

permanent ['pə:mənənt]	*a.* 永久的，持久的 【辨　　析】permanent, perpetual, eternal： permanent 指永久不变的，与"暂时的"相对。perpetual 指动作无休止进行或状态无休止继续。eternal 表示"无始无终的，永恒的"。
permission [pə'miʃən]	*n.* 允许，许可 【反　义　词】refusal 【固定搭配】with your permission 如果你允许的话
permit [pə'mit]	*v.* 允许，许可　*n.* 执照，许可证 【固定搭配】permit of 允许……，容许……
persist [pə'sist]	*vi.* 坚持到底，持续；继续存在 【联想记忆】persistence *n.* 坚持，持续 【固定搭配】persist in doing sth. 坚持做某事；persist with sth. 不畏困难继续做某事
person ['pə:sn]	*n.* 人；人称 【固定搭配】in person 亲自
personal ['pə:sənl]	*a.* 私人的；本人的，亲自的；身体的，容貌的
personality [,pə:sə'næləti]	*n.* 人格，个性
personnel [,pə:sə'nel]	*n.* 全体人员，全体职员；人事部门
phase [feiz]	*n.* 阶段，时期；月相　*v.* 按阶段计划或进行某事 【固定搭配】phase in 逐步采用；phase out 逐步停止；out of phase with 与……不协调；in phase with 与……协调
pick [pik]	*n.* 选择　*v.* 拾，采，摘；挑选 【反　义　词】reject 【固定搭配】pick out 选出，挑选；pick on 找岔子，唠叨，指责；pick up 捡起，拾起；(车、船等)中途搭(人)/带(货)；增加；获得，(通过实践)学会
pitch [pitʃ]	*n.* 投，掷 【固定搭配】pitch in 协力，做贡献
pity ['piti]	*n./v.* 怜悯，惋惜　*n.* 可惜的事，憾事 【固定搭配】feel pity for sb. = take pity on sb. 同情某人
place [pleis]	*n.* 地方，地点，位置；职位，职责；住所，寓所；地位，等级，名次　*vt.* 放，置；安排 【反　义　词】remove 【固定搭配】in place 在适当的位置；in place of 代替；out of place 不适当的，不得其所的；take place 发生；take the place of 代替，取代；in the first place 起初，首先
plain [plein]	*n.* 平原　*a.* 平易的，易懂的；简单的，朴素的 【反　义　词】complicated，fanciful

☐ **plan** [plæn]	*n.* 计划，打算；平面图 *v.* 计划，安排 【固定搭配】plan for/on 拟订……的计划，预订……
☐ **play** [plei]	*vi.* 玩，游玩；演奏，表演；比赛 *n.* 游戏，娱乐；剧本，戏剧；比赛，运动 【固定搭配】bring into play 使活动，使运转，启动；come into play 开始活动，开始运转，投入使用，起作用；play at 玩，做（游戏）等；假扮……玩；play down 降低……的重要性，贬低；play on 利用；play up 强调，突出；play with 不认真地考虑（主意、提议等）；轻率地对待某事物
☐ **point** [pɔint]	*n.* 尖端，头；点，小数点；论点，观点，要点；分数，得分 *v.* 指 【固定搭配】beside the point 离题的，不相关的；make a point of doing sth. 特别注意做某事，重视；on the point of 正要……之际，就要……之时；there is no point (in) doing sth. 做……毫无意义；point out 指出，指明；to the point 切中要害，对准
☐ **popular** ['pɔpjulə]	*a.* 广受欢迎的，有名的；通俗的，流行的，大众的 【固定搭配】be popular with/among... 受……欢迎；popular opinion 舆论
☐ **popularity** [ˌpɔpju'læriti]	*n.* 普及，流行，受欢迎，声望
☐ **portable** ['pɔːtəbl]	*a.* 轻便的，手提（式）的；便于携带的
☐ **portion** ['pɔːʃən]	*n.* 部分，一份
☐ **position** [pə'ziʃən]	*n.* 位置；职务，职位；姿势，姿态，见解，立场 【固定搭配】in position 在适当的位置；out of position 在错误的位置
☐ **possibility** [ˌpɔsi'biliti]	*n.* 可能（性） 【固定搭配】by any possibility 万一，也许
☐ **possible** ['pɔsəbl]	*a.* 可能的，做得到的；合理的，可接受的 【反 义 词】impossible 【固定搭配】if possible 可能的话
☐ **possibly** ['pɔsəbli]	*ad.* 可能，也许
☐ **post** [pəust]	*n.* （支）柱；邮政；哨所；岗位，职位 *vt.* 贴出，宣布，公告；邮寄，投寄 【联想记忆】postage *n.* 邮资，邮票
☐ **postpone** [pəust'pəun]	*vt.* 推迟，延期
☐ **pour** [pɔː]	*v.* 灌，倒，注；泻，流出 【固定搭配】pour out 倾诉
☐ **poverty** ['pɔvəti]	*n.* 贫穷，贫困 【固定搭配】poverty of/in 缺乏，不足 【反 义 词】richness

power ['pauə]	*n.* 能力，力，精力；权力，势力，政权；功率，动力，电力；乘方 【固定搭配】beyond one's power 某人力所不及的，某人不能胜任的；come into/to power 掌握政权，得势
powerful ['pauəfl]	*a.* 强大的，有力的，有权的
practical ['præktikl]	*a.* 实际的，实用的
practically ['præktikəli]	*ad.* 实际上；几乎
practice/-tise ['præktis]	*n.* 实践，实施；练习，实习；业务，开业 *v.* 实践，实行；练习，实习；开业 【固定搭配】in practice 实际上，在实践中；out of practice 久不练习，荒疏；put into practice 实施，施行
praise [preiz]	*n.* 称赞，赞美 *v.* 称赞，表扬 【固定搭配】in praise of 极力赞美……，称赞……；praise sb. for 因……而赞扬某人；sing high praise for 因……而高度赞扬
predict [pri'dikt]	*v.* 预言，预测
prefer [pri'fə:]	*vt.* 更喜欢；宁愿 【固定搭配】prefer sth. to sth. 喜爱……而不喜爱……；prefer doing sth. to doing sth. 喜欢……而不喜欢……；prefer to do sth. rather than do sth. 宁愿做……而不愿做…… 【联想记忆】preference *n.* 偏好
prevent [pri'vent]	*vt.* 预防，防止 【反义词】help 【联想记忆】preventable *a.* 可预防的 【固定搭配】prevent sb. from doing sth. 阻止某人做某事
prevention [pri'venʃən]	*n.* 预防，防止
previous ['pri:vjəs]	*a.* 先前的，以前的 【联想记忆】previously *ad.* 先前，以前 【固定搭配】be previous to 在……之前 【辨析】preceding, previous, prior：preceding 指"此前的"，多用于在时间、顺序、行列上，在……之前；先于……。previous 多指时间发生在前的。prior 是"优先的"的意思。
primary ['praiməri]	*a.* 首要的，主要的，基本的；最初的，初级的
probability [ˌprɔbə'biliti]	*n.* 可能性；概率 【固定搭配】in all probability 十有八九，很可能
produce [prə'dju:s]	*v.* 生产，制造，产生；显示，出示；引起；拍摄 *n.* 农产品 【联想记忆】productive *a.* 多产的，肥沃的；有收获的，很多成果的；productivity *n.* 生产率，生产能力

product ['prɔdʌkt]	*n.* 产品，产物；结果，成果，乘积；创作，作品
production [prə'dʌkʃən]	*n.* 生产，产量；产品，作品
profession [prə'feʃən]	*n.* 职业，自由职业 【固定搭配】by profession 在职业上，就职业而说
professional [prə'feʃənl]	*a.* 职业的，专门的 *n.* 专业人员
professor [prə'fesə]	*n.* 教授 【固定搭配】an associate professor 副教授；a full professor 正教授
profit ['prɔfit]	*n.* 收益，利润，益处 *v.* 得利，获益 【反 义 词】loss 【固定搭配】make profits 获利；profit by/from 从……中获利
profitable ['prɔfitəbl]	*a.* 有利可图的，有益的
program(me) ['prəugræm]	*n.* 计划，规划，大纲；节目，节目单；程序 *v.* 编制程序
progress ['prəugres]	*n./v.* 前进，进步，进 【固定搭配】in progress 在进展中；make progress 进步
progressive [prə'gresiv]	*a.* 不断前进的，渐进的；进步的，先进的；（动词）进行时的 *n.* 进步人士
propel [prə'pel]	*vt.* 推进，驱使
propeller [prə'pelə]	*n.* 推进器，螺旋桨
proper ['prɔpə]	*a.* 适当的，恰当的，适宜的；正确的，真正的；体面的；特有的，固有的 【反 义 词】improper 【固定搭配】be proper to 特有的，固有的 【联想记忆】be specific/peculiar to 特有的，固有的
protect [prə'tekt]	*vt.* 保护，保卫 【反 义 词】attack, threaten 【固定搭配】protect...from/against 保护……，使……免受
protection [prə'tekʃən]	*n.* 保护 【固定搭配】protection for sb./against sth. 保护，护卫
protective [prə'tektiv]	*a.* 保护的，防卫的
provide [prə'vaid]	*vt.* 提供，供给，供应，供养 【反 义 词】demand 【联想记忆】provision *n.* 供应，供应品；预备，准备；规定，条款；provided/providing *conj.* 只要，假如 【固定搭配】provide sth. for sb. = provide sb. with sth. 为某人提供某物

| □ pull [pul] | *v./n.* 拉，拖，牵
【反 义 词】push
【固定搭配】pull down 拉倒，拆毁；pull out 拔出，抽出，取出；pull up 使停下；pull through 渡过难关，摆脱危难 |

| □ punish ['pʌniʃ] | *vt.* 惩罚，处罚
【反 义 词】reward
【联想记忆】punishment *n.* 处罚，惩罚
【固定搭配】punish sb. (for sth.) (by/with sth.) （通过……方式，因……而）惩罚某人 |

| □ purpose ['pə:pəs] | *n.* 目的；意图；企图，打算
【固定搭配】on purpose 故意，有意；for/with the purpose of 为了；to no purpose 无效，毫无结果 |

| □ put [put] | *vt.* 放，置；记下，写下；表达；使……进入（状态）
【固定搭配】put across 解释清楚，说明；put aside 储存，保留 put away 把……收起来，放好；put down 记下，写下；put forward 提出；put off 推迟，拖延；put on 穿上，戴上；上演；增加（体重）；put out 熄灭，消灭；生产，出版，发布；put up with 容忍，忍受；put up 举起，升起，提（价）；为……提供食宿；建造，搭起，支起；张贴 |

| □ puzzle ['pʌzl] | *n.* 难题，谜；疑问 *vt.* 使迷惑
【联想记忆】puzzling *a.* 费解的，使人为难的，莫名其妙的 |

| □ quit [kwit] | *vt.* 离开，退出；停止，放弃，辞职
【固定搭配】quit doing sth. 停止做某事；quit to do 停下来做（另一件事） |

| □ radiate ['reidieit] | *vt.* 闪光，发光，辐射 *vi.* 发光，辐射；流露
【联想记忆】radiation *n.* 辐射，辐射物；radiant *a.* 发光的，发热的 |

| □ raise [reiz] | *vt.* 举起，提高，提升；增加，筹集；引起；抚养，饲养；提出，发起
【固定搭配】raise a family 养家；raise a question 提出一个问题；raise money 筹集资金 |

range [reindʒ]	*n.* 范围，距离，领域；（山）脉 【固定搭配】range from...to... 从……到……不等
rank [ræŋk]	*n.* 排，行，列；等级，地位 *vt.* 评价，分等级，归类 【联想记忆】ranking *n.* 等级，顺序 *a.* 一流的，高级的
rare [rɛə]	*a.* 稀有的，难得的，珍奇的；稀薄的，稀疏的 【反 义 词】common 【辨 析】rare, scarce： 很少见到的东西或很少发生的现象，可用 rare 一词来表达；有些东西，通常为日用品，因匮乏而难以得到，即用 scarce。
rarely [ˈrɛəli]	*ad.* 不常，很少，难得 【反 义 词】usually
rather [ˈrɑːðə]	*ad.* 有些，相当；相反，反而 【固定搭配】rather than 而不是；would rather 宁愿，宁可
ratio [ˈreiʃiəu]	*n.* 比率，比
reach [riːtʃ]	*vt.* 够到，触到；到，到达 *vi.* 达到，延伸；伸手 *n.* 能达到的范围 【固定搭配】reach out 伸出；reach out for 设法抓到；beyond/out of one's reach 无法得到（拿到，联系到等）；reach a decision 做出决定
react [riˈækt]	*vi.* 反应，起作用 【固定搭配】react to 对……做出反应
reaction [riˈækʃən]	*n.* 反应；反作用（力） 【固定搭配】reaction to 对……的反应
recall [riˈkɔːl]	*vt.* 回想；召回；收回
reduce [riˈdjuːs]	*vt.* 缩小，减小，降低；简化；使还原 【反 义 词】increase 【固定搭配】reduce...to sth. 使变成；reduce costs/expenses 降低成本/费用
reduction [riˈdʌkʃən]	*n.* 减少，缩小
refusal [riˈfjuːzl]	*n.* 拒绝，回绝 【反 义 词】acceptance
refuse [riˈfjuːz]	*vt.* 拒绝，推辞
regard [riˈgɑːd]	*vt.* 看作，对待；考虑，认为；尊重 *n.* (*pl.*) 敬重，敬意，问候 【联想记忆】regarding *prep.* 关于；regardless *a.* 不顾一切的 【固定搭配】as regards 关于，至于；in/with regard to 关于；give one's regard to 代某人向……问好
regular [ˈregjulə]	*a.* 有规律的，规则的，规矩的；定时的，定期的；正规的，正式的；匀称的，整齐的 【反 义 词】irregular
relax [riˈlæks]	*vt.* 使放松，使休息；缓和，放宽 *vi.* 放松，休息；松弛

remain [ri'mein]	*vi.* 剩下，遗留；尚需；仍然是，依旧是 *n.* (*pl.*) 余，残余，遗迹；遗体 【联想记忆】remains *n.* 剩余物，残留物；遗体，遗迹 【固定搭配】remain calm/silent 保持冷静/沉默
remark [ri'mɑ:k]	*n.* 评语，意见 *v.* 说，评论，谈论 【固定搭配】remark on/upon 就某事发表意见
remind [ri'maind]	*vt.* 提醒，提示，回想，使想起；意识到 【固定搭配】remind sb. of 使想起，提起；提醒
remote [ri'məut]	*a.* 遥远的，偏僻的；疏远的，边缘的 【反 义 词】near
respect [ris'pekt]	*n./vt.* 尊敬，尊重 *n.* [*pl.*] 方面，细节 【联想记忆】respectable *a.* 可敬的，值得尊敬的 【固定搭配】in some respect 在某些方面；in respect to/of 关于，就……而言；in no respect 决不；with respect to 关于 【反 义 词】contempt
respectful [ris'pektfl]	*a.* 尊敬的，尊重的，恭敬的
respective [ris'pektiv]	*a.* 各自的，各个的 【辨 析】respective, respectable, respectful, respected：respective 各自的。respectable 值得尊敬的。respectful 表示敬意的。respected 受尊敬的
respectively [ri'spektivli]	*ad.* 各自地，独自地，个别地，分别地 【反 义 词】irrespectively *ad.* 整体地
rest [rest]	*v.* 休息；中止；依据 *n.* 剩余部分；(the) 其余的人/物；休息时间 【固定搭配】rest on 依靠
right [rait]	*a.* 正确的；合适的，恰当的；右边的；直角的 *n.* 权利；右面 *ad.* 正确地，笔直地；完全，正好；直接，马上 【固定搭配】all right 好，行；令人满意的，不错的；（健康）良好的；right away 立刻，马上；right now 在此时，在此刻；be in the right 有理的，正当的；put sb. right 使……恢复健康；on the right 在右边
ripe [raip]	*a.* 成熟的 【固定搭配】ripe time for 干……的时机成熟
rise [raiz]	*vi.* 上升，上涨；升起；起床，起立 *n.* 增加，升高；高地 【固定搭配】give rise to 引起，造成；make a rise in life 飞黄腾达
risk [risk]	*n.* 风险 *vt.* 冒险 【固定搭配】at the risk of 冒……风险；face/take/run the risk of 冒……风险
rough [rʌf]	*a.* 粗糙的；粗野的，粗鲁的；大致的，粗略的
routine [ru:'ti:n]	*a.* 常规的，例行的 *n.* 常规，例行公事 【固定搭配】break the routine 打破常规；follow the routine 墨守成规 【反 义 词】unusual

S

sack [sæk]	n. 袋，麻袋；开除，解雇；抢劫 v. 劫掠，掠夺 【固定搭配】get the sack 被解雇；give sb. the sack 解雇某人
sake [seik]	n. 缘故，理由 【固定搭配】for the sake of 为了
same [seim]	a. 同一的，相同的 pron. 相同的人，相同的事情 【固定搭配】all the same 仍然
sample ['sæmpl]	n. 样品，标本 vt. 采样，取样 【辨析】sample, specimen：sample 意为"样品，标本"，指随便挑选出来作为同类事物或整体代表的样品。specimen 意为"标本，样本"，指选出来的有代表性的样品或科研、化验、检验的标本。
scarce [skɛəs]	a. 稀少的，罕见的；缺乏的；不足的 【反义词】abundant
scarcely ['skɛəsli]	ad. 几乎不；勉强 【固定搭配】scarcely...when 一……就……
scare [skɛə]	vt. 惊吓，使害怕 vi. 惊慌，惊恐
scene [si:n]	n. 景色，景象；（戏）场；布景；镜头 【固定搭配】on the scene 在现场；make/have a scene 大吵大闹
scenery ['si:nəri]	n. 舞台布景；风景，景色
schedule ['ʃedju:l; 'skedʒjul]	n. 时间表；进度表，一览表 vt. 安排；预定 【固定搭配】on schedule 按预定时间；ahead of schedule 提前
scholar ['skɔlə]	n. 学者
scholarship ['skɔləʃip]	n. 奖学金；学问，学识 【固定搭配】award/grant a scholarship 授予奖学金；get/receive/win a scholarship 获得奖学金
score [skɔ:]	n. 得分，分数；二十 v. 得分，记分 【固定搭配】scores/dozens of 大量，许多（接可数名词）；on that score 关于那一点，为了这一点
scream [skri:m]	v. 尖声叫喊，放声大笑；（机器、汽笛等）发出尖锐刺耳的声音 n. 尖叫，尖锐刺耳的声音 【反义词】whisper
section ['sekʃən]	n. 章节；部分；地区；截面，剖视图 【联想记忆】sectional a. 组装的，拼凑成的；地区的，区域性的

sector ['sektə]	n. 扇形；部门
see [si:]	vt. 看见；理解，明白；会见，见面；获悉，知道；送行；经历，目睹 【固定搭配】see to 负责，照料；注意，留心；see about 调查，查询；see into 调查，检查；see off 给……送行；see through 看穿，识破
sense [sens]	vt. 感觉到，意识到 n. 感官，官能；辨别力，感觉；意义，意思 【联想记忆】senseless a. 无知觉的，无感觉的；无意义的 【固定搭配】make sense 讲得通，言之有理；in a sense 从某种意义上说
series ['siəri:z]	n. 一系列，一连串；序列；系列节目 【固定搭配】a series of 一系列，一连串
serious ['siəriəs]	a. 严肃的，庄重的；严重的，危急的；认真的
serve [sə:v]	vt. 服务，尽责；伺候，招待；适用，适合；服役 vi. 服务，供职；有用，其作用 【固定搭配】serve as 担任；起……作用；serve sb. right 活该
service ['sə:vis]	n. 服务；公共事业；服役，帮助，服侍；公共设施维护，保养 【固定搭配】at sb.'s service 随时为某人效劳；be of service 能帮忙的，有用的；do sb. a service 帮某人忙；in service 在使用中；正在服役
set [set]	vt. 放，安置；调整，校正；树立，规定；使处于特定状态；使开始 vi.（日、月等）落山，下沉 n. 一套，一副 a. 固定的，规定的 【固定搭配】set about 开始，着手；set aside 宣布无效，驳回，废止；set back 推迟，延缓，阻碍；set off 动身，出发；使爆炸，使爆发；引起；set out 动身，出发，开始；制订，打算；set up 建立，设立，树立；资助，使自立，扶持
sign [sain]	n. 符号，标记，招牌；征兆，迹象 v. 签（名），签署 【固定搭配】sign for 签收 【辨　析】sign, signal, symbol, token： sign 意为"标记；招牌"。signal 意为"信号，暗号"，也可以是"警告的标记"。symbol 意为"象征；符号，记号"，指具有象征意义的符号。token 意为"标志，象征"，常用来代替或证实某种思想或感情的东西。
signal ['signl]	n. 信号，暗号 v. 发信号，打暗号
signature ['signitʃə]	n. 签字，签名
significance [sig'nifikəns]	n. 意义，含义；重要性
significant [sig'nifikənt]	a. 重大的；重要的；意味深长的 【反　义　词】insignificant 【联想记忆】significantly ad. 意味深长地，值得注目地
similar ['similə]	a. 相似的，类似的 【固定搭配】be similar to 与……相似

simple ['sɪmpl]	a. 简单的，朴素的；单纯的，直率的；迟钝的，头脑简单的，容易受到欺骗的
so [səʊ; sə]	conj. 因此，那么；结果是，为的是，以便 ad. 那么，如此；非常，很；也，同样；不错，确实；这样，那样 【固定搭配】so far 迄今为止；so that 以便，为的是；结果是，以致；so as to 为的是；so...as to... 如此……以至于……，如此……以便……；so...that... 如此……以至于……；or so 大约，左右；not so much sth. as sth. 不是……而是…… 【辨　析】so as to, in order to, so...as to...： so as to 与 in order to 用法相同，引导目的状语。so as to 只能放在句后，in order to 既可放在句首，也可放在句后。so...as to... 用来引导结果状语从句。
solid ['sɒlɪd]	n. 固体 a. 固体的；实心的；纯的，结实的，稳固的，可靠的；一致的
somewhat ['sʌm(h)wɒt]	ad. 一点儿，几分
somewhere ['sʌm(h)weə]	ad. 在/到某处；附近，前后，大约
spark [spɑːk]	n. 火花，火星 vi. 发火花，发电花；导致，引起
spread [spred]	vt. 伸展，展开；散布，传播，蔓延；涂，撒 n. 展开，伸展；传开，蔓延 【固定搭配】spread education 普及教育；spread out one's arms 伸开双臂；spread out（人群等）散开；伸展，延伸
stair [steə]	n. [pl.] 楼梯；阶梯 【联想记忆】upstairs 在楼上；downstairs 在楼下
stand [stænd]	n. 抵抗；立场；立足点；看台，架子 v. 站，立，站起；（使）竖立，（使）位于；维持不变，持久，经受 【固定搭配】stand by 站在旁边，袖手旁观；站在一起，支持，帮助；stand for 代表，代替；象征，支持，做……的候选人；stand out 站出来；突出，坚持抵抗；stand up for 为……辩护，维护；stand up to 勇敢地面对，坚决抵抗；stand up 站起来，竖立，站得住脚；坚持，经得起；拥护，抵抗
standard ['stændəd]	n. 标准，规格 【联想记忆】standardize vt. 使标准化 【固定搭配】reach a standard 达到标准 【辨　析】standard, criterion： standard 指被公认为质量、价值、数量或道德水准等的比较基础的准则或典范。criterion 指据判断已经存在的某物的价值、优点或其他品质的准则或测试标准。
stock [stɒk]	n. 树干；库存；股票，股份；托盘；祖先，血统；原料 a. 股票的；普通的；常备的，存货的；繁殖用的 v. 进货；备有 【固定搭配】check a stock 清点存货；in/out of stock 备有现货/没有现货；stock certificate 股票，证券；stock dividend 红利，股息；stock exchange 证券交易所；stock market 股票市场

strength [streŋθ]	*n.* 力量，毅力，力气；人力，兵力，实力 【固定搭配】acquire/gain strength 获得力量；on the strength of 依据，基于
strengthen ['streŋθən]	*v.* 加强，巩固 【反 义 词】weaken
stress [stres]	*n.* 压力；紧迫；强调 *vt.* 强调，着重 【固定搭配】put/lay/place stress on 强调
strict [strikt]	*a.* 严格的；严谨的，精确的 【联想记忆】strictly *ad.* 严格地，确实地 【固定搭配】be strict with 对……严格；in the strict sense 严格说来
strike [straik]	*n.* 罢工；打击，殴打 *vt.* 打，撞击，冲击；划燃；到达，侵袭；给……深刻印象 *vi.* 突击，攻击；罢工；行进 【固定搭配】go on strike 举行罢工 【联想记忆】impress...on/upon 将某事铭刻在某人心中；impress sb. with... 给某人……的印象；be impressed by/at/with 对……印象很深
striking ['straikiŋ]	*a.* 显著的，惊人的
subject ['sʌbdʒikt]	*n.* 主题，题目；学科，科目；试验对象 *a.* 易遭受……的，受……支配的（~ to） 【联想记忆】subjective *a.* 主观的，个人的 【固定搭配】be subject to 易遭受……的；易患……（疾病）的
suburb ['sʌbə:b]	*n.* [*pl.*] 郊外，近郊
subway ['sʌbwei]	*n.* 地铁；地下人行道
such [sʌtʃ]	*a.* 如此的；这样的 *pron.* 这样的人/事物 【固定搭配】such as 像……这样的，诸如，例如；such...that 这样……以致；[such...that... 这样……以致（such 后面接名词）；so...that... 如此……以至于（so 后面接形容词或副词）]
supply [sə'plai]	*vt./n.* 供给，供应，提供；贮备；补给 【固定搭配】in short supply 供应不足；supply sb. with sth./supply sth. to sb. 给某人提供某物；provide sth. for sb.；provide sb. with sth.；offer sb. sth.；give sth. to sb.；give sb. sth. 给某人提供某物
support [sə'pɔ:t]	*vt.* 承受，支撑，支持；鼓励；拥护；供养，资助 *n.* 支撑，支持；支撑物；支援，拥护；生活费 【固定搭配】give/offer/provide support to sb. 支持某人
suppose [sə'pəuz]	*vt.* 猜想，料想，假定，以为 【联想记忆】supposed *a.* 假定的，推测的；supposedly *ad.* 据想象，据推测，大概；supposing *conj.* 万一，假使；supposition *n.* 假定之事；假设 【固定搭配】be supposed to do sth. 应该做某事
switch [switʃ]	*n.* 转换，转变；电闸，开关；突然转向 *v.* 改变，交换 【固定搭配】switch off/on 关上/打开（开关）

| **system**
['sɪstəm] | n. 系统，体系；制度，体制 |
| **systematic**
[ˌsɪstə'mætɪk] | a. 系统的；有计划的，有步骤的；有秩序的，有规则的
【联想记忆】systematically ad. 系统地 |

take [teɪk]	vt. 拿，取；带走；需要；花费；接收，获得；认为，当作；做（一次动作） 【固定搭配】take after 与……相像；take apart 拆开；take down 记下，写下；take for 认为，以为；take in 接受，容纳；领会，理解；欺骗；take off 拿走，脱下；起飞；take on 呈现；具有；接纳，接受；承担，从事；take over 接管，接收；take up 占去，占据；开始从事；拿起，捡起
talk [tɔːk]	vt. 谈论，讨论 vi. 讲话，谈话，交谈 n. 谈话，演讲，讲话 【联想记忆】talker n. 健谈者，空谈者；talkative a. 爱说话的 【固定搭配】talk back 顶嘴；talk into 说服；talk over 商量，讨论
tariff ['tærɪf]	n. 关税，关税表 【联想记忆】duty n. 关税；tax n. 税（款）；value added tax n. 增值税；additional tax 附加税；rate n. 价格，费用；toll n. 通行费；tuition n. 学费；fare n. 车船费；fee n. 费用；expense n. 花费；expenditure n. 支出
temper ['tempə]	n. 情绪，脾气 【固定搭配】be in a good/bad temper 心情好 / 不好；lose one's temper 发脾气，发怒；be in a good temper 心情好；get into a temper 发怒
temporary ['tempərəri]	a. 暂时的，临时的 【反 义 词】permanent 【联想记忆】temporarily ad. 临时地
term [təːm]	n. 学期；任期，期限；词，措辞，术语；[pl.] 条件，条款 vt. 称为，叫作 【联想记忆】terminology n. 术语，术语学 【固定搭配】be on good/bad terms with 与……关系好 / 不好；in terms of 按照，依照；用……措辞；in the long/short term 就长 / 短期而言
terrible ['terəbl]	a. 可怕的；令人生畏的；极度的；厉害的；坏透的，很糟的 【联想记忆】terribly ad. 可怕地；十分，极
terrific [tə'rɪfɪk]	a. 非常的，极度的；很好的，了不起的 【联想记忆】terrifically ad. 极端地，可怕地
terrify ['terɪfaɪ]	vt. 使恐怖，使惊吓 【联想记忆】terrifying a. 极大的，可怕的

□ **terror** ['terə]	*n.* 恐怖；恐怖的人 【联想记忆】terrorist *n.* 恐怖分子；terrorism *n.* 恐怖主义 【固定搭配】quiver in terror 怕得发抖
□ **than** [ðæn; ðən]	*conj.* 比；多于，小于，少于；就 【固定搭配】no more than 仅仅，只是；no other than 只有，正是，就是；no/not any more than 与……一样不；other than 除了……之外；rather than 而不是
□ **that** [ðæt]	*pron.* 那，那个 *conj.*（引出名词从句） *ad.* 那样，那么 【固定搭配】that is 就是说，即；so that 为的是，使得；结果是，以至；in that 因为（引导原因状语从句）；so that 为了（同 in order that），以便（引导目的状语从句）；the moment（that）一……就……
□ **therefore** ['ðɛəfɔː]	*ad.* 因此，所以
□ **thorough** ['θʌrə]	*a.* 彻底的，完全的；精心的 【联想记忆】thoroughly *ad.* 十分，彻底
□ **those** [ðəuz]	*pron.* 那些，那些
□ **though** [ðəu]	*conj.* 尽管，虽然 *ad.* 可是，然而 【固定搭配】as though 好像；even though 即使（though 和 but, however 不能用在同一句中，但可以和 yet, nevertheless 同用。）
□ **threat** [θret]	*n.* 威胁，危险现象；（不详的）预兆
□ **threaten** ['θretn]	*vt.* 威胁，恐吓 【联想记忆】threatening *a.* 威胁的，胁迫的 【固定搭配】threaten sb. with/to do 威胁要……
□ **thus** [ðʌs]	*ad.* 如此，这样；因而，从而
□ **track** [træk]	*n.* 跑道，路线，轨道；足迹，踪迹 *vt.* 跟踪，追踪 【固定搭配】keep track 通晓事态，注意动向
□ **trap** [træp]	*n.* 陷阱，圈套 *vt.* 诱捕，使中圈套 【固定搭配】fall into a trap 陷入圈套
□ **treasure** ['treʒə]	*n.* 财富，珍宝 *vt.* 珍视，珍爱
□ **treat** [triːt]	*v.* 对待；处理，治疗 *n./v.* 款待，请客 【固定搭配】treat...as... 把……当作……
□ **treatment** ['triːtmənt]	*n.* 待遇，对待；治疗，疗法 【辨　析】见 therapy
□ **tremble** ['trembl]	*vi.* 颤抖，颤动

☐ **tremendous** [tri'mendəs]	*a*. 巨大的；了不起的，极好的
☐ **turn** [tə:n]	*n*. 旋转，翻，转动；机会；轮替；变化，改变；转折点 *v*. 旋转，翻，转动；改变方向；回头，转身 *vi*. 变为，变得 【固定搭配】by turns 轮流，交替；in turn 依次轮流；转而，反过来；take turns 轮流；turn down 调低，关小；拒绝；turn in 交出，上缴；进入；turn into 变成；turn off 关，关闭；turn on 打开，拧开；turn out 生产，制造；驱逐，使离开；证明是，结果是；turn over 翻过来，翻倒，移交；turn to 转向；求助于；turn up 出现，发生
☐ **typical** ['tipikəl]	*a*. 典型的，有代表性的；独有的，独特的 【联想记忆】typically *ad*. 有代表性地 【固定搭配】be typical of 代表性的，典型的

☐ **uniform** ['ju:nifɔ:m]	*a*. 清一色的，相同的，一致的；一成不变的，始终如一的，一贯的 *n*. 制服，军服
☐ **unless** [ən'les]	*conj*. 除非，如果不；除……之外
☐ **unlike** ['ʌn'laik]	*a*. 不同的，不相似的 *prep*. 不像……，和……不同 【反义词】like, similar
☐ **unlikely** [ʌn'laikli]	*a*. 未必的，多半不可能的；不大可能发生的 【反义词】likely, possible 【固定搭配】be unlikely to do 不大可能……
☐ **until** [ən'til]	*prep./conj*. 到……为止，在……以前；直到…… 【固定搭配】not... until... 直到……才
☐ **unusual** [ʌn'ju:ʒuəl]	*a*. 不平常的，稀有的；例外的，独特的，与众不同的 【反义词】usual, common
☐ **up** [ʌp]	*ad*. 向上；往北；起床，起来；朝；完全；完结，关闭 *prep*. 向上，向/在高处；沿着 *a*. 向上的 【反义词】down 【固定搭配】up to 一直到；等于；从事，忙于
☐ **urban** ['ə:bən]	*a*. 城市的，市内的 【反义词】rural 【联想记忆】urbanize *vt*. 使都市化；urbanization *n*. 都市化
☐ **used** [ju:st]	*a*. 旧的，用旧了的；习惯于 【固定搭配】used to do sth. 过去常常做某事（接动词不定式）；be/get used to doing sth. 习惯于做某事（接动名词）

V

vague [veig]	*a.* 不明确的，含糊的 【反 义 词】clear 【联想记忆】vaguely *ad.* 含糊地；vagueness *n.* 含糊；模糊 【辨 析】vague, obscure: vague 指言辞不确定或太笼统；使人不能完全猜透其意。obscure 指某物的意思复杂、深奥或未明确地表达出来，使其晦涩难懂。
valuable ['væljuəbl]	*a.* 贵重的；有价值的 *n.* [*pl.*] 贵重物品，财宝 【反 义 词】cheap 【辨 析】invaluable, valueless: invaluable 十分有价值以至无法估价（另见 costly）；valueless 毫无价值的。
value ['vælju:]	*n.* 价值；实用性；重要性 *vt.* 评价，估计；尊重，重视 【固定搭配】place/set value on 重视
victim ['viktim]	*n.* 牺牲者，受害者
victory ['viktəri]	*n.* 胜利，战胜 【固定搭配】achieve/gain/win a victory 赢得胜利
view [vju:]	*n.* 观察，视野，眼界；观点，见解，看法；风景，景色 *vt.* 看待，考虑，观察 【固定搭配】view...as... 把……看作……；in view of 考虑到；由于；come into view 进入视野；on a long view 从长远看 【联想记忆】regard... as/think of ... as/look upon... as 把……看作
viewer ['vju:ə]	*n.* 电视观众，观众
viewpoint ['vju:pɔint]	*n.* 观点，看法，视角
visible ['vizəbl]	*a.* 可见的，有形的 【反 义 词】invisible 【联想记忆】visibly *ad.* 显然；visibility *n.* 可见度，可见性；显著，明显度，能见度
vision ['viʒən]	*n.* 视觉，视力；幻想，幻影；眼力，想象力；远见 【联想记忆】visionary *a.* 幻想的，梦想的 *n.* 有眼力的人 【辨 析】vision, sight, view: vision 指人的视力或视野，引申为远见卓识、美妙景色等。sight 指事物在人视线中的客观映现，引申为奇观、风景名胜等。view 指视线、视野时，可与 sight 互换使用；此外，view 可指运用视力直接观察事物，也可指问题的角度、个人意见、美景等。

visit ['vizit]	v./n. 访问，参观；观察，巡回
	【固定搭配】pay/make a visit to 参观，访问

visitor ['vizitə]	n. 客人，来宾，参观者

visual ['vʒuəl]	a. 视觉的
	【联想记忆】visually ad. 视觉上

vital ['vaitl]	a. 极其重要的，致命的；生命的；有生机的
	【联想记忆】vitality n. 活力，生命力，热情
	【固定搭配】be vital to 对……极其重要

volume ['vɔljuːm]	n.（一）卷，（一）册；体积，容积；音量，响度

volunteer [vɔlən'tiə(r)]	n. 志愿者，志愿兵
	【联想记忆】voluntary a. 志愿的，自愿的

wander ['wɔndə]	vi. 徘徊，漫步；走神，恍惚；迷路，迷失；离开正道，离题
	【固定搭配】wander off the subject 离题

way [wei]	n. 道路，路程；方法，手段，方式；习惯，作风；状态，情况
	【固定搭配】lead the way 带路，引路；make way 开路，让路；in one's way/in the way 妨碍，阻碍；by the way 顺便提一下，另外；by way of 通过……方式；give way to 让路；让步，屈服；坍塌，倒塌；go out of one's way 让开，避开；解决；in a way 从某种程度上；in no way 决不；one way or another 以某种形式；no way 无论如何不；不可能；under way 在进行中

wear [wɛə]	vt. 穿着，佩戴；磨损
	【固定搭配】wear away 磨损，磨去；消磨，流逝；wear down 磨损，损耗，用旧；wear off 渐渐减少，逐渐消失；wear out 穿破，磨损，用坏；（使）疲乏，（使）厌倦，（使）耗尽

weigh [wei]	vt. 称，量；重，重达；考虑，权衡 vi. 重……
	【固定搭配】weigh...against/with 权衡（考虑）……与……

weight [weit]	n. 重量，体重；砝码，秤砣；重压，负担；重要性，价值
	【固定搭配】attach/give/lend weight to 重视；carry weight 有分量，有影响；gain/pick up/put on weight 体重增加；lose one's weight 体重减轻；pull one's weight 干好本分工作；throw one's weight about/around 滥用职权，耀武扬威

welfare ['welfɛə]	n. 福利

well [wel]	*n.* 井，水井 *ad.* 好，令人满意地；有理由地，恰当地；完全地，充分地 *a.* 健康的；良好的 *int.* 好啦，那么 【固定搭配】as well as 既……又……，除……之外；as well 同样，也，不妨；just as well（＋动词原形）没关系，无妨，不妨；may/might as well（＋动词原形）还不如，不妨（as well as 作"既……又……"解时，不能接动词，只能接动名词；may/might as well＋动词原形"不妨，还不如……"）
what [wɔt]	*pron.* 什么，什么东西/事情；[关系代词]……的事物/人 *a.* 什么，怎样的；[表示感叹] 多么，何等；[关系形容词] 所……的，尽可能多的 【固定搭配】what about（对于）……怎么样；what if 如果……将会怎样，即使……又有什么要紧；what's more 更重要的是
whatever [wɔt'evə]	*pron.* 无论什么，不管什么；任何……事物，凡是……的东西 *a.* 不管怎样的，无论什么样的
whatsoever [wɔtsəu'evə(r)]	= whatever
when [wen]	*ad.* 什么时候，何时；[关系副词] 在……时 *conj.* 在……时，当……时；其时，然后；可是，然而 *pron.* 什么时候
whenever [wen'evə]	*ad.* 无论何时，随时；每当
where [wɛə]	*ad.* 在/往/到哪里；在/到什么地方 *conj.* 然而，但是；哪里，什么地方 *pron.* 哪里，什么地方
whereas [wɛər'æz]	*conj.* 鉴于；然而，但是，反之
wherever [wɛər'evə]	*ad.* 无论（去）哪里；究竟在/到哪里 *conj.* 无论在/到哪里
whether ['weðə]	*conj.* 是否，会不会；不管，无论 【固定搭配】whether... or... 是……还是……，不管……还是…… 【辨 析】whether 与 if 的用法区别： ① whether 可引导宾、主、表、同位语从句，if 只能引导宾语从句。 ② whether 可直接接 or not，而 if 不能，如接 or not, or not 只能放在句尾。 ③ whether 引导主语从句时可放在句首，而 if 不能。 ④ whether 可用于介词后，而 if 不能。 ⑤ whether 从句可用于 discuss 等词后，而 if 不能。 ⑥ whether 引导宾语从句时可省略为 whether to do，而 if 不能。
which [witʃ]	*pron./a.* 哪一个，哪一些 *pron.* [限制性关系代词]……的那个，……的那些；[非限制性关系代词] 那个，那些 【联想记忆】which 与 that 引导从句时的用法区别： ① 定语从句的先行词有形容词最高级/序数词或 last, next, only 等修饰时，只能用 that。 ② 定语从句的先行词是不定代词（something 除外）时，只能用 that。 ③ 宾语从句要由 that 引导。 ④ 同位语从句只能由 that 引导。 ⑤ 强调句只能由 that 引导。 ⑥ 非限制性定语从句要用 which 引导。

☐ **whichever** [wɪtʃ'evə]	*pron.* 无论哪个，无论哪些
☐ **while** [waɪl]	*conj.* 当……的时候；和……同时；而，然而；虽然，尽管 *n.* 一会儿，一段时 【固定搭配】after a while 过了一会儿；all the while 始终；for a while 一时，暂时；once in a while 偶尔，有时；while away 消磨时间
☐ **who** [hu:]	*pron.* 谁，什么人；[限制性关系代词]……的人；[非限制性关系代词]表示所指的人
☐ **whoever** [hu:'evə(r)]	*pron.*（引出名词从句）谁；无论谁，不管谁；究竟是谁
☐ **whole** [həʊl]	*n.* 全部，全体，整体 *a.* 全部的，整体的；完好无损的 【反 义 词】partial, part 【固定搭配】as a whole 作为一个整体，整个来看；on the whole 总的来说
☐ **whom** [hu:m]	*pron.* [宾格] 谁，什么人
☐ **whose** [hu:z]	*pron.* 谁的；哪个（人）的，哪些（人）的
☐ **why** [waɪ]	*ad.* 为什么，……的理由 *int.* 咳，哎 【固定搭配】why not 为什么不
☐ **widespread** ['waɪdspred]	*a.* 普遍的；分布/散布广的
☐ **with** [wɪð]	*prep.* 和……一起，用，以；具有，带有；关于，就……而言；因，由于；随着；虽然，尽管
☐ **within** [wɪð'ɪn]	*prep.* 在……里面，在……以内
☐ **without** [wɪð'aʊt]	*prep.* 毫无，没有 *ad.* 在外面 【固定搭配】do without 没有……也行，不需要
☐ **wonder** ['wʌndə]	*n.* 惊异，惊奇；奇迹，奇事 *v.* 诧异，奇怪；想弄明白，想知道 【反 义 词】indifference 【固定搭配】no wonder 难怪，怪不得；wonder at 对……感到惊讶；wonder about 对……感到疑惑 【辨　析】wander, wonder： wander 漫游。wonder 惊异。
☐ **work** [wə:k]	*v./n.* 工作，劳动 *n.* [pl.] 著作，作品；成果，制品 *v.* 运转，开动 【固定搭配】work at/on 从事；work off 消除，去除；work out 解决，算出，设计出，制定出；work up 引起，激起；逐渐向上，向上爬；at work 在工作，忙于；out of work 失业

☐ **worth** [wə:θ]	*a.* 值……的 *n.* 价值 【固定搭配】be worth doing sth.（某事）值得一做 【辨　　析】worth, worthy, worthwhile： worth 意为"值得……的，值……钱"，做表语，后接表示价钱或代价等类似的名词，或接动名词表示被动意义。worthy 做表语时意为"值得的，配得上的"，其后一般接介词 of，或接不定式。做定语时意为"有价值的，可敬佩的"。worthwhile 意为"值得干的，有价值的"，尤指值得花费时间、金钱、劳力等，既可做定语，也可做表语。
☐ **worthless** ['wə:θlis]	*a.* 无价值的，无用的
☐ **worthwhile** [,wə:θ'wail]	*a.* 值得（做）的
☐ **worthy** ['wə:ði]	*a.* 有价值的，可尊敬的；值……的，足以…… 【固定搭配】be worthy of 值得……的；be worthy to do 配得上做…… 【联想记忆】it is worthwhile to do sth., sth. is worth doing 值得做某事 【辨　　析】sth. is worth (doing)（接名词或动名词）；sth. is worthy to be done（接不定式）；sth. is worthy of...（接 of 短语）；it is worthwhile to do sth.（接不定式做主语）；sth. is deserving of（接 of 短语）

☐ **yet** [jet]	*ad.* 还，仍然；更 *conj.* 然而，可是 【固定搭配】and yet 虽然如此，然而；as yet 到目前为止

普通基础词汇

月份和星期

月份	缩写	星期	缩写
January 一月	Jan.	Sunday	Sun.
February 二月	Feb.	Monday	Mon.
March 三月	Mar.	Tuesday	Tue.
April 四月	Apr.	Wednesday	Wed.
May 五月	May.	Thursday	Thu.
June 六月	Jun.	Friday	Fri.
July 七月	Jul.	Saturday	Sat.
August 八月	Aug.		
September 九月	Sep.		
October 十月	Oct.		
November 十一月	Nov.		
December 十二月	Dec.		

季节、节日和其他

spring 春	month 月份
summer 夏	week 星期
autumn 秋	weekday 工作日
winter 冬	weekend 周末
morning 早晨	day 白天
afternoon 下午	dawn 拂晓
evening 傍晚	eve 前夜
midday 中午	midnight 半夜
nightfall 晚上	today 今天
tomorrow 明天	tonight 今晚
easter 复活节	fortnight 两个星期
dusk 黄昏	

地点相关

国家或地域	语言	国民（复数）	国籍（形容词）
America 美国	/	American(-s)	American
Arab 阿拉伯	Arabian	Arabian(-s)	Arabian
Australia 澳大利亚	/	Australian(-s)	Australian
Brazil 巴西	/	Brazilian(-s)	Brazilian
Britain 英国	English	Briton(-s)	British
Canada 加拿大	/	Canadian(-s)	Canadian
China 中国	Chinese	Chinese	Chinese
Egypt 埃及	/	Egyptian(-s)	Egyptian
England 英格兰	English	Englishman(-men)	English
France 法国	French	Frenchman(-men)	French
Germany 德国	German	German(-s)	German
Greece 希腊	Greek	Greek(-s)	Greek
India 印度	/	Indian(-s)	Indian
Italy 意大利	Italian	Italian(-s)	Italian
Japan 日本	Japanese	Japanese	Japanese
Mexico 墨西哥	Mexican	Mexican(-s)	Mexican
Norway 挪威	Norwegian	Norwegian(-s)	Norwegian
Rome 罗马	Roman	Roman(-s)	Roman
Russia 俄罗斯	Russian	Russian(-s)	Russian
Scot 苏格兰	Scottish	Scottish(-es)	Scottish
Thailand 泰国	Thai	Thai(-s)	Thai
Africa 非洲	/	African(-s)	/
Europe 欧洲	/	European(-s)	/
Asia 亚洲	/	Asian(-s)	/
America 美洲	/	American(-s)	/
Antarctica 南极洲	/	Antarctican(-s)	/
Oceania 大洋洲	/	Oceanian(-s)	/
Arctic 北极	/	Arctic	/

地名（n.）	中文	地名（n.）	中文
Jupitor	木星	Neptune	海王星
Mars	火星	Mercury	水星
mainland	大陆	Mediterranean	地中海（的）
Moslem	穆斯林（的）	warehouse	仓库
volcano	火山	trunk	行李箱
tunnel	隧道	temple	寺庙
tanker	油轮	studio	工作室
skyscraper	摩天大楼	plaza	广场

（续）

地名（n.）	中文	地名（n.）	中文
platform	讲台	peninsula	半岛
jail	监狱	hut	小屋
gym/gymnasium	体育馆，健身房	elevator	电梯
delta	三角洲	galary	美术馆
embassy	大使馆	campus	校园
workshop	车间		

数字

基数词	序数词	基数词	序数词
one	first，1st	twelve	twelfth,12th
two	second，2nd	twenty	twentieth,20th
three	third，3rd	twenty-one	twenty-first,21st
four	fourth，4th	one hundred	one hundredth,100th
five	fifth，5th	one thousand	one thousandth,1000th
eight	eighth，8th		

方向

方向（n.）	方向（adj.）	方向（adv.）
east	eastern	eastwards
west	western	westwards
north	northern	northwards
south	southern	southwards

常见动物

家禽、哺乳动物			
cat 猫	kitten 小猫	dog 狗	puppy 小狗
sheep 羊	goat 山羊	lamb 羊羔	goose 鹅
ox 牛	bull 公牛	cow 母牛	calf 小牛
horse 马	donkey 驴	pony 小马	yak 牦牛
mule 骡	mouse 老鼠	rat 鼠	duck 鸭子
pig 猪	piglet 小猪	herd 兽群	duckling 小鸭子
rabbit 兔子	hare 野兔	sheepdog 牧羊犬	turkey 火鸡
cock 公鸡	hen 母鸡	chick 小鸡	bat 蝙蝠

（续）

陆地动物、爬行动物			
tiger 老虎	lion 狮子	leopard 豹	puma 美洲豹
elephant 大象	camel 骆驼	rhinoceros 犀牛	cub 幼兽
giraffe 长颈鹿	deer 鹿	reindeer 驯鹿	antelope 羚羊
monkey 猴子	gorilla 大猩猩	chimpanzee 黑猩猩	frog 青蛙
zebra 斑马	hippo 河马	snake 蛇	wolf 狼
fox 狐狸	polar bear 北极熊	koala 树熊	panda 熊猫
kangaroo 袋鼠	squirrel 松鼠	mole 鼹鼠	
lizard 蜥蜴	tortoise 乌龟	snail 蜗牛	crocodile 鳄鱼
海洋生物			
fish 鱼	sponge 海绵	tuna 金枪鱼	octopus 章鱼
shark 鲨鱼	eel 鳗鱼	whale 鲸鱼	salmon 鲑鱼
shrimp 虾	crayfish 小龙虾	lobster 龙虾	prawn 明虾
crab 蟹	shell 贝类	oyster 牡蛎	penguin 企鹅
coral 珊瑚	jellyfish 水母	dolphin 海豚	seal 海豹
sea lion 海狮	starfish 海星	sea horse 海马	sea turtle 海龟
鸟类			
eagle 雕	condor 秃鹫	hawk 鹰，隼	crane 鹤
crow 乌鸦	cuckoo 布谷鸟	canary 金丝雀	peacock 孔雀
parrot 鹦鹉	sparrow 麻雀	swallow 燕子	pigeon 鸽子
nightingale 夜莺	lark 云雀	seagull 海鸥	swan 天鹅
owl 猫头鹰	ostrich 鸵鸟	robin 知更鸟	
昆虫类			
ant 蚂蚁	mosquito 蚊子	moth 飞蛾	bee 蜜蜂
bug 臭虫	caterpillar 毛虫	fly 苍蝇	cricket 蟋蟀
butterfly 蝴蝶	dragonfly 蜻蜓	beetle 甲虫	flea 跳蚤
grasshopper 蚱蜢	worm 虫子		

常见职业、人物关系和身份

actor 演员	actress 女演员	artist 艺术家	aunt 阿姨
baker 面包师	banker 银行家	barber 理发师	boss 老板

(续)

brother 兄弟	businessman 商人	butcher 屠夫	carrier 搬运工
chairman 主席	cook 厨师	doctor 医生	engineer 工程师
farmer 农夫	fireman 消防员	fisherman 渔夫	gardener 园丁
hairdresser 美发师	headmaster 校长	king 国王	mayor 市长
merchant 商人	miner 矿工	musician 音乐家	novelist 小说家
nurse 护士	officer 职员	painter 画家	nephew 侄子
niece 侄女	cousin 堂兄弟/姐妹	daughter 女儿	grandmother 祖母
grandfather 祖父	grandson 外孙	husband 丈夫	parent 父母
father 父亲	mother 母亲	uncle 叔叔	peasant 农民
poet 诗人	policeman 警察	postman 邮差	queen 皇后
prince 王子	princess 公主	professor 教授	sailor 船员
salesman 销售员	spaceman 宇航员	sportsman 运动员	steward/stewardess 服务员
jury 陪审团	tailor 裁缝	waiter/waitress 服务员	soldier 士兵
worker 工人	writer 作家	clerk 店员	seaman 水手
servant 佣人	singer 歌手	youngster 青年	workman 工人
host 节目主持人	journalist 记者	reporter 记者	retailer 零售商
trainer/trainee 培训者/受训者	technician 技术员	surgeon 外科医生	warden 看守人
landlord 房东	statesman 政治家	staff 工作人员	spy 间谍
spokesman 发言人	scout 侦察兵	referee 裁判	teenager 青少年
orphan 孤儿	offspring 后代	missionary 传教士	mistress 女主人
millionaire 百万富翁	male 男性	female 女性	maid 女佣
housewife 家庭主妇	heir 继承人	grocer 杂货商	infant 婴儿
entrepreneur 企业家	employer 雇主	employee 雇员	editor 编辑
diplomat 外交官	detective 侦探	dentist 牙科医生	dean 教务长，系主任
cyclist 骑自行车的人	creditor 债权人	crew 全体船员	corps 部队
carpenter 木匠	cashier 出纳，收银员	bachelor 学士，单身汉	attorney 律师
athlete 运动员	analyst 分析者	bureaucrat 官僚	chemist 化学家
juvenile 未成年人	physicist 物理学家	physician 内科医生	politician 政客
radiologist 放射专家	psychiatrist 精神科专家	receptionist 接待员	psychologist 心理学家
spouse 配偶	tenant 承租人	usher 引座员	

身体部位

ankle 脚踝	back 背	bone 骨头	brain 头脑
brow 眉毛	cheek 脸颊	chin 下巴	ear 耳朵
eye 眼睛	face 脸	finger 手指	forehead 前额
knee 膝盖	limb 肢，臂，腿	lip 嘴唇	neck 脖子
shoulder 肩膀	throat 喉咙	toe 脚趾	tongue 舌头
tooth 牙齿	body 身体	jaw 颚	heart 心脏
liver 肝	lung 肺	nose 鼻子	wrist 手腕
stomach 胃	kidney 肾脏	waist 腰	vein 静脉
palm 手掌	lap 大腿	muscle 肌肉	joint 关节
gland 腺体	elbow 肘	belly 肚子	breast 胸脯
fist 拳头	hip 臀部	rib 肋骨	

常见食物、蔬菜、水果、植物、酒水等

banana 香蕉	bean 豆子	beef 牛肉	beer 啤酒
chocolate 巧克力	biscuit 饼干	onion 洋葱	carrot 胡萝卜
garlic 蒜	butter 黄油	cream 奶油	fruit 水果
cheese 芝士	coffee 咖啡	egg 鸡蛋	lemon 柠檬
honey 蜂蜜	grape 葡萄	peach 桃	ice-cream 冰淇淋
liquor 烈酒	mushroom 蘑菇	porridge 粥	pudding 布丁
pea 豌豆	pear 梨	salad 沙拉	salt 盐
pork 猪肉	potato 土豆	sausage 香肠	soda 苏打
pumpkin 南瓜	cocaine 可卡因	sugar 糖	tea 茶
sandwich 三明治	sauce 酱料	wheat 小麦	wine 红酒
soup 汤	steak 牛排	dessert 甜食	vegetation 植物
tobacco 烟草	tomato 西红柿	grease 动物脂	mutton 羊肉
jam 果酱	softdrink 饮料	beverage 饮料	vitamin 维生素
cereal 谷物	grain 谷物	cigar 雪茄 /cigarette 香烟	cabbage 卷心菜
cocktail 鸡尾酒	cocoa 可可粉	coke 可乐	peanut 花生
bud 芽，花蕾			

颜色

green 绿色	grey 灰色	black 黑色	blue 蓝色
violet 紫罗兰色	red 红色	pink 粉色	orange 橙色
ivory 象牙色	yellow 黄色	white 白色	

交通工具

bicycle/bike 自行车	helicopter 直升机	cab/taxi 出租车	automobile 交通工具
bus 巴士	train 火车	aircraft 飞机	liner 班机
motorbike 摩托车	airplane 飞机	ambulance 救护车	tractor 拖拉机
spacecraft 宇宙飞船	satellite 人造卫星		

学科名称

Biochemistry 生物化学	Biomedicine 生物医学	Botany 植物学	Chemistry 化学
Ecology 生态学	Economics 经济学	Electronics 电子学	Journalism 新闻学
Politics 政治	Geology 地质学	Geometry 几何学	Geography 地理
Linguistics 语言学	Math/mathematics 数学	Philosophy 哲学	Physics 物理学
Psychology 心理学	Radiology 放射学		

人称代词

	I	you	he	she	it	we	they	you（复数）
主格	I	you	he	she	it	we	they	you
宾格	me	you	him	her	it	us	them	you
形容词性物主代词	my	your	his	her	its	our	their	your
名词性物主代词	mine	yours	his	hers	its	ours	theirs	yours
反身代词	myself	yourself	himself	herself	itself	ourselves	themselves	yourselves

第二部分
核心意义词汇（A-K）

全国医学博士英语
统考词汇巧战通关

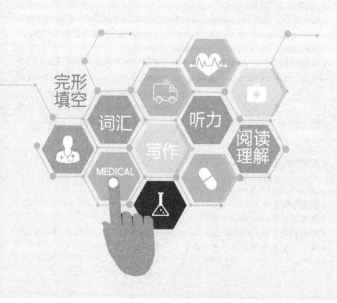

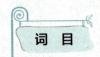

词目

abandon
[əˈbændən]

vt. 放弃，抛弃，离弃 **n.** 放任，放纵

【固定搭配】abandon oneself to 沉溺于；with abandon 放任地，放纵地，纵情地

【联想记忆】give up doing sth., quit doing sth. 放弃做某事

【名师导学】abandon 后接动名词，不接动词不定式，如：abandon doing sth. 放弃做某事。

【经典例题】But even if some disaster meant that the vault was abandoned, the permanently frozen soil would keep the seeds alive.

【译　　文】但是，即使一些灾难意味着储藏室被遗弃了，永远冰冻的土地将使种子仍具有生命力。

abnormal
[æbˈnɔːməl]

a. 不正常的

【名师导学】abnormal, irregular, unnatural 均含有"反常的"之意。abnormal 指因超过适当的限度而显得奇形怪状；irregular 是一般用语，指因偏离风俗习惯、规章制度而不符合常规；unnatural 指由于不合乎人情或天理而使人感到反常。

【经典例题】The so-called Mad Cow Disease is caused by abnormal proteins coming into contact with neurons in the brain.

【译　　文】所谓"疯牛病"，是异常蛋白质侵入脑神经元的结果。

abrupt
[əˈbrʌpt]

a. 突然的，意外的

【名师导学】近义词：sudden, immediate, instantaneous, hurried, hasty, quick, swift, rapid, speedy, precipitate unexpected, surprising, startling, unanticipated, unforeseen, violent, headlong, breakneck, meteoric

【经典例题】*The Day After Tomorrow* is particularly interesting for science students because it focuses on a topic that is currently the subject of considerable scientific research: the possibility of abrupt climate change.

【译　　文】理科学生对《后天》特别感兴趣，原因在于这部电影主要描述了目前许多科学研究所关注的问题：气候突变的可能性。

absence
[ˈæbsəns]

n. 缺席；缺乏

【固定搭配】in the absence of 在（人）不在时；在（物）缺乏或没有时

absent
[ˈæbsənt]

a. 缺席的；缺乏的；漫不经心的

【固定搭配】be absent from 缺席

【联想记忆】be present at 出席

【经典例题】So many directors being absent, the board meeting had to be put off.

【译　　文】由于太多的董事缺席，董事会议不得不推迟。

第二部分　核心意义词汇（A-K）

absolute
['æbsəlu:t]

a. 绝对的；完全的
【派生词汇】absolutely *ad.* 绝对地
【经典例题】Sometimes we buy a magazine with absolutely no purpose other than to pass time.
【译　　文】有时我们买杂志是完全没有目的的，仅仅为了消遣。

absorb
[əb'sɔ:b]

vt. 吸收；吸引，使专心
【派生词汇】absorption *n.* 吸收
【固定搭配】be absorbed in 全神贯注于；distract sb. from doing sth. 使某人做某事时分心
【联想记忆】concentrate / focus / center on, be lost in 全神贯注于
【经典例题】She was so_____ in her job that she didn't hear anybody knocking at the door.
A. attracted　　B. absorbed　　C. drawn　　D. concentrated　　[B]
【译　　文】她完全沉浸在工作当中，没有听到任何敲门声。

abundance
[ə'bʌndəns]

n. 丰富，充足，富裕；多
【派生词汇】abundant *a.* 丰富的

abuse
[ə'bju:z] *v.*
[ə'bju:s] *n.*

n. 滥用；虐待；辱骂；陋习，弊端 *vt.* 滥用；虐待；辱骂
【派生词汇】abusive *a.* 滥用的；abuser *n.* 滥用者
【固定搭配】abuse one's authority 滥用职权
【经典例题】The abuse of alcohol and drugs is also a common factor.
【译　　文】酗酒和吸毒是常见的因素。
【经典例题】It has been revealed that some government leaders_____ their authority and position to get illegal profits for themselves.
A. employ　　B. take　　C. abuse　　D. overlook　　[C]
【译　　文】一些政府领导人已经被揭露出来利用自己的职权和地位获取非法利益。

academic
[ˌækə'demik]

a. 学院的；学术的
【派生词汇】academics *n.* 学术
【经典例题】The effective work of maintaining discipline is usually performed by students who advise the academic authorities.
【译　　文】有效地维持纪律通常是由一些学生来做的，这些学生负责给学校的领导提建议。

accelerate
[ək'seləreit]

vi. 加快；加速；（使）加速
【经典例句】Growth will accelerate to 2.9 per cent next year.
【译　　文】明年的增长会加快到2.9%。

access
['ækses]

n. 通路；访问 *vt.* 访问；存取
【派生词汇】accessible *n.* 可接近的；accessory *a.* 辅助的
【固定搭配】get / gain / have (no) access to （没）有机会或权利得到（接近、进入、使用）
【联想记忆】approach / entrance / admittance to 有（机会、手段、权利）得到 / 接近 / 进入
【经典例题】It doesn't give the person access to ideas.
【译　　文】它也让人们无法有机会接触到那些观点。

accommodate [əˈkɔmədeit]

vt. 为……提供住宿；容纳，接纳；使适应，调节

【名师导学】该词常用短语为 accommodate oneself to，意思是"使自己适应……"。contain, involve, hold 以及 accommodate 都有"容纳"之意。contain 是一般用语，指某物所容纳的东西是其组成的一部分，有时指一大物体容纳着许多小物体；involve 指包含由整体的性质决定的成分或结果，一般用于抽象的意思；hold 指在一定固定空间内能接纳人或物的能力，有时用于比喻；accommodate 与 hold 同义，但指某物很舒适地接纳某人住宿或休息。

【经典例题】The union has made every possible effort to accommodate the management.

【译　　文】工会极力迁就管理方。

accommodation [əˌkɔməˈdeiʃən]

n. (*pl.*) 膳宿供应；住处；适应，调节

accompany [əˈkʌmpəni]

v. 陪伴，伴随；伴奏

【联想记忆】accompany *vt.* 陪伴；company *n.* 陪伴，公司；companion *n.* 同伴，伙伴

【固定搭配】accompany (on / at) 为……伴奏（或伴唱）

【经典例题】The minister was accompanied by his secretary to the hospital.

【译　　文】部长由他的秘书陪同到医院去。

accomplish [əˈkɔmpliʃ]

v. 完成，实现，达到

【派生词汇】accomplishment *n.* 成就

【名师导学】辨析 accomplish, achieve, complete, finish：accomplish 一般指功地完成预期的计划、任务等；achieve 多指完成伟大的功业；complete 指使事物完善、完整；finish 指做完一件事，强调事情的终止、了结。

【经典例题】I accomplished two hours' work before dinner.

【译　　文】我在吃饭前完成了两小时的工作。

accord [əˈkɔ:d]

v. 给予；允许；使一致

【固定搭配】according to 按照，根据；据……所说，按……所载

【经典例题】His opinion accorded with mine.

【译　　文】他的意见与我的一致。

accordance [əˈkɔ:dəns]

n. 一致，相符

【固定搭配】in accordance with 依照，依据，与……一致

according [əˈkɔ:diŋ]

adj. 相应的

【派生词汇】accordingly *ad.* 依照，由此，于是，相应地

【固定搭配】according to 依照，根据

【经典例题】By 2015, those figures are likely to grow to 700 million and 2.3 billion respectively, according to the World Health Organization.

【译　　文】据世界卫生组织估计，到 2015 年，那些数据有可能分别上涨到 7 亿和 23 亿。

account [əˈkaunt]

n. 账，账户；说明，叙述　*vi.* 解释

【派生词汇】accountant *n.* 会计，出纳

【固定搭配】account for 解释；on account of 因为，由于；on no account 决不；on all accounts 无论如何；take into account 考虑，重视

【联想记忆】because of, due to, owing to, in consequence of, on the ground of, in view of, thanks to 基于，由于；not on any account, in no way / respect / sense, in no case, under / in no circumstances, not ever, not at all, by no means 决不；on any / every account, at all events, in any event, at any rate, in any case / way 无论如何；take into consideration 考虑，重视
【经典例题】I am afraid that you'll have to account for the deterioration of the condition.
【译　　文】恐怕你要对状况恶化做出解释。

accountable [əˈkaʊntəbl]
a. 有责任的；应负责的，应对自己的行为做出说明的
【经典例题】The hospital should be held accountable for the quality of care it delivers.
A. practicable　　B. reliable　　C. flexible　　D. responsible　　[D]
【译　　文】医院应该对其提供的护理质量负责。

accumulate [əˈkjuːmjəleit]
v. 积累；积聚；（数量）逐渐增加；（数额）逐渐增长
【派生词汇】accumulation *n.* 积累
【经典例句】None can afford to neglect the accumulated experience of man.
【译　　文】谁也不能忽视人类所积累的经验。

accuracy [ˈækjurəsi]
n. 准确性，精密度

accurate [ˈækjurit]
a. 正确的，精确的
【派生词汇】accurately *ad.* 精确地
【名师导学】辨析 accurate, exact, precise, correct：accurate "精确的，正确无误的"，强调准确性，与事实无出入；exact 意为 "精密的，严密的"，指某人或某事不仅符合事实或标准，而且在细枝末节上也丝毫不差；precise 意为 "精确的，精密的"，在实行、实施或数量上很准确的，强调范围、界限的鲜明性或细节的精密，有时略带 "吹毛求疵" 的贬义；correct 指某人或某事符合事实或公认的标准，没有差错。
【经典例题】Although technically accurate, that is an impersonal assessment.
【译　　文】虽然从技术上说是精确的，但是那是非人性的评估。

accuse [əˈkjuːz]
vt. 谴责；指控，告发
【固定搭配】accuse sb. of 控告某人（做……），为……指责某人
【联想记忆】charge sb. with sth. 控告某人犯有……罪；blame sb. for sth. 因……责备某人；complain to sb. of / about sth. 向某人抱怨……
【经典例题】The shop assistant was dismissed as she was＿＿＿of cheating customers.
A. accused　　B. charged　　C. scolded　　D. cursed　　[A]
【译　　文】这个售货员因被指控欺诈顾客而遭到解雇。

accustom [əˈkʌstəm]
vt. 使习惯
【固定搭配】be accustomed to 习惯于

accustomed [əˈkʌstəmd]
a. 通常的，习惯的，按照风俗习惯的
【联想记忆】be used to (doing) sth. 习惯于

acknowledge [əkˈnɔlidʒ]
vt. 承认；感谢；告知收到（信件等）
【经典例题】I acknowledge the truth of his statement.
【译　　文】我承认他说的是事实。

acquaint
[əˈkweint]

vt. 使熟悉，使认识

【派生词汇】acquaintance *n.* 熟悉的人（物）

【名师导学】该词常与介词 with 搭配，acquaint with 意为"使认识，使了解，使熟悉"。该词用于被动语态中时，过去分词 acquainted 已经失去动作意义，相当于一个形容词。例如："我是去年认识他的。"不能译作："I acquainted him last year." 或 "I was acquainted with him last year." 第一句是语态错误，第二句混淆了"状态"和"动作"，只能译成 "I got/ became acquainted with him last year." 或 "I made his acquaintance last year."。

【经典例题】The leadership at various levels will acquaint itself with the situation through these bulletins and be able to find solutions to problems when they arise.

【译　　文】各级领导接到这样的简报，掌握了情况，有问题就有办法处置了。

acquire
[əˈkwaiə]

vt. 取得，获得；学到

【派生词汇】acquisition *n.* 获得，取得

【名师导学】辨析 acquire, attain, obtain：acquire 指通过不断的学习或逐步获得精神上的东西，如知识、才能等；attain 指通过艰苦努力才使人达到完美境地；obtain 指通过努力，尤其是相当的努力、恳请或要求才得到。

【经典例题】It is through learning that the individual＿＿＿many habitual ways of reacting to situations.

A. retains　　B. gains　　C. achieves　　D. acquires　　[D]

【译　　文】人是通过学习来获得处理事情的惯常方式的。

activate
[ˈæktiveit]

vt. 使活动起来，使开始起来

【经典例题】Research discovered that plants infected with a virus give off a gas that activates disease resistance in neighboring plants.

【译　　文】研究发现，感染了病毒的植物会散发出一种气体，来激活周围植物的疾病抵抗能力。

【名师导学】近义词：stimulate, initiate, arouse, actuate

activist
[ˈæktivist]

n. 积极分子，活动分子

activity
[ækˈtiviti]

n. 活动；活力；行动

acute
[əˈkjuːt]

a. (头脑或五官) 灵敏的，敏锐的；急性的

adapt
[əˈdæpt]

vt. 使适应；改编

【派生词汇】adaptation *n.* 适应，改变

【固定搭配】adapt oneself to 使自己适应或习惯于某事；adapt...to 使……适应

【联想记忆】adopt *vt.* 采纳

【经典例题】In spite of the wide range of reading material specially written or adapted for language learning purposes, there is yet no comprehensive systematic program for the reading skills.

【译　　文】虽然有大量的为了语言学习而编写或改编的阅读材料，但是在阅读技巧方面仍然还没有全面系统的方案。

addict
['ædikt]

n. 吸毒成瘾的人，瘾君子
【派生词汇】addiction *n.* 成瘾
【经典例题】Many people mistakenly believe the term "drug" refers only to some sort of medicine or an illegal chemical taken by addicts.
【译　　文】很多人错误地认为，"药物"这个术语仅仅指某些药品或是吸毒成瘾者服用的违禁化学品。

addicted
[ə'diktid]

a. 对……上瘾的，入迷的
【固定搭配】be addicted to 对……上瘾，入迷

address
[ə'dres]

n. 地址；称呼；演说；通信处　*v.* 称呼；演说；写姓名地址；向……说话；没法解决，处理
【经典例题】The most serious behaviors are relatively easy to spot and address.
【译　　文】最严重的行为相对来说容易发现和解决。

adequate
['ædikwit]

a. 足够的，充分的
【名师导学】辨析 adequate, enough, sufficient：adequate 指"足够的"，满足要求或需求的，也指"恰当的，胜任的"；enough 指"充足的"，数量上足以满足需要或愿望的；sufficient 比 enough 正式，尤指程度上能满足或达到某种需要。
【经典例题】you are bound to have nights where you don't get an adequate amount of sleep.
【译　　文】你一定会经历睡眠不足的夜晚。

adhere
[əd'hiə]

vi. 依附，附着；坚持
【名师导学】该词常用短语是 adhere to，意为"黏附，附着，遵守，坚持"。近义词：bond, cleave, cling, cohere, stick,connect; abide by, carry out, comply, conform, follow, keep, mind, obey, observe
【经典例题】Adhere to the principle of coordinated development between the economy, society and the environment.
【译　　文】坚持经济、社会和环境协调发展的方针。

administer
[əd'ministə]

vt. 管理，经营
【名师导学】近义词：conduct, direct, control, govern,command , manage; furnish, dispense, regulate, apply, authorize
【经典例题】In the 3rd International Mathematics and Science Study, 13-year-olds from Singapore achieved the best scores in standardized tests of maths and science that were administered to 287,896 students from 41 countries.
【译　　文】在第三届国际数学与科学研究中，来自新加坡的 13 岁年龄组在标准化考试中获得最好成绩，参加该项测试的共有来自 41 个国家的 287896 名学生。

admonish
[əd'mɔniʃ]

v. 劝告，训诫，告诫，提醒，敦促
【经典例题】The witness was ＿＿＿ by the judge for failing to answer the question.
　　A. sentenced　　　　　　　B. threatened
　　C. admonished　　　　　　D. jailed　　　　　　　　　　[C]
【译　　文】由于回答不上问题，这位目击者被法官催促。

	【名师导学】advise, caution, warn, admonish, counsel 均有"劝告，忠告，警告"之意。advise 是普通用词，泛指劝告，不涉及对方是否听从劝告。caution 主要指针对有潜在危险提出的警告，有"小心从事"的意味。warn 的含义与 caution 相同，但语气较重，尤指较严重后果。admonish 一般指年长者或领导对已犯错误的或有过失的人提出的忠告或警告，目的是避免类似错误。counsel 是正式用词，语气比 advise 强一些，侧重指对重要问题提出的劝告、建议或咨询。
□ **adjust** [əˈdʒʌst]	*v.* 调整，调节；校准 *vt.*（to）适应于 【派生词汇】adjustment *n.* 调整，调节 【固定搭配】adjust...to 使……适应于 【联想记忆】adapt...to, make...suitable for 使……适应于 【经典例题】As a teacher you have to ____ your methods to suit the needs of slower children. A．adopt　　B．adjust　　C．adapt　　D．acquire　　[B] 【译　　文】作为一名教师，你应该调整你的方法去适应反应速度慢的孩子的需求。
□ **administration** [əd,minisˈtreiʃən]	*n.* 管理；行政，行政机关，政府 【联想记忆】minister *n.* 部长；ministry *n.* 部委
□ **adolescence** [,ædəuˈlesəns]	*n.* 青春期，青少年
□ **adolescent** [,ædəˈlesnt]	*a.* 青春期的，青少年的　*n.* 青少年 【联想记忆】adolescence 青春期；childhood 童年，幼年时代；adulthood 成年期，成人 【经典例题】New research confirms what parents have known all along: simply lack the ability to make smart decisions consistently. A．adolescents　B．adults　　C．parents　　D．intellects　　[A] 【译　　文】新研究表明，父母亲一直都清楚年轻人还不具备长久做出明智决定的能力。
□ **adopt** [əˈdɔpt]	*vt.* 收养；采用，采纳；通过 【派生词汇】adoption *n.* 采纳，收养 【固定搭配】the adopted children 养子 【联想记忆】step mother / father 继母 / 继父；half sister 异母 / 父姐妹；ex-wife / husband 前妻 / 夫 【名师导学】此词（adopt）在历年词汇题中以选项形式出现过多次，而在阅读中则以它的扩展词出现。 【经典例题】Since pollution control measures tend to be money consuming, many industries hesitate to adopt them. 【译　　文】因为污染控制措施会增加开销，很多行业在采取这些措施时都很犹豫。
□ **adore** [əˈdɔːr]	*vt.* 崇拜；爱慕，喜爱
□ **adult** [ˈædʌlt, əˈdʌlt]	*n.* 成人　*a.* 成年的，成熟的 【联想记忆】adulthood *n.* 成年人阶段

【名师导学】辨析 adult, grown-up：adult 指已成熟或达到法定年龄的人，较为正式；grown-up 指身体发育成熟的人。
【经典例题】Given that we can not turn the clock back, adults can still do plenty to help the next generation cope.
【译　　文】虽然我们不能令时光倒流，但成年后仍能够帮助下一代处理很多事情。

advantage
[əd'vɑ:ntidʒ]

n. 优点，有利条件；利益，好处
【固定搭配】take advantage of 乘……之机，利用；be of advantage to 利于
【名师导学】辨析 advantage, benefit, interest, profit：advantage 多指优越条件或有利地位，优势；benefit 是常用词，指任何"利益，好处"，在"利润"时只能用 profit 而不能用 benefit；interest 做可数名词与 benefit 同义，做不可数名词指"利息"；profit 指金钱上获得的好处，有时也指在精神上获得的有价值的东西。

advent
['ædvent]

n.（尤指不寻常的人或事）到来
【名师导学】近义词：approach, coming, appearance, arrival
【经典例题】People are much better informed since the ＿＿ of the Internet.
A. convenient　　B. advent　　C. interface　　D. aftermath　　[B]
【译　　文】互联网面世以来，人们的见识广了。

adverse
['ædvə:s]

a. 不利的；有害的；逆的；相反的
【名师导学】记忆技巧：ad 去 +vers 转 +e → 再转 → 逆反的
【经典例题】Chronic high-dose intake of vitamin A has been shown to have ＿＿ effects on bones.
A. adverse　　B. prevalent　　C. instant　　D. purposeful　　[A]
【译　　文】维生素 A 的长期高剂量摄入被证明对骨骼有不利影响。

advocate
['ædvəkit] n.
['ædvəkeit] v.

vt. 提倡，鼓吹 n. 提倡者，鼓吹者
【经典例题】At the same time, those advocates must not overstate their case.
【译　　文】同时，那些提倡者也不能夸大其词。

aesthetic
[i:s'θetik]

a. 美学的，审美的；艺术的
【经典例题】The more one is conscious of one's political bias, the more chance one has of acting politically without sacrificing one's aesthetic and intellectual integrity.
【译　　文】一个人越是意识到自己的政治态度，他越是可能按政治行事而又不牺牲自己美学和思想上的气节。

affect
[ə'fekt]

vt. 影响，作用；感动；（疾病）侵袭
【名师导学】辨析 affect, effect, influence：affect 指产生的影响之大足以引起反应，着重影响的动作，有时含有"对……产生不利影响"的意思；effect 指实现、达成，着重造成一种特殊的效果；influence 指间接地、以一种无形的力量去潜移默化地影响、同化人的行为或观点等。
【经典例题】We are interested in the weather because it ＿＿ us so directly — what we wear, what we do, and even how we feel.
A. affects　　B. benefits　　C. guides　　D. effects　　[A]
【译　　文】我们对天气十分感兴趣，因为它直接影响了我们——穿衣、行为，甚至感受。

affection [əˈfekʃən]	n. 爱，感情；作用，影响 【固定搭配】have an affection for sb. 热爱某人 【经典例题】We know the kiss as a form of expressing affection. 【译　文】我们知道亲吻是表达感情的一种方式。
affirm [əˈfəːm]	vt. 断言，肯（确）定 【名师导学】近义词 assert, repeat, insist, declare
affirmative [əˈfəːrmətiv]	a. 肯定的，赞成的
afflict [əˈflikt]	vt. 使苦恼，折磨
affluent [ˈæfluənt]	a. 富裕的，富足的
afford [əˈfɔːd]	v. 负担得起；提供；买得起；（有时间）做，能做；承担得起（后果）；给予 【派生词汇】affordable a. 负担得起的 【经典例题】If there is a good drug available, it is everyone's responsibility to make sure patients can ＿＿＿ it. A. afford　　B. demand　　C. tolerate　　D. supply　　[A] 【译　文】如果有好药，那么社会就有责任让病人都用得起。
agency [ˈeidʒənsi]	n. 代理（处），代办（处） 【经典例题】The agency developed a campaign that focused on travel experiences such as freedom, escape, relaxation and enjoyment of the great western outdoors. 【译　文】这个代理商开展了一个活动，这个活动主要是关于旅行经验的，如在广阔的西部户外旅行的自由、逃离现实的生活、放松和乐趣。
agenda [əˈdʒendə]	n. 议事日程，记事册 【固定搭配】put on the agenda 提到议事日程上来
agent [ˈeidʒənt]	n. 代理人，经办人 【经典例题】The Hong Kong agent stressed the need to fulfill the order exactly. 【译　文】那个代理人强调要严格按照要求完成订单。
aggravate [ˈæɡrəveit]	vt. 加重；加剧；[口] 使恼火，激怒；使……恶化
aggregate [ˈæɡriɡeit]	vt. 结合；集结；（使）聚集 n. 集合体；总数，总计 a. 合计的，总计的，聚集的
aggression [əˈɡreʃən]	n. 侵略，攻击
aggressive [əˈɡresiv]	a. 侵略的，侵犯的；爱挑衅的，放肆的；有进取心的，敢作敢为的 【经典例题】They turn people with expendable income into consumers of aggressively marketed foods. 【译　文】他们将拥有可支配收入的人变成强势营销食品的消费者。

agony
['æɡəni]

n. (极度的)痛苦，创痛

【名师导学】agony, distress, misery, suffering 都有"苦痛"之意。agony 指全身的、连续的、剧烈的痛苦；distress 指因不幸发生而带来的精神上的痛苦；misery 指巨大的痛苦和不幸；suffering 强调对痛苦的感受和忍耐。

【经典例题】Nobody can stand for long agony of a severe toothache.
A. sufferance　　B. suppuration　C. plague　　D. torment　　[D]
【译　文】没有人能够忍受强烈的牙痛带来的长期煎熬。

aid
[eid]

vi. 援助，救援　*n.* 援助，救护；助手，辅助物

【名师导学】辨析 aid, assist, help：做动词时，aid 指提供帮助、支援或救助；assist 指"给……帮助"或"支持"，尤指作为隶属或补充；help 的含义较多，表示"给予协助、救助，对……有帮助，(在商店或餐馆中)为……服务，促进，(治疗、药物等)缓解、减轻(疼痛、病症)"；help 为普通词，常可代替 aid、assist。做名词时，aid 指帮助的行为或结果，也指助人者，辅助设备；assist 指助人行为；help 指帮助的行动或实例，或指补救的办法，也指助手、雇工。

alert
[ə'lə:t]

a. 警觉的　*n.* 警惕　*vt.* 使警觉；使意识到

alien
['eiljən]

a. 外国的，外国人的；陌生的；性质不同的，不相容的　*n.* 外国人；外星人

【名师导学】alien 与 foreign 都含有"外国人"的意思。alien 指住在一个国家，但不是该国公民的人；foreigner 指生于或来自他国者，尤指有不同语言、文化的人。

【经典例题】There are more than 1,000 alien species in China.
【译　文】中国约有 1 000 多种外来物种。

alienate
['eiliəneit]

vt. 离间，使疏远，挑拨；让渡(财产等)

【经典例题】By adopting this cunning policy, the clinic risks_____ many of its patients.
A. acquitting　B. allocating　　C. alleviating　D. alienating　　[D]
【译　文】通过采用这个狡猾的政策，诊所冒了得罪很多病人的风险。

alike
[ə'laik]

a. 相同的，相似的

【经典例题】Exercise seems to benefit the brain power of healthy and sick, young and old alike.
【译　文】锻炼似乎有益于健康人和病人的智力，无论是年轻人还是老年人。

allegation
[,æli'geiʃən]

a. 断言，主张，见解

allege
[ə'ledʒ]

vt. 断言，声称

【名师导学】近义词：assert, affirm, testify, claim, declare

【经典例题】It was alleged that the restaurant discriminated against black customers.
【译　文】据称那家饭店歧视黑人顾客。

allergic [ə'lə:rdʒik]	*a.* 对……过敏的,极反感的 【派生词汇】allergy *n.* 过敏 【固定搭配】be allergic to... 对……过敏 【名师导学】allergic reaction 过敏反应;be allergic to 对……有过敏反应,厌恶;allergic to 对……过敏;allergic antibody 变应性抗体;allergic arteritis 变应性动脉炎;allergic asthma 变应性哮喘
alleviate [ə'li:vieit]	*vt.* 减轻(痛苦等),缓和(情绪) 【经典例题】Rheumatologist advises that those with ongoing aches and pains first seek medical help to ____ the problem. A. affiliate　　B. alleviate　　C. aggravate　　D. accelerate　　[B] 【译　　文】风湿病学家建议,那些持续疼痛和痛苦的人首先应该借助医疗来缓解问题。
alliance [ə'laiəns]	*n.* 结盟,联盟,联姻
allied [ə'laid, 'ælaid]	*a.* 联合的,同盟的,联姻的
allocation [,ælə'keiʃən]	*n.* 配置,分配,安置 【派生词汇】allocate *v.* 分配,分派 【经典例题】Twelve hours a week seemed a generous ____ of your time to the nursing home. A. affliction　　B. alternative　　C. allocation　　D. alliance　　[C] 【译　　文】您每周将12个小时分配给护理之家,这好像很慷慨了。 【名师导学】近义词 admeasurement, assignment, apportionment, dispensation, distribution, division
allowance [ə'lauəns]	*n.* 津贴;零用钱 【名师导学】辨析 pay, wage, income, salary:pay 表示"支付",wage 侧重计时计件工资,income 为各种收入的综合,salary 则强调"薪水"。 【经典例题】His mother gives him a monthly ____ of ¥450. A. income　　B. allowance　　C. wages　　D. pay　　[B] 【译　　文】他母亲每月给他450元的零用钱。
alloy ['ælɔi]	*n.* 合金 【经典例题】Brass is an alloy of copper and zinc. 【译　　文】黄铜是铜和锌的合金。
ally [ə'lai, 'ælai]	*n.* 同盟者;伙伴;同类
alternative [ɔ:l'tə:nətiv]	*a.* 两者选一的　*n.* 供选择的东西;取舍 【经典例题】The person needs to explore alternatives for thoughts and actions and learn to care for himself or herself enough to modify his or her own behavior. 【译　　文】人需要为自己寻求其他思维及处事的方式,以此修正自身行为。

alter
[ˈɔːltə]

vt. 改变，变更

【名师导学】辨析 alter, change, convert, modify, shift, transform, vary：alter 指局部、表面的改变，不影响事物的本质或总体结构，如修改衣服的大小等；change 指全部、完全的改变；convert 指由一种形式或用途变为另一种形式或用途；modify 指做小的修改，只能用于改变方法、计划、制度、组织、意见、条款等；shift 指位置或方向的移动、改变；transform 指外貌、性格或性质的彻底改变；vary 多指形式、外表、本质上的繁多而断续的变化或改变，使其多样化。

【经典例题】With the tools of technology he has altered many physical features of the earth.

【译　文】通过一些技术手段，他已经改变了泥土的许多物理特征。

alternate
[ɔːlˈtəːnit] *a.*
[ˈɔːltəneit] *v.*

v. 交替，轮流　*a.* 交替的，轮流的

【名师导学】近义词：vary, fluctuate, vacillate, oscillate, waver, seesaw, teeter, shift, sway, totter; rotate, substitute

【经典例题】Conversation calls for a willingness to alternate the role of speaker with that of listener, and it calls for occasional "digestive pauses" by both.

【译　文】会话要求说话人与听话人都愿意交换角色，并且要求双方偶尔做出停顿，让对方有时间"消化吸收"说话一方的意思。

altitude
[ˈæltitjuːd]

n. 高，高度

amaze
[əˈmeiz]

vt. 使惊愕，使惊叹

【名师导学】辨析 amaze, astonish, surprise, shock：前三个词中，amaze 语气最强，尤其在被认为不可能之事实际上已发生时使用，也可表示"惊奇，惊叹"；astonish 语气稍强，意为"使大吃一惊，使惊愕"，指事情的发生不可思议而"难以置信"；surprise 是一般用语，指对事出突然或出乎意料而"吃惊，惊奇"；shock 意为"使……震惊，使……惊讶"，指事物的发生出乎意料，使人感到震惊。

amazing
[əˈmeiziŋ]

a. 令人惊讶的，令人吃惊的

【名师导学】It's amazing that 从句中的动词用原形或"should+ 原形"表示虚拟语气。

【经典例题】Some people apparently have an amazing ability to come up with the right answer.

【译　文】很明显，一些人有惊人的得出正确答案的能力。

ambiguity
[ˌæmbiˈɡjuːiti]

n. 模棱两可，含义模糊；不确定

ambiguous
[æmˈbigjuəs]

a. 模棱两可的，意思含糊的；引起歧义的

【名师导学】obscure, vague 和 ambiguous 都含有"不明确的"的意思。obscure 指因某事的意思含糊不清或因知识缺乏而难解；vague 指"模糊的，不明确的"；ambiguous 表示有两种或两种以上的解释而意义不明确的。

【经典例题】You need to rewrite this sentence because it is ambiguous; the readers will have difficulty in understanding it.

【译　文】你需要把这个句子改写一下，因为它模棱两可，读者不易理解。

ambition
[æm'biʃən]

n. 雄心；野心

【经典例题】These diplomatic principles completely laid bare their ＿＿＿ for world conquest.
A. admiration　　　　　　B. ambition
C. administration　　　　D. orientation　　　　　　[B]

【译　　文】这些外交政策使他们想征服世界的野心暴露无遗。

ambitious
[æm'biʃəs]

a. 有雄心的，有抱负的

【固定搭配】be ambitious to do sth. 有抱负做某事

【经典例题】She's ambitious and eager to get on (in the world).

【译　　文】她雄心勃勃，一心要（在世上）出人头地。

amend
[ə'mend]

vt. 修正，修订

【名师导学】correct, rectify 和 amend 均有"改正"之意。correct 是一般用语，指按一定标准或规则，把不正确的、不真实的、不完善的、有错误的、有缺点的东西变成正确、完善的东西。rectify 语气较强，指不仅改正了过失或错误，使其变得正当，而且还强调不再犯类似的过失。amend 语气最强，用于人时，指改邪归正，含有积极的意味；用于物时，指既改正缺点又弥补不足，使其变得更加完美。

【经典例题】The Secret Act has been amended to prevent further leaks.

【译　　文】《保密法案》已得到修订，以防止进一步泄漏。

amendment
[ə'mendmənt]

n. 改正，修正，改善；修正案

amount
[ə'maunt]

n. 数据，数额，总数　*vt.* (to) 合计，相当于，等同

【固定搭配】a large amount of（+不可数名词）大量的

【名师导学】辨析 number, total, amount：number 和 total 均为及物动词；amount 是不及物动词，须加 to 再跟宾语。

【经典例题】Getting a proper amount of rest is absolutely essential for increasing your energy.

【译　　文】适量的休息绝对是增加体能所必需的。

ample
['æmpl]

a. 足够的；宽敞的，面积大的

【名师导学】近义词：sufficient, adequate, abundant, plentiful; spacious, roomy, extensive; broad

amplify
['æmplifai]

vt. 放大，增大，扩大

【经典例题】By turning this knob to the right you can amplify the sound from the radio.

【译　　文】朝右边拧一拧旋钮，你就能放大收音机的声音。

analyse
['ænəlaiz]

vt. 分析，分解

【固定搭配】in the final / last analysis 归根结底

analytical
[ˌænə'litikl]

a. 分析的，解析的

【联想记忆】动词 analyze；名词 analysis；名词 analyzer（分析器，分析者）

第二部分 核心意义词汇（A-K）

【经典例题】Or we may be interested in an <u>analytical</u> technique but not enough to stay at its cutting edge.
【译　　文】或许我们会对一项分析技术感兴趣，但还没达到划时代的地步。
【名师导学】analytic center 分析中心；analytic chemistry laboratory 分析化学试验室；analytic control 分析控制；analytic demonstration 分析论证，解析证明

analogy
[əˈnælədʒi]

n. 类似，相似；类比，类推
【名师导学】该词常用短语是 by analogy，意为"用类比的方法"。
【经典例题】If you understand this point, you can understand the rest by analogy.
【译　　文】如果懂得这点，其他的就可以触类旁通了。

analysis
[əˈnælisis]

n. 分析，解析
【固定搭配】in the final (last) analysis 归根结底；on / upon analysis 经分析
【名师导学】该词复数形式为 analyses。
【联想记忆】单复数形式转换：basis — bases 基础；crisis — crises 危机；thesis — theses 论题；hypothesis — hypotheses 假设；diagnosis — diagnoses 诊断；emphasis — emphases 强调
【经典例题】At the same time bispectral analysis recorded the depth of anesthesia.
【译　　文】同时，双频分析记录了麻醉的深度。

anchor
[ˈæŋkə]

n. 锚　*v.* 抛锚，停泊
【固定搭配】anchor...to 把……固定在

anguish
[ˈæŋgwiʃ]

n. 极度痛苦　*v.* 使极度痛苦，感到极度痛苦
【联想记忆】
【经典例题】I am just <u>fed up with</u> his excuses for not getting his work done.
A. anguished at　B. annoyed at　C. agonized by　D. afflicted by　[ ]
【译　　文】我已经厌烦他用各种借口搪塞工作了。
【名师导学】agony, anguish, torment, torture, grief, misery, distress, sorrow 均有"苦恼，痛苦"之意。
agony：侧重指精神或身体痛苦的剧烈程度。
anguish：指精神方面令人难以忍受的极度痛苦；用于身体时，多指局部或暂时的痛苦。torment：强调烦恼或痛苦的长期性。
torture：语气比 torment 强，指在精神或肉体上受到的折磨所产生的痛苦。
grief：指由某种特殊处境或原因造成的强烈的感情上的苦恼与悲痛。
misery：着重痛苦的可悲状态，多含不幸、可怜或悲哀的意味。
distress：多指因思想上的压力紧张、恐惧、忧虑等所引起的精神上的痛苦，也可指某种灾难带来的痛苦。
sorrow：语气比 grief 弱，指因不幸、损失或失望等所产生的悲伤。

animate
[ˈænimeit]

vt. 使有生气，赋予生命

annoy
[əˈnɔi]

vt. 使烦恼，使生气，打搅
【名师导学】辨析 annoy, worry：annoy 强调由于受到干扰而使人烦躁或恼火；worry 常指使人产生焦虑不安或忧愁的情绪。
【经典例题】At this time of the year, university admission offices are annoyed with inquiries from anxious applicants.
【译　　文】每逢此时，大学录取办公室都会被考生焦虑的咨询所困扰。

annual
['ænjuəl]

a. 每年的，年度的 *n.* 年刊，年鉴

【联想记忆】daily *n.* 日刊；weekly *n.* 周刊；monthly *n.* 月刊；quarterly *n.* 季刊；yearly，annual *n.* 年刊

【经典例题】The fruit account for more than half the country's annual exports, according to a recent report.

【译　　文】根据最新的报告，水果出口量占该国年度出口总量的一半以上。

anonymous
[əˈnɔninəs]

a. 匿名的；无名的

【经典例题】The individual TV viewer invariably senses that he or she is nothing more than an anonymous, statistically insignificant part of a huge and diverse audience.

【译　　文】单个电视观众总是感到自己仅仅是个在巨大的、形形色色的观众群中默默无闻的、在统计数字上无关紧要的一员。

anxiety
[æŋɡˈzaiəti]

n. 挂念，焦虑，担心；渴望，热望

【名师导学】后面常接不定式做定语，不接动名词，如：the anxiety to go home 对回家的渴望。

【经典例题】He was waiting for his brother's return with anxiety.

【译　　文】他焦虑不安地等着兄弟归来。

apart
[əˈpɑːt]

ad. 分离，隔开；相距，相隔

【固定搭配】apart from (=besides) 除……之外

【联想记忆】except for 除……之外；in addition to 除……之外；fall apart 土崩瓦解；take apart 分离，破开

【经典例题】He had taken apart the wall oxygen unit.

【译　　文】他将墙上的氧气装置分开了。

apparatus
[ˌæpəˈreitəs]

n. 器械；装置；仪器

【名师导学】apparatus, machine, machinery 均有"器械"之意。apparatus 指比较复杂而又精密的机械装置；machine 指能代替人工作、全自动或半自动的机械装置；machinery 与 machine 同义，指机器的总称，不能用复数。

【经典例题】It took us half an hour to fit up the apparatus.

【译　　文】安装这台仪器花了我们半小时的时间。

apparent
[əˈpærənt]

a. 明显的；表面的

【固定搭配】apparent to 对……是显而易见的

【名师导学】辨析 apparent, evident, clear, obvious：apparent 意为"显露，表面看起来很明显"，表示表面上看来是怎样的，暗含实际情况未必如此之意；evident 表示考虑到各种事实、条件或迹象后而显得很明显；clear 意为"清楚的，明白的"，指不存在使人迷惑或者把问题搞复杂的因素；obvious 意为"显而易见的"，表示被觉察的事物具有显著特点，不需要很敏锐的观察力就能觉察到。

【经典例题】It is apparent that the watches that finally arrived have been produced from inferior materials

【译　　文】很明显，最后到货的那批手表是用劣等材料制成的。

appeal
[əˈpiːl]

vi. (to) 请求，呼吁；吸引；上诉　求助　*n.* 呼吁；吸引力；上诉

【经典例题】On the positive side, emotional appeals may respond to a consumer's real concerns..

【译　　文】在积极的一面，（广告的）情感的鼓动也能反映消费者真正的需求。

第二部分 核心意义词汇（A-K）

appendix
[ə'pendiks]
n. 附录
【名师导学】注意 appendix 的复数形式可以是 appendixes 或 appendices。
【经典例题】The dictionary has several appendices including one on irregular verbs.
【译　　文】这本词典后有好几个附录，包括一个不规则动词表。

applaud
[ə'plɔːd]
vt. 鼓掌，欢呼或喝彩（以示赞许等）
【经典例题】The school master applauded the girl's bravery in his opening speech.
【译　　文】在开场演说中，校长表扬了那个女孩子的勇敢。

applause
[ə'plɔːz]
n. 鼓掌，喝彩，赞许
【固定搭配】give sb. applause for 因……而夸奖某人
【经典例题】There was a storm of applause when he entered the hall.
【译　　文】当他走进大厅时，里面响起了暴风雨般的掌声。

appetite
['æpitait]
n. 食欲，胃口；欲望
【固定搭配】have no appetite for work 不想工作
【联想记忆】have a desire for, have inclination for, long for, be hungry / thirsty for 渴望

appliance
[ə'plaiəns]
n. 用具，设备，器械，装置
【联想记忆】equipment *n.* 设备（不可数）；instrument *n.* 仪器；facilities *n.* 设施

applicant
['æplikənt]
n. 申请者

application
[,æpli'keiʃən]
n. 申请，申请书；运用，应用

apply
[ə'plai]
vi. 申请 *vt.* 运用，应用
【固定搭配】apply for 申请；apply...to 将……应用于，涂，抹；apply oneself to (doing) sth. 致力于
【联想记忆】devote oneself to，be dedicated to 致力于
【经典例题】I want to apply for the job.
【译　　文】我想申请这份工作。

appoint
[ə'pɔint]
vt. 任命，委派；约定
【固定搭配】appoint sb.（后面接名词）任命某人为……职
【经典例题】To their surprise, she has been nominated as candidate for the Presidency.
A. recognized　　　　　　B. defined
C. appointed　　　　　　 D. promoted　　　　　　　　　　　　[C]
【译　　文】出乎他们意料的是，她被提名为总统选举的候选人。

appointment
[ə'pɔintmənt]
n. 约会，约见；任命，委派
【固定搭配】keep / make / cancel an appointment 守约 / 约会 / 取消约会

appraisal
[ə'preizəl]
n. 评价，估价
【名师导学】appraisal, estimation 以及 evaluation 皆有"估计，评估"之意。estimation 指凭自己经验和知识对某种事物的性质、数量做大概的推断；

appraisal 语气比 estimation 强，用于物时指内行对某物的真伪或好坏的辨别，并确定其准确的价值和价格，用于人时指对某人的优缺点的鉴别；evaluation 与 appraisal 同义，但只能指对人的品质或物的价值给予评定，而不能评定物的价格。
【经典例题】She gave a detailed appraisal of the current situation.
【译　　文】她对当前的局势做出了详细的评估。

appreciate
[ə'pri:ʃieit]

vt. 感激，感谢；评价；欣赏，赏识
【名师导学】后面接动名词，不接动词不定式，如：appreciate (one's) doing。
【经典例题】I appreciate President Castro's invitation for us to visit Cuba, and have been delighted with the hospitality we have received since arriving here.
【译　　文】我们一行承卡斯特罗主席的邀请访问古巴，我不胜感激。我们来到这里后受到了热情接待，我一直沉浸在喜悦之中。

approach
[ə'prəutʃ]

v. 接近 vt. 处理；对待 n. 走进；方法；探讨；观点
【固定搭配】approach to=access to 接近
【经典例题】They must change their institutional and legal approaches to water use.
【译　　文】他们必须从制度和法规的方式上改变对水资源的使用。

appropriate
[ə'prəupriət]

a. 适当的，恰当的
【固定搭配】be appropriate to 对……适合
【名师导学】It's appropriate that... 从句中的谓语用原形或 should+原形结构。
【经典例题】For many patients, institutional care is the most appropriate and beneficial form of care.
【译　　文】对于许多病人来说，机构看护是最适当也是最有益的护理方式。

appropriation
[ə,prəupri'eiʃn]

n. 拨款；挪用
【经典例题】Faculty members don't need to commit egregious acts such as sexual harassment or appropriation of students' work to fail in their responsibility to their charges.
【译　　文】教职员工不用犯下诸如性骚扰或侵占学生成果等令人发指的罪行来表明自己失职。

approval
[ə'pru:vəl]

n. 赞成，同意；批准

approve
[ə'pru:v]

v. 赞成，赞许，同意；批准，审议，通过
【固定搭配】approve sth. 批准某事；approve of sth. 赞许、同意某事；approve of sb. doing sth. 同意某人做某事
【名师导学】前缀 ap-（ab- 的变体）表示运动的方向、朝向、变化。
【经典例题】Mike Foster is trying to get Parliament to approve a new law.
【译　　文】迈克·佛斯特正努力使国会通过一项新的法律。

aptitude
['æptitju:d]

n. 才能，资质，天资

apt
[æpt]

a. 易于，有……倾向；恰当的；聪明的

【名师导学】apt, liable, prone 均有 "易于……的" 的意思，只能做表语，不能做定语，后面都接动词不定式。apt 为常用词，尤其是用于口语中；liable 表示易于产生某种（对主语的）后果的（常用于警告）；prone 侧重主语（往往是人，极少用物）的本性，使之 "倾向于（某种弱点、错误或不良行为）"。

【经典例题】Shoes of this kind are apt to slip on wet ground.

【译　　文】这种鞋在潮湿的地上容易打滑。

arbitrary
[ˈɑːbitrəri]

a. 任意的，武断的；专断的，专横的

【经典例题】This is the sort of case in which judges must exercise the arbitrary power.

【译　　文】这就是法官必须使用专断权力的案例。

arduous
[ˈɑːdjuəs]

a. 费力的，辛勤的；险峻的

【经典例题】The doctor advised Ken to avoid strenuous exercise.
A. arduous　　B. demanding　　C. potent　　D. continuous　　[A]

【译　　文】医生建议肯避免激烈运动。

【名师导学】近义词 difficult, severe, strenuous, laborious

arise
[əˈraiz]

vi. 出现，发生；(from) 由……引起，由……产生

【名师导学】辨析 arise, arouse, raise, rise：arise 是不及物动词，意为 "出现，产生，发生"，后常跟介词 from，表示 "由……引起，由……产生"，其主语常常是 an argument, a problem, a quarrel, a doubt, a question, a storm, a difficulty, a disagreement 等；arouse 只能做及物动词，意为 "唤醒，引起"，常用固定搭配有 interest, sympathy, curiosity, excitement, criticism, suspicion 等；raise 是及物动词，意为 "举起，增加，提高"，尤指人或人体某部分的抬高，如举杯、举手等；rise 是不及物动词，意为 "升起，上升，增高"。

【经典例题】A completely new situation will＿＿＿＿ when the examination system comes into existence.
A. arise　　B. rise　　C. raise　　D. arouse　　[A]

【译　　文】当考试体系形成的时候，一个全新的状况就会出现。

arrange
[əˈreindʒ]

vt. 整理，布置；安排，筹备

【固定搭配】arrange for sb. to do sth. 安排某人做某事

arrangement
[əˈreindʒmənt]

n. 安排，准备工作；整理，布置

array
[əˈrei]

n. 一系列，大量；排列，数组

【经典例题】When the Council gets an enquiry from a member about a particular product or market, we provide the member with an array of services.

【译　　文】当我协会中的会员询问关于某种特殊产品或市场的情况时，我们会为其提供一系列的服务。

arrest
[əˈrest]

vt. / n. 逮捕；扣留

【固定搭配】arrest sb. for 因……而逮捕某人；under arrest 被捕

【经典例题】I realize that our medical resuscitation of this child was futile, as has been shown in children who present to the emergency department in full cardiac arrest.

【译　　文】我意识到我们对于这个孩子的医疗救援是无效的，因为孩子送到急诊室的时候心脏已经骤然停了。

arrogance
['ærəgəns]

n. 傲慢态度，自大

【联想记忆】形容词 arrogant

【名师导学】近义词群：bigheaded 自负的，自大的；boastful 自夸的；bold 大胆的；conceited 极其自负的；contemptuous 轻视的；disdainful 鄙视的；domineering 专横的；egotistic 自我本位的；haughty 傲慢的；overconfident 自负的；proud 自豪的；self-important 妄自尊大的

arrogant
['ærəgənt]

a. 傲慢的，自大的

【名师导学】arrogant, conceited, proud, vain 都有"骄傲的，傲慢的"的意思。arrogant 一般为贬义，表示"傲慢无礼的"；conceited 一般为贬义，表示"自负的，自大的"；proud 可褒可贬，表示"自豪的（褒），傲慢的（贬）"；vain 一般为贬义，表示"无益的，爱虚荣的"。

【经典例题】Often these children realize that they know more than their teachers, and their teachers often feel that these children are arrogant, inattentive, or unmotivated.

【译　　文】这些孩子常常觉得他比老师知道得多，老师们常常感到这些孩子自大、不用心或者缺乏学习动机。

articulate
[ɑːˈtikjulət] *a.*
[ɑːˈtikjuleit] *vt.*

a. 发音清晰的，善于表达的；表达清晰有力的　*vt.* 明确有力地表达；清晰地吐（词），清晰地发音

【经典例题】With no friends nearby, he finds it very difficult to articulate his distress.

【译　　文】没有一个朋友在身边，他感到很难表达清楚自己的痛苦。

artificial
[ˌɑːtiˈfiʃəl]

a. 人工的，人造的；人为的，做作的

【名师导学】辨析 artificial, fake, false：artificial 指由人工制成的而非自然的；fake 指"伪造的，冒充的"；false 是指与真理或事实相反的，故意造假的。

【经典例题】The colors in these artificial flowers are guaranteed not to come out.

【译　　文】这些假花保证不会褪色。

ascend
[əˈsend]

v. 上升，升高；登上

【名师导学】climb, ascend, mount 以及 scale 均有"登上"之意。climb 是一般用语，用于人时，指用手足攀登着东西往上爬；用于物时，指很费力地往高处移动；有时可做比喻，指社会地位的上升。ascend 是正式用语，指一直往上升。用于人时，指用脚很不费力地逐步上升到较高处；用于物时，指通过水或空气垂直向上运动；用于比喻时指某人的地位达到了极点。mount 指人攀着某物上升到最高处，有时指跨到某物上，用于比喻时指数量提高了。scale 指人用梯子或有阶梯的东西爬上某物顶部或爬过某物，有时用于比喻数字按比例增大。

【经典例题】The path started to ascend more steeply at this point.

【译　　文】这条路从这里向上就更陡了。

ascertain
[ˌæsəˈtein]

vt. 查明，弄清，确定

【名师导学】近义词：learn, find out, determine, discover

【经典例题】We shall probably never be able to ascertain the exact nature of these sub-atomic particles.

【译　　文】我们可能将永远不能确定这些亚原子颗粒的确切本质。

ascribe
[əˈskraib]

vt.（常与 to 连用）归于，归因于

【联想记忆】形容词 ascribable；名词 ascription，注意拼写变化。类似的词还有 describe, prescribe 等。

【名师导学】attribute, ascribe 这两个动词均有"把……归于"之意。
attribute：指出于相信而把……归于某人或某物，含较多的客观性。
ascribe：指根据推论或猜想把……归于某人或某物，含主观臆断成分较重。

aspect
[ˈæspekt]

n. 样子，面貌；方面

【联想记忆】respect *v.* 尊敬；inspect *v.* 视察；prospect *n.* 前景；expect *v.* 期望；perspective *n.* 洞察力

【经典例题】Most national news has an important financial aspect to it.
【译　　文】绝大多数的国内新闻都会涉及重要的金融信息。

aspire
[əsˈpaiə]

vi. 追求，渴求，渴望（to, after）

aspirin
[ˈæspərin]

n. 阿司匹林

aspiration
[ˌæspəˈreiʃən]

n. 强烈的愿望，志向，抱负

【经典例题】But as useful as computers are, they are nowhere close to achieving anything remotely resembling these early aspirations for humanlike behavior.
【译　　文】但是，尽管计算机非常有用，但它们离早期期望的类似人类行为的愿望还相差万里。

assassinate
[əˈsæsineit]

vt. 暗杀，行刺

assassination
[əˌsæsiˈneiʃən]

n. 暗杀，刺杀

【经典例题】Two members of a UN team investigating the February assassination of former Lebanese Prime Minister on Friday interviewed Lebanon's President.
【译　　文】负责调查黎巴嫩前总理二月遭暗杀事件的两名联合国调查小组成员于周五会见了黎巴嫩总统。

assemble
[əˈsembl]

vt. 集合，集会；装配，组装　*vi.* 集会，聚集

【名师导学】辨析 assemble, converge, collect, accumulate, gather：assemble 表示集合或召集到一起成为一组或整体，或指"装配"，把配件或零件装配在一起；converge 指从不同方向汇聚到一起、向或靠拢于某一交叉点，多指线条聚集于一点或河流等的汇合；collect 指按计划进行收集整理，其对象往往是物。偶尔也用于人，意为"集合"；accumulate 指从无到有累积的过程；gather 是一般用语，指将分散的东西聚集在一起，或指"收获，采摘"，指人时表示"聚集，集中"。

【经典例题】Everybody＿＿＿＿＿ in the hall where they were welcomed by the minister.
A. assembled　　　　　　　B. accumulated
C. piled　　　　　　　　　D. joined　　　　　　　[A]
【译　　文】所有集聚在大厅的人都受到了部长的欢迎。

assembly
[ə'sembli]

n. 集会，会议；装配，组装

【名师导学】辨析 assembly, conference, congress, convention, meeting：assembly 指"集会"；conference 指磋商或讨论的会议；congress 指代表大会，正式的代表举行会议讨论问题；convention 指某一团体或政党的正式会议；meeting 是常用词，表示"会议，大会"，也表示"会合，会面"。

assert
[ə'sə:t]

vt. 宣称，断言；维护，坚持（权利等）

【名师导学】assert, asseverate, declare, affirm, aver, avow 这些动词的意思是"肯定地提出……"。assert 是指自信地讲出自己的观点，但常常是没有证据来支持；asseverate 指郑重真诚地断言；declare 有接近于 assert 所表述的力量，但含有表示讲话者有礼节和权威的意思；affirm 和 aver 强调讲话人对所讲东西正确性的自信；avow 指坦诚地、坦率地承认或确认。

【经典例题】Why does the author assert that all things from American are fascinating to foreigners? Because they have gained much publicity through American media?

【译　　文】为什么作者断言美国所有的东西对外国人都有吸引力？因为它们通过美国的媒体已经获得了巨大的知名度。

assertive
[ə'sə:tiv]

a. 断言的；武断的；过分自信的

assess
[ə'ses]

vt. 估计，估算；评估，评价，评定

【派生词汇】assessment *n.* 评估，估算

【联想记忆】access *n.* 接近；excess *n.* 超额量；asset *n.* 资产

【名师导学】辨析 assess, estimate, evaluate：assess 指为征税估定（财产）的价值，确定或决定（某项费用，如税或罚款）的金额，评估某事物的价值、意义或程度；estimate 指估计，恰当地推测；evaluate 指确定……的数值或价值，对……评价，仔细地考查和判断。

【经典例题】The researchers say hippocampus could help with assessing geometry or remembering whether they have already visited a location.

【译　　文】研究者说，海马体在评估几何形状、回忆曾经去过的位置方面会起作用。

asset
['æset]

n. 资产，财产；有用的资源，宝贵的人／物；优点，益处

【经典例题】He misled management by giving it the idea that the older and more experienced men were not an asset but a liability.

【译　　文】他认为年长者和有经验的人不是财产，而是累赘，这一观点误导了管理部门。

assign
[ə'sain]

vt. 派给，分配；选定，指定（时间、地点等）

【经典例题】In your first days at the school you'll be given a test to help the teachers to assign you to a class at your level.

【译　　文】在刚入学的几天你会参加一个测试，以帮助老师们为你选定一个适合你的水平的班级。

assignment
[ə'sainmənt]

n. （分派的）任务，（指定的）作业；分配，指派

assimilate
[ə'simileit]

vt. 吸收，消化；使同化 *vi.* 同化，融入

【经典例题】One of the reasons why children resemble their parents is that they assimilate the characteristics of their parents.
【译　　文】孩子往往长得像父母，其原因之一就是孩子吸取并同化了父母的各种特征。

assist
[ə'sist]

vi. 援助，帮助

【固定搭配】assist in doing sth. 帮助做某事；assist sb. in doing sth. 帮助某人做某事；assist sb. to do sth. 帮助某人做某事
【经典例题】The clerk assisted the judge by looking up related precedent.
【译　　文】这位书记官协助那位法官查阅相关的判决先例。

assistance
[ə'sistəns]

n. 帮助，援助

associate
[ə'səuʃieit] *vt.*
[ə'səuʃiət] *n.*

vt. 联系；联合 *vi.* 交往 *n.* 合作人，同事

【固定搭配】associate...with 把……与……联系在一起
【联想记忆】associate...with, link...to, relate...with / to, combine / connect...with 把……与……联系在一起；have association with 与……交往
【经典例题】What do you associate with such a heavy snow?
【译　　文】对这样一场大雪你有什么联想？

association
[ə,səusi'eiʃən]

n. 协会，团体；交往；联合，合伙

【固定搭配】have association with 与……交往

assume
[ə'sju:m]

vt. 假定，设想；假装；承担

【联想记忆】consume *v.* 消费；presume *v.* 推测；resume *v.* 重新开始
【经典例题】Researchers conclude that any effect of money on happiness is smaller than most daydreamers assume.
【译　　文】研究者得出结论，即金钱对幸福的影响要比空想家假设的小。

assumption
[ə'sʌmpʃən]

n. 假定，设想；担任，承当；假装

assure
[ə'ʃuə]

vt. 使确信；向……保证

【名师导学】辨析 assure, ensure：两者皆意为"保证"，但用法有些区别，具体用法有 assure sb. that / assure sb. of；ensure that / ensure sb. against / from；assure / ensure sth.。
【联想记忆】insure 保险，投保；guarantee 提出担保
【经典例题】He was proud of being chosen to participate in the game and he ＿＿ us that he would try as hard as possible.
　　A. assured　　B. insured　　C. assumed　　D. guaranteed　　[A]
【译　　文】他为被选上参加比赛而感到骄傲，并且向我们保证他会竭尽全力。

astonish
[əs'tɔniʃ]

vt. 使惊讶，使吃惊

【经典例题】The researchers were astonished to find that brain tissue surrounding the original injury had also died.
【译　　文】研究者们很惊讶地发现，原始伤口周围的脑组织也死亡了。

atmosphere
['ætməsfiə]
n. 空气；大气，大气层；气氛

atmospheric
[ætməsˈferik]
a. 大气的，空气的

atom
[ˈætəm]
n. 原子
【固定搭配】be blown / broken / smashed to atoms=be blown / broken / smashed into pieces 炸（打）得粉碎；an atom of 一点儿……

atomic
[əˈtɔmik]
a. 原子的，原子能的
【联想记忆】molecule *n.* 分子；particle *n.* 粒子；electron *n.* 电子；nucleus *n.* 原子核

attach
[əˈtætʃ]
vt. 贴上，系上，附上；使依附
【固定搭配】be attached to 喜爱，依恋，附属于；attach importance to 重视……
【联想记忆】pay attention to, lay stress / emphasis on 重视
【经典例题】I've attached my contact information in the recommendation letter.
【译　　文】我已经把我的联系信息附在了推荐信中。

attain
[əˈtein]
vt. 达到；取得
【派生词汇】attainable *a.* 可达到的

attachment
[əˈtætʃmənt]
n. 附属物，附件；依恋；依附

attitude
[ˈætitjuːd]
n. 态度，看法

attraction
[əˈtrækʃən]
n. 吸引；吸引力
【经典例题】Niagara Falls is a great tourist＿＿, drawing millions of visitors every year.
A．attention　B．attraction　C．appointment　D．arrangement　　[B]
【译　　文】尼亚加拉大瀑布是一个著名的旅游景点，每年都会吸引数百万的游客。

attractive
[əˈtræktiv]
a. 有吸引力的；有魅力的，动人的

attributable
[əˈtribjutəbl]
a. 可归于……的

attribute
[ˈætribjuːt] *n.*
[əˈtribju(ː)t] *vt.*
n. 属性，特征；*vt.*（to）把……归因于
【名师导学】辨析 attribute, owe：attribute...to... 意为"把……归因于……"；owe...to... 意为"把……归功于"。
【联想记忆】contribute *v.* 贡献；distribute *v.* 分发
【经典例题】How large a proportion of the sales of stores in or near resort areas can be＿＿to tourist spending?
A．contributed　B．applied　　C．attributed　D．attached　　[C]
【译　　文】在旅游点或者旅游点附近商店的销售中，有多大比例与旅游者的消费有关？

auction
['ɔːkʃən]

n. 拍卖　*vt.* 拍卖

【经典例题】His car is certain to fetch a good price at the auction.
【译　　文】他的那部车在这次拍卖会上一定能卖个好价钱。

audience
['ɔːdjəns]

n. 听众，观众

【名师导学】audience 做主语时，看作整体则谓语用单数，看作个体则谓语用复数。

audio
['ɔːdiəu]

n. / a. 声音（的），听觉（的）；音频（的）；音响（的）

【经典例题】The school's audio-visual apparatus includes a new set of multi-media device, not to mention films, records, etc.
【译　　文】这所学校的视听设备包括一套新的多媒体装置，更不用说电影、录音等设备了。

authentic
[ɔːˈθentik]

a. 真的，真正的；可靠的，可信的

author
['ɔːθə]

n. 作者

【名师导学】辨析 author, writer：author 指某作品的作者；writer 多指职业性作家。

authoritative
[əˈθɔːrəteitiv]

a. 有权威的，可信的

authority
[ɔːˈθɔriti]

n. 权力，权威；权威人士；（*pl.*）当局

【经典例题】This can lead to a reduction in parental authority.
【译　　文】这会导致父母权威的降低。

authorize
['ɔːθəraiz]

vt. 授权，委托；许可，批准

【名师导学】该拼法是美式拼法，英式英语拼法为 authorise。重要短语有 authorize sb. to do sth.。-rize 是很重要的后缀，意思是"使……"，名词/形容词 +ize 变为相应动词，如：realize, urbanize 等。相关近义词都有"给某人以行动的职权"的意思：accredit（信任，授权，归于）；commission（委任，任命，委托）；empower（授权予，使能够）；licensed to（授权给）。
【经典例题】I authorized him to act for me while I was away.
【译　　文】我曾委托他在我不在的时候做我的代理人。

automate
['ɔːtəmeit]

vt. 使自动化，自动操作

automatic
[ˌɔːtəˈmætik]

a. 自动的

【经典例题】The factory is equipped with two fully automatic assembling lines, and the control room is at the center.
【译　　文】这座工厂里有两条全自动生产线，控制室就在正中央。

autonomy
[ɔːˈtɔnəmi]

n. 自治，自治权；自主权

【名师导学】该词的形容词是 autonomous。the autonomous region 自治区
【经典例题】The authors of the United States Constitution attempted to establish an effective national government while preserving autonomy for the states and liberty for the individuals.
【译　　文】美国宪法的缔造者们试图建立一个有效的全国政府，而同时保护各州的自治权和个人的自由权利。

available [ə'veiləbl]

a. 可利用的；可得到的
【名师导学】常做表语，做定语要放在所修饰词后面，如：These data are readily available. 这些资料易于得到。
【经典例题】Humanity uses a little less than half the water available worldwide.
【译　　文】人类使用了全球可利用水资源的一小部分，不足一半。

avenue ['ævinju:]

n. 林荫路，大街
【经典例题】My parents took me to Constitution Avenue to see the parade.
【译　　文】我父母带我到宪法大街去看游行。

avert [ə'və:t]

vt. 防止，避免；转移（目光、思想等）（常与 from 搭配使用）
【名师导学】近义词 avoid

avoid [ə'vɔid]

vt. 避免，逃避
【名师导学】后面接动名词，不接动词不定式，如：avoid doing sth. 避免做某事。
【经典例题】They often try to avoid feeling unpleasant emotions, such as loneliness, worry, and grief.
【译　　文】他们经常尽量避免产生不愉快的情绪，例如孤独、担心和悲伤。

award [ə'wɔ:d]

n. 奖，奖品　*vt.* 授予，奖给
【联想记忆】reward *n.* 回报
【名师导学】辨析 award, reward：award 指因优点奖励或授予的东西；reward 指为某些特殊服务提供或给予的酬劳。award sb. sth., award sth. to sb. 奖赏某人某物；reward sb. for sth. 因某事奖赏某人；reward sb. with sth. 用某事酬劳某人。
【经典例题】An example of the second type of house won an Award of Excellence from the American Institute of Architects.
【译　　文】第二种房子的一个设计样本赢得了美国建筑学院的优秀奖。

aware [ə'wɛə]

a. 知道的，意识到
【固定搭配】be aware of 意识到
【经典例题】Coaches and parents should be aware, at all times, that their feedback to youngsters can greatly affect their children.
【译　　文】教练们和父母们应该随时意识到他们的反应将会极大地影响到他们的孩子。

awful ['ɔ:fəl]

a. 糟糕的，极坏的，可怕的
【经典例题】She had put a good three miles between herself and the awful hitchhiker.
【译　　文】在她和那个吓人的旅行者之间保持了恰好三英里的距离。

awkward ['ɔ:kwəd]

a. 粗笨的，笨拙的；尴尬的，棘手的
【经典例题】The shy girl felt ＿＿＿＿ and uncomfortable when she could not answer her teacher's questions.
A. amazed　　B. awkward　　C. curious　　D. amused　　[B]
【译　　文】这个害羞的女孩在回答不上来老师的问题时感到尴尬和不安。

bacteria
['bæk'tiəriə]

n. (*pl.*) 细菌

【名师导学】bacteria 是 bacterium 的复数，但此词往往以复数形式在文章中出现。
【经典例题】The bacteria which make the food go bad prefer to live in the watery regions of the mixture.
【译　文】能使食物变坏的细菌更喜欢在有水的混合物区域生存。

balance
['bæləns]

vt. 使平衡　*n.* 平衡；差额，结余；天平，秤
【固定搭配】off balance 不平衡
【经典例题】They throw out all ideas about a balanced diet for the grandkids.
【译　文】他们将孩子的平衡饮食思想完全抛于脑后。

bald
[bɔːld]

a. 光秃的，秃的；不加掩饰的，明显的

ban
[bæn]

n. / vt. 禁止，取缔
【经典例题】If the law is passed, wild animals like foxes will be protected under the ban in Britain.
【译　文】如果这项法律通过了，像狐狸这样的野生动物在英国就会得到禁令的保护。

band
[bænd]

n. 条，带；乐队，军乐队；一群，一伙；波段
【联想记忆】violin *n.* 小提琴；piano *n.* 钢琴；trumpet *n.* 小号；horn *n.* 号角；guitar *n.* 吉他
【名师导学】band 做主语时，若看作整体，则谓语用单数；若看作个体，则谓语用复数。

bankrupt
['bæŋkrʌpt]

a. 破产的　*vt.* 使破产　*n.* 破产者

bare
[bɛə]

a. 赤裸的，光秃的，空的；极少的，仅有的
【固定搭配】a bare possibility 一点点可能性；万一
【名师导学】辨析 bare, blank, empty, hollow, vacant：bare 表示赤裸的，没有通常的或适当的覆盖物的；blank 指空白的，未填写的，没有字迹、图像或标记的；empty 指的是无人居住的，内无一物的，未载东西的，还指含义上空洞的；hollow 指中空的，凹的，挖空的；vacant 指空缺的，没有现任者或占有者的。
【经典例题】We'd better take the bare necessities.
【译　文】我们最好只带极少的必需品。

barely
['bɛəli]

ad. 仅仅；几乎不能

barrier
['bæriə]

n. 栅栏；障碍，屏障
【经典例题】Some people prefer the original English text whereas others feel a translation into their native language removes a barrier to understanding.
【译　文】有人更喜欢英语原版，也有人觉得翻译成母语消除了理解上的障碍。

beam [bi:m]	*n.* 一束；一道横梁 *vi.* 发光，发热 【联想记忆】flame *v.* 燃烧；spark *v.* 发火花，发电花
bear [beə(r)]	*n.* 熊；（在证券市场等）卖空的人 *v.* 承受，忍受；不适于某事（或做某事）；承担责任 【名师导学】bear 做动词时，过去式和过去分词形式是不规则的 bore, born。常见的形容词形式为 bearable "可忍耐的"，unbearable "不可忍受的"，比如 unbearable arm pain "难以忍受的胳膊剧痛"。
behalf [bi'hɑ:f]	*n.* 代表，利益 【固定搭配】on behalf of 代表
behave [bi'heiv]	*vi.* 举动，举止，表现 【固定搭配】behave oneself 规规矩矩地 【经典例题】They still seemed to make people behave more honestly. 【译　　文】他们仍然好像能使人们举止坦诚。
behavio(u)r [bi'heivjə]	*n.* 行为，举止
being ['bi:iŋ]	*n.* 存在，生存；存在物，生物，人 【固定搭配】come into being 产生，形成，成立；for the time being 暂时
beneficial [beni'fiʃəl]	*a.* 有利的，有益的 【固定搭配】be beneficial to... 对……有益
beneficiary [ˌbeni'fiʃəri]	*n.* 受惠者，受益人 *a.*（封建制度下）受封的；采邑的；臣服的 【联想记忆】动词和名词形式均为 benefit，形容词 beneficial 有益的，有好处的；名词 benefactor 捐助者，恩人 【名师导学】advantage, benefit, interest, favour, profit, gain 这些名词均有"利益、好处"之意。 advantage：指因某方面占优势或利用某机会以及对方弱点而获得利益与好处。 benefit：普通用词，指通过正当手段从物质或精神方面得到的任何好处或利益。 interest：作"利益"解时，多用复数形式，既可指集团、群体的利益，又可指个人的利益。 favour：指在竞争中获得的 advantage，也可指狭隘的个人利益。 profit：着重收益，尤指从物质、钱财等方面获得的利益。 gain：指获得的物质利益，也暗示不损坏他人利益而得的无形好处。 avail, benefit, profit 这些动词均含有"有益于，有益"之意。 avail：较文雅，常见于历史小说、演说或讲道中，较少用于日常话语，侧重功效或效力。 benefit：通常既可指个人情况（如身体、智力或精神状态等）的好转或改善，又可指对实现某个目标等带来的好处。 profit：着重于物质方面的受益，常用于财富或知识等方面的得益。
benefit ['benifit]	*n.* 利益，恩惠 *vt.* 有利于，受益于 *vi.* 得益于 【固定搭配】benefit from 受益于
besides [bi'saidz]	*ad.* 而且，还有 *prep.* 除……之外 【名师导学】辨析 besides, except, except for：besides 表示"除……之外（也/还）"；except 指"除此以外"，除去的是同类、同等的人或事；except for 表示除去的是整体的一部分。

第二部分 核心意义词汇（A-K）

bestow [bi'stəu]
vt. 授予，献给
【名师导学】近义词：accord, award, confer, grant, present; contribute, donate, give, hand out
【经典例题】The country's highest medal was＿＿＿ upon him for heroism.
A. earned B. bestowed C. credited D. granted [B]
【译　　文】由于英勇，他被授予国家的最高奖项。

bet [bet]
vt. 以……打赌，与……打赌 *vi.* 赌，打赌 *n.* 打赌；赌注，赌金

betray [bi'trei]
vt. 出卖，背叛

beware [bi'wɛə]
v. 谨慎，当心

bewilder [bi'wildə]
vt. 使迷惑，使糊涂
【名师导学】近义词：addle, befuddle, confound, confuse, discombobulate, dizzy, fuddle, jumble, mix up, muddle, mystify, perplex, puzzle

bias ['baiəs]
n. 偏见，偏心，偏袒 *vt.* 使有偏见

bibliography [,bibli'ɔgrəfi]
n. 参考书目
【经典例题】The scholar compiled a bibliography of the unpublished writings of Emerson.
【译　　文】这位学者整理了一系列爱默生未发表的作品书目。

bid [bid]
vt. 出价，投标 *n.* 出价，投标

bilateral [bai'lætərəl]
a. 双边的，双方的

bile [bail]
n. 胆汁
【联想记忆】biliary *a.* 胆汁的

bind [baind]
vt. 绑，包扎；束缚
【名师导学】bind 过去式和过去分词均为 bound。辨析 bind, fasten, tie：bind 意为"捆，扎"，指缠绕周围；fasten 指"捆紧，拴牢"；tie 指用绳等捆紧。

biography [bai'ɔgrəfi]
n. 传记

bionics [bai'ɔniks]
n. 仿生学

biotechnology [,baiəutek'nɔlədʒi]
n. 生物技术

bizarre [bi'zɑ:]
a. 稀奇古怪的，异乎寻常的
【名师导学】近义词 unconventional

blank [blæŋk]
n. 空白；空白表格 *a.* 空白的，空着的；茫然的，无表情的

119

blaze
[bleiz]

vi. 熊熊燃烧，着火；发（强）光，放火焰 *n.* 火焰，烈火；迸发，爆发；灿烂，炫耀

【名师导学】相关近义词辨析：blaze 强调燃烧强度并暗示发光的光辉；flame 指喷火或一道火舌；flare 指耀眼但不稳定的光；flash 意指突发瞬间的爆发；glare 强调强烈、让人难以忍受的强光；glow 强调一种无焰光，它尤其暗示无强光下辐射的稳定性。

【经典例题】The fire blazed away and destroyed the whole hotel.
【译　　文】大火继续燃烧，最终把整个旅馆烧毁。

blast
[blɑ:st]

vt. 炸掉，摧毁 *n.* 爆炸，爆破；一阵（风）
【经典例题】The blasting work still goes on.
【译　　文】爆破工作仍然在继续。

bleach
[bli:tʃ]

v. 漂白 *n.* 漂白剂

bleak
[bli:k]

a. 萧瑟的，严寒的，阴郁的
【经典例题】The company still hopes to find a buyer, but the future looks bleak.
A. chilly　　B. dismal　　C. promising　　D. fanatic　　[B]
【译　　文】公司仍然希望找到买主，但未来不容乐观。

bleed
[bli:d]

vi. 出血，流血
【联想记忆】blood *n.* 血；bleed/bled（bleed 的过去式和分词）*vi.* 流血；food *n.* 食物　feed/fed（feed 的过去式和分词）*v.* 喂养；speed/sped（speed 的过去式和分词）*v.* 加速；breed/bred（breed 的过去式和分词）*v.* 繁殖

blend
[blend]

vi. 混在一起，混合；交融
【经典例题】Sunny periods will be interspersed with occasional showers.
A. interrupted　　　　　　B. blocked
C. blended　　　　　　　D. intersected　　　　　　[C]
【译　　文】晴朗的天气总是时不时地有几场雷阵雨。

blink
[bliŋk]

n. 眨眼，瞬间 *v.* 闪亮，闪烁；微微闪光；惊愕地看（at）；无视，假装不见
【固定搭配】in a blink 一瞬间；blink at 惊愕地看，睁一只眼闭一只眼

bloom
[blu:m]

vi. 开花；繁荣 *n.* 花，开花期
【固定搭配】bloom into 长成……；be in full bloom 盛开；be out of bloom 凋谢；come into bloom 开花
【经典例题】What beautiful blooms!
【译　　文】多么美丽的花啊！

blossom
['blɔsəm]

n.（果树的）花 *vi.*（植物）开花

blueprint
['blu:ˌprint]

n. 蓝图，设计图，计划 *vt.* 制成蓝图，计划

blunder
['blʌndə]

n.（因无知、粗心造成的）错误 *vt.* 犯愚蠢的错误
【名师导学】常用搭配：make a blunder 犯错误；blunder about / around 跌跌撞撞；blunder into 撞上某物。带有"笨拙而跌跌地移动"的意思的相近词有：bumble（爬行，跟跑，笨拙地做）；flounder（挣扎，笨重地移动）；lumber（笨重地行动），lurch（举步蹒跚）；stumble（跌跌撞撞地走）。

【经典例题】I think that I committed a blunder in asking her because she seemed very upset by my question.
【译　　文】我认为问她是一个错误，因为她似乎被我的问题弄得不安。

blur [blə:]
n. 模糊，模糊的东西　*v.* (使)变模糊
【经典例题】The houses appeared as a blur in the mist.
【译　　文】房屋在雾霭中呈现出一片模糊的景象。

boost [bu:st]
n./v. 提升，增加，提高
【经典例题】Millions of dying trees would soon lead to massive forest fires, boosting global warming.
【译　　文】数百万棵枯树会很快导致大规模的森林火灾，加速全球变暖。

border ['bɔ:də]
n. 边缘；边界，边境　*v.* (on, upon) 交界，与……毗邻
【固定搭配】border on / upon 交界，与……毗邻；与……近似
【名师导学】辨析 border, boundary, frontier：border 指政治划分或地理区域的分隔线或边界；boundary 指标识边界或范围的某物，如河流、山脉等；frontier 指边境，沿国界的地区。

bore [bɔ:]
vt. 钻洞，打眼，钻探；使厌烦　*n.* 令人讨厌的人／物
【派生词汇】boring *a.* 令人讨厌的　bored *a.* 感到厌烦的
【固定搭配】be bored to death 厌烦得要死
【经典例题】These were vital decisions that bore upon the happiness of everybody.
A. ensured　B. ruined　C. achieved　D. influenced　　　[D]
【译　　文】这些是关乎所有人幸福的重大决定。

bored [bɔ:d]
a. 觉得无聊的，无趣的，烦人的
【名师导学】近义词：wearied, fatigued, uninterested, jaded, dull, irked, annoyed
【固定搭配】be bored with ... 对……不耐烦或感到厌烦

botanical [bə'tænikl]
a. 植物学的，植物的

bounce [bauns]
vi. 弹起来，跳起　*vt.* 使弹起，使弹回　*n.* 弹，反弹

bound [baund]
a. 必定，约定；受约束的；开往
【固定搭配】be / feel bound to do sth. 一定；必须；be bound for 准备起程开往……；在赴……途中
【经典例题】She seemed unwilling to acknowledge that this might not be wise and would be bound to cause her husband concern.
【译　　文】她看起来很不愿意承认这样是很不明智的，而且还会引起她丈夫的担心。

boundary ['baundəri]
n. 界线，边界

bow [bau]
n. 弓，弓形；点头，鞠躬　*vi.* 鞠躬，点头 (以示招呼、同意等)
【固定搭配】bow sb. in / out 鞠躬迎进／送出；exchange bows 相互鞠躬行礼；make a slight bow 微微点头

bowel
['baul]

n. (常用 *pl.*) 肠

【联想记忆】bowl 是"碗",bowel 意为"肠",用碗吃东西后进入到"肠道"
【经典例题】All this time you have been prescribing tablets for heart burn, and it turns out that I got cancer of the bowel?
【译　文】你一直给我开的是治疗心脏灼烧的药,现在你告诉我检查结果是我得了肠癌?

boycott
['bɔikɔt]

vt. (联合) 抵制,拒绝参与

【经典例题】It can be inferred from the passage that women should boycott the products of the fashion industry.
【译　文】从文章中可以推断出,女人们需要联合抵制时装业的产品。

brake
[breik]

v. / *n.* 刹车　*n.* 闸,制动器

【名师导学】在构词法中,其中之一就是转化,本词是动词和名词之间的转化。而在英文中,很多单词就含有动词和其意思相同或相近的名词,大家在学习中有所注意,就会在不知不觉中增加词汇量。

brand
[brænd]

n. 商品;(商品的)牌子

【名师导学】辨析 brand, trademark:brand 指商标、标志,一种产品或制造商的商标或特有名称,或指品牌;trademark 指商标、牌号,标明产品的名字、符号或其他设计,经过正式注册,并只合法地限于其拥有者或制造商使用。

breach
[bri:tʃ]

v. 破坏,违反,不履行　*n.* 违犯(法纪);毁约

【固定搭配】breach of sth. 违背,违反,破坏;in breach of sth. 违犯
【经典例题】Your action is a breach of our agreement.
【译　文】你的行为破坏了我们的协议。

breakthrough
['breikθru:]

n. 重大发现,突破

【名师导学】来自于词组 break through(突破)。常和 breakdown,outbreak 放在一起作为辨析题。outbreak 意思是"(战争的)爆发,(疾病的)发作"。
【经典例题】While a full understanding of what causes the disease may be several years away, a breakthrough leading to a successful treatment could come much sooner.
【译　文】尽管要完全理解这种疾病的病因还要好几年时间,但距离治疗方法的突破性进展已为时不远。

breed
[bri:d]

vt. 生殖,繁殖;生产,饲养　*n.* 品种,种类

【名师导学】breed 过去式和过去分词均为 bred。辨析 breed, class, kind, sort, species, type:breed 意为"种类,品种",指一组有共同的祖先的动物,而且这些动物在某一方面都很相像;class 也可指"种类",指事物按照相同性质所归的类;kind 意为"种类",指任何一组由于具有相同的兴趣或特征而综合在一起的事物;sort 意为"种类",指具有相同的一般特征的一群人或事,可与 kind 换用,但有时有轻蔑意味;species 意为"种,属",指一组在各方面都很相像的动物或植物;type 指"类型",一定数量的人或事物,具有把他们与一个集体或种类区分开的共同特征或特点。
【经典例题】These nutrients can contribute to the breeding of the organisms.
【译　文】这些营养物质能够促进生物体的繁殖。

breeze
[bri:z]

n. 微风,和风

【联想记忆】wind *n.* 风;blast *n.* 一阵风;storm *n.* 风暴

brief
[bri:f]

a. 简短的,简洁的;短暂的 *vt.* 简单介绍
【固定搭配】in brief 简单地说
【经典例题】There is not much time left so I'll tell you about it____.
A. in detail　B. in brief　C. in short　D. in all　[B]
【译　文】没有多少剩余时间了,所以我就简单地跟你说一下。

briefing
['bri:fiŋ]

n. 简要指示,情况简介

brood
[bru:d]

vi. 沉思;孵蛋 *n.* (雏鸡等的)一窝;(一个家庭的)所有孩子
【名师导学】常考词组 brood on / over / about 考虑,沉思。
【经典例题】People do brood over bygone wrongs sometimes.
【译　文】人们有时候对于过去的冤屈总是无法忘却的。

browse
[brauz]

v. / n. 浏览

browser
['brauzə]

n. 浏览器;吃嫩叶的动物;浏览书本的人

bruise
[bru:z]

n. 青肿,擦伤,挫伤,擦痕 *v.* 使出现伤痕,擦伤
【经典例题】He was covered with bruises as a result of a fall from his bicycle.
【译　文】由于从自行车上跌下来,他全身伤痕累累。

brutal
['bru:tl]

a. 残忍的,野蛮的
【名师导学】近义词:pitiless, harsh, unmerciful, cruel
【经典例题】His behavior was so____that even the most merciful people could not forgive him.
A. unique　B. unconventional　C. brutal　D. brilliant　[C]
【译　文】他的行为十分残暴,哪怕是最仁慈的人都不会原谅他。

brutality
[bru:'tæləti]

n. 兽性,残忍,蛮横,粗野

bubble
['bʌbl]

n. 泡,水泡,气泡 *vi.* 冒泡,起泡,沸腾
【固定搭配】bubble over 达到顶点

budget
['bʌdʒit]

n. 预算 *vi.* 做预算,编入预算
【经典例题】The government has devoted a larger slice of its national____to agriculture than most other countries.
A. resources　B. potential　C. budget　D. economy　[C]
【译　文】在农业上,这个政府比其他国家投入了更多的国家财政预算。

buffer
['bʌfə]

n. 缓冲,缓冲区 *vt.* 减轻,缓冲
【经典例题】Humor can also be a powerful____against stress and misfortune.
A. bravery　B. blossom　C. buffer　D. buffet　[C]
【译　文】幽默也可以是对抗压力和不幸的强大的缓冲器。

bully
['buli]

n. 恃强欺弱者 *vt.* 威吓,欺侮
【经典例题】Our survey indicates that one in four children are bullied at school.
【译　文】我们的调查表明,四分之一的孩子在学校受到欺负。

burden
['bə:dn]

n. 担子,重担,负担;义务,责任
【名师导学】辨析 burden, load:burden 一般用于表示烦恼、责任、工作等精神上的"负担";load 指人、动物、船只、车轮、飞机等负荷运送的东西,借喻精神上的负担。

| **burdensome** ['bə:dnsəm] | *a.* 沉重的；麻烦的；难于负担的 |

| **bureau** ['bjuərəu] | *n.* 局，司，处，部，所，署
【固定搭配】The Political Bureau 政治局 |

| **bureaucracy** [bjuə'rɔkrəsi] | *n.* 官僚，官僚主义，官僚机构
【经典例题】Many an old firm was replaced by a limited liability company with a bureaucracy of salaried managers.
【译　文】许多老商行被责任有限公司所取代，这种公司有一个由领薪经理们组成的官僚机构。 |

| **bust** [bʌst] | *v.* 使爆裂，击破
【经典例题】I dropped my smartphone on the pavement and bust it.
【译　文】我把手机掉在人行道上摔坏了。 |

C

| **calamity** [kə'læmiti] | *n.* 灾难，灾祸
【经典例题】Losing his job was a financial catastrophe for his family.
A. calamity　B. accident　　C. frustration　D. depression
【译　文】他的失业对于整个家庭来说是一场噩耗。
【名师导学】disaster, calamity, catastrophe, misfortune 这些名词均表示"灾难"或"不幸"之意。
disaster 普通用词，指大破坏、痛苦或伤亡。
calamity 多指个人的不幸，比 disaster 严重，强调灾难引起的悲痛及对于损失的感觉。
catastrophe 语气最强，指可怕的灾难，强调最终的结局。
misfortune 多指较为严重的不幸，强调不幸多由外界因素所致。 |

| **calcium** ['kælsiəm] | *n.* 钙 |

| **calculation** [ˌkælkju'leiʃn] | *n.* 计算，统计，估计，预测 |

| **calculate** ['kælkjuleit] | *vt.* 计算，推算；估计，推测；计划，打算
【派生词汇】calculator *n.* 计算器
【名师导学】辨析 calculate, count, figure：calculate 表示通过计算或运算以解决疑难题目或问题，还可以表示"估计，推算，考虑"；count 指一个接一个地说出或列出以得其总数；figure 指用数字来计算。
【经典例题】The tuition is too high to be calculated.
【译　文】学费太高了，无法计算。 |

calorie
['kæləri]

n. 卡（热量单位）

【经典例题】I would like to have a cup of black coffee. I am counting my calories at the moment.

【译　文】我想要一杯不加糖和奶的咖啡（黑咖啡）。我目前正在控制所摄取的热量。

callous
[kæləs]

a. 麻木的，无情的，硬结的，起老茧的

【经典例题】We were shocked at the physician's callous disregard for the human dimension of medicine.

A. involuntary　　　　　B. apparent
C. deliberate　　　　　 D. indifferent　　　　　[D]

【译　文】对于医生对用药的尺度把握的漠不关心，我们非常震惊。

campaign
[kæm'pein]

n. 战役；运动

【经典例题】All kinds of extravagant promises were made during the election ＿＿＿＿.

A. struggle　　　　　B. campaign
C. battle　　　　　　D. conflict　　　　　[B]

【译　文】在选举运动中出现了各式各样过分的承诺。

cancel
['kænsəl]

vt. 取消，撤销，删去

【经典例题】All flights having been canceled because of the snowstorm, they decided to take the train.

【译　文】因为暴风雪，所有的航班都取消了，他们决定坐火车。

cancer
['kænsə]

n. 癌

cancerous
['kænsərəs]

a. 癌的；像癌的；得癌症的；不治的

【经典例题】In the 38 missed cancers, 15 were the result of interpretation error (identifying an image but dismiss it as noncancerous).

【译　文】在38例漏掉的癌症病患中，15例是解释错误的结果（影像显示为癌症，但却被当成非癌来搁置了）。

candidate
['kændidit]

n. 候选人；报考者；求职者

【经典例题】A second language isn't generally required to get a job in business, but having language skills gives a candidate the edge when other qualifications appear to be equal.

【译　文】掌握第二门语言通常不是在贸易方面找到一份工作的条件，但是有语言方面的技能则能使候选人在其他条件同等的情况下比其他人具有更大的优势。

canvas
['kænvəs]

n. 帆布；油画

【名师导学】习惯用语：under canvas 在帐篷里

【经典例题】The priceless canvas was stolen from the art gallery.

【译　文】那幅珍贵的油画被人从艺术馆偷走了。

capability
[,keipə'biliti]

n. 能力，才能；性能，容量

【固定搭配】have the capability of 有……的才能；beyond / above one's capability 超过某人的能力范围

【联想记忆】have the ability to do, have the capacity for / to do 有能力做……

capable [ˈkeipəbl]	*a.* 能干的，有能力的，有才能的
capacity [kəˈpæsiti]	*n.* 容量，容积；能力；能量；接受力 【经典例题】The memory capacity of bees means they can distinguish among more than 50 different smells to find the one they want. 【译　　文】蜜蜂的记忆能力意味着它们能在50多种不同的味道中找到它们想要的那种。
capsule [ˈkæpsjuːl]	*n.* 胶囊；太空舱
caption [ˈkæpʃən]	*n.*（图片、漫画等的）说明文字 【经典例题】I didn't understand the drawing until I read the caption. 【译　　文】直到我看了这幅画的说明才理解了它的含义。
captive [ˈkæptiv]	*a.* 被俘虏的，被俘获的　*n.* 俘虏 【经典例题】The pirates took many captives and sold them as slaves. 【译　　文】海盗抓了许多俘虏并把他们当作奴隶卖掉了。
capture [ˈkæptʃə]	*vt.* 捕获，捉拿；夺得，攻占 【经典例题】The decline in moral standards — which has long concerned social analysts — has at last captured the attention of average Americans. 【译　　文】社会学家一直关注的道德滑坡问题，最终引起了美国大众的关注。
carbon [ˈkɑːbən]	*n.* 碳
cardinal [ˈkɑːdinəl]	*a.* 极其重要的，主要的，基本的 【名师导学】近义词：capital, chief, first, foremost, key, leading, main, major, number one, paramount, premier, primary, prime, principal 【固定搭配】cardinal numbers 基数词；ordinal numbers 序数词 【经典例题】Having clean hands is one of the cardinal rules when preparing food. 【译　　文】做饭之前把手洗干净非常重要。
career [kəˈriə]	*n.* 生涯，经历；专业，职业 【名师导学】career, position, profession 都有"职业"的意思，辨析：career 既可指一般工作，也可指专业性较强的职业；position 主要指工作岗位；profession 尤指从事脑力劳动或受过专门训练的工作，如医生、教师、律师等工作。 【经典例题】A lateral move that hurt my feelings and blocked my professional progress, promoted me to abandon my relatively high profile career. 【译　　文】一次侧面的打击伤害了我的感情，阻碍了我事业的发展，使我放弃了我那份引人注目的工作。
cargo [ˈkɑːgəu]	*n.* 船货，货物
carve [kɑːv]	*vt.* 雕刻；切割，切开 【经典例题】She carved up the roast beef and gave us each a proportion. 【译　　文】她切碎烤牛肉，给我们每人一份。

☐ **casual** ['kæʒuəl]	*a.* 随便的；偶然的；临时的 【名师导学】辨析 accidental, casual, occasional：accidental 意为"偶然的，意外的"，指事先没想到而突如其来，有时还能给人带来不愉快或灾难性后果；casual 意为"偶然的，碰巧的"，指一反常态发生的事情；occasional 意为"偶尔的，不时"，指没有规律的事。 【经典例题】Friendships among Americans tend to be casual. 【译　　文】美国人之间的友谊趋向于随便。	
☐ **casualty** ['kæʒuəlti]	*n.* 伤亡人数，死伤者；受害人，损失的东西 【名师导学】近义词：accident, mishap, calamity, fatality; catastrophe, disaster, misfortune; fatalities, losses, death toll, the injured, dead, victims 【经典例题】Though we often hear about air crashes and serious casualties, flying is still one of the safest ways to travel. 【译　　文】尽管我们经常听到飞机失事或严重人员伤亡事故，但是飞行仍然是最安全的旅行方式之一。	
☐ **category** ['kætigəri]	*n.* 种类，类别；（逻）范畴	
☐ **cater** ['keitə]	*v.* 满足，迎合，投合 【名师导学】catering 公共饮食业；酒席承办；cater for / to sb. / sth. 满足需要，迎合。 【经典例题】TV programmes usually cater for all tastes. 【译　　文】电视节目一般是为了迎合大众的口味。	
☐ **catastrophe** [kə'tæstrəfi]	*n.* 大灾难，大祸 【名师导学】近义词群：disaster, calamity, mishap, mischance, misadventure, failure, fiasco, misery, accident, trouble, casualty, misfortune, infliction, affliction, contretemps, stroke, havoc, ravage, wreck, fatality, grief, crash, devastation, desolation, avalanche, hardship, blow, visitation, ruin, reverse, emergency, scourge, cataclysm, convulsion, debacle, tragedy, adversity, bad luck, upheaval	
☐ **caution** ['kɔːʃən]	*n.* 谨慎，小心；警告 【固定搭配】do sth. with caution 谨慎小心地做；caution sb. against / about sth. 警告某人某事 【经典例题】Others viewed the findings with caution, noting that a cause-and-effect relationship between passive smoking and cancer remains to be shown. 【译　　文】其他人谨慎地看待这些发现，因为他们注意到在被动吸烟和癌症之间的因果关系仍然有待观察。	
☐ **cautious** ['kɔːʃəs]	*a.* 谨慎的，小心的 【经典例题】He started by cautiously "chewing" on people. 【译　　文】他开始小心翼翼地打量人们。	
☐ **cease** [siːs]	*v. / n.* 停止，终止	
☐ **celebrity** [si'lebriti]	*n.* 著名人士，名人	
☐ **cell** [sel]	*n.* 细胞；电池	

cellular
['seljulə(r)]

a. 【生】细胞的,细胞质(状)的;多孔的
【联想记忆】cell 为名词,"细胞"的意思。
【经典例题】The case is built on several studies that bring together cellular biology, biochemistry and epidemiology.
【译　　文】这个研究集合了几种不同学科。如细胞生物学、生物化学和传染病学的研究。

censorship
['sensəʃip]

n. 审查机构,审查制度;审察员(检查员)的职权

census
['sensəs]

n. 人口普查
【经典例题】Emerging from the 1980 census is the picture of a nation developing more and more regional competition, as population growth in the Northeast and Midwest reaches a standstill.
【译　　文】1980 年的人口普查表明,随着东北和中西部地区人口增长停止,国家内部的地区之间竞争加剧了。

centigrade
['sentigreid]

n. 摄氏温度
【联想记忆】Fahrenheit *n.* 华氏

centimeter
['senti,mi:tə(r)]

n. 厘米

ceremony
['seriməni]

n. 典礼,仪式,礼节
【固定搭配】wedding ceremony 婚礼;opening/closing ceremony 开/闭幕式

certificate
[sə'tifikit]

n. 证书;凭证;执照

certification
[s:tifi'keisn]

n. 证明,证明书;合格证

certify
['sə:tifai]

vt. 证明;证实;宣称
【名师导学】近义词群:guarantee, accredit, vouch for, endorse; attest, verify, swear, confirm; declare

challenge
['tʃælindʒ]

n. 挑战,挑战书;艰巨任务,难题　*vt.* 向……挑战
【固定搭配】challenge sb. to do sth. 向某人挑战做某事;challenge sb. to sth. 向某人挑战某事

change
[tʃeindʒ]

vt. 改变,变更,变革;交换,更迭,替换;把……变成……(into) *n.* 改变,变化;找回的零钱;调换(口味);换衣服
【经典例题】The average quality of his works did not change.
【译　　文】他的作品的平均质量没有变化。

chant
[tʃɑ:nt]

vt. 反复有节奏地喊或叫(唱);咏唱　*n.* 反复有节奏的喊叫;赞美诗,圣歌
【经典例题】They chanted "Equal rights for all".
【译　　文】他们反复高喊"人人平等"。

chaos
['keiɔs]

n. 混沌,混乱
【经典例题】The desk was a chaos of papers and unopened letters.
【译　　文】桌上杂乱地堆放着一些纸张和未拆的信。

chaotic
[kei'ɔtik]

a. 混乱的;无秩序的

character
['kærɪktə]

n. 性格，品质；特性，特征；人物，角色；（书写或印刷）符号，（汉）字

【名师导学】辨析 character, nature, personality：character 指性格、品性、人格，尤指是非观念、品德等；nature 指性格、天性、气质等的总称，与生俱来的，也指事物的性质或人类的通性；personality 指个性、个人魅力，强调感情因素。

characteristic
[,kærɪktə'rɪstɪk]

a. 特有的，独特的 *n.* 特征，特性

【名师导学】辨析 characteristic, feature, property, quality：characteristic 指人、物或抽象的特点或特征，是识别他人或他物的明显标志；feature 指显著的非常突出的特点，具有足以引人注目的部分或细节，常用于生理、自然条件、物品等；property 性质、特征，通常指事物的基本特征；quality 指个人的品行、品质。

characterize
['kærɪktəraɪz]

vt. 描绘……的特性，刻画……的性格

【经典例题】Our society is characterized with the "knowledge economy".
【译　　文】我们的社会以"知识经济"为特征。

charm
[tʃɑːm]

vt. 使着迷，使陶醉 *n.* 招人喜欢之处，魅力

chase
[tʃeɪs]

v. / n. 追逐，追赶

chemical
['kemɪkəl]

a. 化学的 *n.* 化学制品 / 产品 / 物质 / 成分

【经典例题】The carbon dioxide would then be extracted and subjected to chemical reactions.
【译　　文】二氧化碳然后被提取出来，并将其进行化学反应。

cherish
['tʃerɪʃ]

vt. 珍惜，珍爱；爱护；抱有（信念、希望）

【名师导学】该词是出现频率较高的词。词义在不同语境下有不同的意思。最后一项意思也出现过（怀有……希望）。常用短语：cherish the memory of... 意为"怀念……"。

【经典例题】He still cherishes the memory of his carefree childhood spent in that small wooden house of his grandparents.
【译　　文】他依旧怀念他在爷爷奶奶的小木屋子里度过的无忧无虑的童年。

cholesterol
[kə'lestərɔːl]

n. 胆固醇

chorus
['kɔːrəs]

n. 合唱；齐声，异口同声地说

【固定搭配】in chorus 一起，一齐，同时；chorus girl 合唱团女成员

【经典例题】Due to the serious corruption of the government, it has aroused a chorus of voices calling for the Prime Minister's resignation.
【译　　文】由于政府严重的腐败问题，引起了人们一致要求首相辞职的呼声。

chronic
['krɔnɪk]

a. 长期的，慢性的

【经典例题】Many observers believe that country will remain in a state of chaos if it fails to solve its chronic food shortage problem.
【译　　文】许多观测者都认为，如果不能解决长期的食品短缺问题，这个国家仍将处于混乱状态。

circuit
['sə:kit]

n. 电路,线路

circular
['sə:kjulə]

a. 圆形的;循环的

circulate
['sə:kjuleit]

v. (使)循环,(使)流通

【经典例题】This local evening paper has a＿＿ of twenty-five thousand.
A. number　B. contribution　C. circulation　D. celebration　[C]
【译　文】当地晚报的发行量为 25 000 份。

circulation
[,sə:kju'leiʃən]

n. 循环;发行量

【名师导学】in circulation (观念)流行中,流通中。与之相反的意思是:out of circulation 不再流通(流行)。表示发行量的常用表达方式为 have a circulation of。
【经典例题】The circulation of rumour is common in wartime.
【译　文】在战争时期谣言流传是常事。

circumstance
['sə:kəmstəns]

n. (*pl.*) 情形,环境;条件

【固定搭配】under the circumstances 在这种情况下,情况既然如此;under / in no circumstances 在任何情况下都不(放在句首要倒装)
【名师导学】辨析 circumstances, environment, setting, surroundings: circumstances 指某事或某动作发生时的情况,形势;environment 指周围的状况或条件,可以是自然环境,也可以是社会环境,可以是物质上的,也可以是精神上的;setting 指某一情形的背景或环境;surroundings 指围绕物,周围的事物。
【经典例题】We have been told that under no circumstances＿＿ the telephone in the office for personal affairs.
A. may we use　　　　　B. we may use
C. we could use　　　　　D. did we use　　　　　[A]
【译　文】我们被告知在任何情况下我们都不允许为了私人的事情而使用办公室的电话。

cite
[sait]

vt. 举(例),引证,引用

civic
['sivik]

a. 城市的;市民的,公民的

civil
['sivl]

a. 市民的,公民的,国民的;民间的;民事的,根据民法的;文职的

【经典例题】He left the army and resumed civil life.
【译　文】他脱离了军队,恢复了平民生活。

civilian
[si'viljən]

a. 平民的,民用的,民众的

civilization
[,sivilai'zeiʃən]

n. 文明,文化

【经典例题】Both civilization and culture are fairly modern words, having come into use during the 19th century by anthropologists.
【译　文】文明和文化都是相当时髦的词汇,人类学家从 19 世纪开始使用。

第二部分 核心意义词汇（A-K）

civilize ['sivilaiz]
vt. 使开化，使文明，教化

claim [kleim]
n.（根据权利提出）要求，要求权，主张，要求而得到的东西 vt.（根据权利）要求，认领，声称，主张，需要
【名师导学】辨析 claim, proclaim：claim 一般指声称对某物的拥有权；proclaim 常为官方正式宣布。

clamp [klæmp]
vt.（用夹具等）夹紧，夹住，固定 n. 夹头，夹具，夹钳
【固定搭配】clamp A and B (together) 把 A 和 B 夹紧，固定；clamp down (on sb./sth.) 严厉打击（犯罪等）
【经典例题】Clamp the two parts together until the glue dries.
【译　文】把两部分夹紧，直到胶水干了再松开。

clarification [,klærifi'keiʃən]
n. 澄清（作用），澄清法；净化；说明，解释

clarify ['klærifai]
vi. 澄清，阐明 vt. 使明晰
【名师导学】辨析 clarify, clear, clean：clarify 指使清晰或易懂，详细阐明，澄清混乱或疑惑；clear 指去除物体或障碍，使明确，使明朗，去除困惑、疑问或模棱两可，也指天空变晴；clean 指扣除，清除，去除垃圾或杂质。

clarity ['klæriti]
n. 清楚，明晰

classic ['klæsik]
n. 杰作，名著 a. 第一流的

classical ['klæsikəl]
a. 经典的，古典的

classification [,klæsifi'keiʃən]
n. 分类，分级

classify ['klæsifai]
vt. 分类，分级
【经典例题】Stereotypes seem unavoidable, given the way the human mind seeks to categorize and classify information.
【译　文】习惯性做法似乎不可避免，这种做法为人类进行信息的归类和分类提供了方法。

client ['klaiənt]
n. 顾客；委托人，当事人

climate ['klaimit]
n. 气候；风气，思潮
【名师导学】辨析 climate, weather：climate 指某地区的气候；weather 指每日的天气。

climax ['klaimæks]
n. 顶点，极点；高潮 v.（使）达到顶点，（使）达到高潮
【名师导学】该词属于常考词汇，经常是在词汇选择、阅读部分。考生要注意常用的相关同义词：culmination（顶峰，结局），highlight（最精彩部分，最重要的部分），summit（顶点，峰会）。
【经典例题】They believed that this was not the climax of their campaign for equality but merely the beginning.
【译　文】他们相信，这不是这场争取平等的运动的高潮，相反，它仅仅是一个开头。

cling
[kliŋ]

vi. 缠住，粘住；依恋，依靠；坚信，坚持

【名师导学】该词属于常考词汇。考生要注意常用的一组相关同义词 adhere to（黏附，坚持），attach to（依附），stick to（坚持），以及另一组常用的相关同义词 grasp（抓住，抓紧），hold（拿住，抓住，抱住，托住）。该词以固定搭配 cling to 出现居多，并且该搭配后均为名词，意为"紧抓住或抱住某人（某物），紧靠着某人或物"。需要重点注意的是此固定搭配 cling to something 还可以表示"舍不得放弃某事物；拒绝放弃某事物"。

【经典例题】At the party we found that the shy girl was clinging to her mother all the time.

【译　　文】在宴会上，我们发现那个害羞的女孩子一直紧贴着她的母亲。

clip
[klip]

vt. 剪短，修剪；夹住　*n.* 曲别针，夹，钳

【名师导学】考生要注意区分这一组词：clip（既可指剪掉不需要的部分，也可指剪下要保留的部分），crop（修剪），pare（除掉某物的外层或边缘），shave（剃毛发，通常指身体上的毛发），trim（为了使某物整齐而修剪，整理）。

【经典例题】The letters were held together with a paper clip.

【译　　文】这些信是用一枚回形针夹在一起的。

clockwise
[ˈklɔ:kwaiz]

a. / ad. 顺时针方向转动的（地），正转的（地）

clog
[klɔg]

n. 累赘；有木跟的鞋子　*vt.* 阻塞，妨碍，超载　*vi.* 阻塞，结块；跳木屐舞

【经典例题】During rush hour, downtown streets are＿＿＿with commuters.
A. scattered　　　　　　B. condensed
C. clogged　　　　　　 D. dotted　　　　　　　　　　　　[C]

clot
[klɔt]

n. 凝块，血块；一群　[非正式]笨蛋，傻瓜

v. 凝结，使……凝结，阻塞

clone
[kləun]

n. 克隆，无性繁殖（的个体）；复制品，翻版

【名师导学】考生要注意常用的相关同义词：duplicate（复制，重复），copy（复印，模仿，仿效，抄写），reproduce（繁殖，生殖）。

clue
[klu:]

n. 线索，提示

【名师导学】考生要注意常用的相关同义词：cue（暗示，提示），evidence（迹象，证据，证物），hint（暗示，提示，线索），proof（证据），sign（征兆，迹象）。

【经典例题】I have not a clue how to compose a waltz.

【译　　文】对于创作华尔兹舞曲我是一窍不通。

cluster
[ˈklʌstə]

n.（果实、花等的）串，簇；（人、物等的）群，组　*vi.* 群集，丛生　*vt.* 使集群，集中

【名师导学】该词属于常考词汇。考生要注意常用的一组相关同义词 assemble（集合，聚集，装配）batch（集中，挤在一起），gather（集合，聚集，渐增），muster（聚集，召集，集合），swarm（云集，挤满），以及另一组相关同义词有 bunch（串，束），group（组，团，群，批），set（一副，一批）。注意用法 cluster / be clustered (together) round sb. / sth.（聚集在某人或某物的周围；丛生，群聚）。

【经典例题】When we go abroad, we tend to cluster in hotels and restaurants where English is spoken.

【译　　文】当我们去国外时，我们一般会聚集在说英语的旅馆和餐馆。

clutch
[klʌtʃ]

v. 抓住，攫取 *n.* 抓紧，紧握；离合器

【名师导学】考生要注意常用的相关同义词：clasp（紧抱，紧握，抱紧，握紧），clench（捏紧，紧握，牢牢地抓住），grasp（抓住，抓紧，掌握）。该词经常以固定搭配 clutch at 出现。其复数形式 clutches 表示"势力范围，控制"，用于以下示例：be in one's clutches（在某人控制下），fall into the clutches of sb. / sth.（落入某人或某物的势力范围）。

【经典例题】Just when man thinks he can do everything, he finds himself helpless in the clutch of some unknown force.

【译　文】正当人类认为自己无所不能时，却发现自己受制于某种不可知的力量而陷于无助。

coach
[kəutʃ]

n. 客车，长途汽车；私人教练，教练 *v.* 训练，辅导，指导

coalition
[ˌkəuəˈliʃən]

n. 联合，盟军

【名师导学】考生要注意常用的相关同义词：alliance（联盟，联合），union（联合，联盟，协会）。

【经典例题】It took five months for the coalition to agree on and publish an economic program.

【译　文】这个同盟花了五个月的时间达成了协议并发布了一个经济计划。

coarse
[kɔːs]

a. 粗的，粗糙的，粗劣的；粗鲁的，粗俗的

【经典例题】Usually you will be more likely to find insects if you examine finer twigs rather than the coarser parts of trees.

【译　文】如果你仔细查看树木的较细的树枝而并非粗糙树干，通常你更有可能找到昆虫。

cognitive
[ˈkɔgnətiv]

a. 认知的

【经典例题】Our soul possesses two cognitive powers.

【译　文】我们的灵魂具有两种认知力量。

coherent
[kəuˈhiərənt]

a. 一致的，连贯的

【名师导学】下列同义词同样值得关注：articulate（发音清晰的，清楚的），logical（合理的），lucid（明晰的，清晰的）。该词的反义词是在该词的基础上加前缀"in"构成"incoherent"（不连贯的，语无伦次的）。

【经典例题】My head hurt so much I could not give a coherent answer.

【译　文】我的头疼得很厉害，我无法给出一个有条理的回答。

cohesion
[kəuˈhiːʒn]

n. 黏着，附着；黏合（力）；结合，连结；内聚性；凝聚性（力）

coil
[kɔil]

vi. 卷，盘绕 *n.*（一）卷，（一）圈，圈线

【经典例题】The lady coiled her hair at the back head for the ball.

【译　文】这位女士为参加舞会把头发盘在了头后。

coincide
[ˌkəuinˈsaid]

vi. 同时发生；一致，相符

【名师导学】近义词：correspond, agree, concur, co-occur, occur simultaneously, fall together, tally, match, accord, harmonize;

【经典例题】It is fortunate for the old couple that their son's career goals and their wishes for him coincide.

【译　文】儿子的职业目标和他们对他的期望不谋而合，这真是老两口的幸运。

coincidence
[kəu'insidəns]
n. 一致，符合；同时发生（存在），巧合

collaborate
[kə'læbəreit]
v. 合作，协作

collaboration
[kə,læbə'reiʃn]
n. 合作，协作；通敌，勾结

collaborative
[kə'læbərətiv]
a. 合作的；协作的；协力的
【经典例题】This newly established fund has a range of medical programs undertaken by universities, industrial labs, or university-industry collaborative projects.
A. cooperative   B. innovative
C. lucrative   D. representative   [A]
【译　　文】这个新成立的基金拥有一系列由大学、工业实验室或大学-工业合作项目承担的医疗项目。

collapse
[kə'læps]
vi. / n. 倒塌；崩溃

collection
[kə'lekʃən]
n. 收藏，收集；收藏品
【根源词汇】collect *vt.* 收集
【经典例题】This book is a _____ of radio scripts, in which we seek to explain how the words and expressions become part of our language.
A. collection   B. publication
C. volume   D. stack   [A]
【译　　文】这本书是一本广播稿集，在这本书里面，我们试图阐述词汇和措辞是如何成为语言的一部分的。

collective
[kə'lektiv]
a. 集体的；共同的 *n.* 集体

collide
[kə'laid]
vi. 碰撞，抵触
【名师导学】该词属于常考词汇。考生要注意常用的相关同义词：bump（撞击，颠簸），clash（冲突，不协调），crash（碰撞，砸碎，碰撞，坠落，坠毁），conflict（冲突，抵触）。注意固定搭配 collide with（与……相撞），后面接名词，是该词的常用搭配。
【经典例题】The morning news says a school bus collided with a train at the junction and a group of policemen were sent there immediately.
【译　　文】早间新闻报道，一辆校车和火车在交叉路口相撞，一队警察立即赶赴现场。

collision
[kə'liʒən]
n. 碰撞，冲突，抵触
【固定搭配】come into collision with 和……相撞（冲突，抵触）；in collision with 和……相撞（冲突）
【名师导学】辨析 collision, combat, conflict, contradiction：collision 指"（车、船的）碰撞"或"（利益、意见的）冲突"；combat 指"战斗，格斗"，尤指"武装斗争"；conflict 指公开的、长期的战斗冲突的状态；contradiction 指"矛盾，不一致"。
【经典例题】But there are also thousands of planets whose orbits put them on a collision course with Earth.
【译　　文】但也有成千上万的行星的轨道处于冲撞地球的线路上。

colony
['kɔləni]
n. 殖民地；聚居地

colonial
[kə'ləunjəl]
a. 殖民地的 *n.* (同类人的) 聚居地
【经典例题】The imperialists plunder and exploit the people of the colonial countries.
【译　　文】帝国主义者掠夺和剥削殖民地国家的人民。

colossal
[kə'lɑ:sl]
a. 巨大的；[口] 异常的
【经典例题】The whole holiday was a colossal waste of money.
A. consecutive　　　　B. conductive
C. considerate　　　　D. considerable　　　　[D]
【译　　文】整个假期是对钱的巨大浪费。

column
['kɔləm]
n. 柱，柱状物；栏，专栏 (文章)

combat
['kɔmbæt]
v. 与……战斗，搏斗 *n.* 战斗，斗争，搏斗

combination
[,kɔmbi'neiʃən]
n. 结合，联合

combine
[kəm'bain]
v. 结合，联合，化合
【固定搭配】combine with 与……联合 (化合、结合)
【经典例题】This combined effects of degrading collagen more rapidly and producing less new collagen is probably what cause premature skin ageing in smokers.
【译　　文】降解胶原质速度增加，生产新胶原质减少，这一双重结果或许正是烟民皮肤提前衰老的原因。

comedy
['kɔmidi]
n. 喜剧
【联想记忆】comic *adj.* 滑稽的，喜剧的；comedy *n.* 喜剧．喜剧性的事情；tragic *adj.* 悲惨的，悲剧的；tragedy *n.* 悲剧；悲惨的事，灾难

comic
['kɔmik]
a. 喜剧的；滑稽的
【名师导学】考生要注意常用的联想词 tragic（悲剧的，悲惨的，可悲的）。
【经典例题】The song provides some comic relief from the intensity of the scene.
【译　　文】这首歌给紧张的画面提供了喜剧性的氛围。

commemorate
[kə'meməreit]
vt. 纪念，庆祝
【名师导学】该词属于常考词汇。考生要注意常用的相关同义词：acclaim（欢呼，喝彩），celebrate（庆祝，颂扬），honor（给以荣誉）。
【经典例题】To commemorate important dates in history, countries create special holidays.
【译　　文】为纪念历史上的重要日子，各国家分别创立了一些特别的节日。

commence
[kə'mens]
vt. 开始；着手

commend
[kə'mend]
vt. 表扬，称赞；推荐
【名师导学】考生要注意常用的一组相关同义词：approve（赞成，满意），compliment（称赞，褒扬，致意），praise（赞扬，歌颂，称赞）。
【经典例题】An order was issued to commend them.
【译　　文】他们被通令嘉奖。

comment ['kɔment]	*n. / v.* 解说,评论 【固定搭配】comment on / upon 评论,谈论,对……提意见 【联想记忆】observe on / upon, remark on / upon 评论 【经典例题】The range of news is from local crime to international politics, from sport to business to fashion to science, and the range of comment and special features as well, from editorial page to feature articles and interviews to criticism of books, art, theatre and music. 【译　文】新闻的范围从当地的犯罪到国际政治,从体育到经济,从时尚到科学,从评论到特写,从社论到专栏文章,以及对书籍、艺术、戏剧和音乐的评论。
commentary ['kɔmentəri]	*n.* 评论,评注;实况广播报道,现场口头评述 【名师导学】该词属于常考词汇。考生要注意常用的相关同义词:explanation(解释,说明,阐述),remark(谈论,评论)。该词后面通常接介词 on 或者 of,意为"对……报道"。 【经典例题】Stop shouting! I can't hear the football commentary. 【译　文】别嚷了!我听不见足球赛的现场解说了。
commentator ['kɔmenteitə]	*n.* 评论员;实况广播员
commerce ['kɔmə(:)s]	*n.* 商业,贸易
commercial [kə'mə:ʃəl]	*a.* 商业的,商务的　*n.* 商业广告
commission [kə'miʃən]	*n.* 委员会,调查团;佣金,酬劳金 【经典例题】As a salesman, he works on a(n) commission basis, taking 10% of everything he sells. 【译　文】作为销售人员,他以佣金的形式工作,他卖出的任何东西都能提成10%。
commissioner [kə'miʃənə]	*n.* 专员,委员,政府部门大官
commitment [kə'mitmənt]	*n.* 承担义务,许诺 【根源词汇】commit *v.* 犯错(commit to 犯错误) 【经典例题】It was felt that he lacked the＿＿＿＿to pursue a difficult task to the very end. 　A. petition　　　　　　　　B. engagement 　C. commitment　　　　　　D. qualification　　　　　　[C] 【译　文】人们感觉到他缺少完成艰巨任务的责任心。
committee [kə'miti]	*n.* 委员会,全体委员
commodity [kə'mɔditi]	*n.* 商品,有用的东西 【名师导学】该词属于常考词汇。考生要注意常用的相关同义词:article(物品,商品),commerce(商业,贸易),merchandise(商品,货物),stock(现货,库存)。 【经典例题】I lead a very busy life, so spare time is a very precious commodity to me. 【译　文】我的生活非常繁忙,所以空余时间对我来说是非常珍贵的东西。

第二部分 核心意义词汇（A-K）

commonplace
['kɔmənpleis]
a. 普通的，平庸的 *n.* 寻常的东西，平庸的东西
【名师导学】该词属于常考词汇。考生要注意常用的相关同义词：common（平常的，普通的），customary（习惯上的，惯常的），routine（例行的，常规的），stale（不新鲜的，陈腐的，疲倦的，陈旧的）。
【经典例题】Men substantially outnumber women, and heavy drinking is a commonplace.
【译　　文】男人数量比女人多得多，酗酒现象司空见惯。

commonwealth
['kɔmənwelθ]
n. 联邦，英联邦
【名师导学】该词属于常考词汇。考生要注意常用的相关词：colony（殖民地），federation（联邦），union（联盟，工会）。
【经典例题】The island country didn't join the commonwealth, thinking it could do better on its own.
【译　　文】这个岛国认为自力更生可以发展得更好，因此没有加入联邦。

communicate
[kə'mju:nikeit]
vt. 传达；交流；通信 *vi.* 传达，传播
【固定搭配】communicate with 和……联系，和……通信；communicate sth. to sb. 把……传达给某人

communication
[kə,mju:ni'keiʃn]
n. 通讯；通信；交际，交流；传达，传送

community
[kə'mju:niti]
n. 社区
【经典例题】A hero has a story of adventure to tell and a community who will listen.
【译　　文】英雄总有冒险的故事可讲，而公众又愿意去听。

commute
[kə'mju:t]
vi. 乘公交车上下班，经常乘车（或船等）往返 *n.* 上下班路程
【名师导学】该词属于常考词汇。考生要注意常用的相关同义词：communication（交通或通信工具，交流，交际），transportation（运输，运输系统，运输工具）。
【经典例题】Urban Japanese have long endured commutes and crowded living conditions, but as the old group and family values weaken, the discomfort is beginning to tell.
【译　　文】都市里的日本人长期忍受着漫长的上下班来回交通和拥挤不堪的居住条件，但随着旧的群体和家庭价值观的削弱，令人不舒服的结果开始显现。

compact
['kɔmpækt]
a. 紧密的，结实的；紧凑的，体积小的
【名师导学】该词属于常考词汇。考生要注意常用的一个相关同义词：dense（压紧的，压缩的），以及另一组相关同义词：brief（简短的），concise（简明的，简练的），succinct（简洁的）。注意 compact disc 表示激光唱片。
【经典例题】As the market develops, the compact family car is becoming more common while the price continues to decrease.
【译　　文】随着市场的发展，紧凑型家庭轿车日益普及化，价格门槛不断降低。

compassionate
[kəm'pæʃinet]
a. 有同情心的，深表同情的
【联想记忆】com "一起，共同" +passion "激情，情感" +ate（形容词后缀之一）=compassionate 有同情心的

【经典例题】I have never seen a more caring,＿＿＿＿group of people in my life.
A. emotional　　B. impersonal　C. compulsory　D. compassionate
【译　　文】在我一生中还从没见过比这群人更体贴更富有同情心的。
【名师导学】pity, mercy, sympathy, compassion 这些名词均有"同情，怜悯"之意。
pity：指对弱者、不幸者所表示的怜惜之情。
mercy：侧重指对应受惩罚或地位卑下者的慈悲或怜悯。
sympathy：普通常用词，含义广。指志趣、看法上的一致，也指感情相投，带有深深的恻隐之心的亲切之情。
compassion：较正式较庄重用词，指对同等人的同情与理解，常含急切愿意帮忙的意味。

compatible
[kəmˈpætəbl]
a. 兼容的
【名师导学】该词属于常考词汇。该词及其衍生词在历年考试中出现频率非常高，尤其是在阅读和词汇部分。考生要注意常用的相关词：appropriate（适当的，恰当的），fitting（适合的，恰当的），suitable（合适的，适宜的）。该词的反义词是在该词的基础上加前缀"in"构成 incompatible（不调和的，不共戴天的），在历年的考试中出现的次数不少于五次。注意固定搭配 be compatible with（与……相兼容），是该词的常用搭配。
【经典例题】Don't trust the speaker any more, since the remarks he made in his lectures are never compatible with the facts.
【译　　文】再也别相信那个演讲者，因为他演讲时说的和事实从来就不一致。

comparable
[ˈkɔmpərəbl]
a. 可比较的，比得上的
【固定搭配】be comparable with 可与……相比的，与……类似的；be comparable to 可与……比拟的，与……匹敌的
【经典例题】Nevertheless, children in both double-income and "male breadwinner" households spent comparable amount of time interacting with their parents.
【译　　文】然而，在双收入家庭和父亲为收入来源的家庭中，孩子都能够花大量的时间和父母进行交流。

comparative
[kəmˈpærətiv]
a. 比较的，相当的

comparison
[kəmˈpærisn]
n. 比较；对比
【固定搭配】in comparison with 与……比较；by comparison 比较起来

compel
[kəmˈpel]
vt. 强迫，迫使
【固定搭配】compel sb. / sth. to do sth. 强迫某人或某物做某事

compete
[kəmˈpi:t]
vi. 比赛，竞赛
【固定搭配】compete with / against sb. 与某人竞争
【联想记忆】rival with sb., contest with / against sb. 与某人竞争
【名师导学】辨析 compete, rival：compete 意为"竞争，比赛"，不直接跟宾语；rival 意为"与……竞争，比得上"，可直接跟宾语，作为名词时意为"敌手"。
【经典例题】Graduates used to compete with each other for a good job in Hong Kong.
【译　　文】过去，香港的毕业生常常为得到一份好工作相互竞争。

compensate
['kɔmpənseit]

vt. 补偿，偿还，酬报（for）；给……付工钱；赔偿

【固定搭配】compensate sb. for 因……而赔偿某人；compensate for 弥补

【名师导学】该词属于常考词汇。注意固定搭配 compensate for（弥补，偿），后面接名词，是该词的常用搭配。考生要注意常用的相关同义词 repay（归还，欠款；报答，回报）。常用的相关同义词有 make up for（补偿），offset（弥补，抵消）。

【经典例题】To compensate for his unpleasant experiences he drank a little more than was good for him.

【译　　文】为了借酒消愁，他喝得有点过了头。

compensation
[ˌkɔmpen'seiʃən]

n. 补偿，赔偿

【名师导学】该词属于常考词汇，经常出现在阅读和词汇部分。

【经典例题】The insurance company paid him $10,000 in compensation after his accident.

【译　　文】事故之后，保险公司支付给他一万美元作为赔偿。

competence
['kɔmpitəns]

n. 能力，胜任

【名师导学】该词属于常考词汇。考生要注意常用的相关同义词：ability（能力，才能），capacity（才能，能力）。注意用法 competence in doing sth. 或者 competence to do sth. 表示"胜任，有能力做，称职"。

【经典例题】I assure you of his honesty and competence.

【译　　文】我向你保证他的诚实和能力。

competent
['kɔmpitənt]

a. 称职的，胜任的，有能力的

【经典例题】The truly competent physician is the one who sits down, senses the "mystery" of another human being, and offers the simple gifts of personal interest and understanding.

A. imaginable　　B. capable　　C. sensible　　D. humble　　[B]

【译　　文】真正称职的医生，能坐下来，感受他人的"秘密"，并表现出个人兴趣和理解。

competition
[ˌkɔmpi'tiʃən]

n. 比赛，竞争

【根源词汇】compete *vi.* 竞争

【固定搭配】keen / fierce competition for a job 求职的激烈竞争

competitor
[kəm'petitə]

n. 竞争对手

compile
[kəm'pail]

vt. 编辑，汇编

【名师导学】考生要注意常用的相关同义词 edit（编辑，校订，主编，选辑）。

【经典例题】The computers can quickly compile the weather information.

【译　　文】计算机能够快速编辑这些气象信息。

complain
[kəm'plein]

vi. 抱怨，诉苦，申诉

【固定搭配】complain to sb. of / about sth. 向某人抱怨某事　complain of doing sth. 抱怨做某事

【名师导学】complain 后面只接 that 从句做宾语，不直接跟 sb. 或 sth. 做宾语。

complaint
[kəm'pleint]

n. 抱怨，怨言；控告

complement
['kɔmplimənt]

n. 补足物，补充物；补语

【名师导学】该词属于常考词汇。考生要注意常用的相关同义词：supplement（补充，增补），supply（补给，供给）。

【经典例题】Movie directors use music to complement the action on the screen.

【译　文】电影导演运用音乐与屏幕上的情节相配合。

complex
['kɔmpleks]

a. 复杂的，复合的

【固定搭配】a complex situation 复杂的情况；a complex sentence 复合句

complexion
[kəm'plekʃən]

n. 面色

【名师导学】考生要注意常用的相关同义词：appearance（外貌，外表，外观），hue（色彩，色调）。

【经典例题】Drinking lots of water is good for the complexion.

【译　文】多喝水对面色有好处。

complexity
[kəm'pleksiti]

n. 复杂（性），复杂的事物

complicate
['kɔmplikeit]

vt. 使复杂化，使混乱，使难懂

complicated
['kɔmplikeitid]

a. 错综复杂的，难懂的

【名师导学】考生要注意常用的相关同义词：ambivalent（矛盾的），intricate（复杂的，错综的，难以理解的），complex（复合的；复杂的，难懂的）。

【经典例题】This is too complicated a matter to settle all by myself.

【译　文】这事太复杂，我一人难以对付。

complication
[,kɔmpli'keiʃ(ə)n]

n. 错杂；新增的困难，新出现的问题；并发症

【经典例题】His broken arm healed well, but he died of the pneumonia which followed as a _____.
A. complement　B. compliment　C. complexion　D. complication　[D]

【译　文】他的断臂愈合得很好，但最终死于肺炎这一并发症。

compliment
['kɔmplimənt]

赞美（话），恭维（话）；（复）致意，问候　*vt.* 赞美，恭维

complementary
[,kɔmpli'mentri]

a. 互补的；互相补足的

comply
[kəm'plai]

vi. 遵守，照办

【名师导学】考生要注意下列常用意义相近词和词组：abide by（坚持，遵守），adhere to（遵守，坚持），conform to（符合，遵照），obey（服从，顺从），observe（遵守）。常用相关反义词：disobey（违反，不服从），resist（抵抗，反抗）。注意固定搭配 comply with（遵从，服从），后面接名词。注意 comply with = conform to = abide by，注意介词的不同。

【经典例题】If you want to set up a company, you must comply with the regulations laid down by the authorities.
A. abide by　　B. work out　　C. check out　　D. succumb to　[A]

【译　文】如果你想成立一家公司，你就必须遵守政府的各项规定。

component
[kəm'pəunənt]

n. 组成部分，成分；部件，元件

compose
[kəm'pəuz]

v. 写作，作曲

【固定搭配】be composed of 由……构成

【联想记忆】be made up of 由……构成；consist of 由……构成（不能用被动语态）

composer
[kɔm'pəuzə]

n. 作曲家，创作者

composite
['kɔmpəzit]

a. 复合的，合成的，集成的 *n.* 混合物

composition
[,kɔmpə'ziʃən]

n. 写作，作文，习作；成分，合成物

compound
['kɔmpaund]

n. 混合物，（化）化合物 *a.* 复合的 *v.* 混合，配合

comprehend
[,kɔmpri'hend]

vt. 理解，领会，了解

comprehension
[,kɔmpri'henʃən]

n. 理解（力），领悟；理解力测验

comprehensive
[,kɔmpri'hensiv]

a. 综合的；全部的；所有的；（几乎）无所不包的；详尽的；综合性的（接收各种资质的学生）

n. （英国为各种资质的学生设立的）综合中学

【名师导学】要注意区分 comprehensive 和 comprehensible，前者为"综合性的，详尽的"，比如 comprehensive reading，意思是"综合阅读"，comprehensive university"综合大学"；后者意思是"可理解的"，比如 comprehensible speech，意思是"易懂的演讲"。

compress
[kəm'pres]

v. 压缩，紧缩

comprise
[kəm'praiz]

vt. 包括，包含，由……组成

compulsory
[kəm'pʌlsəri]

a. 强制的，必修的；规定的，义务的

【名师导学】该词属于常考词汇。考生要注意常用的相关同义词：forced（被迫的，强迫的），mandatory（命令的，强制的），obligatory（强制性的，约束的，有义务的）。相关的反义词：optional（可选择的，随意的），selective（选择的，选择性的），voluntary（自愿的，志愿的）。需要注意其衍生词使用范围更广。

【固定搭配】compulsory subject 必修学科；optional subject 选修学科

【经典例题】In front of the platform, the students were talking with the professor over the quizzes of their _____ subject.
A. compulsory B. compulsive C. alternative D. predominant   [A]

【译　文】学生们在讲台前与教授谈论他们选修课程的测试。

compute
[kəm'pju:t]

vt. 计算；估计

【名师导学】该词属于常考词汇。考生要注意常用的相关同义词 calculate（计算，核算）。需要注意其衍生词。

【经典例题】Scientists have computed the probable course of the rocket.

【译　文】科学家们用计算机计算了火箭可能运行的轨道。

☐ **computerize** [kəm'pju:təraiz]	*vt.* 用计算机处理，使计算机化
☐ **conceal** [kən'si:l]	*vt.* 隐瞒，隐藏，隐蔽 【固定搭配】conceal sth. from sb. 对某人隐瞒某事物 【经典例题】John's mindless exterior concealed a warm and kindhearted nature. 【译　　文】约翰漫不经心的外表掩盖了他热情和善良的本性。
☐ **concede** [kən'si:d]	*v.* 承认；给予，割让
☐ **conceited** [kn'si:tid]	*a.* 骄傲的，自高自大的，自负的
☐ **conceive** [kən'si:v]	*vt.* 设想，构想出（主意、计划等） 【名师导学】该词属于常考词汇。考生要注意常用的相关同义词：contrive（设计，想出，谋划，策划），devise（设计，发明，图谋），envisage（想象，设想），imagine（想象）。注意固定搭配 conceive of（构想出，设想），后面接名词，是该词的常用搭配。 【经典例题】Even after reading it for three times he couldn't ＿＿＿ the meaning of that letter. A. conceive　　B. consult　　C. contrast　　D. concern　　[A] 【译　　文】即使读了三遍，他也想不出那封信的意思。
☐ **concentrate** ['kɔnsentreit]	*vt.* 集中；聚集；浓缩　*vi.* 集中，专心 【固定搭配】concentrate on / upon 集中在，专心于 【联想记忆】be absorbed in 集中精力于；pay attention to 注意；focus / center on 专心于 【经典例题】Rejecting the urging of his physician father to study medicine, Hawking chose to ＿＿＿ on math and theoretical physics. A. impose　　B. center　　C. overwork　　D. concentrate　　[D] 【译　　文】霍金拒绝了他做内科医生的父亲让他学习医药的要求，选择了专攻数学和理论物理。
☐ **concentration** [ˌkɔnsen'treiʃən]	*n.* 专注，专心；集中；浓度
☐ **concept** ['kɔnsept]	*n.* 概念，观念
☐ **conception** [kən'sepʃən]	*n.* 构思，构想；概念，观念
☐ **concern** [kən'sə:n]	*vt.* 涉及，关系到；使挂念，使担心　*n.* 关心，挂念 【固定搭配】as far as...be concerned 就……而言；be concerned with 与……有关；concern oneself about, be concerned about 关心，挂念；show concern for sb. 关心某人 【联想记忆】have sth. to do with, relate to, be in connection with 与……有关；have no concern with, have nothing to do with 与……无关
☐ **concerning** [kən'sə:niŋ]	*prep.* 关于，涉及，就……来说

concession [kənˈseʃən]
n. 让步，妥协

concise [kənˈsais]
a. 简明的，简要的
【名师导学】考生要注意常用的相关同义词：brief（简短的，简练的），compact（紧凑的，紧密的），succinct（简洁的），terse（简洁的，简练的）。
【经典例题】The new secretary has written a remarkably concise report within a few hundred words but with all the important details included.
【译　　文】新来的秘书写了一份十分简洁的报告，只用几百个字就概括了所有重要的细节。

conclude [kənˈkluːd]
vt. 结束，完结；下结论，断定
【经典例题】Steele concludes that the Mozart effect doesn't exist.
【译　　文】斯蒂尔断定，莫扎特效应并不存在。

conclusion [kənˈkluːʒən]
n. 结束，终结，结局；推论
【固定搭配】come to / arrive at / reach / draw a conclusion 得出结论；in conclusion 最后，总之

concrete [ˈkɔnkriːt]
n. 混凝土 *a.* 具体的，实质性的

concurrent [kənˈkʌrənt]
a. 同时发生的
【经典例题】Reading a book and listening to music simultaneously seems to be on problem for them.
A. intermittently　　　　B. constantly
C. concurrently　　　　D. continuously　　　　[C]
【译　　文】在读书的时候听音乐对他们来说似乎有点问题。
【名师导学】近义词群：simultaneous, parallel, coexisting, side-by-side; concomitant, converging, coinciding, coterminous, convergent, meeting, uniting, confluent

condemn [kənˈdem]
vt. 谴责，指责；宣判，判刑
【固定搭配】condemn sb. to sth. 判处某人……罪

condemnation [ˌkɔndemˈneiʃən]
n. 谴责，非难，指责

condense [kənˈdens]
vt. 压缩，浓缩，精简

condole [kənˈdəul]
vt. 慰问

condolence [kənˈdəuləns]
n. 吊唁，吊慰；哀悼，悼词；追悼

conduct [ˈkɔndʌkt] *n.* [kənˈdʌkt] *v.*
n. 行为，品行　*vt.* 引导，指挥；传电，传热

conduction [kənˈdʌkʃən]
n. 传导

conductor [kən'dʌktə]
n. 领导者，经理，（管弦乐队、合唱队的）指挥，（市内有轨电车或公共汽车）售票员，＜美＞列车长，导体

confer [kən'fə:]
vt. 商谈，商议 vt. 授予，赋予
【名师导学】考生要注意常用的相关同义词 award（给予，授予），bestow（赠予，授予），consult（商量，商议，请教），discuss（讨论）。注意固定搭配 confer on（赋予，授予），是该词的常用搭配。
【经典例题】She withdrew to confer with her advisers before announcing a decision.
【译　　文】她先去请教顾问，然后再来宣布决定。

confess [kən'fes]
vt. 坦白，供认，承认

confidence ['kɔnfidəns]
n. 信任，信心
【固定搭配】in confidence 秘密地；with confidence 充满自信地；have confidence in 对……有信心

confident ['kɔnfidənt]
a. 确信的，有自信的
【固定搭配】be / feel confident in / of 确信某事
【联想记忆】be / feel certain of, be / feel sure of , be convinced of, have confidence in 确信某事
【经典例题】He is confident that scientists can block transmission of malaria to humans.
【译　　文】他确信科学家能够阻止疟疾向人类的传播。

confidential [,kɔnfi'denʃəl]
a. 秘密的，机密的；表示信任（或亲密）的

configuration [kən,figjə'reiʃn]
n. 配置，布局，结构，构造

confine [kən'fain]
vt. 限制，限于；监禁

confirm [kən'fə:m]
vt. 证实，进一步确定，确认；批准

confirmation [,kɔnfə'meiʃn]
n. 确定，确立，证实；确认，批准
【联想记忆】形容词 firm "紧紧的，牢固的"，动词 confirm "确认，证实，批准"
【经典例题】Wainwright found confirmation that Morrell gave Hitler antibiotics as a precaution in a recent translation of Morrell's own diary.
【译　　文】怀恩怀特在最近翻译莫雷尔的私人日记时确认莫雷尔给希特勒注射了抗生素预防针。

conform [kən'fɔ:m]
vi. 遵守，适应，顺从；相似，一致，符合
【名师导学】该词属于常考词汇。考生要注意常用的相关同义词：abide（遵守，履行），accord（符合），adhere（遵守，坚守），comply（遵从，依从，服从），follow（遵循，跟随）。该词的固定词组有 conform to 与 comply with。

conformity [kən'fɔ:miti]
n. 相似；一致；遵从；顺从

第二部分 核心意义词汇（A-K）

conflict ['kɒnflikt]
n. 争论，抵触，冲突 vi. 抵触，冲突
【固定搭配】in conflict with 与……相冲突；conflict with sb. / sth. 与……相冲突

confront [kən'frʌnt]
vt. 使面对，使遭遇
【经典例题】China Daily never loses sight of the fact that each day all of us a tough, challenging world.
A. encounter B. acquaint C. preside D. confront [D]
【译　文】《中国日报》对每天我们面对的这个既艰难又有挑战性的世界的方方面面都有深刻的见解。

confrontation [ˌkɒnfrʌn'teiʃn]
n. 面对；对峙（抗）；对质

confuse [kən'fju:z]
vt. 使混淆，搞乱
【固定搭配】confuse A with B 把 A 与 B 混淆
【经典例题】We tried to confuse the enemy.
【译　文】我们试图迷惑敌人。

confusion [kən'fju:ʒən]
n. 混淆，搞乱

conjunction [kən'dʒʌŋkʃən]
n. 联合，连接，结合；连接词

conquest ['kɒŋkwest]
n. 攻占，占领，征服；战利品

conscience ['kɒnʃəns]
n. 良心，道德心

conscientious [ˌkɒnʃi'enʃəs]
a. 认真（负责）的，真心实意的，小心谨慎的

conscious ['kɒnʃəs]
a. 意识到的；有知觉的；有觉悟的，自觉的
【固定搭配】be conscious of 意识到
【名师导学】该词属于常考词汇。考生要注意常用的相关同义词 aware（知道，明白的，意识到的）。该词的反义词是在该词的基础上加前缀"un"构成 unconscious（不省人事，未发觉的，无意识的），或者 unaware（不知道的，没觉察到的）。注意固定搭配 be conscious of（知道）和 become conscious（恢复知觉，意识），都是该词的常用搭配。
【经典例题】I am conscious of your thoughts, and of your violent purposes against me.
【译　文】我知道你们的想法，以及陷害我的计谋。

consecutive [kən'sekjutiv]
a. 连续的，依顺序的；连贯的

consensus [kən'sensəs]
n. （意见等）一致，一致同意
【名师导学】该词属于常考词汇，经常出现在阅读部分。考生要注意常用的相关同义词：concord（和谐，一致），consent（准许，同意，赞同），unanimity（全体一致，一致同意）。
【经典例题】The executives believed that consensus rather than conflict enhanced financial indicators.
【译　文】经理们相信，是意见一致，而不是相互争论，促进了金融指标的上升。

consequent
['kɔnsikwənt]
a. 作为结果的，随之发生的
【名师导学】考生要注意常用的相关同义词：following（接着的，下面的），ensuing（随后的，继而发生的）。
【经典例题】The warming of the Earth and the consequent climatic changes affect us all.
【译　　文】全球升温以及由此带来的气候变化影响着我们大家。

conserve
[kən'sə:v]
vt. 保存，保护；节约，节省
【派生词汇】conservation *n.* 保存，保护
【名师导学】辨析：conserve, protect, reserve, preserve：conserve 指保护从而使其不受损失或伤害，也指节约，谨慎或节省地使用，避免浪费；protect 指保护使免于受到损坏、攻击、偷盗或伤害；reserve 指收藏保留，如用于将来使用或某个特殊的目的，也指"预订，预约"；preserve 意为"保存，保持，收藏"，指保护某物不受破坏，使之完好无损。
【经典例题】We must conserve our famous scenic spots for future generations.
【译　　文】我们必须为子孙后代保护好风景胜地。

considerable
[kən'sidərəbl]
a. 相当的；可观的
【名师导学】considerable 相当多（或大、重要等）的；considerate 体贴的。
【经典例题】The visit to the country received considerable attention at this time.
【译　　文】此次访问该国引起了相当大的关注。

considerate
[kən'sidərit]
a. 考虑周到，体谅的，体贴的
【根源词汇】consider *v.* 考虑
【经典例题】It is ____ of you to turn down the radio while your sister is still ill in bed.
A. considerable　B. considerate　C. concerned　D. careful　[B]
【译　　文】你妹妹生病卧床的时候你能把收音机调小，这真是考虑周到。

consideration
[kən,sidə'reiʃən]
n. 考虑；要考虑的事；体贴，关心
【固定搭配】take...into consideration 顾及……，考虑到……
【经典例题】Although architecture has artistic qualities, it must also satisfy a number of important practical ____.
A. obligations　B. regulations　C. observations　D. considerations　[D]
【译　　文】虽然建筑具有艺术特质，但是它也要满足一些重要的实际需要。

considering
[kən'sidəriŋ]
prep. 就……而论，照……说来；鉴于

consist
[kən'sist]
vi. 由……组成，由……构成；在于
【固定搭配】consist in 在于，存在；consist of 由……构成，由……组成
【名师导学】consist 是不及物动词，没有被动态。
【经典例题】The Chinese community there, consisting of 67,000 adults, is the largest concentration of Chinese outside Asia.
【译　　文】那里的华人社区由 67 000 名成年人组成，是亚洲以外华人最大的集聚地。

consistency
[kən'sistənsi]
n. 一致性，连贯性；坚持

consistent
[kən'sistənt]
a. 一致的，符合的；坚持的；相容的
【固定搭配】consistent with 与……一致

【经典例题】This statement is not consistent with what you said at yesterday's meeting.
【译　　文】这个说法与你昨天会上的发言不一致。

console
[kən'səul]

vt. 安慰，慰问　*n.* 控制台，操作台
【名师导学】考生要注意常用的相关同义词：comfort（安慰，使痛苦缓和），solace（安慰），soothe（安慰，使平静）。常用的相关反义词：torment（折磨），torture（折磨）。该词的衍生词应该多加注意。
【经典例题】He consoled himself with the thought that it might have been worse.
【译　　文】他聊以自慰的是，幸亏事情没有更糟。

consolidate
[kən'sɔlideit]

v. 加固，巩固
【名师导学】该词属于常考词汇，尤其出现在词汇部分。考生要注意常用的相关同义词：solidify（使……凝固，使……团结，巩固），strengthen（加强，巩固），unify（使联合，统一）。
【经典例题】Consolidate and develop socialist relations characterized by equality, unity and mutual assistance among all ethnic groups for common prosperity and progress.
【译　　文】巩固和发展平等、团结、互助的社会主义民族关系，实现各民族共同繁荣和进步。

conspicuous
[kn'spikjus]

a. 显著的，显眼的

conspiracy
[kən'spirəsi]

n. 阴谋，密谋，共谋

constant
['kɔnstənt]

a. 不断的，持续的；始终如一的；坚定的，忠实的；恒定的，经常的
【名师导学】辨析 constant, continual, continuous：constant 表示连续发生的，在性质、价值或范围上持久不变的，始终如一的；continual 表示有规律地或经常地再发生，强调中间有间断的连续；continuous 表示不间断的连续。
【经典例题】The newly-designed machine can help the room maintain a constant and steady temperature.
【译　　文】这种新设计的机器能够帮助房间保持一个稳定不变的温度。

constitute
['kɔnstitju:t]

vt. 构成；制定

constitution
[ˌkɔnsti'tju:ʃən]

n. 法规，宪法，章程；组织，构造；体质，素质

constrain
[kən'strein]

vt. 限制，约束；克制，抑制
【名师导学】近义词：necessitate, compel, hold back, stifle; force, restrain
【经典例题】The mayor was asked to constrain his speech in order to allow his audience to raise questions.
【译　　文】市长被要求压缩他的讲话，以便听众有时间提问题。

constrict
[kən'strikt]

vt. 压缩，使收缩；妨害，阻碍
【联想记忆】con "合力，一起" + strict "紧的，严厉的" = constrict，压缩，阻碍
【经典例题】They are known to have antioxidant properties and other beneficial effects on aging bodies, such as dilating constricted coronary arteries.
【译　　文】它们具有抗氧化属性，对于抗衰老也有其他的有效作用，比如扩大狭隘的冠状动脉。
【名师导学】近义词群：compact 紧密的，compress 压缩，constrain 强迫，constringe 使收缩，crush 压碎

construct
[kən'strʌkt]
vt. 建造，建设
【派生词汇】construction *n.* 建筑，建造

consult
[kən'sʌlt]
vt. 请教，咨询；查阅；就诊 *vi.* 商量，会诊
【固定搭配】consult...about... 向……讨教某事；consult with...about... 跟某人商量某事
【名师导学】辨析 consult, consult with：consult 指"向……请教或咨询"，或指"参考，查阅"；consult with 指"磋商，交换意见"。

consultant
[kən'sʌltənt]
n. 顾问
【名师导学】辨析 consultant, guide：consultant 指提供专家意见或专业意见的人；guide 指在方法或道路上引导或指导另一人的人，或在行为等方面堪称他人楷模的人。
【经典例题】I think we need to see all investment＿＿＿＿ before we make an expensive mistake.
A. guides　　　　　　B. entrepreneurs
C. consultants　　　　D. assessors　　　　　　　　[C]
【译　　文】我认为我们需要拜访所有的投资顾问以免付出昂贵的代价。

consume
[kən'sju:m]
vt. 消耗，消费
【经典例题】They consume around 40 megawatt hours of electricity in the US every year.
【译　　文】在美国，他们每年大约消耗 40 兆瓦时的电。

consumer
[kən'sju:mə]
n. 用户，消费者

consumption
[kən'sʌmpʃən]
n. 消费（量）；结核病

contact
['kɔntækt]
n. / vt. 接触，联系，交往
【固定搭配】be in (out of) contact with 与……有（失去）联系
【联想记忆】keep in touch with sb. 与某人保持联系

container
[kən'teinə]
n. 容器，集装箱

contaminate
[kən'tæmineit]
vt. 弄脏，污染
【名师导学】该词属于常考词汇。考生要注意常用的相关同义词：foul（弄脏，污染），pollute（弄脏，污染；腐蚀），taint（弄脏，污染；使感染）。常用的相关反义词：purify（使纯净）。
【经典例题】Now a paper in *Science* argues that organic chemicals in the rock come mostly from contamination on earth rather than bacteria on Mars.
【译　　文】最近《科学》上的一篇文章宣称：岩石中的有机化学物质主要来自地球本身的污染，而并非来自火星上的细菌。

contemplate
['kɔntempleit]
v. 沉思，仔细考虑
【名师导学】考生要注意常用的相关同义词：consider（考虑，细想），ponder（思索，考虑，沉思），reflect（反省，细想），think（想，思索），survey（调查，全面审视）。该词的衍生词应该多加注意。
【经典例题】Every inhabitant of this planet must contemplate that it may no longer be habitable.
【译　　文】世界上每个人都必须思考到地球上可能不再适合人住的那一天。

☐ **contemporary** [kən'tempərəri]	*a.* 当代的；同龄的，同时代的 *n.* 同代人，同龄人	
☐ **contempt** [kən'tempt]	*n.* 轻视，蔑视；受辱，丢脸 【名师导学】该词属于常考词汇。考生要注意常用的相关同义词：disdain（蔑视，鄙视，不屑），disgrace（使丢脸，使耻辱），dishonor（使丢脸，使耻辱），scorn（轻蔑，藐视）。常用的相关反义词：admiration（钦佩，赞美，羡慕），respect（尊敬，尊重，敬意）。注意词组 beneath contempt, 表示"不齿"。 【经典例题】She looked at him with contempt. 【译　文】她轻蔑地看着他。	
☐ **contend** [kən'tend]	*vi.* 竞争；争夺 *vt.* 争论；主张；声称 【名师导学】近义词：contest, battle, dispute, fight , quarrel 【固定搭配】contend with / against sb. / sth. 与对手竞争，与他人争夺，与困难搏斗	
☐ **contented** [kən'tentid]	*a.* (与 with 连用) 满足的，满意的 【联想记忆】contented 和 content 都有"满意的，知足的"意思，但用法有别：contented 既可以做表语又可以做定语，而 content 只能做表语不能做定语。	
☐ **contention** [kən'tenʃən]	*n.* 斗争，竞争；争论，辩论	
☐ **contestant** [kən'testənt]	*n.* 竞争者；竞赛参加者；争论者	
☐ **contest** ['kɔntest] *n.* [kən'test] *v.*	*v. / n.* 竞争，比赛；争夺，争辩 【固定搭配】contest with / against 与……对抗	
☐ **context** ['kɔntekst]	*n.* 上下文；(事情等的) 前后关系，情况	
☐ **continual** [kən'tinjuəl]	*a.* 连续不断的，频繁的 【根源词汇】continue *v.* 继续 【名师导学】注意区分 continual 和 continous 的区别：continual 的意思是"不间断地连续"，后者含有"间断性地连续"。 【经典例题】Continual practice, through guided participation, is needed. 【译　文】在指导下，进行不断的实践是必需的。	
☐ **continuance** [kən'tinjuəns]	*n.* 保持；停留，逗留；继续，延续	
☐ **continuity** [ˌkɔnti'nju:lti]	*n.* 连续性；继续性	
☐ **continuous** [kən'tinjuəs] *n.* [kən'trækt] *v.*	*a.* 连续的，继续的，持续的 【经典例题】It rained continuously from Monday to Friday. 【译　文】雨连续不断地从周一下到周五。	
☐ **contract** ['kɔntrækt] *n.* [kən'trækt] *v.*	*n.* 契约，合同，包工 *v.* 收缩；感染；订约 【固定搭配】enter into / make a contract (with sb.) (for sth.) (与某人) (为某事) 订立和约；sign a contract 签订合同；contract with 与……签订合同	

contradict
[ˌkɔntrə'dikt]

vt. 反驳，反对，否认；与……矛盾，与……抵触，与……相反
【名师导学】近义词：differ, confront, oppose; disclaim, repudiate, deny

contradiction
[ˌkɔntrə'dikʃən]

n. 反驳，矛盾
【固定搭配】be in contradiction with 与……互相矛盾
【经典例题】As skies fill with millions of migrating birds, European scientists say the seasonal miracle appears to depend on a seeming contradiction: The fatter the bird, the more efficiently it flies.
【译　　文】当天空上满是迁徙的鸟时，欧洲的科学家们认为这个季节性奇观似乎建立在一个矛盾基础上，即鸟越胖，飞的效率越高。

contrary
['kɔntrəri]

a. 相反的，矛盾的 *n.* 反面，相反
【固定搭配】on the contrary, 反之，；contrary to 与……相反
【名师导学】辨析 on the contrary, on the other hand, in contrast: on the contrary 引出与前述情况完全相反的观点；on the other hand 补充说明事物的另一方面；in contrast 对比同一事物的两个方面。辨析 contrary, opposite: contrary 表示相反的意见、计划、目的等抽象意义，有时带有矛盾或敌对的意味；opposite 指相反的位置、方向、性质、结果等静态含义，但不一定有敌对的含义。
【经典例题】____ popular belief, she is a warm-hearted person.
　A. Subject to　　　　　B. Contrary to
　C. Familiar to　　　　　D. Similar to　　　　　[B]
【译　　文】与一般的观点不同，她实际上是一个热心肠的人。

contrast
['kɔntræst] *n.*
[kən'træst] *v.*

v. / n. 对比，对照
【固定搭配】in contrast with / to 和……形成对比（对照）contrast A with B 把 A 与 B 对照
【经典例题】Preliminary estimation puts the figure at around $110 billion,____ the $160 billion the president is struggling to get through the Congress.
　A. in proportion to　　　B. in rely to
　C. in relation to　　　　D. in contrast to　　　　[D]
【译　　文】预先估算的款项在 1 100 亿美元左右，而总统正尽力通过议会获得 1 600 亿美元。

contribute
[kən'tribjuːt]

v. 捐助，捐献（与 to 连用，后接某种公益事业；与 for 连用，后接目的）；投稿
【固定搭配】contribute to 为……出力 / 贡献
【经典例题】Eating too much fat can contribute to heart disease and cause high blood pressure.
【译　　文】摄入过多的脂肪会导致心脏病和高血压。

contribution
[ˌkɔntri'bjuːʃən]

n. 贡献，捐助，捐助之物

contrive
[kən'traiv]

vi. 计划，发明；设计；设法，图谋
【名师导学】近义词群：improvise, devise; manage, compass, negotiate, afford, engineer, manipulate, shift, arrange, execute, carry out, effect, bring about, maneuver

controversial
[ˌkɔntrə'vəːʃəl]

a. 争论的；引起争论的；被议论的；可疑的
【经典例题】The idea of correcting defective genes is not particularly controversial in the scientific community.
【译　　文】在科学界，对于矫正缺陷基因的想法并没有什么争议。

第二部分 核心意义词汇（A-K）

convene [kən'vi:n]
vt. 召集，集合；召唤，叫出
【名师导学】近义词 congregate, collect, convoke; assemble, gather

convention [kən'venʃən]
n. 习俗，惯例；大会，会议；公约
【固定搭配】break established conventions 打破成规；sign a convention of peace with a neighbouring country 与邻国签订一项和平协定
【经典例题】The North American states agreed to sign the <u>agreement</u> of economical and military union in Ottawa.
A．convention B．conviction
C．contradiction D．confrontation [A]
【译　文】北美各国同意在渥太华签署经济和军事联盟协议。

converge [kən'və:dʒ]
vi. 会合，相互靠拢；会聚，集中；（思想、观点等）趋势
【名师导学】考生要注意常用的相关同义词：approach（靠近，接近），concentrate（集中，聚集），focus（聚集，集中，聚焦）。
【经典例题】If the fire alarm is sounded, all residents are requested to converge in the courtyard.
【译　文】如果火警响起来，所有居民就应到院子里集合。

converse [kən'və:s] *vi.* ['kɔnvə:s] *n.*
vi. 谈话，交谈（with, on, upon）*n.* 相反的事物；反面

conversion [kən'və:ʃən]
n. 转化，转换，转变
【名师导学】考生要注意常用的相关词：modification（更改，修改），transformation（改变，改革，改造）。
【经典例题】He used to support monetarist economics, but he underwent quite a conversion when he saw how it increased unemployment.
【译　文】他一向赞同货币经济理论，然而当他看到这种理论加重了失业现象之后，他彻底改变了看法。

conventional [kən'venʃənl]
a. 普通的，常见的；习惯的，常规的

convert [kən'və:t] *vi.* ['kɔnvə:t] *n.*
vi. 使转变，更改 *n.* 改变信仰者

convertible [kən'və:təbl]
a. 可转换的；可转变的；可改装的；可兑换的

convey [kən'vei]
vt. 传达，表达；传送，运输
【经典例题】Gestures are an important means to _____ messages.
A．convey B．study C．exploit D．keep [A]
【译　文】手势是一种传达信息的重要手段。

convict ['kɔnvikt] *n.* [kən'vikt] *v.*
vt. 证明……有罪，宣判……有罪；使……知罪 *n.* 罪犯
【经典例题】Tom was _____ of a crime he didn't commit. He fought for many years to clear his name.
A．convicted B．convinced C．conceived D．condemned [A]
【译　文】汤姆被误判为有罪，他用了很多年洗清罪名。

151

conviction
[kən'vikʃən]

n. 坚信；定罪，证明有罪

【经典例题】Mrs. Brown couldn't shake the conviction that these kids were in deep trouble and it was up to her to help them.

【译　　文】布朗夫人认为这些孩子遇到了极大的麻烦，并且需要她的帮助，她的这种信念是不会动摇的。

convince
[kən'vins]

vt. 使信服，使确信

【固定搭配】convince sb. of 使某人相信；be convinced of 确信

【名师导学】convince 是及物动词，必须跟 sb. 做宾语。convince sb. that / of sth. 说服某人相信某事。

【经典例题】He is eager to convince us of his brother's innocence.

【译　　文】他急切地想让我们相信他兄弟是清白的。

cooperate
[kəu'ɔpəreit]

vi. 合作，协作，相配合

【固定搭配】cooperate with sb. in doing sth. 与某人合作做某事

【经典例题】The British cooperated with the French in building the new craft.

【译　　文】英、法两国合作制造这种新式飞船。

coordinate
[kəu'ɔ:dinit]

v. （使）协调，调整；（使）互相配合

【固定搭配】coordinate with each other 互相配合

cope
[kəup]

vi. 对付，应付

【固定搭配】cope with 应付，对付，克服

【名师导学】辨析 cope with, deal with, handle：cope with 指成功地对付困难或困境；deal with 指"与……交往（有生意往来）"，也指"安排，处理，涉及，研究"；handle 含有"管理，操纵，（用手）操作"的意思，表示掌握了工具或方法，能应付各种情况。

【经典例题】Her husband's left her and the kids are running wild, so it's not surprising that she can't cope.

【译　　文】她丈夫离开了她，孩子们又不听管教，难怪她束手无策。

copper
['kɔpə]

n. 铜，铜币，铜制品

【联想记忆】aluminum *n.* 铝；bronze *n.* 青铜

copyright
['kɔpirait]

n. 版权，著作权

cordial
['kɔ:diəl]

a. 热情友好的，热诚的

【名师导学】考生要注意常用的相关同义词：friendly（友好的，友谊的），hearty（亲切的），gracious（亲切的，和蔼的），hospital（好客的，热情的），sincere（诚挚的，真诚的，诚恳的），warm（热情的）。

【经典例题】The letter you wrote me is very cordial.

【译　　文】你写给我的信很诚恳。

core
[kɔ:]

n. 核心，要点；果心

【经典例题】The central portion of the earth below the mantle is made up of a liquid outer core and solid inner core.

【译　　文】地幔下面的中心部分是由液体的外核和一个固体的内核构成的。

cornerstone
['kɔ:nəstəun]

n. 奠基石，基石

第二部分 核心意义词汇（A-K）

corporate
['kɔːpərit]
a. 公司的；法人组织的；社会团体的；共同的；自治的

corporation
[ˌkɔːpəˈreiʃən]
n. 公司，团体

corpse
[kɔːps]
n. 尸体，死尸
【名师导学】考生要注意常用的相关同义词 remains（残骸，遗体）。
【经典例题】A corpse was found in the park early this morning.
【译　　文】今天一大早，公园里发现了一具尸体。

correlate
['kɔrileit]
vt. 使相互有关　*vi.* (to, with) 相关，关联
【名师导学】注意固定搭配 correlate to / with（相关，关联），后面接名词，是该词常用的搭配。
【经典例题】It is true that being overweight correlates with an increased risk of heart and blood vessel disease.
【译　　文】确实如此，超重和增加患心血管疾病的风险是紧密相关的。

correlation
[ˌkɔriˈleiʃən]
n. 关联，（相互）关系，相关，相应，交互作用
【联想记忆】co "相互，一起，共同" +relate "联系" +tion（名词后缀之一）=correlation 关联，相关
【经典例题】He doubts there is a correlation between the Internet and depression.（2004）
【译　　文】他质疑网络和抑郁之间的相关性。
【名师导学】join, combine, unite, connect, link, attach, couple, associate, relate 这些动词均有"连接，结合，联合"之意。
join：侧重把原来不相连接的物紧密地连接在一起，但仍可再分开。也指把分散的人或几个部分的人联合起来，或加入到某团体中去。
combine：指两个或两个以上的人或物结合在一起。
unite：指联合、团结、结合在一起，构成一个整体。
connect：指两事物在某一点上相连接，但彼此又保持独立。
link：指连环式的连接，或用接合物或其他方式连接，还可指一事物与另一事物的联系或关系。
attach：指把局部连接在整体上，小的接在大的上面，活动的接在固定的上面。
couple：专指连接两件东西，或把事物成对进行连接。
associate：指人与人友好和平、平等地联合在一起；用于物时，指两事物因历史或其他原因，很自然被人们联系在一起，即产生联想。
relate：指人与人有亲戚或婚姻关系；也指人或物之间尚存的实际或假想的联系。

correspond
[ˌkɔriˈspɔnd]
vi. 相当，对应；符合；通信
【固定搭配】correspond to sth. 相当的，相似的；correspond closely / exactly / precisely to sth. 完全相一致，相符合；correspond with sb. 通信
【联想记忆】agree with, coincide with, match with, conform to 符合；与……一致
【经典例题】Mark the corresponding letter on your answer sheet.
【译　　文】在你的答题纸上画出相应的字母。

correspondence
[ˌkɔrisˈpɔndəns]
n. 相当（应，称）；符合，一致；通信，信件

correspondent [ˌkɔrisˈpɔndənt]	n. 通信员，记者
corresponding [ˌkɔrisˈpɔndiŋ]	a. 相应的，相当的；符合的，一致的
corrode [kəˈrəud]	vt. 腐蚀，侵蚀；损害，损伤
corrupt [kəˈrʌpt]	a. 腐败的，贪污的 vt. 使腐化，使堕落 【经典例题】It is corrupt friends who lead him astray. 【译　文】近墨者黑。
corruption [kəˈrʌpʃən]	n. 腐败，堕落；贪污，贿赂
cosmic [ˈkɔzmik]	a. 宇宙的，外层空间的；无比巨大的，无尽的
costume [ˈkɔstjuːm]	n. 服装；剧装 【经典例题】We were greatly impressed by her national costume at the anniversary last night. 【译　文】在昨晚的周年聚会上她身着民族服饰，给我们留下了深刻的印象。
council [ˈkaunsil]	n. 理事会，委员会；议事机构
counsel [ˈkaunsəl]	n./v. 劝告，建议
countdown [ˈkaunt,daun]	n. 倒数计秒
counter [ˈkauntə]	n. 计算器，计数器，计算者；柜台；筹码 ad./a. 相反地（的）
counterpart [ˈkauntəpɑːt]	n. 职位（或作用）相当的人；对应的事物 【名师导学】该词属于常考词汇，主要出现在词汇选择和阅读部分。其中 counter 原指"柜台"，可想象成顾客和服务生面对面的场景，转义为"相对的"。 【经典例题】Your right hand is the counterpart of your left hand. 【译　文】你的右手是你左手的相对物。
courtesy [ˈkəːtisi]	n. 礼貌，客气
coverage [ˈkʌvəridʒ]	n. 范围，总额；保险额，保证金；新闻报道（范围） 【名师导学】该词在翻译时容易直译成"覆盖面"，但它在特定语境下还表示观察、分析、报道事物的范围或程度，比如和 news 搭配译为"新闻报道"，意指新闻所覆盖的范围。 【经典例题】They must reflect that diversity with their news coverage or risk losing their readers' interest and their advertisers' support. 【译　文】报纸行业必须展现其新闻报道的多样性，否则就有失去读者的关注以及广告商的支持的风险。

coward
['kauəd]

n. 胆小鬼，懦夫

【名师导学】该词在近十年考试中共出现 3 次，主要出现在词汇选择和阅读部分。
【经典例题】I'm a real coward when it comes to going to the dentist.
【译　　文】我一去看牙医就胆战心惊。

cozy
['kəuzi]

a. (暖和) 舒适的；亲切友好的
【名师导学】常同 cosy。
【经典例题】Things are cozy enough around here for Nelson.
【译　　文】这里的一切对纳尔逊来说已够舒适的了。

crack
[kræk]

v. (使) 破裂，砸开；发爆裂声 *n.* 裂纹，龟裂；爆裂声
【名师导学】辨析 crack, break：crack 指"破裂，裂缝"，没有完全分离部分的破裂；break 指"打破，击碎"，使突然或猛烈地分裂成碎片。

crackdown
[kræk'daun]

n. 压迫，镇压，打击

cradle
['kreidl]

n. 摇篮，发源地
【经典例题】He was in the company of poverty from cradle to grave.
【译　　文】从生到死，贫穷一直伴随着他。

crash
[kræʃ]

v. / n. 摔坏，坠毁
【名师导学】辨析 crash, crush, smash：crash 指"坠毁"，碰撞中造成的突然损毁；crush 指"压碎"，把（石头或矿石等）挤压、捣碎或碾成小碎块或粉末；smash 指"打碎"，或突然地、大声地、猛力地把某种东西毁成碎片。
【经典例题】After our computer network＿＿＿for the third time that day, we all went home.
A. crashed　B. collided　C. smashed　D. fell　　　　　[A]
【译　　文】那天当我们的电脑网络系统第三次崩溃后，大家都回家了。

crawl
[krɔːl]

n. 爬行，慢行
【名师导学】辨析 crawl, creep：crawl 指用手或膝盖拖曳身体在地上缓慢移动；creep 指蹑足前进，秘密地或谨慎地移动，非常缓慢地移动或前进。

credible
['kredəbl, -ibl]

a. 可信的，可靠的
【名师导学】近义词：probable, believable, conceivable; trustworthy, dependable, sincere; reliable
【经典例题】He will be a credible witness when needed.
【译　　文】如果需要的话，他会是一位可信的证人。

creep
[kriːp]

n. 爬，徐行，蠕动 *vi.* 爬，蔓延，潜行

crime
[kraim]

n. 罪，罪行，犯罪

criminal
['kriminl]

a. 犯罪的，刑事的 *n.* 罪犯，刑事犯

cripple
['kripl]

n. 残疾的人，跛子 *vt.* 使残疾

crisis
['kraisis]

n. 危机；决定性时刻

【名师导学】crisis 复数形式为 crises（参见 analysis）。辨析 crisis, emergency, urgency：crisis 指关键时刻，决定性时刻，转折点；emergency 指突然发生并要求马上处理的严重情况或事件；urgency 指紧要、紧迫的特征或状态。

crisp
[krisp]

a. 脆的，易碎的；新鲜的；爽快的，明快的

【名师导学】该词主要用来形容食物松脆。如：crisp potato chips（松脆土豆片），crisp noodle（干脆面）。

【经典例题】The reason why so many children like to eat this new brand of biscuit is that it is particularly sweet and crisp.

【译　文】如此多的儿童喜欢吃这个新牌子的饼干，是因为这种饼干又甜又脆。

criterion
[kraiˈtiəriən]

n. 标准，准则

【名师导学】该词经常用于指代各类赛事的评分标准，常见的近义词：rule（准则），standard（标准），regulation（规则）等。

【经典例题】The most important criterion for assessment in this contest is originality of design.

【译　文】这次比赛最重要的评判标准就是设计的原创性。

critic
['kritik]

n. 批评家，评论家

critical
['kritikəl]

a. 批评的，批判的；危急的，紧要的

【固定搭配】be critical of 挑剔，不满

【经典例题】We are at a critical point in our nation's history.

【译　文】我们现在正处于我们国家历史上的一个关键时刻。

criticism
['kritisiz(ə)m]

n. 批评，评论

criticize
['kritisaiz]

vt. 批评，评论

【经典例题】Yet they have been criticized as a monumental waste of money.

【译　文】但是，他们遭到了谴责，说他们浪费了很多钱。

crucial
['kruːʃəl]

a. 关键的，决定性的

【经典例题】Social identity and motivational factors can be crucial.

【译　文】社会身份和动机也是关键因素。

crumble
['krʌmbl]

vt. 弄碎，粉碎

cue
[kjuː]

n. 提示，暗示

【经典例题】One involved using visual and spatial cues, such as posters on a well, to learn to find a platform hidden under murky water.

【译　文】一个任务是使用视觉和空间的线索，比如墙上的海报等，来尝试找到昏暗水中的台子。

culminate
['kʌlmineit]

vi. 达到极点，达到最高潮

【固定搭配】culminate in... 以……而终结，以……而达到顶峰

【名师导学】近义词群：finish, crown, consummate, result in; climax, complete

第二部分 核心意义词汇（A-K）

□ cumulative
['kju:mjulətiv]
a. 累积的，渐增的；附加的

□ cultivate
['kʌltiveit]
vt. 耕作，栽培，养殖；培养，陶冶，发展
【派生词汇】cultivation *n.* 培养，栽培
【经典例题】They have enough money and leisure time to cultivate an interest in the arts.
【译　　文】他们有足够的金钱和空闲时间来培养艺术方面的兴趣。

□ culture
['kʌltʃə]
n. 文化，文明；教养
【经典例题】Smiles convey a wide range of meanings in different areas and cultures.
【译　　文】微笑在不同的地区和文化中，承载着极为广泛的意义。

□ curb
[kə:b]
vt. 控制，约束 *n.* 控制，约束；（街边和人行道）路缘
【经典例题】You have to curb your laughter when you are in church.
【译　　文】在教堂里你得收敛你的笑声。

□ curious
['kjuəriəs]
a. 好奇的，爱打听的

□ curiosity
[,kjuəri'ɔsiti]
n. 好奇（心）

□ curl
[kə:l]
n. 卷曲，鬈 *vt.* 弄卷 *vi.* 卷曲，弯曲

□ currency
['kʌrənsi]
n. 货币，通货

□ current
['kʌrənt]
n. 水流，气流，电流；潮流，趋势 *a.* 通用的，流行的，当前的
【经典例题】There is currently no evidence that mobile phones harm users or people living near transmitter masts.
【译　　文】目前没有证据表明手机会伤害手机使用者或是发射站附近的居民。

□ curriculum
[kə'rikjuləm]
n. （学校、专业的）全部课程；（取得毕业资格的）必修课程

□ curve
[kə:v]
v. 弄弯，使成曲线 *n.* 曲线，弯曲

□ cyberspace
['saibəspeis]
n. 网控空间，赛百空间

□ cyclist
['saiklist]
n. 骑自行车/摩托车的人

□ cynical
['sinikəl]
a. 愤世嫉俗的，（对人性或动机）怀疑的
【经典例题】Popularly, one refers cynically to "human nature" in accepting the inevitability of such undesirable human behavior as greed, murder, cheating and lying.
【译　　文】生活中会出现贪婪、谋杀、作弊、撒谎等种种令人不悦的行为，而人们往往对发生诸如此类行为的必然性欣然接受，在谈到这种"人性"时也总是显得玩世不恭。

D

dash
[dæʃ]

vt. 猛冲，撞破 *vi.* 猛冲 *n.* 猛冲，短跑，破折号
【经典例题】The boat was dashed against the rocks.
【译　　文】那艘船猛地撞到礁石上。

data
[ˈdeitə]

n. (datum 的复数) 资料，材料
【名师导学】做主语时，谓语可以是单数，也可以是复数。
【经典例题】There are more than 2.5 million workers who need help, according to Labour Department data.
【译　　文】根据劳动部的数据，有 250 多万名工人需要帮助。

database
[ˈdeitəbeis]

n. 数据库
【名师导学】该词在历年考题中均出现在阅读部分。需要注意的是，data 一词来源于 datum，表达复数概念。
【经典例题】This information is combined with a map database.
【译　　文】这一信息同地图数据库结合在一起。

dazzle
[ˈdæzl]

vt. 使目眩，耀眼；使惊叹不已，使倾倒 *n.* 耀眼的光，令人赞叹的东西
【名师导学】该词的词形容易和下列词语混淆，如：drizzle (*n.* 细雨), dizzy (*a.* 眩晕的) 等。在记忆单词时应加以辨别。
【经典例题】The dazzle of the spotlights made him ill at ease.
【译　　文】聚光灯的耀眼强光使他局促不安。

deadlock
[ˈdedlɔk]

n. 僵局

deadly
[ˈdedli]

a. 致命的，致死的；极有害的
【名师导学】辨析 deadly, fatal, mortal：deadly 意为"可能致死的"(likely to cause or able to produce death)，表示能够或可能引起死亡，但不一定有导致死的结果；fatal 意为"导致死亡的"(causing or resulting in death)，多指已经或将导致死亡，强调死亡是不可避免的；mortal 意为"死亡的"，指未能永存。
【经典例题】It was the worst tragedy in maritime history, six times more deadly than the Titanic.
【译　　文】这是航海史上一次空前的灾难，所造成的损失超过泰坦尼克号的六倍。

deaf
[def]

a. 聋的；不愿听的，装聋的
【固定搭配】turn a deaf ear to 充耳不闻，对……根本不听；be deaf to 不听
【经典例题】Helen is deaf and dumb, but she continues to study.
【译　　文】海伦又聋又哑，但她仍然坚持学习。

debate
[diˈbeit]

vt. 争论，辩论
【经典例题】We debated the advantages and disadvantages of filming famous works.
【译　　文】我们就把著名的作品拍成电影的优点和缺点进行了辩论。

debt
[det]

n. 债，欠债
【固定搭配】in debt 欠债，欠情
【经典例题】If I pay all my debts I shall have no money left.
【译　　文】如果我偿清了所有的债，我就一分钱不剩了。

decade
['dekeid]

n. 十年
【经典例题】For the past decade or so, practical courses, such as computer and business, have gained tremendous development on college campuses.
【译　　文】过去十年来，实用性课程，诸如计算机和商业课程已在大学校园中得到极大的发展。

decay
[di'kei]

n. 衰退，腐烂　*v.* 衰退，腐烂
【经典例题】Dr. Li of the U.S. Department of Agriculture, has found that oranges can be prevented from decaying by the use of certain chemicals containing sulfur compounds.
【译　　文】美国农业部的李博士发现，使用某种含硫的化合物能防止橘子腐烂。

deceive
[di'si:v]

v. 欺骗，蒙蔽
【固定搭配】deceive sb. into doing sth. 骗某人做某事
【经典例题】The secret agent concealed her real mission, therefore many local people were ＿＿＿ into thinking that she was a good person.
A. betrayed　B. driven　C. deceived　D. convinced　[C]
【译　　文】这个特务隐瞒了她的真实使命，因此许多当地人都误认为她是一个好人。

deceit
[di'si:t]

n. 欺骗，欺诈

decent
['di:snt]

a. 庄重的，正派的，大方的；（服装等）相称的，体面的
【经典例题】My friend Ling has no education, so it's hard for her to find a decent job and earn enough money for her family.
【译　　文】我的朋友玲没有受过教育，因此对于她来说找一个体面的工作并赚钱来养家是很困难的。

deception
[di'sepʃən]

n. 欺骗；受骗，上当
【联想记忆】动词 deceive, de "不再，远离" +ceive "收到，接收" =deceive 欺骗
【名师导学】deceit, deception, fraud 这3个名词均含有"欺骗"之意。
deceit：指歪曲实情，惯于说谎或蓄意欺骗。
deception：语气较弱，一般用词，侧重于具体的骗人行为。但有时并无欺骗行为，只是玩弄把戏，故弄玄虚而已。
fraud：一般用于犯罪行为的欺骗，通常指政治或经济活动中的舞弊行为。

decline
[di'klain]

vi. 减少，下降；衰落；婉言拒绝　*n.* 降低，消减
【名师导学】辨析 decline, refuse, reject：decline 表示"（委婉）拒绝，谢绝"；refuse 是表示"拒绝"这一概念的最普通用词，含有非常坚决地、不客气地拒绝的意味；reject 指"拒不接受，不采纳"，语气比 refuse 强，有抵制的意思。
【经典例题】The percentage of the population in the workforce declines when there is either a rapid increase in births or a falling birth rate.
【译　　文】无论出生率是快速增长或者下降，都会导致劳动力人口的百分比的减少。

【经典例题】Does brain power_____as we get older? Scientists now have some surprising answers.
A. decline B. descend C. deduce D. collapse [A]
【译　文】智力会随着年龄的增长而下降吗？现在科学家给出了惊人的答案。

decode
[ˌdiːˈkəud]
vt. 解码，译解

decorate
[ˈdekəreit]
v. 装饰，装潢，布置
【经典例题】The hall is decorated with flowers and lights.
【译　文】大厅里装饰着鲜花和彩灯。

decoration
[ˌdekəˈreiʃən]
n. 装饰，装饰品

decrease
[ˈdiːkriːs] n.
[diːˈkriːs] v.
v. / n. 减少，减小

decree
[diˈkriː]
n. 法令，命令，政令 v. 颁布

dedicate
[ˈdedikeit]
vt. 奉献
【经典例题】I want to see all of us dedicate ourselves to the principles for which we fought.
【译　文】我希望看到所有的人献身于我们为之奋斗的道义中去。

deduce
[diˈdjuːs]
vt. 推论，推断，演绎
【名师导学】近义词：infer, conclude, reason, gather, assume
【经典例题】His conclusion is deduced from the facts and evidence presented by the court.
【译　文】他的结论是从法庭提供的事实和证据中推断出来的。

deduct
[diˈdʌkt]
vt. 扣除，减除；演绎

deduction
[diˈdʌkʃən]
n. 缩小，减小；演绎

deductive
[diˈdʌktiv]
a. 推论的，推断的；演绎的

deem
[diːm]
vt. 认为，视为
【名师导学】表示"认为，想"的意义时单词较多，不一定总是使用 I think..., 还包括 consider, assume, believe, suppose 等等。
【经典例题】Being thin is deemed as such a virtue.
【译　文】身材瘦削竟被视为优点。

default
[diˈfɔːlt]
n. 假设值，默认（值），不履行责任，缺席
v. 默认，不履行义务，缺席，拖欠；　[计算机] 缺省
【经典例题】Mortgage_____had risen in the last year because the number of low-income families was on the increase.
A. defects B. deficits C. defaults D. deceptions [C]
【译　文】去年抵押拖欠提高了，因为低收入家庭的数量在增长。

defect ['di:fekt]	*n.* 缺点；瑕疵 【经典例题】Is it true that is the major drawback of the new medical plan? A. defect　　B. assistance　　C. culprit　　D. triumph　　[A] 【译　文】那就是新的医疗计划的主要缺陷，这是真的吗？
defection [di'fekʃən]	*n.* 缺点；背信，背叛，变节
defective [di'fektiv]	*a.* 有缺陷（缺点）的，不完美的，有故障的（常与 in 连用）
defendant [di'fendənt]	*n.* 被告 【经典例题】He stood there as a defendant, dull and wordless. 【译　文】他作为被告站在那里，目光呆滞，一言不发。
defer [di'fə:]	*vt.* 推迟，拖延　*vi.*(to) 遵从，听从，服从
defiance [di'faiəns]	*n.* 挑战，挑衅；蔑视
deficient [di'fiʃənt]	*a.* 缺乏的，欠缺的；不足的，不完善的 【联想记忆】名词 deficiency 【经典例题】The recent deterioration in the economy is of great concern to the government. A. depression　B. deficiency　　C. degeneration　D. deformity　　[B] 【译　文】最近经济衰退引起了政府的极大关注。
deficiency [di'fiʃənsi]	*n.* 缺乏，不足；缺点，缺陷 【名师导学】近义词：scarcity, insufficiency, paucity, lack, loss 【经典例题】He looked pale because of nutrient deficiency. 【译　文】由于营养不足，他看上去脸色苍白。
deficit ['defisit]	*n.* 不足，缺陷；亏损，亏空（额）；赤字，逆差，欠缺
define [di'fain]	*vt.* 下定义，解释
definite ['definit]	*a.* 明确的，确定的，限定的
definition [,defi'niʃən]	*n.* 定义，解释
definitive [di'finitiv]	*a.* 限定的；明确的 【联想记忆】动词 define，限定，下定义；definitive 形容词，限定的，据定性的，最后的；finite 有限的，限定的；indefinite 无限的
defy [di'fai]	*vt.* 公然反抗，蔑视；无法（相信、解释等） 【经典例题】He challenged the tradition, defied the law and was exiled to the north at the end of 18th century. 【译　文】他不循规蹈矩，不服从法律，于18世纪末被流放到北方。
degeneracy [di'dʒenərəsi]	*n.* 堕落，退化，退步

degrade [di'greid]
v. 分解，降级，使受屈辱

dehydration [ˌdi:hai'dreiʃn]
n. 脱水

delegate ['deligeit]
n. 委员，代表　*vt.* 派……为代表；委任

delegation [ˌdeli'geiʃən]
n. 代表团；派遣

delete [di'li:t]
vt. 删除
【固定搭配】delete...from 从……除去

deliberate [di'libəreit] *v.* [di'libərət] *a.*
a. 故意的；深思熟虑的　*v.* 仔细考虑
【经典例题】Sometimes the messages are conveyed through deliberate, conscious gestures.
【译　　文】有时，信息是通过故意的、下意识的手势表达的。

delicacy ['delikəsi]
n. 娇嫩，优美；精致

delicate ['delikit]
a. 纤弱的，娇嫩的，易碎的；优美的，精美的，精致的；微妙的，棘手的；灵敏的，精密的
【经典例题】Delicate plants must be protected from cold wind and frost.
【译　　文】娇弱的植物必须妥善保护，以避免风霜的侵袭。

delivery [di'livəri]
n. 递送，交付，分娩，交货，引渡，发送，传输；（法律）财产等的正式移交

democracy [di'mɔkrəsi]
n. 民主，民主制；民主国家

democrat ['deməkræt]
n. 民主主义者，民主人士

democratic [ˌdemə'krætik]
a. 民主的，有民主精神（作风）的

demolish [di'mɔliʃ]
vt. 拆毁，毁坏；驳倒（论点等），推翻
【名师导学】近义词群：destroy, wreck, devastate, obliterate

demonstrate ['demənstreit]
vt. 表明；论证；演示　*vi.* 示威
【固定搭配】demonstrate against 示威反对
【名师导学】辨析 demonstrate, prove, testify：demonstrate 意为"证实，说明，示范"，指某人用例证、实验等实物证明某人或某物的真实性；prove 意为"证明，证实"，指某人用可靠的材料或事实来断定事物的真实性；testify 意为"作见证"，指某人用其耳闻目睹的事实来为他人提供证据，该词常用于在法庭上作证。
【经典例题】History has demonstrated that countries with different social systems can join hands in meeting the common challenges.
【译　　文】历史表明，不同社会体制的国家能够联手迎接共同的挑战。

demonstration
[ˌdemənsˈtreiʃən]
n. 展示;示威

dense
[dens]
a. 密的,稠密的;浓密的
【经典例题】I had trouble getting through the dense crowd of people.
【译　　文】我在穿过密集的人群时遇到了麻烦。

density
[ˈdensiti]
n. 稠密;密度
【经典例题】Britain has the highest＿＿of road traffic in the world over 60 cars for every mile of road.
A. density　　B. intensity　　C. popularity　　D. prosperity　　[A]
【译　　文】英国的道路车流量是世界上最大的,平均每英里的路面上有超过60辆汽车。

dental
[ˈdentl]
a. 牙齿的

denial
[diˈnaiəl]
n. 否认
【名师导学】表达"拒绝"含义的名词有很多,但各有侧重点,如:refusal 强调推却,rejection 强调抵制,declination 强调婉言谢绝,而 denial 在下述真题例句中强调拒绝颁发的意义。
【经典例题】Failure in a required subject may result in the denial of a diploma.
【译　　文】如果有一门必修课程不及格,就拿不到毕业证书。

denote
[diˈnəut]
vt. 意思是;表示,是……的标志
【经典例题】A red face often denotes embarrassment or shyness.
【译　　文】脸儿通红经常意味着尴尬或害羞。

denounce
[diˈnauns]
vt. 指责;告发
【名师导学】近义词:condemn, charge, blame, accuse, censure, criticize, indict, implicate, vilify, prosecute, revile, stigmatize, reproach, castigate, rail at, brand, boycott, rebuke
【经典例题】Would you rather denounce your stepmother?
【译　　文】你愿意揭发你的继母吗?

deny
[diˈnai]
v. 否定,否认;拒绝,谢绝
【固定搭配】deny doing sth. 否认做某事;deny oneself 节制,克己,拒绝;deny sb. sth. 拒绝给予某人某物
【名师导学】deny 后接动名词,不接动词不定式。
【经典例题】Some teenagers harbor a generalized resentment against society, which denies them the rights and privileges of adults, although physically they are mature.
【译　　文】一些青少年对社会怀有普遍的怨恨,因为尽管他们在生理上已经成熟,但社会仍不给予他们成人的权利。

depart
[diˈpɑːt]
v. 出发,离开
【固定搭配】depart for, make for 动身去

departure
[diˈpɑːtʃə]
n. 离开,出发

☐ **dependent** [di'pendənt]	*a.* (on / upon) 依靠的，依赖的，从属的 【固定搭配】be dependent on 依靠；be independent of 独立于 【经典例题】Food production is dependent on water. 【译　　文】食物的生产离不开水。
☐ **depict** [di'pikt]	*v.* 描绘，描写，描述 【名师导学】表达"描述"意义的单词还有 describe（描述，形容），如：The driver described the accident to the police.（司机向警方描述了这起事故。）picture（构想，生动描绘），如：It is hard to picture the life of the old days.（很难想象过去人们的生活是什么样的。）portray（描绘，扮演），如：She successfully portrayed Jones and won her an Oscar.（她成功地扮演了琼斯的角色并为自己赢得了一次奥斯卡奖。） 【经典例题】The artist tried to depict realistically the Battle of Waterloo. 【译　　文】这位画家试图逼真地刻画滑铁卢战役。
☐ **deplore** [di'plɔː]	*vt.* 悲悼，痛惜
☐ **deploy** [di'plɔi]	*v.* 部署，调动
☐ **deport** [di'pɔːt]	*vt.* 把……驱逐出境
☐ **deposit** [di'pɔzit]	*vt.* 存放，寄存；储蓄；使沉淀 *n.* 存款，押金，保证金；沉淀物 【固定搭配】deposit sth. with sb. 把某物寄放在某人处
☐ **depress** [di'pres]	*vt.* 压抑；降低 【经典例题】When business is depressed, there is usually an obvious increase in unemployment. 【译　　文】当经济下滑时，失业率就会有明显的上升。
☐ **depression** [di'preʃən]	*n.* 不景气，萧条，沮丧，消沉 【经典例题】Many people lost their jobs during the business depression. 【译　　文】经济不景气时，许多人都失去了工作。
☐ **deprive** [di'praiv]	*vt.* 剥夺，夺去，使丧失 【名师导学】该词最常见的用法为 be deprived of。 【经典例题】They were imprisoned and deprived of their basic rights. 【译　　文】他们遭到监禁并被剥夺了基本权利。
☐ **deputy** ['depjuti]	*n.* 代理人，代表；副职 *a.* 代理的，副的
☐ **derivative** [di'rivətiv]	*n.* 派生物，衍生物 *a.* 非独创性的，模仿他人的
☐ **derive** [di'raiv]	*vi.* 起源 *vt.* 得自 【经典例题】The symbols were derived from Chinese. 【译　　文】这些符号来自中文。
☐ **descend** [di'send]	*vi.* 下来，下降 【经典例题】We managed to reach the top of the mountain, and half an hour later we began to descend. 【译　　文】我们努力到达了山顶，半个小时之后我们开始下山。

descendant
[di'send(ə)nt]

n. 后裔，子孙
【经典例题】Some descendants of Confucius were said to dwell in this small southern village for ages.
【译　　文】据说在这座南方的小山村里老早就居住着孔老夫子的一些子孙。

descent
[di'sent]

n. 降下；血统，出身
【经典例题】He was born an Asian descent but spoke British English because he was brought up by a British family.
【译　　文】他具备亚洲血统，但因为在一个英国家庭被抚养长大，所以他说的语言是英语。

deserve
[di'zə:v]

vt. 应受，值得
【联想记忆】preserve *v.* 保藏，保存；reserve *v.* 保留
【名师导学】deserve 后可接动名词和不定式：deserve doing=deserve to be done。
【经典例题】One thing, however, is certain: your chances of getting the raise you feel you deserve are less if you don't at least ask for it.
【译　　文】然而这一点是肯定的：如果你甚至都不去争取，那么你得到的你觉得应得的加薪机会就会更少。

designate
['dezigneit]

v. 指明，标明，指出；指派，指定
【经典例题】Junior Peter was designated as his only successor.
【译　　文】小彼得被指定为他的唯一继承人。

desolate
['desəlit] *a.*
['desəleit] *v.*

a. 荒凉的，荒芜的；孤独的，凄凉的　*v.* 使荒芜，使孤寂

despatch
[dis'pætʃ]

vt. 派遣，发送　*n.* （公文）急件，快信；（记者发回的）新闻报道；派遣，调遣　*a.* 衰退的，堕落的

despair
[dis'pɛə]

vi. / n. 失望，绝望
【固定搭配】in despair 绝望地；despair of 对……丧失信心

desperate
['despərit]

a. 绝望的，危急的；不顾一切的，铤而走险的
【经典例题】Thousands of Mexicans arrive each day in this city, desperate for economic opportunities.
【译　　文】每天都有成千上万的墨西哥人到达这个城市，渴望获得发财的机会。

despise
[dis'paiz]

vt. 鄙视，看不起
【名师导学】近义词：scorn, disdain, hate, look down on, spurn, sneer at, flout, dislike, loathe, detest, abhor
【经典例题】Certainly the last thing an Englishman should despise is poetry.
【译　　文】英国人是绝不会轻视诗歌的。

despite
[dis'pait]

prep. 不管，不顾
【名师导学】despite=in spite of，两者都是介词，后接名词性结构。although / though 是连词，接从句。
【经典例题】Despite all our efforts to save the museum, the authorities decided to close it.
【译　　文】尽管我们竭尽全力挽救这个博物馆，当局还是决定关闭它。

☐ **destination** [ˌdestiˈneiʃən]	*n.* 目的地，终点；目的，目标
☐ **destined** [ˈdestind]	*a.* 注定的，预定的
☐ **destiny** [ˈdestini]	*n.* 命运，定数
☐ **destruction** [disˈtrʌkʃən]	*n.* 破坏，毁灭

☐ **destructive** [disˈtrʌktiv]

n. 破坏（性）的

【名师导学】近义词：adverse, negative, unfavorable; ruinous, noxious, fatal, deleterious, pestilential, catastrophic, calamitous, disastrous, devastating, dire, lethal, mortal, mischievous, detrimental, annihilative, hurtful, harmful, subversive, murderous, disruptive, suicidal, evil, injurious, toxic, baleful, disintegrative, corrosive, corroding, erosive, eroding, damaging

【经典例题】The electronic economy made possible by information technology allows the haves to increase their control on global markets with destructive impact on the have-nots.

【译　　文】信息技术所带动的电子经济使得富国增强了对国际市场的掌控能力，而给贫穷国家带去了毁灭性的影响。

☐ **detach** [diˈtætʃ]	*v.* 分开，分离，分派，解开
☐ **detail** [ˈdiːteil, diˈteil]	*n. / vt.* 细节；说情；枝节，琐事；详述，详谈 【固定搭配】in detail 详细地
☐ **detailed** [ˈdiːteild]	*a.* 详细的
☐ **detain** [diˈtein]	*v.* 拘留，扣押 【经典例题】One man has been detained for questioning. 【译　　文】一个男人被拘留审问。
☐ **detect** [diˈtekt]	*vt.* 察觉，发觉
☐ **detection** [diˈtekʃən]	*n.* 察觉，发觉；侦察；探测

☐ **deter** [diˈtəː(r)]

v. 制止；阻止；威慑；使不敢

【经典例题】Fluoride <u>deters</u> tooth decay by reducing the growth of bacteria that destroy tooth enamel.
A. inhibits　　B. loosens　　C. hastens　　D. triggers　　[A]
【译　　文】氟化物通过减少破坏牙釉质的细菌的生长来阻止蛀牙。

☐ **deteriorate** [diˈtiəriəreit]

v. （使）恶化，变坏，蜕变

【经典例题】Some scientists are dubious of the claim that organisms deteriorate with age as an inevitable outcome of living.

【译　　文】有机组织随着年龄的增长而退化是不可避免的自然生理现象，对这一论断有些科学家持怀疑态度。

【联想记忆】动词 deteriorate 使恶化，变坏；
【经典例题】The recent deterioration in the economy is of great concern to the government.
A. depression　　　　　B. deficiency
C. degeneration　　　　D. deformity　　　　　　　　　　[C]
【译　　文】近期的经济恶化成了政府的关注点。

determination
[diˌtəːmiˈneiʃən]

n. 决心，决定

detrimental
[ˌdetriˈmentl]

a. 有害的，不利的
【经典例题】The chemical was found to be detrimental to human health.
A. toxic　　　B. immune　　　C. sensitive　　D. allergic　　[A]
【译　　文】人们发现这种化学品对人类健康有害。

devastate
[ˈdevəsteit]

v. 使荒芜，破坏；压倒
【经典例题】It will be a devastating blow for the patient, if the clinic closes.
A. permanent　B. desperate　C. destructive　D. sudden　　[C]
【译　　文】如果关闭门诊，对病人将是毁灭性的打击。
【名师导学】ravage, desolate, waste; overwhelm, confound, crush

develop
[diˈveləp]

vt. 发展，发达，发扬，进步，逐步展开（情节，音乐主题，方程式等）；洗印，显影 *vi.* 发展，生长，发育，逐步显示出来
【经典例题】The child may develop physically but will begin to show signs of emotional disturbance at an early age.
【译　　文】孩子身体会成长，但是很小就会开始显示情绪不稳定的症状。

development
[diˈveləpmənt]

n. 发展

deviate
[ˈdiːvieit]

vi. 背离，偏离

device
[diˈvais]

n. 设备，装置；方法，设计
【经典例题】Her husband is interested in designing electronic _____.
A. management　B. safety　　C. devices　　D. routine　　[C]
【译　　文】她的丈夫对设计电子设备很感兴趣。

devise
[diˈvaiz]

vt. 设计，想出，发明
【经典例题】The function of teaching is to create the conditions and the climate that will make it possible for children to devise the most efficient system for teaching themselves to read.
【译　　文】教育的作用是创造条件和气氛，使孩子们能够摸索出对于他们自学阅读最有效率的方法。

diagnose
[ˈdaiəgnəuz]

v. 诊断；判断
【经典例题】One of my neighbors caught a bad cold and went to his doctor, who diagnosed his cold as SARS.
【译　　文】我的一个邻居感冒得很厉害，看病时被医生诊断为非典型性肺炎。

diagnosis
[ˌdaiəgˈnəusis]

n. 诊断；调查分析
【名师导学】diagnosis 复数形式为 diagnoses（参见 analysis）。

dialect [ˈdaiəlekt]	*n.* 方言
diameter [daiˈæmitə]	*n.* 直径
dictate [dikˈteit]	*v.* 听写，口授，口述
diet [ˈdaiət]	*n.* 饮食，食物 【固定搭配】be / go on a diet 节食
dietary [ˈdaiətəri]	*a.* 饮食的；规定食物的 *n.* 规定食物
differentiate [ˌdifəˈrenʃieit]	*v.* 区别，区分 【名师导学】近义词：contrast, set apart, separate, discriminate, distinguish; modify, adapt, alter, change 【经典例题】This company does not differentiate between men and women—they employ both equally. 【译　　文】这家公司对男女职工一视同仁——男女职工都雇用。
dignity [ˈdigniti]	*n.* 威严，尊严 【经典例题】Poverty failed to make her lose her dignity. She stood there with head upward, confident as usual. 【译　　文】贫穷没能让她丧失尊严，她总是站在那儿，头高高地昂起，一如既往地自信。
digestive [diˈdʒestiv]	*a.* 消化的；有助消化的 【联想记忆】动词 digest；名词 digestion 【名师导学】absorb, suck, digest, incorporate 这些动词均有"吸收"之意。 absorb：普通用词，词义广泛，既可指吸收光、热、液体等具体东西，又可指吸收知识等抽象概念的东西。 suck：作"吸收"解时，可与 absorb 换用，但还可有"吮吸"之意。 digest：侧重在消化道内改变食物的化学结构后被人体吸收。 incorporate：指一物或多物与它物相融合，形成一整体。 summary, abstract, digest, outline, resume 这些名词均含"摘要，概要，概括"之意。 summary：普通用词，指将书籍或文章等的内容，用寥寥数语作简明扼要的说明。 abstract：指论文、书籍等正文前的内容摘要，尤指学术论文或法律文件的研究提要。 digest：侧重对原文融会贯通，重新谋篇布局，以简明扼要的语言，简短篇幅成文，展现原作精华。 outline：指配以释义文字的提纲。 resume：源于法语，与 summary 极相近，通常可互换使用。
dilemma [diˈlemə, dai-]	*n.* 困境，进退两难 【名师导学】该词在历年考题中均为词汇题选项。 【经典例题】The issue raises a moral dilemma. 【译　　文】这个问题引发了一个道德上的两难抉择。

第二部分 核心意义词汇（A-K）

□ diligent
['dilidʒənt]
a. 勤奋的，勤勉的
【名师导学】近义词：industrious, hard-working, assiduous, sedulous, studious, pertinacious, persevering, persistent, keen, tireless
【经典例题】I have nothing but one key to success: be diligent, whenever and wherever.
【译　　文】我成功的秘诀只有一个：无论何时何地，都要用功。

□ dilute
[dai'lju:t, di'l-]
v. 稀释，冲淡；*a.* 稀释的，冲淡的
【经典例题】Dilute wine with water.
【译　　文】掺水把酒冲淡。

□ dim
[dim]
a. 昏暗的；模糊不清的

□ dimension
[di'menʃən]
n. 尺寸，长（宽，厚，高）度；维（数）；(*pl.*) 容积，面积，大小

□ diminish
[di'miniʃ]
v. 减少，缩小
【名师导学】近义词：decrease, wane, abate, decline; decrease, lessen, reduce, abbreviate
【经典例题】Environmental worries and diminishing oil reserves would prohibit mass car use anywhere.
【译　　文】对环境恶化的担忧以及原油储备的减少将使得大量汽车上路的现象不复存在。

□ dioxide
[dai'ɔksaid]
n. 二氧化物

□ diploma
[di'pləumə]
n. 文凭，证书

□ diplomatic
[ˌdiplə'mætik]
a. 外交的

□ directory
[di'rektəri]
n. （规则、指令等）指南；通讯录；电话簿
【经典例题】I found the address and telephone number of this advertisement company in the directory.
【译　　文】我在地址簿上找到了这家广告公司的地址和电话号码。

□ disabled
[dis'eib(ə)ld]
a. 残疾的

□ disadvantage
[ˌdisəd'vɑ:ntidʒ]
n. 不利，不利条件；缺点，劣势

□ disarm
[dis'ɑ:m]
vt. 解除武装，裁军

□ disaster
[di'zɑ:stə]
n. 灾害，灾难，灾祸

□ disastrous
[di'zɑ:strəs]
a. 损失惨重的，灾难性的

discard [dis'kɑ:d]	vt. 丢弃，舍弃，抛弃
discern [di'sə:n]	v. 看出，觉察出；识别，认出 【经典例题】The child finds it hard to discern between blue and green. 【译　　文】那孩子对于分辨蓝绿二色感到有困难。
discharge [dis'tʃɑ:dʒ]	v. / n. 卸（货），解除，排出；释放，允许离开；放电
discipline ['disiplin]	n. 纪律，风纪；学科；训练　vt. 训练，训导；惩罚 【经典例题】Students must learn to discipline themselves. 【译　　文】学生必须学会自律。
disclose [dis'kləuz]	v. 透露，泄露 【名师导学】近义词：uncover, unveil, expose; confess, reveal, publish 【经典例题】The witness refuses to disclose his name and address. 【译　　文】这名目击者拒绝透露自己的姓名和住址。
disclosure [dis'kləuʒə]	n. 揭发，败露，透漏
discontent [,diskən'tent]	n. 不满
discount ['diskaunt]	n. 折扣，贴现（率）　vt. 打折扣 【经典例题】Students receive a 20 percent discount when they buy the book. 【译　　文】学生买这本书时给他们打八折。
discourage [dis'kʌridʒ]	vt. 使泄气，使失去信心 【固定搭配】discourage sb. from 劝阻某人做；persuade / encourage sb. to do 说服某人做某事 【名师导学】discourage 只能做及物动词，但不能说 discourage (sb.) to do，可以说 discourage doing sth.
discourse [dis'kɔ:s, 'diskɔ:s]	n. 论文，演说，讲道；谈话，交谈；语段，话语　v.（on, upon）讲述，著述
discreet [dis'kri:t]	a. 小心的，慎重的
discrepancy [dis'krepənsi]	n. 矛盾；偏差；亏损
discrete [dis'kri:t]	a. 不连续的，离散的
discriminate [dis'krimineit]	v.（between）区分，辨别；（against）歧视 【名师导学】使用该词时多搭配介词 from "将……同……区分开来"，between "区分，辨别" 以及 against "歧视，排斥"。 【经典例题】When do babies learn to discriminate voices? 【译　　文】婴儿什么时候学会辨别声音呢？
disguise [dis'gaiz]	n. 假装；化妆服　vt. 假装，扮作；隐瞒 vt. 假装；掩饰；隐瞒 【经典例题】They surface, heavily disguised, only in our dreams. 【译　　文】它们常常大力伪装后，只在我们的睡梦中显现。

disgust
[disˈgʌst]
n. 厌恶，反感

disgusting
[disˈgʌstiŋ]
a. 令人厌恶的，令人厌烦的

disillusion
[ˌdisiˈluːʒən]
n. 觉醒；幻灭

dismal
[dizml]
a. 阴沉的，凄凉的，暗的
【经典例题】The company still hopes to find a buyer, but the future looks bleak.
A. chilly　　B. dismal　　C. promising　　D. fanatic　　[B]
【译　文】公司仍然希望找到买主，但未来不容乐观。

dismay
[disˈmei]
n. 失望，气馁，惊愕　*vt.* 使失望，使惊愕
【经典例题】I was dismayed at Professor Smith's comment on my paper.
【译　文】听到史密斯教授对我的论文的评价，我感到沮丧。

dismiss
[disˈmis]
vt. 不再考虑；免职，解雇，开除；解散
【经典例题】The company was losing money, so they had to lay off some of its employees for three months.
A. owe　　B. dismiss　　C. recruit　　D. summon　　[B]
【译　文】公司正在亏损，因此他们不得不让部分员工停工3个月。

disorder
[disˈɔːdə]
n. 紊乱，混乱；骚动，骚乱；疾病，失调

dispatch / despatch
[disˈpætʃ]
v. 分派特定任务　*n.* 派遣

disperse
[disˈpəːs]
vi. 散开，分散　*vt.* 使消散，驱散
【名师导学】近义词：scatter, break up, separate, disband
【经典例题】The police dispersed the crowd and arrested two of the political activists.
【译　文】警察疏散了人群，并逮捕了两名政治激进分子。

displace
[disˈpleis]
vt. 取代，替代；迫使……离开家园，使离开原位
【经典例题】Television have displaced motion picture as America's most popular form of entertainment.
【译　文】电视取代了电影的地位，成了美国最为普遍的娱乐方式。

display
[diˈsplei]
vt. / n. 陈列，展览；显示
【固定搭配】on display 正在展览中
【经典例题】The museum displays the tools and clothes of the native Chinese.
【译　文】这个博物馆陈列着土生土长的中国人的生产工具和服饰。

disposal
[disˈpəuzəl]
n. 配置，布置，排列；处置，处理
【经典例题】The three disrespectful sons began to feel worried about the ultimate _____ of the family's property.
A. proposal　　B. disposal　　C. removal　　D. salvation　　[B]
【译　文】这三个不孝之子开始担心对家庭财产的最终处理问题。

□ **dispose** [dis'pəuz]	*vt.* 处置，布置；使倾向于，使有利于 *vi.* (of) 去掉，丢掉，除掉；处理，解决 【固定搭配】dispose of 处理，安排；排列；安放 【经典例题】He disposed of the problem quickly. 【译　　文】他很快解决了这个问题。
□ **disposition** [,dispə'ziʃən]	*n.* 性情，性格；意向，倾向；处置，布置，部署 【名师导学】在历年考题中该词均以词汇选择题干扰项出现，常见用法为 at sb.'s disposition，意为"随某人支配"；易混淆的词有：temper（脾气），personality（个性），以及 temperament（气质）。 【经典例题】Whether a person likes a routine office job or not depends largely on disposition. 【译　　文】一个人是否喜欢程式化的办公室工作很大程度上取决于性情。
□ **disputable** [dispjutbl]	*a.* 有争议的，可疑的 【经典例题】The idea of correcting defective genes is not particularly controversial in the scientific community. A. inevitable　B. applicable　C. disputable　D. incredible　　　　[C] 【译　　文】在科学界，矫正缺陷基因并没有什么争议。
□ **dispute** [dis'pju:t]	*v.* 争论，辩论，争吵 *n.* 争论，争端
□ **disregard** [,disri'ga:d]	*vt.* 忽视，忽略，漠视，不顾 *n.* 忽视，漠视
□ **disrupt** [dis'rʌpt]	*vt.* 使混乱，使崩溃，使分裂，使瓦解 【经典例题】The successive storms seriously disrupted the transportation in Beijing and consequently brought a series of car accidents. 【译　　文】连续不断的暴风雪严重干扰了北京的交通秩序，并随之导致了一系列的交通事故。
□ **disseminate** [di'semineit]	*vt.* 散布，传播
□ **dissolve** [di'zɔlv]	*v.* 溶解，融化；解除，解散，取消 【名师导学】辨析 dissolve, melt：dissolve 指固体被溶解于液体中；melt 指固体受热后熔化。
□ **distill** [di'stil]	*vt.* 蒸馏，提取，精炼
□ **distinct** [dis'tiŋkt]	*a.* 不同的；清楚的，明显的，显著的 【固定搭配】be distinct from 与……不同的
□ **distinction** [dis'tiŋkʃən]	*n.* 区别 【经典例题】We should make a clear　　　　between the two scientific terms for the purpose of our discussion. A. distinction　B. discrimination　C. deviation　　D. separation　　　[A] 【译　　文】我们应该对这两个科学术语进行明确的区分，这样才能有利于我们的讨论。

distinctive
[dis'tiŋktiv]

a. 明显不同的，特别的，突出的

【联想记忆】distinct 明显的，独特的；distinctive 有特色的，与众不同的
【经典例题】And more is being learned about its distinctive pathology.
【译　　文】人们对它独特病理学的认知不断加深。
【名师导学】distinct, distinctive 是两个形近单词。

distinct：意思是"分明的，明了的，清楚的"（well-marked, clearly defined or easily discernible）。distinct 还可用以表示"不同的，有区别的"

distinctive：The photo you took in the Hong Kong Cultural Centre is not distinct enough. 你在香港文化中心拍的那张照片不够清晰。

distinctive 意思是"表示差别的，有特色的，特殊的"（marking or showing a difference）。如 Can you find the distinctive watermarks of this stamp? 你能找到这枚邮票上有明显的水纹吗？

peculiar, characteristic, individual, distinctive 这些形容词均含"特有的，显示特征的"之意。

peculiar：侧重指某人或某物本身与众不同；也可指种族、民族或性别有其无可争议的特点。

characteristic：侧重指具有区别能力的，典型的或本质的特征。

individual：指特指的人或物，着重其与众不同，强调可将其区别出的品质与特性。

distinctive：突出与众不同的或令人称赞的个性或特征。

distinguish
[dis'tiŋgwiʃ]

v. 区别，辨别，辨认出

【固定搭配】distinguish...from 区分，辨别；distinguish oneself 使自己出名
【经典例题】The microscope enables scientists to distinguish an incredible number and variety of bacteria.
【译　　文】科学家通过显微镜能够辨别出大量的很多种类的细菌。
【经典例题】The factor that＿＿＿＿this company from the competition is customer service.
　A．keeps　　B．separates　　C．distinguishes　D．prevents　　　　　[C]
【译　　文】这家公司在竞争中脱颖而出的关键在于他们的客户服务。

distort
[dis'tɔ:t]

v. 曲解，歪曲

【名师导学】该词主要为阅读和词汇选择题，动词后加 ed 变成形容词词形，意为"被扭曲的，被误解的"。
【经典例题】Many Americans harbor a grossly distorted and exaggerated view of most of the risks surrounding food.
【译　　文】许多美国人对食品周遭暗藏的多数危险因素怀着非常扭曲和夸大的态度。

distract
[dis'trækt]

vt. 使……分心，使分散注意力

【经典例题】Although we tried to concentrate on the lecture, we were distracted by the noise from the next room.
【译　　文】尽管我们试图将注意力集中在讲座上，但隔壁房间传来的噪声还是让我们分了神。

distracted
[dis'træktid]

a. 分神的，心烦意乱的

distress
[dis'tres]

n. 苦恼，悲痛；危难，不幸　*vt.* 使苦恼，使痛苦

【经典例题】Yet occurrences of shortages and droughts are causing famine and distress in some areas, and industrial and agricultural by-products are polluting water supplies.

【译　　文】然而水资源的短缺和干旱正使一些地方面临着饥荒和贫困，而工业和农业的副产品正在污染水资源。

distribute
[dis'tribju(:)t]

vt. 分发，分送，配给；分布

【经典例题】Local government officials skim money off the top as they distribute funds and business owners pay them brides to win contacts and inflate project costs.

【译　　文】当地政府官员在发放基金的时候就把钱抽走，一些企业乘机向他们行贿从而争取到合同并同时哄抬项目的成本。

diverge
[dai'və:dʒ]

vi. 分歧；分开，叉开；偏离，背离　*vt.* 使发散；使偏离

【经典例题】These included ignoring those whose interests diverged from their own and belittling colleagues in front of students.

【译　　文】这些（行为）包括忽视那些与自己的研究方向有分歧的人，在学生面前贬低同事。

diverse
[dai'və:s]

a. 不同的，多种多样的

【固定搭配】be diverse / different from 与……不同

【经典例题】It is equally true that, in studying the diverse wisdom of others, we learn how to think.

【译　　文】同样正确的是，在学习其他人不同的智慧的时候，我们学会了如何去思考。

diversion
[dai'və:ʃən]

n. 偏离，转向；注意力分散

【联想记忆】动词 diverge，转移，分散注意力；diverse 不同的，多种多样的；diversity 多样性；

【经典例题】One of the most noticeable features of U.S. society is the diversity of its people.

A. liberty　　B. democracy　　C. variety　　D. origin

【译　　文】美国社会的一个最显著的特征是人群的多样化。

【名师导学】diverge deviate 这两个动词都有"偏离，离轨"之意。
diverge：指从一主道分成 Y 形。
deviate：强调离开思想、行动或规则的惯例。
DNA *abbr.* 脱氧核糖核酸

divert
[dai'və:t]

vt. 使转向，使转移

【经典例题】The government planned to divert the water from rivers into fields.

【译　　文】政府部门计划将水从河里引向田间。

dividend
['dividend]

n. 红利

divine
[di'vain]

a. 神的，神圣的，神授的

【经典例题】Divine songs flew in the air when Christmas was approaching.

【译　　文】圣诞节来临之际，到处都能听到圣歌。

divorce
[di'vɔ:s]

v. / *n.* 离婚，离异；分离

第二部分 核心意义词汇（A-K）

dizzy ['dizi]
a. 头昏眼花的
【经典例题】Climbing so high made me feel dizzy.
【译　　文】爬那么高使我感到头晕目眩。

document ['dɔkjumənt]
n. 文件，文献

domain [də'mein]
n.（活动、思想等）领域，范围；领地，势力范围
【名师导学】该词源于拉丁语 dominium，意为"财产"，常见用法有 out of one's domain，意为"不是某人的专长"；the domain of sth.，意为"在某个领域"。
【经典例题】If you do not confirm this Internet domain change with your ISP, you will not be able to send or receive E-mail.
【译　　文】如果不与 ISP 确认该 Internet 域的更改，你将无法收发电子邮件。

domestic [də'mestik]
a. 家里的，家庭的；国内的，国产的；驯养的
【经典例题】Instead, for all uses except the domestic demand of the poor, governments should price water to reflect its actual value.
【译　　文】政府应该将除了国内的穷人使用外的用水进行定价收费，以表明水的实际价值。

dominant ['dɔminənt]
a. 支配的，统治的，居高临下的；显性的

dominate ['dɔmineit]
vt. 支配，统治，控制；高出于，居高临下 *vi.* 居支配地位，处于最重要的地位
【经典例题】For the past two years, Audi cars have＿＿＿＿ Germany's Touring Car Championship.
　A. dominated　　　　　　B. conquered
　C. determined　　　　　　D. contested　　　　　　　　　[A]
【译　　文】在过去的两年中，奥迪汽车一直是德国房车冠军赛的冠军。

donate [dəu'neit]
v. 捐赠，馈赠
【经典例题】The president donated thousands of books to the local library and visited the local schools with his wife.
【译　　文】总统向当地的图书馆捐赠了成千上万本图书，并和夫人一起参观了当地的几所学校。

donation [dəu'neiʃən]
n. 捐献，捐款
【经典例题】The television station is supported by＿＿＿＿ from foundations and other sources.
　A. donations　　　　　　B. pensions
　C. advertisements　　　　D. accounts　　　　　　　　　　[A]
【译　　文】电视台是由基金会及其他资金来源的捐款支持的。

doom [du:m]
vt. 注定，命定 *n.* 厄运，劫数
【名师导学】表达"命运，定数"意义的单词还有 fortune，fate，lot，destiny 等；用作动词时，doom 的用法为 be doomed to sth.。
【经典例题】A sense of impending doom gripped her.
【译　　文】她有一种大难临头的压迫感。

dose [dəus]
n. 剂量，一服，一剂

175

dot [dɔt]
n. 点，圆点
【固定搭配】on the dot 准时；to a / the dot 丝毫不差地

doubtful ['dautful]
a. 怀疑的，不相信的；可疑的；难料的
【固定搭配】be / feel doubtful of / about sth. 对某事有怀疑

download ['daunləud]
n. / v. 下载

doze [dəuz]
n. / v. 打瞌睡

draft [drɑːft]
n. 草稿，草案，草图 *vt.* 起草，草拟

drain [drein]
n. 耗竭，消耗，排水管，水沟，下水道 *vt.* 排（水），放（水），放干
【经典例题】After ten years in the same job her enthusiasm finally _____.
A. deteriorated   B. dispersed
C. dissipated   D. drained   [D]
【译　文】经过10年的重复工作，她的热情最终消失殆尽。

drainage ['dreinidʒ]
n. 排水；排泄设备

drama ['drɑːmə]
n. 戏剧，剧本
【名师导学】辨析 drama, opera：drama 指在舞台上演的戏剧；opera 指歌剧，在戏院上演的配有音乐的戏剧表演。

dramatic [drə'mætik]
a. 戏剧的，戏剧性的；引人注目的 *n.* (*pl.*) 戏剧，戏曲

drastic ['dræstik]
a. 激烈的，强有力的，彻底的

drawback ['drɔːbæk]
n. 因难，缺点，不足之处
【经典例题】Is it true that this is the major drawback of the new medical plan?
【译　文】那就是新的医疗计划的主要缺点，这是真的吗？

dread [dred]
n. 恐惧，恐怖，可怕的人（或物）*v.* 惧怕，担心

dreadful ['dredfəl]
a. 可怕的
【名师导学】近义词：terrible, appalling, fearful, frightful, offensive
【经典例题】They told us the dreadful news.
【译　文】他们告诉了我们那糟糕透顶的消息。

dreary ['driəri]
a. 沉闷的，枯燥的，无味的，令人沮丧的

drip [drip]
vi. 滴下；漏水 *n.* 滴，水滴，点滴
【名师导学】辨析 drip, drop：drip 指液体的"滴，滴下"；drop 指"落下，降落"，从较高地方或位置落到低地方或位置。
【经典例题】The rain was dripping from the trees.
【译　文】雨水从树上滴落。

drizzle ['drizl]
vi. 下毛毛雨 *n.* 毛毛雨

dropout
['drɔpaut]

n. 退学学生；中途退学

drought
[draut]

n. 旱灾

【经典例题】The soil is fertile, productive and drought-enduring.
【译　　文】这是一片肥沃的土地，多产且耐旱。

drowsy
['drauzi]

adj. 昏昏欲睡的；沉寂的；催眠的；呆滞的

【经典例题】Inform the manager if you are on medication that makes you drowsy.
A. uneasy　　B. sleepy　　C. guilty　　D. fiery　　　[B]
【译　　文】如果你服用的药物让你昏昏欲睡，就告诉经理。

dual
['dju(:)əl]

a. 双的；二重的；二元的

【经典例题】In the past, American colleges and universities were created to serve a dual purpose.
【译　　文】过去，美国高校都是为了双重目的而设立。

dubious
['dju:biəs]

n. 怀疑的，犹豫不决的，无把握的；有问题的，靠不住的

【经典例题】Why people are prepared to tolerate a four-hour journey each day for the dubious privilege of living in the country is beyond my ken.
【译　　文】为了追求在农村生活的所谓好处，人们甘愿忍受每天在路上花四个小时，真是让我大跌眼镜。

dumb
[dʌm]

a. 哑的，无声的

【联想记忆】deaf *a.* 聋的
【经典例题】During the war, soldiers remained dumb despite torture.
【译　　文】在战争期间，士兵们忍受刑罚而不开口。

duplicate
['dju:plikeit] *vt.*
['dju:plikət] *n.*

vt. 复制　*n.* 复制品，副本

【经典例题】His task will be to duplicate his success overseas here at home.
【译　　文】他在海外取得了成功，现在的任务就是要在国内再创辉煌。

durable
['djuərəbl]

a. 耐久的

【经典例题】They are often more comfortable and more durable than civilian clothes.
【译　　文】它们要比平时穿的衣服更舒适耐磨。

duration
[djuə'reiʃən]

n. 持续，持续时间

dwarf
[dwɔ:f]

n. 个头矮小的人　*vt.* 使矮小，阻碍发育

dwell
[dwel]

vi. 居住

【名师导学】该词在历年考题中多数为词汇选择题。dwell 为"居住"的含义，而 dwell on 则表示"详细描述，仔细研究；停留，驻足于"。
【经典例题】I'd rather not dwell on the past.
【译　　文】我不想再沉湎于过去了。

dynamic
[dai'næmik]

a. 有活力的；动力的

【经典例题】He was such a ＿＿＿ teacher that he held our attention every minute of the two-hour class.
A. ambitious　B. dynamic　　C. heroic　　D. diplomatic　　[B]
【译　　文】他是一个有活力的老师，在两小时的课程中他一直紧紧地吸引着我们的注意力。

earnest ['ə:nist]	*a.* 认真的，热心的 【名师导学】辨析 earnest, sincere：earnest 指表现出高度真诚和认真的；sincere 指真诚的，不虚伪的或不假装的。 【经典例题】It is my earnest wish that you use this money to continue your study of music. 【译　　文】我真挚地希望你能用这笔钱继续学习音乐。
earthquake ['ə:θkweik]	*n.* 地震 【经典例题】Most of the houses in the city were destroyed in the earthquake. 【译　　文】城里大多数的房子在地震中毁了。
ease [i:z]	*n.* 容易，轻易；安逸，安心 *v.* 减轻，放松，缓和 【固定搭配】at ease 自由自在地，舒服地；with ease, easily 容易地；ease sb. of 减轻某人
easy-going [i:zi'gəuiŋ]	*a.* 随和的
eccentric [ik'sentrik]	*a.* （人、行为、举止等）古怪的，怪癖的，异乎寻常的 *n.* 古怪的人，有怪癖的人 【经典例题】It is generally known that New York is a city and a center for eccentric odd bits of information. 【译　　文】众所周知，纽约这座城市就是个蕴藏着各种离奇古怪见闻的信息中心。
echo ['ekəu]	*n.* 回声，反响 *v.* 发出回声，共鸣 【经典例题】The valley was filled with the echoes of our voices. 【译　　文】山谷中充满了我们自己声音的回声。
eclipse [i'klips]	*n.* （日、月）食 *vt.* 使暗淡，使失色，使相形见绌
ecology [i(:)'kɔlədʒi]	*n.* 生态学；生态系统 【名师导学】可遵循构词法记忆此类单词，如以 -ology 结尾的单词大多为某一门学科，如 biology（生物学），geology（地质学）等。 【经典例题】Chemicals in the factory's sewerage system have changed the ecology of the whole area. 【译　　文】这座工厂排出的化学物质改变了整个地区的生态。
economic [,i:kə'nɔmik]	*a.* 经济的，经济学的 【联想记忆】financial *a.* 财政的，金融的；commercial *a.* 商业的 【经典例题】At first, the exchange has been confined to culture but extended to the economic and other fields. 【译　　文】开始这种交流仅限于文化领域，但是后来延伸到了经济和其他领域。

economical
[ˌiːkəˈnɔmikəl]

a. 节俭的，节省的，经济的

【名师导学】辨析 economic, economical：economic 表示经济的或与之有关的，经济学的或与之有关的；economical 表示节俭的，不浪费或不挥霍的，节约的，通过高效率的运作和削减不必要的性能来节省费用的。

economy
[i(ː)ˈkɔnəmi]

n. 经济，经济制度；节约，节省

【经典例题】In the information economy, value has shifted rapidly from tangible to intangible assets.

【译　文】在知识经济中，价值已经快速从有形资产向无形资产转移。

edible
[ˈedibl]

a. 可以吃的，可食用的

【经典例题】Such kind of flower is edible and on sale in supermarkets.

【译　文】此类花卉可供食用，超市里均有销售。

edit
[ˈedit]

vt. 编辑

edition
[iˈdiʃən]

n. 版，版本，版次

editorial
[ediˈtɔːriəl]

n. 社论

educate
[ˈedju(ː)keit]

vt. 教育，培养，训练

【经典例题】An educator must first educate himself.

【译　文】教育者必须自己先受教育。

effective
[iˈfektiv]

a. 有效的，生效的

【名师导学】辨析 effective, efficient, valid：effective 表示"有效的，具有预期或先见效果的"，既强调产生满意的效果，又注重不浪费时间、精力等因素，因此往往带有"有效率的"意味；efficient 意为"有能力的；高效率的"；valid 表示（法律上）有效的，正当的，或在一段时间、某种情况下有效的。

【经典例题】A proven method for effective textbook reading is the SQ3R method.

【译　文】经过证明的一种有效的阅读课本的方法是 SQ3R 方法。

efficiency
[iˈfiʃənsi]

n. 效率，功效

efficient
[iˈfiʃənt]

a. 效率高的，有能力的

ego
[ˈiːgəu]

n. 自我，自己，自尊

eject
[iˈdʒekt]

vt. 驱逐，逐出；喷射，排出

【经典例题】Many types of rock are ejected from volcanoes as solid, fragmentary material.

【译　文】火山喷发的岩石中有许多都是坚硬而碎裂的。

elaborate
[iˈlæbərət] *a.*
[iˈlæbəreit] *v.*

a. 精细的，详尽的　*v.* 详细描述

【经典例题】Elaborate preparations were being made for the Prime Minister's official visit to the four foreign countries.

【译　文】就总理对四国的正式访问作了详尽的准备。

elapse
[i'læps]
vi. 时间消逝

elastic
[i'læstik]
n. 橡皮圈，松紧带　*a.* 有弹性的，弹力的；灵活的，可伸缩的
【经典例题】Our plans are still very elastic.
【译　　文】我们的计划仍然是有弹性的。

elasticity
[ilæs'tisiti]
n. 弹性，弹力

elderly
['eldəli]
a. 上了年纪的，垂老的

elegant
['eligənt]
a. 优雅的，高雅的，漂亮的

element
['elimənt]
n. 元素；成分，要素
【经典例题】There are three elements to hydrotherapy: heat, buoyancy, and motion.
【译　　文】水疗三大要素为：热、浮力和运动。

elementary
[,eli'mentəri]
a. 初等的；基本的

elevate
['eliveit]
vt. 提升……的职位，提高，改善；使情绪高昂，使兴高采烈；举起，使上升
【名师导学】近义词：hoist, heave, tilt, levitate, raise; advance, upgrade, further, promote
【经典例题】Will male-dominated companies elevate women to higher-paid jobs as they elevate men?
【译　　文】男士主宰的公司会像他们提拔男士一样提拔女士到高薪岗位吗？

elevation
[,eli'veiʃn]
n. 提拔，海拔，提高；　[计算机] 标高
【经典例题】The temperature of the atmosphere becomes colder as elevation increases.
A. altitude　　B. aptitude　　C. latitude　　D. longitude　　[A]
【译　　文】海拔越高，大气温度越低。

elicit
[i'lisit]
vt. 诱出，引出，探出

eligible
['elidʒəbl]
a. 有资格的；合格的，适宜的
【名师导学】本词属于常考词汇，考生要注意相关短语：eligible for something（符合），eligible to do something（有资格去做）。
【经典例题】Only native-born citizens are eligible for the U.S. presidency.
A. obliged　　B. intelligible　　C. competent　　D. qualified　　[D]
【译　　文】只有本国出生的公民才有资格担任美国总统的职务。

eliminate
[i'limineit]
vt. 消灭，除去，排出
【经典例题】She has been eliminated from the swimming race because she did not win any of the practice races.
【译　　文】她已被取消了参加游泳比赛的资格，因为她在训练中没有得到名次。

elite [ei'li:t]
n. 精华，名流
【经典例题】We have a political elite in this country.
【译　　文】我们国家有一群政治精英。

eloquent ['eləkwənt]
a. 雄辩的，有口才的，动人的，意味深长的

elsewhere ['els,hwer]
ad. 在别处
【经典例题】Better to join forces with the military for this trial and spend the money saved elsewhere.
【译　　文】最好能与军方联合行动进行实验，把节省下来的钱用于其他地方。

emaciate [i'meiʃieit]
v. （使）消瘦，（使）憔悴

emancipate [i'mænsipeit]
vt. 解除（束缚），解放（from）；解脱，摆脱（思想上疑虑、偏见等）

embark [im'bɑ:k]
v. 乘船，上船，搭乘
【名师导学】本词属于常考词汇，考生要注意相关短语 embark on（着手，开始做）。作为"上船""上飞机"的意思时，既可用作及物动词也可用作不及物动词。
【经典例题】We have embarked on the most important and wide-ranging reforms since 1992.
【译　　文】1992年以来，我们着手进行了最重大、涉及领域最广泛的改革。

embarrass [im'bærəs]
vt. 使窘迫，使困惑，使为难
【固定搭配】to one's embarrassment 让某人尴尬的是
【经典例题】To our embarrassment, my friend and I discover that neither of us has cash, and my credit card is not good here.
【译　　文】让我们尴尬的是，我和我的朋友发现，我俩都没带现金，信用卡在这里也无法使用。

embody [im'bɔdi]
vt. 使具体化，具体表现，体现；包括，包含
【经典例题】Such institutions embody the value of solidarity and the duty of mutual help, without which a society cannot survive.
【译　　文】这种体系体现了团结的价值观和相互帮助的责任感，没有这些，一个社会是难以存续的。

embrace [im'breis]
vt. 抱，拥抱；包括，包含；包围，环绕

emerge [i'mə:dʒ]
vi. 出现；浮现，显露
【经典例题】Advanced figures are emerging in multitude in this era of ours.
【译　　文】在我们这个时代先进人物正在大量地涌现出来。

emergency [i'mə:dʒənsi]
n. 紧急情况，突然事件
【经典例题】Mexicans are able to adapt themselves to the current emergency.
【译　　文】墨西哥人能够很好地适应目前的紧急情况。

emigrate ['emigreit]
vi. 移居外国，移民

emigrant
['emigrənt]
a. 移居的；移民的，侨居的

eminent
['eminənt]
adj.（尤指在某专业中）卓越的，著名的，显赫的；非凡的；杰出的
【联想记忆】prominent, remarkable, distinguished, obvious, clear, noted, renowned, famous
【经典例题】I would like to thank this eminent scholar and friend for his valuable contribution to the debate on this issue.
【译　　文】我要感谢这位杰出的学者和朋友对这个问题的辩论做出的宝贵贡献。
【经典例题】A group of eminent scientists from around the world have voted *Blade Runner* the best science fiction movie of all time.
【译　　文】来自世界各地的一群杰出科学家将《银翼杀手》评为有史以来最好的科幻电影。

emit
[i'mit]
vt. 发出，发射；散发（光、热、气味等）
【经典例题】The report is expected to call for the mobile phone industry to refrain from promoting phone use by children, and to start labeling phones with data on the amount of radiation they emit.
【译　　文】这份报告可能会倡导手机行业禁止儿童使用移动电话，并且开始将手机散发的辐射量数据用标签的形式展示出来。

emotion
[i'məuʃne]
n. 情感，情绪
【名师导学】emotion, feeling, passion：emotion 一般指比较强烈、深刻且能感动人的感情或情绪，多含精神上的反应，如爱、惧、哀、乐等；feeling 泛指人体的一切感觉、情绪和心情；passion 意为"激情"，往往指由于正确的判断受其影响而表现出强烈的或激烈的情绪，有时不能自持，甚或失去理智。
【经典例题】Love, hatred, and grief are emotions.
【译　　文】爱、恨、悲伤都是感情。

emotional
[i'məuʃənl]
a. 情绪的，情感的

emphasis
['emfəsis]
n. 强调，重点
【固定搭配】lay / put / place emphasis on / upon 注重，着重于，强调
【名师导学】emphasis 复数形式为 emphases（参见 analysis）。

emphasize
['emfəsaiz]
vt. 强调，着重
【经典例题】Advertisements showed pictures of the beautiful scenery that could be enjoyed along some of the more famous western routes and emphasized the romantic names of some of these trains (Empire Builder, etc).
【译　　文】广告展示了在沿途能够欣赏的一些有名的西部线路美丽景色的图片，而且还着重点强调了一些火车浪漫的名字（帝国建造者等）。

empirical
[em'pirikəl]
a. 经验主义的
【名师导学】本词属于常考词汇，记住它的反义词 theoretical（理论上的），就可以很好地理解 empirical 的含义。
【经典例题】His theory is inconsistent with the empirical evidence.
【译　　文】他的理论与以经验为根据的证据不一致。

employ
[im'plɔi]
vt. 雇用，使用

employment
[im'pləimənt]

职业，就业；雇用

【固定搭配】in the employment of 受雇于；be out of employment 失业

【经典例题】The father had arrived from his place of employment to the emergency department.

【译　　文】父亲从工作的地方赶到了急诊室。

emulate
['emjuleit]

vt. 同……竞赛（竞争）；努力赶上（超过）

enable
[i'neibl]

vt. 使能够，使可能

【固定搭配】enable sb. to do 使某人能做

enclose
[in'kləuz]

vt. 围住，圈起；封入，附上

【经典例题】The football field is enclosed by a wall.

【译　　文】足球场被一道墙围了起来。

encounter
[in'kauntə]

v. 遭遇，遇到

【经典例题】They encounter many principles of science daily.

【译　　文】他们每天都会遇到很多科学的原则。

encumber
[in'kʌmbə]

v. 妨害，阻碍

【经典例题】The biggest engineering project that they undertook was encumbered by lack of funds.

A. hampered　B. propelled　C. cancelled　D. haunted　[A]

【译　　文】他们接手的这项最大的工程由于缺乏资金而被耽搁了。

endeavour
[in'devə]

vi. 努力，尽力，尝试

【名师导学】近义词：attempt, aim, essay, strive, try, effort

【经典例题】Apart from philosophical and legal reasons for respecting patients' wishes, there are several practical reasons why doctors should endeavor to involve patients in their own medical care decisions.

【译　　文】除了在道义上和法律方面要求尊重病人的愿望之外，医生之所以努力让病人参与自己的医疗护理决策也有不少现实的原因。

ending
['endiŋ]

n. 终止，终了

endless
['endlis]

a. 无限的，无穷的

endorse
[in'dɔ:s]

v. 在（票据）背面签名，签注（文件），认可，签署

【经典例题】When the former President_____ her candidacy, she knew she had a good chance of being elected.

A. enforced　B. endorsed　C. followed up　D. put forward　[B]

【译　　文】当前总统支持她的时候，她就知道她当选的机会很大。

endow
[in'dau]

v. 捐赠，赋予

endurance
[in'djuərəns]

n. 忍耐（力），持久（力），耐久（性）

endure [in'djuə]	*vt.* 忍受，容忍 *vi.* 忍受，忍耐；持久，持续 【经典例题】He studied in detail Robert Schumann, the great composer, who was known to endure bouts of manic depression that drove him to attempt suicide. 【译　文】他仔细研究了伟大的作曲家罗伯特·舒曼，众所周知，他长期忍受精神抑郁的痛苦，甚至试图自杀。
enforce [in'fɔ:s]	*vt.* 实行，执行；强制，强迫 【固定搭配】enforce sth. on sb. 迫使某人干某事
enforcement [in'fɔ:smənt]	*n.* 执行，强制
engage [in'geidʒ]	*vt.* 使从事，使忙于；占用（时间等）；雇用，聘用；使订婚 *vi.* 从事于，参加 【固定搭配】be engaged in 正忙于，从事于；be engaged to 与……订婚
engagement [in'geidʒmənt]	*n.* 约会；婚约，诺言；交战，接站；雇用
engine ['endʒin]	*n.* 发动机，引擎；火车头，机车
engineering [,endʒi'niəriŋ]	*n.* 工程，工程学
engross [in'grəus]	*v.* 使全神贯注，独占，大量收购，正式誊写，用大字体书写 【经典例题】I was so absorbed in my work that I completely forgot the time. A. engraved　B. engrossed　C. enforced　D. enveloped　　[B] 【译　文】我太专注于工作，完全忘记了时间。
enhance [in'hɑ:ns]	*vt.* 提高，增强 【经典例题】Neuroscientists and psychologists at several universities have now enhanced understanding of just how the arts might improve thinking, memory, and language skills. 【译　文】几所大学里的神经科学家们和心理学家们深化了对艺术如何提升思维、记忆及语言技能的认识。
enlarge [in'lɑ:dʒ]	*vt.* 扩大，放大，增大 【名师导学】辨析 enlarge, expand, extend：enlarge 指尺寸、范围、能力的扩大；expand 表示膨胀，扩张，指的是增加尺寸、体积、数量或范围；extend 指伸长或扩展（某物）到较大程度或最大长度。
enlighten [in'laitn]	*vt.* 启发，开导 【经典例题】I see teaching as an opportunity to enlighten students, not just inform them. 【译　文】我认为教育是启迪学生的良机，而不只是传授他们知识。
enlist [in'list]	*v.* 征募，征召，参军
enormous [i'nɔ:məs]	*a.* 巨大的，庞大的 【名师导学】辨析 enormous, huge, immense, massive, vast：enormous 指在大小、范围、数目或程度上很大的；huge 一般指体积，也可指空间、距离、程度、容量等，强调体积之大超过一般标准；immense 强调大而不强调重量，所指

体积、数量、程度等大到无法用尺度衡量；massive 既强调大又强调重，有分量；vast 指范围的广大和数量的大，侧重于面积的极为开阔，但一般不用于体积的大小。

【经典例题】It brings us not only the enormous pressure, but also great opportunities.
【译　　文】这不仅给我们带来了巨大的压力，也带来了极大的机遇。

enquire [in'kwaiə]
v. =inquire 打听，询问；调查，查问

enrich [in'ritʃ]
vt. 使富裕，使丰富
【经典例题】It is important to enrich the soil prior to planting.
【译　　文】在种植前给土壤增肥很重要。

enroll [in'rəul]
vt. 登记；编入，招收
【经典例题】The club will enroll new members in the first week of September.
【译　　文】九月的第一个星期这家俱乐部将要招收新会员。

enrollment [in'rəulmənt]
n. 登记，注册；入伍，入会，入学

ensue [in'sju:]
vi. 跟着发生，继起

ensure [in'ʃuə]
vt. 确保，保证
【固定搭配】ensure (sb.) against sth. 使（某人）安全，避免
【经典例题】The government must＿＿＿＿ that the price of oil is controlled as rapidly as possible.
A. assure　　B. secure　　C. ensure　　D. issue　　[C]
【译　　文】政府必须确保石油的价格尽快得到控制。

entail [in'teil]
vt. 使承担，使成为必要，需要
【经典例题】I didn't want to take on a job that would entail a lot of traveling.
【译　　文】我不想做需要经常出差的工作。

enterprise ['entəpraiz]
n. 企业，事业

entertain [,entə'tein]
vt. 使欢乐，使娱乐；招待，款待

entertainment [,entə'teinmənt]
n. 娱乐，文娱节目，表演会；招待，款待，请客

enthusiasm [in'θju:ziæzəm]
n. 热情，热心，积极性

entitle [in'taitl]
vt. 给……题名；给……权利（资格）

entity ['entiti]
n. 实体，独立存在体，实际存在
【经典例题】Fish resources are diminishing because they are not owned by any particular entity.
【译　　文】鱼类资源逐渐枯竭是由于这种资源不属于任何企业和个人。

entrust [in'trʌst]
vt. 委托，托付

entry ['entri]
n. 进入，入场；入口，河口；登记，登录
【经典例题】This music film is Mrs. Wilson's entry in the competition.
【译　文】这部音乐片是威尔森夫人的参赛作品。

enzyme ['enzaim]
n. 酶

epidemic [,epi'demik]
n. 传染病，流行病　a. 流行的，传染性的
【经典例题】This year mark the 100th anniversary of the deadliest event U.S. history: the Spanish influenza epidemic of 1918.
【译　文】今年是美国历史上最致命的事件——1918年西班牙流感爆发100周年。

episode ['episəud]
n. 插曲，片段
【经典例题】Most episode of absent-mindedness — forgetting where you left something or wondering why you just entered a room — are caused by a simple lack of attention.
【译　文】许多健忘的生活小插曲，如忘记东西放在哪里或奇怪为什么进入一个房间等，都是仅仅由于没有用心的缘故。

equation [i'kweiʃən]
n. 方程式，等式
【经典例题】$x+2y=7$ is an equation.
【译　文】"$x+2y=7$"是方程式。

equator [i'kweitə]
n. 赤道
【经典例题】The Northern Hemisphere is the part of the world north of the equator, and the Southern Hemisphere is south of the equator.
【译　文】北半球是地球赤道以北的部分，南半球是赤道以南的部分。

equivalent [i'kwivələnt]
a. 相等的；等价的，等量的　n. 同等物，等价物，对等
【经典例题】A mile is equivalent to about 1.6 kilometers.
【译　文】1英里大约等于1.6千米。

era ['iərə]
n. 时代，年代，阶段

eradicate [i'rædikeit]
v. 根除
【名师导学】近义词群：extirpate, exterminate, annihilate; abolish, destroy

erase [i'reiz]
vt. 抹去，擦掉

erect [i'rekt]
a. 直立的，竖立的，笔直的　vt. 使竖立，使直立，树立，建立
【名师导学】辨析 erect, straight, upright, vertical：erect 形容事物或身体挺拔而不倾斜；straight 只有直的概念，并不表示直立的；upright 指与倾斜物相比几乎垂直；vertical 意为"垂直的"。
【经典例题】Angry owners have called on the government to erect sea defenses to protect their homes.
【译　文】愤怒的业主呼吁政府建立海上防护墙，以保护他们的家园。

erode
[i'rəud]
vt. 侵蚀，腐蚀，使变化

erosion
[i'rəuʒən]
n. 腐蚀，侵蚀
【经典例题】The sea has an important earth-shaping power, producing erosion through the action of the waves and tides.
【译　　文】通过波浪和潮汐的运动而产生侵蚀，海洋便有了造地的力量。

erupt
[i'rʌpt]
v. (火山等) 迸发，爆发
【经典例题】Violence erupted after police shot a student during the demonstration.
【译　　文】警察射杀了一名示威学生后，暴力活动爆发了。

essence
['esns]
n. 本质，实质；精华，精粹
【名师导学】近义词：core, gist, root, nature, basis, essential quality, spirit, reality, quintessence, constitution, substance
【经典例题】For most thinkers since the Greek philosophers, it was self-evident that there is something called human nature, something that constitutes the essence of man.
【译　　文】不言而喻，对于希腊哲学家及其后的思想家来说，有种叫作人性的东西；一种构成人的本质的东西。

essential
[i'senʃəl]
a. 必不可少的，必要的；本质的，实质的；基本的
【固定搭配】be essential to 对……是必要的
【名师导学】辨析 essential, necessary, indispensable：essential 指本质的，基本的或绝对必要的，强调基本性、本质性；necessary 指必不可少的，为达到某种目的而必须具备的，强调必需性；indispensable 强调不可或缺的。It's essential that 从句要用（should）+动词原形的虚拟语气
【经典例题】These concepts are essential to safe, efficient travel.
【译　　文】要安全高效地旅行，这些原则是必要的。

establish
[is'tæbliʃ]
n. 建立，设立，创办；确立，使确认
【经典例题】The Minister established a commission to suggest improvements in the educational system.
【译　　文】部长组织了一个委员会，为改进教育制度提供建议。

establishment
[is'tæbliʃmənt]
n. 建立，设立，确立；建立的机构（组织）

estate
[i'steit]
n. 不动产，财产

esteem
[is'ti:m]
n. / vt. 尊重，珍重

esthetic
[i:s'θetik]
a. 美学的，审美的；悦目的；雅致的

estimate
['estimeit] *vt.*
['estimət] *n.*
vt. / n. 估计，估价，评价
【经典例题】At the moment, doctors estimate fat content from knowing body volume and water content.
【译　　文】目前，医生从身体体积和含水量来估计脂肪含量。

ethnic ['eθnik]
a. 人种的

eternal [i(:)'tə:nl]
a. 永久的，不朽的

【名师导学】本词属于常考词汇，相关近义词有：everlasting（永恒的，持久的，无止境的，耐用的），infinite（无穷的，无限的，无数的，极大的），permanent（永久的，持久的），perpetual（永久的）。相关反义词有：momentary（瞬间的，刹那间的），temporary（暂时的，临时的，临时性的）。
【经典例题】Seeking perfection is the eternal theme of our factory.
【译　　文】追求完美是我厂永恒的主题。

evacuate [i'vækjueit]
vt. 转移，撤离，疏散

evade [i'veid]
v. 规避，逃避，躲避

evaluate [i'væljueit]
vt. 评价，评估

【派生词汇】evaluation *n.* 评估，评价
【经典例题】The proposal could not be evaluated because the details had not been published.
【译　　文】还不能评估这个建议，因为细节还没有披露。

evaporate [i'væpəreit]
v. 蒸发，气化

【派生词汇】evaporation *n.* 蒸发

evidence ['evidəns]
n. 证据，证物

【固定搭配】in evidence 明显的，显而易见的
【联想记忆】evidence *n.* 抽象意义的证据；proof *n.* 实物证据
【名师导学】辨析 evidence, proof, witness：evidence 一般指"物证"；proof 则强调构成事实的结论性的东西；witness 通常指"人证"。

evident ['evidənt]
a. 明显的，明白的

【经典例题】The cyclic preference for masculine faces was evident among 23 British women.
【译　　文】对男性特征脸庞周期性的偏好在 23 名英国女性中是很明显的。

evidently ['evidəntli]
ad. 明显地，显而易见地

evoke [i'vəuk]
vt. 唤起，引起，使人想起

【名师导学】近义词：elicit, provoke
【经典例题】"Yuppies" usually evokes a negative image.
【译　　文】雅皮士通常让人想起反面形象。

exacerbate [ig'zæsəbeit]
vt. 加重（使……恶化，激怒）

【经典例题】The symptoms may be ＿＿＿＿ by certain drugs.
A. exaggerated　B. exacerbated　C. exceeded　D. exhibited　　　　[B]
【译　　文】某些药品可能加剧症状。

exaggerate [ig'zædʒəreit]
v. 夸张，夸大

【经典例题】They exaggerated the function of the medicine.
【译　　文】他们夸大了这个药品的功能。

exasperate
[igˈzæspəreit]

vt. 使……恼怒，激怒，使恶化

【经典例题】The physician was becoming exasperated with all the questions they were asking.
A. frustrated　B. perplexed　C. irritated　D. crippled　　[C]
【译　　文】医生开始被他所问的问题激怒了。

exceed
[ikˈsi:d]

vt. 超过，胜过

exceedingly
[ikˈsi:diŋli]

ad. 非常，极度地

excel
[ikˈsel]

v. 优秀，胜过他人

excerpt
[ˈeksə:pt]

n. 摘录

excess
[ikˈses] *n.*
[ˈekses] *a.*

n. 超过；过分，过量　*a.* 过度的，额外的

【固定搭配】in excess of 超过；to excess 过度，过分
【经典例题】Her excess behavior leads to the break up of her marriage.
【译　　文】她过分的行为导致了她婚姻的破裂。

excessive
[ikˈsesiv]

a. 过度的，过分的，极度的

【名师导学】辨析 excessive, excess：excessive 表示过度的，极端的，超过正常的、通常的、合理的或正当界限的；excess 表示多余的，额外的。
【经典例题】Excessive consumption of fried foods has serious consequences.
【译　　文】过度食用油炸食品会有很严重的后果。

exclaim
[ikˈskleim]

v. 大叫，呼喊，大声叫

exclude
[ikˈsklu:d]

vt. 把……除外，排斥

exclusively
[ikˈsklu:sivli]

ad. 唯一地；专门地，特定地；专有地；排外地

【经典例题】Catalase activity reduced glutathione and Vitamin E levels were decreased exclusively in subjects with active disease.
A. definitely　B. truly　C. simply　D. solely　　[D]
【译　　文】过氧化氢酶活性降低了谷胱甘肽，维生素 E 水平仅在具有活动性疾病的受试者中降低。

excursion
[ikˈskə:ʃən]

n. 远足，短途旅行

execute
[ˈeksikju:t]

vt. 实行，执行，实施；处死，处决

【名师导学】辨析 execute, perform：execute 指执行计划、命令等；perform 多指执行一项费时、费力、需要技巧的工作。
【经典例题】The national government is to make every effort to execute the will of the people.
【译　　文】国家政府将竭尽全力执行人们的意愿。

execution
[ˌeksiˈkju:ʃən]

n. 实行，完成，执行；死刑

executive [ig'zekjutiv]	*a.* 执行的，实施的 *n.* 执行者，行政官；高级官员 【经典例题】The executive committee tells me we may not even have enough money to build the new critical care wing this year. 【译　　文】执行委员会告诉我，我们今年连修建重要的护理区域的资金都不够。
exemplify [ig'zemplifai]	*vt.* 例证，例示；作为……例子 【名师导学】近义词群：illustrate, typify, embody, epitomize; explain, represent
exempt [ig'zempt]	*v.* 免除 *a.* 被免除的
exert [ig'zə:t]	*v.* 尽（力），发挥，运用
exhaust [ig'zɔ:st]	*vt.* 用尽，耗尽，竭力；使衰竭，使精疲力竭 *n.* 排气装置，废气 【经典例题】Anyone who is faced with a serious and painful illness or the loss of a limb, is exhausted by repeated narrow escapes from death. 【译　　文】任何一个身患重疾，或是四肢残缺的人，都会因为常常濒临死亡边缘而筋疲力尽。
exhaustion [ig'zɔ:stʃən]	*n.* 耗尽，枯竭，疲惫，筋疲力尽，竭尽
exhaustive [ig'zɔ:stiv]	*a.* 详尽的；彻底的；全面的 【名师导学】要注意 exhausitve 和 exhausting/exhausted 的区分。后者的意思是"令人精疲力竭的 / 感到疲力竭的"。 【固定搭配】exhaustive list 详尽的清单
exile ['eksail, 'egz-]	*n.* 流放，放逐，充军；被流放者 *vt.* 流放，放逐，把……充军 【经典例题】The house was raided and the family was forced into exile. 【译　　文】房子被袭击后，这家人被迫流亡了。
exotic [ig'zɔtik]	*a.* 奇异的，异乎寻常的；异国情调的 【经典例题】These girls are wild, exotic creatures. 【译　　文】这些女孩性情奔放，又有异国情调。
exit ['eksit, -zit]	*n.* 出口；太平门 *vi. / n.* 退出，退场
expectancy [ik'spektənsi]	*n.*（常与 of 连用）期望，期待
expedition [,ekspi'diʃən]	*n.* 远征（队），探险（队），考察（队） 【经典例题】The purpose of the expedition was to explore the North American coastline. 【译　　文】这次远征的目的是探索北美洲的海岸线。
expel [ik'spel]	*vt.* 把……除名，把……开除；驱除，赶走，放逐 【经典例题】We've just installed a fan to expel cooking smells from the kitchen. 【译　　文】我们刚才安装了一个排气扇用来排出厨房里的气味。

expenditure
[ik'spenditʃə, eks-]

n. (时间、劳力、金钱等)支出；使用，消耗

【名师导学】本词属于常考词汇，在词汇题中多次出现，比较选项有：nutrition（营养），routine（惯例），provision（供应；预备），dissipation（挥霍），disposal（处置；安排）和 consumption（消费）等。各词词义差别较大，主要根据语境选择通顺的选项。

【经典例题】The budget provided for a total expenditure of $27 billion.

【译　　文】预算规定支出总额为 270 亿美元。

experimental
[ik,speri'mentl]

a. 试验（上）的

expert
['ekspə:t]

n. 专家，能手　*a.* 专家的，内行的

expertise
[,ekspə'ti:z]

n. 专门知识，专长

【名师导学】来自 expert。expertise 可以理解为专家的意见。相关近义词有：specialization（特殊化，专门化），profession（职业，专业），specialty（专业；特色菜）。

【经典例题】Additionally we continued to show our expertise in technology and project management.

【译　　文】此外，我们继续在技术与项目管理方面表现出我们的优势。

expire
[ik'spaiə, eks-]

v. 期满，失效；去世

【经典例题】In addition to their mastery of forging passports, at least three of the 19 Sept. 11 hijackers（劫机者）were here on expired visas.

【译　　文】除了善于伪造护照，19 名 911 劫机者中至少三人持有已经过期的签证。

explicit
[ik'splisit]

a. 详述的，明确的；直言的，毫不隐瞒的，露骨的

【名师导学】本词属于常考词汇，考生要注意的相关近义词有：definite（明确的，一定的），direct（径直的，直接的，直率的），distinct（清楚的，明显的，截然不同的），express（急速的，特殊的，明确的）。相关反义词有：ambiguous（暧昧的，不明确的），implicit（暗示的，含蓄的），vague（含糊不清的，茫然的，暧昧的）。

【经典例题】Creating so much confusion, Mason realized he had better make explicit what he was trying to tell the audience.

【译　　文】造成如此大的混乱，梅森意识到他最好把他想要告诉观众的讲清楚。

explode
[ik'spləud]

v. (使)爆炸，爆发，破裂

【派生词汇】explosion *n.* 爆炸；explosive *a./n.* 易爆炸的，爆炸物

【固定搭配】explode with anger 勃然大怒，大发脾气；explode with laughter 哄堂大笑

【经典例题】It was during the morning rush hour that the bomb exploded.

【译　　文】爆炸是在早高峰时发生的。

exploit
[ik'sploit]

vt. 使用，利用；开采，开发

【经典例题】The new TV stations are fully＿＿＿＿the potential of satellite transmission.

A. exposing   B. exhausting   C. exhibiting   D. exploiting   [D]
【译　　文】这些新的电视台将要全面开发卫星传播的潜力。
【经典例题】The Chinese government summoned people to exploit the Western China.
【译　　文】中国政府号召人民开发西部。

explore
[ik'splɔ:]
vt. 探险；探索，探究；勘探
【派生词汇】exploration *n.* 探索
【经典例题】Play is the most powerful way a child explores the world and learns about himself.
【译　　文】玩耍是孩子探索世界和了解自身的最有效的方法。

explosion
[ik'spləuʒən]
n. 爆炸，爆发

explosive
[ik'spləusiv]
a. 爆炸（性）的 *n.* 炸药

exposition
[ˌekspə'ziʃən]
n. 解释；讲解，说明（文）；展览，陈列；暴（显）露；曝光

expose
[ik'spəuz]
vt. 暴露，揭露
【固定搭配】be exposed to 暴露在……之下，受……影响
【名师导学】辨析 expose, reveal, uncover, disclose：expose 指"暴露，使……被看见"，或"揭露（罪恶或错误的行为）"；reveal 指"泄露，使（某些隐藏的事或秘密）为人所知"；uncover 指"揭开……的盖子，揭示"；disclose 意为"透露"，指某人把不愿意让人知道的事主动让人知道。
【经典例题】It is feared that people living near the power station may have been _____ to radiation.
A. revealed   B. uncovered   C. disclosed   D. exposed   [D]
【译　　义】住在核电站附近的居民可能会受到辐射，这是非常可怕的。

exposure
[ik'spəuʒə]
n. 暴露；揭露；曝光
【经典例题】More international trend for business and pleasure brings greater _____ to other societies.
A. exchange   B. exposure   C. expansion   D. contribution   [B]
【译　　文】在商业和娱乐方面，更多趋于国际化的潮流使之受到更多社会的影响。

exquisite
['ekskwizit]
a. 精美的，精致的；敏锐的，有高度鉴赏力的；剧烈的，感觉剧烈的
【名师导学】本词属于常考词汇，考生要注意的相关近义词有：delicate（精巧的，精致的；病弱的，脆弱的），elegant（文雅的，端庄的，雅致的），superb（极好的）。
【经典例题】The sets and costumes for the dance performance were exquisite.
【译　　文】这场舞蹈表演的布景和服装十分精美。

extend
[ik'stend]
vt. 伸，延伸；扩大；致，给予
【固定搭配】extend...to 给予，向某人提供（帮助、友谊等）

extension
[ik'stenʃən]
n. 延长部分，扩大部分；伸展，扩大，延长；电话分机

extensive [ik'stensiv]

a. 广博的；广泛的

【经典例题】The Adult Vocational College is an opportunity to gain the right qualifications for various careers, for it offers an ____ range of subjects and courses.
A. additional B. excessive C. adequate D. extensive [D]
【译　文】成人职业大学为从事各个行业的人获得职业资格提供了机会，因为该大学教授很多学科和课程。

extent [ik'stent]

n. 广度，宽度，长度；范围，程度

【固定搭配】to a certain extent, to a certain degree 在一定程度上；to a great / large extent 在很大程度上；to some extent=to some degree 在某种程度上；to the extent of 到……地步

【名师导学】这是个重点词，除在词汇选择和完形填空中以词义辨析出现外（见练习），在阅读中出现的次数也较多。

【经典例题】The newspaper did not mention the extent of the damage caused by the flood.
【译　文】报纸没有提及洪水带来的损失程度。

exterior [ek'stiəriə]

a. 外部的，外在的；表面的

【经典例题】The exterior structure of the architecture is perfect.
【译　文】这幢建筑的外部结构是完美的。

exterminate [ik'stə:mineit]

vt. 扑灭，消灭，根绝

【经典例题】The whole area of the national and local governments tried to wipe out rats to prevent the spread of disease.
A. exterminate B. dominate C. determinate D. contaminate [A]
【译　文】为阻止疾病的扩散，整个国家和地方政府都尽力全力灭鼠。

【名师导学】destroy, exterminate, extinguish 这 3 个动词均有"消灭"之意。
destroy：指通过杀戮或终止某人某物的机能，使之无用或毁灭。
exterminate：指大量地、成批地杀害、消灭。
extinguish：原义指灭火，转义后暗示生命、希望像灭火一样地被消灭、熄灭。

external [ek'stə:nl]

a. 外部的，外面的

【经典例题】They also need significant increases in external financing and technical support.
【译　文】他们也需要大幅度增加外部资助和技术支持。

extinct [ik'stiŋkt]

a. 濒临灭绝的

【名师导学】本词及其变形 extinction 在词汇选择和阅读部分都有出现。

【经典例题】If we continue to destroy the countryside many more animals will become extinct.
【译　文】我们若继续破坏自然环境，将会有更多的动物绝种。

extinguish [ik'stiŋgwiʃ]

vt. 熄灭，扑灭

【经典例题】The news extinguished all hope of his return.
【译　文】这些消息让他返回的希望破灭了。

extract [ik'strækt] *vt.* ['ekstrækt] *n.*

vt. 取出，抽出，拔出；提取，提炼，榨取；获得，索取；摘записать抄写 *n.* 摘录，选段；提出物，精华，汁

【经典例题】It is one thing to locate oil, but it is quite another to extract and transport it to the industrial centers.
【译　文】找到石油是一回事，提炼并把石油运送到工业中心却完全是另一回事。

全国医学博士英语统考词汇巧战通关

□ **extraordinary**
[ik'strɔ:dnri, ik'strɔ:dinəri]

a. 非常的，特别的
【经典例题】But we know that people go to extraordinary lengths to get it.
【译　　文】但是我们知道，人们为了得到它，无所不用其极。

□ **extravagant**
[ik'strævəgənt]

a. 奢侈的，浪费的，过分的，放纵的

□ **extreme**
[ik'stri:m]

a. 极度的，极端的；尽头的，末端的　*n.* 极端
【固定搭配】in the extreme 极，非常；go to extremes 走极端
【经典例题】It is not necessary to establish yourself as top dog or leader of the dog pack by using extreme measures. You can teach your dog its subordinate role by teaching it to show submission to you.
【译　　文】没有必要用极端的方法将你自己塑造成狗群的领导，你可以教你的狗表现出依附于你，从而确定它的从属地位。

□ **fabric**
['fæbrik]

n. 织物，纺织品；结构，组织

□ **fabricate**
['fæbrikeit]

vt. 制造，建造，装配，伪造
【名师导学】考生要注意相关近义词：invent（发明，创造，编造），contrive（设计，想出；谋划，策划），manufacture（制造，产生，编造）等。
【经典例题】The woman said she fabricated her testimony because she thought she was going to get a $10,000 reward.
【译　　文】这个妇女说她编造了证词，因为她认为她会获得一万美元的酬劳。

□ **fabrication**
[,fæbrikeiʃn]

n. 制造，建造，虚构的谎言
【经典例题】Her story was a complete ＿＿＿ from start to finish, so nobody believed in her.
A. facility　　B. fascination　　C. fabrication　　D. faculty　　　　[C]
【译　　文】她的故事从头至尾都是假的，没有人相信她。

□ **facilitate**
[fə'siliteit]

vt. 使容易；促进，帮助
【名师导学】考生要注意相关近义词有：assist（援助，帮助），ease（使安心，减轻）等。
【经典例题】Technology has facilitated the sharing, storage and delivery of information, thus making more information available to more people.
【译　　文】科学技术已经促进了信息的共享、储存和传递，因此，更多的人就可以获得更多的信息了。

□ **facility**
[fə'siliti]

n. 便利；（*pl.*）设备，工具
【名师导学】意为"设施"时，要用复数形式。
【经典例题】In the meeting, the government officer promised an improvement in hospital and other health care facilities.
【译　　文】在会上，政府官员许诺对医院和其他医疗健康设备进行改善。

factor
['fæktə]

n. 因素，要素

faculty
['fækəlti]

n. 才能，本领，能力；全体教师；院，系
【固定搭配】have a faculty for sth. 有做某事的才能
【名师导学】做主语时，看作整体，谓语用单数形式；看作个体，谓语用复数形式。
【经典例题】The average number of the faculty of law in every city is forty-five.
【译　文】在每个城市中平均有45所法学院。

fade
[feid]

vi. 褪色；逐渐消失

fake
[feik]

n. 假货，赝品；骗子，冒充者　*a.* 假的，伪造的，冒充的　*vt.* 伪造，捏造；伪装，假装
【名师导学】近义词：false, pretended, fraudulent, bogus, artificial; deception, counterfeit, copy, cheat, imitation, fraud, pretense, fabrication, forgery
【经典例题】Some criminals were printing fake dollar bills until they were arrested.
【译　文】一些罪犯在被捕前一直在印制假美钞。

fascinate
['fæsineit]

vt. 使着迷，强烈地吸引
【名师导学】近义词群：charm, entrance, captivate, enthrall, intrigue, interest, enchant, bewitch, ravish, enrapture, beguile, delight, overpower, subdue, enslave, please, attract, compel, lure, allure, seduce, entice, tempt, ensnare

fascinating
['fæsineitiŋ]

a. 迷人的，醉人的

fasten
['fɑ:sn]

v. 扣紧，结牢，闩上
【固定搭配】fasten / tie...to 把……拴在 / 系在 / 固定在……上；fasten one's eyes on 盯着

fatality
[fə'tæliti]

n. 命运决定的事物，不幸，灾祸，天命

fatal
['feitl]

n. 致命的，毁灭性的
【经典例题】It has been proved that the chemical is lethal to rats but safe for cattle.
A. fatal　　B. reactive　　C. unique　　D. vital　　[A]
【译　文】经证实，这种化学药品对于鼠类是致命的，而对家禽则无害。

fate
[feit]

n. 命运
【名师导学】辨析 fate, destiny：fate 指不可避免的命运，尤指不幸的命运；destiny 指预先注定的命运，宿命。

fatigue
[fə'ti:g]

n. 疲乏，劳累
【经典例题】This pill will work wonders for fatigue.
【译　文】这种药片对（缓解）疲劳有神奇的效果。

feasibility
[,fi:zə'biləti]

n. 可行性，可能性

feasible
['fi:zəbl]
a. 可行的，可能的

feast
[fi:st]
n. 盛宴，筵席
【经典例题】All the guests were invited to attend the wedding feast and had a very good time.
【译　文】所有的客人都被邀请参加婚宴，大家都玩得很愉快。

feature
['fi:tʃə]
n. 面貌，容貌；特征，特色；特写
【名师导学】辨析 feature，mark，trace，appearance，characteristic：feature 指的是让某物有辨识度的局部特点，mark 意为"记号，标记"，trace"踪迹"，appearance"面部整体，外表"，characteristic 强调整体特征。
【经典例题】A peculiarly pointed chin is his most memorial facial ＿＿＿.
A. mark　　　B. feature　　　C. trace　　　D. appearance　　　[B]
【译　文】他那特别尖的下巴是最让人记忆犹新的面貌特征。

federal
['fedərəl]
a. 联邦的，联盟的，联合的

federation
[,fedə'reiʃən]
n. 联合会；联邦
【经典例题】He is now chairman of the British Olympic Federation.
【译　文】他目前是英国奥委会主席。

fee
[fi:]
n. 酬金；手续费；学费

feeble
['fi:bl]
a. 虚弱的，衰弱无力的；无效的，无益的
【名师导学】本词属于常考词汇。辨析：feeble 指体质虚弱，意志薄弱；weak 为普通用词，指身体、精神和意志上缺乏力量；fragile 指人容易生病。
【经典例题】The heartbeat was feeble and irregular.
【译　文】心搏无力，心律不齐。

feedback
['fi:dbæk]
n. 反馈

fellowship
['feləuʃip]
n. 社团；（常指学术团体的）会员资格；（大学中的）研究员职位，研究员薪金；伙伴关系，交情
【经典例题】Regular outings contribute to a sense of fellowship among co-workers.
【译　文】经常户外旅行有助于增强同事之间的友谊。

feminine
['feminin]
a. 女性的；娇柔的
【经典例题】His long, feminine eyelashes were very noticeable.
【译　文】他那长长的女人似的睫毛很引人注意。

fertile
['fə:tail; 'fə:til]
a. 肥沃的，富饶的；多产的，丰富的
【经典例题】All the flowers are grown in the fertile soil.
【译　文】所有的花都生长在肥沃的土壤里。

fertilizer
['fə:ti,laizə]
n. 化肥，肥料

fiber
['faibə]
n. 纤维，纤维质

fierce
[fiəs]

a. 猛的，凶恶的；猛烈的，强烈的

【名师导学】辨析 fierce, violent, savage：fierce 指有野蛮和残忍的性质的，或极其可怕的、极为猛烈的；violent 指显示巨大力量的，由巨大力量产生的，或暴力、强力（非自然力）所致的；savage 指野蛮的，未驯服或培养过的，或残暴的、易怒的。

【经典例题】Owing to _____ competition among the airlines, travel expenses have been reduced considerably.
A. fierce　　B. violent　　C. eager　　D. critical　　[A]
【译　文】由于航空业的激烈竞争，乘飞机旅行的费用大幅下降。

file
[fail]

n. 文件夹，卷宗；（计算机）文件　*vt.* 把……归档

【固定搭配】on file 存档

【经典例题】It makes sense to keep such information on _____ for quick reference.
A. pile　　B. segment　　C. sequence　　D. file　　[D]
【译　文】现在把这些信息存档以便今后快速查询，这是十分有意义的。

finance
[faiˈnæns]

n. 财政，金融　*vt.* 提供资金，接济

【经典例题】One U.S. dollar is comparable to 131 Japanese yen according to *China Daily's* finance news report yesterday.
【译　文】据昨天《中国日报》财经新闻报道，1美元可兑换131日元。

financial
[faiˈnænʃəl]

a. 财政的，金融的

finite
[ˈfainait]

a. 有限的，有限制的；限定的

【经典例题】The world's resources are finite.
【译　文】世界的资源是有限的。

flare
[flɛə]

vi.（火焰）闪耀，（短暂地）烧旺；突发，突然发怒（或激动）　*n.* 闪光信号，照明弹

【经典例题】A match flared in the darkness.
【译　文】一根火柴的光线在黑暗中一闪。

flash
[flæʃ]

n. 闪光，一闪，闪光灯　*vi.* 发闪光；闪现，闪过；飞驰，掠过

【名师导学】辨析 flash, shine, spark, sparkle：flash 意为"闪光"，指突然闪亮而又瞬间即逝的光；shine 意为"发光，照耀"，是指因物体表面光滑而闪亮；spark 指冒出火花或电花；sparkle 意为"闪烁，闪耀"，指射出火花般微小、短暂的闪光。

flatter
[ˈflætə]

vt. 向……献媚，奉承；使满意，使高兴，使感到荣幸；使显得（比实际）好看，使（某优点）显得突出

【名师导学】本词属于常考词汇，考生要注意相关短语：flatter oneself 自以为是，自鸣得意。

【经典例题】I cannot flatter myself that I am better than him.
【译　文】我不能自夸比他好。

flaw
[flɔː]

n. 缺点，裂纹，瑕疵

【经典例题】The statue would be perfect but for a few small <u>defects</u> in its base.
A. faults　　B. weaknesses　　C. flaws　　D. errors　　[C]
【译　文】要不是基底部分有一些小的瑕疵，这座雕塑就很完美了。

【名师导学】近义词群：defect, imperfection, blemish, stain。

flesh [fleʃ]

n. 肉,肉体,肌体

【名师导学】辨析 flesh, meat, muscle:flesh 指人和动物身上的肉,或水果、蔬菜的果肉;meat 指可食用肉,尤指(与鱼或家禽不同的)哺乳动物的肉;muscle 指肌肉组织,它能够使身体的某个部位产生运动。

flexible ['fleksəbl]

a. 柔软的,易弯曲的;灵活的,可变通的
【经典例题】Goals should be measurable but flexible.
【译　文】目标应该可估量并且非常灵活。

fling [fliŋ]

vt. (用力地)扔,掷
【经典例题】The excited fans had a fling at the lost team.
【译　文】情绪激动的球迷们嘲弄输球的球队。

flock [flɔk]

n. 兽群,鸟群
【名师导学】辨析 flock, crowd, pack, swarm:flock 指禽、畜的群;crowd 指人群;pack 指狼群或狗群等,或有共同兴趣的有组织的群体、一帮人;swarm 指正在行进中的一大群昆虫,成群出动的一大批人或动物。

flourish ['flʌriʃ]

v. 繁荣,茂盛,兴旺
【经典例题】All industries flourish when people eat more.
【译　文】当人们吃得更多时,所有的行业都兴盛繁荣。

flu [flu:]

n. 流行性感冒

fluctuate ['flʌktjueit]

vi. 变动,波动,涨落,动摇　*vt.* 使波动,使起伏,使动摇
【派生词汇】fluctuation *n.* 波动
【名师导学】本词属于常考词汇。辨析:vibrate (使)振动;flutter 拍翅膀,飘动;swing 摇摆。
【经典例题】With prices fluctuating so much, it is difficult for the school to plan a budget.
【译　文】物价起伏这么大,给学校做预算带来了一些困难。

fluent ['flu(:)ənt]

a. 流利的,流畅的

fluid ['flu(:)id]

a. 流动的,流体的;液体的　*n.* 流体,液体

focus ['fəukəs]

n. 中心,焦点,焦距　*vi.* 聚焦,集中
【固定搭配】focus on 集中于
【名师导学】focus 复数形式为 foci 或 focuses。
【经典例题】All her energies are＿＿＿ upon her children and she seems to have little time for anything else.
A. guided　　B. aimed　　C. directed　　D. focused　　[D]
【译　文】她所有的精力都放在孩子身上,她看起来没有时间做别的事儿。

folk [fəuk]

n. 人们　*a.* 民间的
【名师导学】folk 作为名词时有两个复数形式 folk 和 folks。

folklore ['fəuklɔ:(r)]

n. 民间传说;民俗学

foremost ['fɔ:məust]

a. 最好的,最著名的,最重要的

forerunner ['fɔː,rʌnə]	n. 先驱（者）；预兆
foresee [fɔː'siː]	vt. 预见，预料到 【名师导学】本词属于常考词汇，考生要注意相关近义词有：anticipate（预期，期望），forecast（预想，预报），foretell（预言，预示，预测），predict（预知，预言，预报），prophesy（预言，预报）。 【经典例题】We don't foresee any difficulties in completing the project so long as we keep within our budget. 【译　文】只要我们不超出预算，完成项目应该不会有什么困难。
foresight ['fɔːsait]	n. 先见，预见；深谋远虑
foretell [fɔː'tel]	v. 预言，预示，预测
formal ['fɔːməl]	a. 正式的；礼仪上的；形式的
formality [fɔː'mæliti]	n. 拘谨，礼节，仪式，拘泥形式
format ['fɔːmæt, -maːt]	n. 版式，（计算机的）格式；编排　vt. 设计，（计算机上）将……格式化
formation [fɔː'meiʃən]	n. 构成；组织，形成物；地岩层
former ['fɔːmə]	a. 在前的，以前的　n. 前者 【固定搭配】the former...the latter 前者……后者 【经典例题】The girl was formally a shop assistant; she is now a manager in a large department store. 【译　文】这个女孩曾经是个售货员，但现在她已经是一家大型百货公司的经理了。
formidable ['fɔːmidəbl]	a. 强大的；令人敬畏的，可怕的；艰难的
formula ['fɔːmjulə]	n. 公式，程式 【固定搭配】formula for... ……的配方 【名师导学】formula 复数形式有：formulas, formulae。
formulate ['fɔːmjuleit]	vt. 制订，规划；做简洁陈述，阐明 【经典例题】Their role is not to formulate policy. 【译　文】他们的角色不是出台政策。
forth [fɔːθ]	ad. 向外 【固定搭配】and so forth 等等
forthcoming [,fɔːθ'kʌmiŋ]	a. 即将来临的；可得到的，乐于提供消息的
fortnight ['fɔːtnait]	n. 两星期 【联想记忆】decade n. 10年　score n. 20年　century n. 100年
fortunately ['fɔːtʃənətli]	ad. 幸亏

forum
['fɔːrəm]
n. 论坛，讨论会

fossil
['fɒsl]
n. 化石
【经典例题】Several dinosaur fossils were found in Montana.
【译　　文】在蒙大拿州发现了一些恐龙化石。

foster
['fɒstə(r)]
v. 促进，助长；培养；鼓励；抚育；照料（他人子女一段时间）a. 与某些代养有关的名词连用（如 foster parents 代养父母）
【经典例题】Policymakers have long regarded electronic medical records as a way to foster patient engagement and improve patient safety.
【译　　文】长期以来，决策者一直将电子病历视为促进患者参与和提高患者安全的一种方式。

fraction
['frækʃən]
n. 碎片，小部分，一点儿；分数
【名师导学】fraction, part, portion, section, segment, share：fraction 意为"小部分，碎片"，常表示可以略去不计的微小部分；part 纯粹为部分，并无比例内涵；portion 意为"一部分，一份"，指某物中所占的份额、比例；section 指通过或似乎通过切割或分离而形成的部分，如书、文章或城市的某一部分；segment 可与 section 换用，但更强调某物以自然的分裂线分开的部分，或因其结构性质而分裂的部分；share 指所分享、分担的一部分，强调共性。

fracture
['fræktʃə]
n. 破裂，骨折 v.（使）破碎，（使）破裂

fragile
['frædʒail]
a. 脆的；虚弱的；易碎的
【名师导学】本词属于常考词汇。辨析：fragile, breakable, frangible, delicate, brittle。这些形容词的意思都是"易打碎"或"易损坏的"。fragile 指那些由于原料的轻薄易损而应该轻拿轻放的物品，例如：a collection of fragile porcelain plates（一堆易碎的瓷盘）。breakable 和 frangible 词义一致，都指能被打碎的但不一定是易碎品。例如：Even earthenware pottery is breakable. 甚至陶器也易碎。The museum stored all frangible articles in a locked showcase. 博物馆的陈列橱里贮藏了所有的易碎物品。delicate 指柔软、纤弱或精致以至于极易受损，例如：The peach is a delicate fruit. 桃子是种易受损的水果。brittle 指在受到压力时易折断的物体。

fragment
['frægmənt]
n. 碎片；片断
【经典例题】Up to 1,500 fungally-infected skin fragments per square meter have been found in some leisure facilities.
【译　　文】在一些休闲设施中，每平方米发现多达 1500 块真菌感染的皮肤碎片。

fragrance
['freigrəns]
n. 香味，芳香；香气

fragrant
['freigrənt]
a. 芬芳的，香味的

fraud
[frɔːd]
n. 欺骗；假货
【经典例题】Harold claimed that he was a serious and well-known artist, but in fact he was a fraud.
【译　　文】哈罗德自称是个有名的技艺精湛的艺术家，但是事实上他是个骗子。

freight [freit]	n. 货运，客货；运费 【联想记忆】express n. 快运；airfreight n. 空运
fright [frait]	n. 惊骇，吃惊
fringe [frindʒ]	n. 边缘；(头发的)刘海 v. 在……加上边饰 a. 边缘的，附加的
frontier ['frʌntiə]	n. 边界，国境；边疆；尖端新领域
frost [frɔst, frɔ:st]	n. 霜，降霜；严寒 【联想记忆】coolness n. 凉爽；chill n. 寒气；cold n. 寒冷；warmth n. 温暖；heat n. 热
frown [fraun]	vi. 皱眉头 【经典例题】He frowned as he tried to work out the sum. 【译　　文】当他试图算出总数的时候，他皱起了眉头。
fruitful ['fru:tful]	a. 结果实的，产量多的
frustrate [frʌs'treit]	vt. 破坏，阻挠；使失败，使泄气 【经典例题】After three hours' frustrating delay, the train at last arrived. 【译　　文】经过3个小时令人心烦的耽搁后，火车终于到达了目的地。
fry [frai]	v. 油煎，油炸 【联想记忆】heat v. 加热；boil v. 煮；steam v. 蒸；bake v. 烘烤；fry v. 油煎；toast v. 烤（面包片）
fuel ['fju:əl]	n. 燃料；（尤指使争论等继续或更加激烈的）刺激性言行 v. 给……提供燃料；给（交通工具）加油；增加；加强；刺激 【经典例题】The push for portals has been fueled by several factors. 【译　　文】对门户网站的推动是由几个因素造成的。
fulfil(l) [ful'fil]	v. 完成；履行；达到 【经典例题】I had been a university student for three years, but not until afternoon had I felt the thrill of fulfillment. 【译　　文】我都成为大学生三年了，但是直到今天下午才有成就感。
function ['fʌŋkʃən]	n. 机能，职能，功能；职务，职责；函数；活动，运行，起作用 【经典例题】The human ear has two main functions: hearing and maintaining balance. 【译　　文】人类耳朵有两大主要功能：听和维持身体平衡。
fund [fʌnd]	n. (pl.) 资金；基金，专款；储备
fundamental [,fʌndə'mentl]	a. 基础的，根本的，重要的 n. (pl.) 基本原则，基本原理 【固定搭配】be fundamental to 对……必不可少 【联想记忆】be essential to, be vital to 对……至关重要的 【经典例题】These experts say that we must understand the fundamental relation between ourselves and wild animals. 【译　　文】这些专家说，我们必须明白我们自己和野生动物之间的重要关系。

funeral
['fju:nərəl]

n. 葬礼，丧葬

【联想记忆】bury *v.* 埋葬；burial *n.* 埋葬，葬礼；grave *n.* 坟墓，墓穴；tomb *n.* 坟墓

fungus
['fʌŋɡəs]

a. 真菌（如蘑菇和霉）；霉菌；霉

【名师导学】这是医学文章中常出现的一个词，复数形式为 fungi ['fʌŋɡi:]，形容词形式为 fungal ['fʌŋɡl]，fungal infection 的意思是"真菌感染"。

【经典例题】30% of Britons, Germans and Belgians had some form of fungal infection.

【译　　文】30% 的英国人、德国人和比利时人有真菌感染。

fur
[fə:]

n. 软毛；毛皮，裘皮，皮衣

【联想记忆】fabric *n.* 织物；wool *n.* 羊毛；leather *n.* 皮革；cotton *n.* 棉布；feather *n.* 羽毛

furious
['fjuəriəs]

a. 狂怒的；猛烈的

【名师导学】近义词：enraged, raging, infuriated; violent, agitated, tumultuous

【经典例题】Although John completed his assignments quickly and successfully, he was furious when he learned that the boss had deliberately assigned him a difficult client.

【译　　文】虽然约翰迅速并顺利地完成了任务，但是当他知道老板是有意给他安排了一个棘手的客人时，他愤怒了。

furnish
['fə:niʃ]

v. 供应，提供；陈设，布置

【固定搭配】furnish sb. / sth. with sth., furnish sth. to sb. 为某人 / 某事提供某物

【联想记忆】provide sb. with sth., provide sth. for sb., supply sth. to / for sb., supply sb. with sth., arm sb. with sth., offer sb. sth. 为某人提供某物

【名师导学】辨析 furnish, equip, supply, arm：furnish 指供生活所必备的或为生活舒适所需的家具；equip 常表示装备工作所需要的东西；supply 可用于在任何环境下供给什何东西；arm 表示以武器或知识、信息等武装或备装。

【经典例题】These finds can_____more information on prehistoric man.

A. rectify　　B. prolong　　C. minimize　　D. furnish　　　　[D]

【译　　文】这些发现能够提供更多有关史前人类的信息。

fury
['fjuəri]

n. 愤怒，怒气；激烈，猛烈

【派生词汇】furious *a.* 愤怒的，激烈的

【经典例题】In their fury, they went through the streets wrecking cars.

【译　　文】他们在狂怒中沿街捣毁汽车。

fuse
[fju:z]

n. 保险丝；导火线，引线　*v.* 熔化，熔合

【经典例题】I taught him how to change a fuse.

【译　　文】我教他如何换保险丝。

fusion
['fju:ʒən]

n. 熔化，熔解，熔合，熔接

fuss
[fʌs]

n. 大惊小怪，小题大做，忙乱

【派生词汇】fussy *a.* 大惊小怪的

【固定搭配】make a fuss 大惊小怪，小题大做，无事自扰；make a fuss of / over 对……过分关心

galaxy
['gæləksi]

n. 星系，银河系
【经典例题】She was awarded a galaxy of medals for her bravery.
【译　　文】由于她的勇敢行为，她被授予了一系列奖牌。

gang
[gæŋ]

n. 一（群），一（帮）
【固定搭配】a gang of 一伙 / 群

gap
[gæp]

n. 缺口，间隔；隔阂，差距
【固定搭配】bridge the gap between 弥合（……之间的）差别；消除隔阂；bridge / fill / stop / close a gap 弥补不足；填补空白
【经典例题】There are wide gaps in my knowledge of history.
【译　　文】我很缺乏历史知识。

garbage
['gɑ:bidʒ]

n. 垃圾
【经典例题】Their advice turned out to be nothing but garbage.
【译　　文】他们的意见都是废话。

gas
[gæs]

n. 煤气；气体；汽油

gasoline
['gæsəli:n]

n. 汽油

gasp
[gɑ:sp]

vi. 喘气，喘息，倒抽气　*vt.* 喘着气说出（或发出喘气声）　*n.* 喘气，喘息，倒抽气
【经典例题】"Do you think you can walk?" I asked. "I'll try." he gasped.
【译　　文】"你能走吗？"我问。"我试试吧。"他喘着气说。

gauge
[geidʒ]

v. 精确计量；估计　*n.* 标准量度；计量器
【名师导学】fuel / temperature / pressure gauge 油表，温度计，气压计。
【经典例题】My car's gas gauge indicated that there was little gas left.
【译　　文】我车上的汽油表显示剩下的油不多了。

gaze
[geiz]

vi. / n. 凝视，盯
【固定搭配】gaze at / on / upon / into 凝视，注视
【联想记忆】stare at 盯，凝视；glance at 快速地扫一眼；glimpse at 瞥见
【名师导学】辨析 gaze, glance, glare, stare, peer：gaze 强调由于惊奇、喜好或兴奋而目不转睛地凝望；glance 意为"一瞥"，表示在匆忙中迅速地看一眼；glare 表示热切地、往往是凶狠地或生气地怒目而视；stare 表示盯着看，直接或固定地看，常指张大眼睛瞪视；peer 指眯着眼睛或从某物后面偷看。
【经典例题】She turned her head away, feeling too ashamed to meet his gaze.
【译　　文】因为害羞而不敢和他凝视的目光相遇，她把头扭开了。

gear
[giə]

n. 齿轮，传动装置；用具，装备　*v.* 开动，连接
【固定搭配】gear up（使）准备好，（使）做好安排　gear...to 使……适合
【经典例题】Education should be geared to children's needs.
【译　　文】教育应适合学生们的需要。

gender
['dʒendə]

n. 性别，性

gene
[dʒi:n]

n. 基因

【经典例题】Most of us inherit half our genes from our mothers and half from our fathers.
【译　　文】我们大多数人继承一半母亲的基因，一半父亲的基因。

generalize
['dʒenərəlaiz]

v. 概况，归纳，推断

【根源词汇】general *a.* 大概的，一般的
【名师导学】本词属于常考词汇，考生要注意 generalized 是形容词，意为"广泛的，普及的"。

generally
['dʒenərəli]

ad. 一般，通常

generate
['dʒenə,reit]

vt. 产生，发生；引起，导致

【经典例题】When coal burns, it generates heat.
【译　　文】煤燃烧时，产生热量。
【经典例题】This procedure describes how suggestions for improvements to the systems are ＿＿＿.
A. celebrated　B. proceeded　C. generated　D. established　[C]
【译　　文】这个过程描述了改进这些体系的建议是如何产生的。

generator
['dʒenəreitə]

n. 发电机，发生器

generosity
[,dʒenə'rɔsiti]

n. 慷慨，宽大

generous
['dʒenərəs]

a. 慷慨的，大方的；丰盛的，丰富的；宽厚的

【固定搭配】be generous to sb. 对某人宽大；be generous with sth. 用某物大方
【经典例题】He made such a ＿＿＿ contribution to the university that they are naming one of the new buildings after him.
A. genuine　B. minimum　C. modest　D. generous　[D]
【译　　文】他给学校如此慷慨的捐助，所以他们将以他的名字给其中一座新楼命名。

genetic
[dʒi'netik]

a. 遗传的，起源的

【经典例题】The human population contains a great variety of genetic variation, but drugs are tested on just a few thousand people.
【译　　文】人类具有各种各样的遗传变异，可是药品的试验只在数千人中进行。

genial
['dʒi:niəl]

a. 和蔼的，亲切的，宜人的

【经典例题】The ＿＿＿ climate of Hawaii attracts visitors from all over the world every year.
A. genial　B. frigid　C. genuine　D. foul　[A]
【译　　文】夏威夷宜人的气候每年都吸引世界各地的游客来到这里。
【名师导学】近义词群：cordial, affable, cheerful, warmhearted; amiable, friendly; warm, agreeable, cheering, cheerful

genius ['dʒi:njəs]

n. 天才

【联想记忆】have a faculty for, have a gift for, have a talent for, have a capacity for 具有……的才能/天赋

【名师导学】辨析 genius, gift, talent：genius 指天赋，超常的智力和创造力，具有这种天赋的人极为罕见；gift 指天资，才能，通常被认为是生来就有的某一方面突出的才能；talent 指生来即有的天分或能力，通常需要加以培养和发展。

【经典例题】I was going to be a complete engineer, technical genius and sensitive humanist all in one.

【译　文】我想做一个真正意义上的工程师，那种技术上的天才和敏感的人文学者集于一身的工程师。

genome ['dʒi:nəʊm]

n. 基因组，染色体组

genuine ['dʒenjuin]

a. 真实的，真正的；真心的，真诚的

【经典例题】The questions usually grow out of their genuine interest or curiosity.

【译　文】问题通常来自他们真正的兴趣或好奇。

germ [dʒə:m]

n. 微生物，细菌

【固定搭配】germ weapon 细菌武器

gesture ['dʒestʃə]

n. 姿势，手势；姿态

【经典例题】He gestured angrily at me.

【译　文】他气愤地对我做手势。

giant ['dʒaiənt]

n. 巨人　*a.* 大的，巨大的

【经典例题】Shakespeare is a giant among writers.

【译　文】莎士比亚是一位文坛巨匠。

gigantic [dʒai'gæntik]

a. 巨人般的，巨大的

glamour ['glæmə]

n. 魅力，诱惑力

【经典例题】Forget all you read about the glamour of television.

【译　文】把你读到的有关电视的魅力都忘了吧。

glare [glɛə]

vi. (at) 怒目而视；发射强光，发出刺眼的光　*n.* 强光；怒视，瞪眼；炫耀，张扬

【经典例题】He didn't shout; he just glared at me silently.

【译　文】他没有喊叫，只是默默地怒视着我。

gleam [gli:m]

vi. 闪亮，闪烁；(with) 闪现，流露　*n.* 闪光，闪亮；闪现，流露

【经典例题】A Rolls Royce was parked outside, gleaming in the sunshine.

【译　文】一辆劳斯莱斯停在外面，在阳光下熠熠生辉。

glide [glaid]

n./vi. 溜，滑行

【经典例题】A swan glided across the surface of the lake.

【译　文】一只天鹅滑翔过湖面。

glimpse [glimps]

n. 一瞥，一看　*v.* 见

【固定搭配】catch / get a glimpse of 瞥见；glimpse at 看一看，瞥见

【联想记忆】stare at 盯，凝视；glance at 快速地扫一眼；catch / get / have / take a glimpse of 瞥见；give / cast / take a glance at 瞥一眼；have / get / catch (a) sight of 发现，看出；take notice of 注意到，觉察到

【名师导学】辨析 glance, glimpse：glance 指匆匆一瞥，强调动作；glimpse 则是瞥见，表示匆匆一瞥中所看到的，强调结果。
【经典例题】A brief glimpse at a daily newspaper vividly shows how much people in the United States think about business.
【译　　文】只要随便翻翻美国的日报就能生动地看出美国人是如何看待经济的。

glitter ['glitə]
vi. 一闪一闪地发光　n. 闪光，光辉，灿烂
【经典例题】Her jewelry glittered under the spotlights which made her become the dominant figure at the ball.
【译　　文】她戴的珠宝在灯光下闪闪发光，让她在舞会上光彩照人。

global ['gləubəl]
a. 地球的，全球的；全局的
【固定搭配】global villag 地球村
【派生词汇】globalize 全球化

globe [gləub]
n. 地球；地球仪，球体
【经典例题】We believe it is a reasonable real-world test of good manners around the globe.
【译　　文】我们相信这是一个世界范围的、合理的、现实的关于礼貌的测试。

gloom [glu:m]
n. 黑暗；阴沉，朦胧；愁闷，忧郁
【名师导学】辨析：gloom 指"忧伤，忧郁，阴暗"，表示不开心的状态；sadness 为普通用词，指"悲哀，悲伤"；blues 为非正式用词，常用于口语，表示"忧郁，沮丧"；depression 则比较正式，表示"精神沮丧，意志消沉"。
【经典例题】He couldn't read in the dim gloom of the warehouse.
【译　　文】在昏暗的仓库里，他无法读书。

glorious ['glɔ:riəs]
a. 光荣的

glory ['glɔ:ri]
n. 光荣，荣誉
【固定搭配】be a glory to 是……的光荣
【联想记忆】be a credit to 是……的荣耀；be a disgrace / dishonor / shame to 是……的耻辱

gorgeous ['gɔ:dʒəs]
a. 华丽的，漂亮的
【名师导学】相关近义词有：beautiful，brilliant，dazzling（眼花缭乱的，耀眼的）；divine（神的，神圣的；非凡的，超人的；非常可爱的）；glorious（光荣的，显赫的）；splendid，stunning（足以使人倾倒的，极好的）。
【经典例题】I love your dress! It's such a gorgeous color!
【译　　文】我喜欢你的衣服！颜色太美了！

gossip ['gɔsip]
n. 闲话，流言；闲谈之人　vi. 搬弄是非，闲聊
【名师导学】gossip 的前身是古英语的复合词 godsib，其中 god 即上帝，而 sib 则意为 relatives（亲属），故 godsib 原意为 godparent（教父或教母），由于教父或教母一般都是受洗者父母的较亲密的朋友，他们之间有许多共同感兴趣的事情可谈，因此 gossip 的意思逐渐演变为"爱说长道短的人"和"闲谈"。
【经典例题】George enjoys talking about other people's private affairs. He is a gossip.
【译　　文】乔治喜欢谈论别人的私事，他是个爱说长道短的人。

grand [grænd]

a. 重大的，主要的；宏大的，盛大的；伟大的，崇高的

【名师导学】辨析 grand, magnificent, splendid：grand 指超凡的成就或品质使人感到崇高而伟大，也可指规模宏大，使人感到庄严雄伟；magnificent 指风景、宝石、建筑物的壮丽堂皇；splendid 指才能、成就出众的人，雄伟、辉煌的物或事。

【经典例题】At that time, a grand ceremony will be held according to traditional customs.

【译　文】届时，还要按照传统风俗举行盛大的活动。

grant [grɑ:nt]

n. 拨款；准许　*v.* 准予，授予，同意

【固定搭配】take...for granted 认为……理所当然

【名师导学】此单词在历年的词汇题中作为选项出现，请大家注意它的各种含义和搭配。

【经典例题】The government gave us a grant to build another classroom.

【译　文】政府给了我们一笔补助，用来盖另外一间教室。

graphic ['græfik]

a. 生动的，形象的；绘画的，文字的，图表的

【名师导学】以 ph 或 phy 结尾的名词，变成形容词时往往都是在名词后面加后缀 ic 或 ical，例如 geographic(al) 地理的，biographic(al) 传记的。

【经典例题】He kept telling us about his operation in the most graphic detail.
A. verifiable　　　　　　B. explicit
C. precise　　　　　　　D. ambiguous　　　　[B]

【译　文】他不停地向我描述他的手术细节，非常详尽（用图解式的语言）。

gratitude ['grætitju:d]

n. 感激，感谢

【经典例题】I would like to express my gratitude to you all for supporting me this summer as a visiting scholar in your department.

【译　文】我向你们表示感激，感谢今年夏天我作为访问学者对贵系进行访问期间你们对我的支持。

greenhouse ['gri:nhaus]

n. 温室

grieve [gri:v]

vt. 使悲哀，使伤心

【派生词汇】grief *n.* 悲哀，伤心

【名师导学】grieve 后面常跟介词 for 或 over，表示"为……感到伤心"，例如：She is still grieving for / over her dead husband. 她仍在为死去的丈夫伤心。另外请注意以 -eve 结尾的动词变为名词时，去掉"ve"变成"f"，例如：believe → belief, relieve → relief, grieve → grief。

近义词：lament, bewail, regret, sorrow for, mourn

【经典例题】I grieve very much for what I have done.

【译　文】我为自己的行为感到痛心。

grin [grin]

vi. / n. 露齿笑

【名师导学】熟记：on the (broad) grin 笑嘻嘻，咧着嘴笑，sardonic grin 冷笑，grin and bear it 逆来顺受。另外应区分该词与其他几个近义词在表示笑的状态时有何差异，如：chuckle, giggle, sneer, snigger。

【经典例题】He was grinning from ear to ear.

【译　文】他笑得合不拢嘴。

grind [graind]
v. 碎，磨，碾

【固定搭配】grind out 机械地做出，用功做出；grind / crush...into 把……碾压成

【联想记忆】bind 捆，包扎—bound 注定，受约束　find 找到—found 成立　grind 研，磨—ground 地面，根据　wind 弯曲—wound 伤害　lie 躺—lay 平放　shoot 射击—shot 发射　think 想—thought 思想

grip [grip]
vt. 紧握，抓牢　*n.* 紧握，抓牢；掌握，控制

【固定搭配】come / get to grips with 努力对付；认真处理；be at grips with 在与……搏斗；在认真对付 / 处理；lose one's grip 失去控制

【名师导学】辨析 grasp, grip：grasp 表示抓住了，但没有用整个手攥紧；grip 是用了肌肉所允许的力量抓紧。

groan [grəun]
n. 呻吟，叹息

【经典例题】After the house collapsed, groans could be heard from the people trapped in the rubble.

【译　文】房屋倒塌后，能听到困在废墟中的人们的呻吟声。

grope [grəup]
n. 摸索，探索　*v.*（暗中）摸索，探索

guardian ['ɡɑːdjən]
n. 监护人，保护人

【经典例题】As the legal guardian of you, I must protect you against being hurt.

【译　文】作为你的合法监护人，我必须保护你，让你免受伤害。

guarantee [ˌɡærən'tiː]
n. 保证，保证书　*vt.* 保证，担保

【名师导学】辨析 guarantee, pledge, warranty：guarantee 意为"担保，保证，抵押品"，指对事物的品质或人的行为提出担保，常暗示双方有法律上或其他方式的默契，保证补偿不履行所造成的损失；pledge 意为"保证，誓约，抵押品"，为普通用语，可泛指保证忠实于某种原则或接受并尽忠某一职责的庄严保证或诺言，但这都是以跟人的信誉做保证的承诺；warranty 指"（商品的）保证书，保单，保证"，如修理或退还残缺货物等。

【经典例题】Nuclear power, with all its inherent problems, is still the only option to guarantee enough energy in the future.

【译　文】虽然核动力还存在它固有的问题，但它仍然是将来有足够能源的唯一保证。

【经典例题】Every camera we sell comes with a two-year ＿＿＿.
A. guarantee　　　　　　B. safety
C. confirmation　　　　　D. conservation　　　　　　　　[A]

【译　文】我们出售的每一台照相机都有 2 年的质保。

guidance ['ɡaidəns]
n. 引导，指导

【根源词汇】guide *v.* 指导　*n.* 指南，指导

【固定搭配】under the guidance of 在……领导之下

guideline ['ɡaidlain]
n. 指南，方针

guilty ['gilti]

a. 有罪的，犯罪的，自觉有罪的；内疚的
【根源词汇】guilt *n.* 愧疚，犯罪
【固定搭配】be guilty of 犯有……罪；be guilty for 因……而内疚
【经典例题】The main function of criminal courts is to determine who is guilty under the law.
【译　　文】刑事法庭的主要作用就是判定按照法律规定谁是有罪的。

gymnastics [dʒim'næstiks]

n. 体育，体操

habitat ['hæbitæt]

n. （动植物的）产地，栖息地

hacker ['hækə]

n. 砍伐工；电脑黑客

halt [hɔ:lt]

v. / n. （使）止步，（使）停住，（使）停

hamper ['hæmpə]

vt. 阻碍，妨碍；牵制，危害
【名师导学】近义词：impede, thwart, embarrass, hinder
【经典例题】The biggest engineering project that they undertook was encumbered by lack of funds.
A. hampered　　B. propelled　　C. cancelled　　D. haunted　　[A]
【译　　文】他们接手的这项最大的工程由于缺乏资金而被耽搁了。

handbook ['hænd,buk]

n. 手册
【名师导学】hand 常常与其他词组合成新词，在词中表示"手的，与手有关的"，例如：hand-knit 用手编织，hand-launder 用手搓洗，handmade 手工的，手制的，handprint 手印。
【经典例题】The software came with a handbook, but David still doesn't know how to use it.
【译　　文】虽然软件买来时带有使用手册，但大卫还是不知道怎么用它。

handicap ['hændikæp]

n. 伤残，障碍，不利条件 *vt.* 妨碍
【名师导学】近义词：hindrance, obstacle, block, impediment; disability, impairment, affliction, chronic disorder
【经典例题】A history of long and effortless success can be a dreadful handicap, but, if properly handled, it may become a driving force.
【译　　文】一段漫长而不费力的成功史有可能成为一道可怕的障碍，但如果处理得当，它也许会成为一股推动力。

- **handle** [ˈhændl] n. 柄，把手，拉手 vt. 触，摸，抚弄；操纵；处理，应付
- **handy** [ˈhændi] a. 手边的，近处的；方便的
- **harden** [ˈhɑːdn] vt. 硬化，变硬
- **hardship** [ˈhɑːdʃip] n. 艰难，困苦
- **harmonious** [hɑːˈməuniəs] a. 和谐的，协调的，和睦的，悦耳的
- **harmony** [ˈhɑːməni] n. 和谐，和睦，融洽
  【固定搭配】in harmony with（与……）协调一致；（与……）和睦相处
  【联想记忆】in accordance with, in agreement with（与……）协调一致，（与……）和睦相处
  【经典例题】Design criteria include harmony of colour, texture, lighting, scale, and proportion.
  【译　　文】设计的准则包括色彩、材质、照明、比例的协调。
- **harness** [ˈhɑːnis] vt. 治理，利用
- **harass** [həˈræs] vt. 使疲乏，困扰，反复袭击
  【经典例题】A number of black youths have complained of being harassed by the police.
  【译　　文】许多黑人青年抱怨被警察骚扰。
- **harassment** [ˈhærəsmənt] n. 骚扰，侵袭；烦恼
- **harsh** [hɑːʃ] a. 粗糙的；刺耳的，刺目的；严厉的，苛刻的
- **haste** [heist] n. 急忙，急速
  【固定搭配】in haste, in a hurry 急忙，慌忙
  【经典例题】More haste, less speed.
  【译　　文】欲速则不达。
- **hatch** [hætʃ] v. 孵，孵化
  【名师导学】注意两个常用的短语：hatch out 孵化出来，想出计划；hatch up 发明，设计，计划。
  【经典例题】Don't count the chickens before they are hatched.
  【译　　文】（谚语）鸡蛋还未孵，别忙数鸡雏。
- **haul** [hɔːl] v./n. 拖，拉
  【名师导学】注意与该词相关的短语，例如：a good haul 一大网鱼，一大笔收获；a long haul 长途旅行，相当长的时间；short haul 短途旅行，短时间；haul in 拉进；haul off 改变航向以躲避某物，退却，撤退；haul up 船迎风行驶，把……拖上来，停止。
  【经典例题】At each night's encampment, we all hauled supplies and cleaned dishes.
  【译　　文】在每晚的露营地，我们都拖运物资，清洗碗碟。

haunt
['hɔ:nt]

n. 常到之处，出没处 *vt.* (鬼魂)出没；(不快的事)萦绕于脑际

【名师导学】haunt 可以指思想、回忆等"萦绕于心头"，此意常被忽略，请注意它的用法，例如：I was haunted by his last words to me. 他向我说的最后的话萦绕在我的心头。

【经典例题】A headless rider haunts the country lanes.

【译　　文】一个无头骑士常出没于乡间的小路上。

hazard
['hæzəd]

n. 危险，危害，公害

【固定搭配】at hazard, in danger 在危险中；at all hazards 不顾一切危险；on the hazard 受到威胁；take a hazard to do 冒险做；run the hazard /risk of doing 冒险

hazardous
['hæzədəs]

a. 危险的；冒险的；危害的

【名师导学】近义词：perilous, uncertain, precarious, dangerous

headline
['hedlain]

n. 大标题

【名师导学】辨析 heading, headline：heading 指文章定的标题、题目，也指谈话的论题、话题；headline 指报刊的大字标题、页头题目等。

headquarters
['hed,kwɔ:təz]

n. 总部，司令部，指挥部

【名师导学】headquarters 单复数同形。

heal
[hi:l]

v. 治愈，愈合

【固定搭配】heal sb. of sth. 治愈某人的病

【联想记忆】cure sb. of sth. 治愈某人

healthcare
['helθkεə]

n. 医疗保健，健康护理

heap
[hi:p]

n. (一)堆；大量，许多 *v.* 堆积

【固定搭配】a heap / heaps of 许多，大量；heap praises / insults on (upon) 大肆赞扬/污蔑

【经典例题】Though her parents heap praises upon her musical ability, Jerrilou's piano playing is really terrible.

【译　　文】尽管她父母极力赞扬她的音乐才能，但杰瑞罗的钢琴演奏实在是糟透了。

heave
[hi:v]

n. 举起，升降

v. 举起，抛，投掷；有规律地起伏，喘息，发出叹息，呻吟

hemisphere
['hemisfiə]

n. 半球

【名师导学】前缀 hemi- 表示"一半的，部分的"，例如：hemicycle 半圆形；hemiidentic 半相同的，近似的；hemistich 诗的半句，半行。

hence
[hens]

ad. 因此；今后

【名师导学】辨析 hence, therefore：两词均为连接副词，表示因果关系；两词后均可接句子，但 hence 后可直接跟名词，therefore 通常不能。

【经典例题】They have the same atomic number and hence nearly identical chemical behaviour but different atomic masses.

【译　　文】它们有相同的原子数，因此化学行为几乎完全一样，但原子质量不同。

herb [hə:b]
n. 草药，草本植物
【经典例题】A large range of herbs and spices are used in Indian cookery.
【译　　文】印度人在烹调时使用各种香草和调味品。

heritage ['heritidʒ]
n. 世袭财产，遗产
【经典例题】They also visit China regularly in order to imbibe its splendors and rich heritage.
【译　　文】他们也不时走访中国，欣赏壮观的自然风景和认识丰富的文化遗产。

hesitant ['hezitnt]
a. 踌躇的，犹豫的

hesitate ['heziteit]
vi. 犹豫，踌躇；含糊，支吾
【固定搭配】hesitate about / at / in / over 对……犹豫不决；hesitate to do 迟疑于做
【经典例题】He hesitated before he answered because he didn't know what to say.
【译　　文】他在回答之前犹豫了一下，因为他不知道该说什么。

hibernate ['haibəneit]
vi. 过冬，冬眠，避寒

hierarchical [ˌhaiə'rɑ:kikəl]
a. 分等级的

hierarchy ['haiərɑ:ki]
n. 等级制度；统治集团，领导层
【经典例题】The lack of importance attached to human-resource management can be seen in the corporate hierarchy.
【译　　文】可以从公司等级制度看出其缺乏对人力资源管理部门的重视。

highlight ['hailait]
n. 最重要的部分，最精彩的场面　vt. 使显著，使突出
【经典例题】Kennedy's term of office was highlighted by appeals to idealism.
【译　　文】肯尼迪在当政期间，突出表现了对理想主义的呼吁。

hike [haik]
vi. 徒步旅行，步行　n. 徒步旅行，步行
【经典例题】It's a four-kilometer hike from my house to the school.
【译　　文】从我家到学校要步行4公里。
【名师导学】熟记：go on a hike 徒步旅行，on the hike 流亡，流浪。另外 hike 还可以表示"提高，增加"，例如：a hike in living expenses 生活费用高涨，a price hike 物价猛涨。

hinder ['hində]
vt. 阻碍，妨碍
【经典例题】His career was not noticeably hindered by the fact that he had never been to college.
【译　　文】他的事业没有因为他从未上过大学受到明显的阻碍。

hinge [hindʒ]
n. 合页，折叶，铰链　v. 以……而转移；取决于，依……而定
【名师导学】以下动词意思相近，注意区分：
rely v. （与 on 或 upon 连用）依赖，依靠，信赖，信任
lie v. （与 with 连用）由……决定，取决于，视……而定
rest v. （与 on 连用）使依赖，建立在……之上，以……为基础或根据
hinge v. （与 on 连用）取决于，随……而定，以……为转移

hollow ['hɔləu]
a. 空的，中空的；空洞的，空虚的
【经典例题】Their plea of national poverty rings a little hollow.
【译　　文】他们关于国家贫困的托词听上去有些空洞。

hook [huk]
n. 钩，钩状物　*vt.* 钩住
【经典例题】He hung his coat on the hook behind the door.
【译　　文】他把外套挂在门后的挂钩上。

hop [hɔp]
vi.（人）单足跳跃，单足跳行；（鸟、昆虫等）齐足跳跃，齐足跳行　*vt.* 跳上（汽车、火车、飞机等）
【经典例题】She hopped across the room because she had her foot hurt.
【译　　文】她单脚跳着穿过房间，因为她的脚受伤了。

horizon [hə'raizn]
n. 地平线；眼界，见识
【固定搭配】on the horizon 即将发生的

horrible ['hɔrəbl]
a. 恐怖的，吓人的

horror ['hɔrə]
n. 恐怖；战栗
【经典例题】He is the stereotyped monster of the horror films.
【译　　文】他是恐怖电影中老一套的怪物。

hospitable [hɔ'spitəbl]
a. 热情好客的；好客的；殷勤的；热情友好的；（作物生长条件）适宜的；（环境）舒适的
【经典例题】Sweaty socks and warm, damp sports shoes provide equally hospitable environments.
【译　　文】出汗的袜子和温暖潮湿的运动鞋提供了同样友好的环境。

hospitality [ˌhɔspi'tæləti]
n.（对客人的）友好款待，好客
【名师导学】以 -able 结尾的形容词变成名词时，往往只需将 -able 变为 -ability，例如：able（能……的，有才能的）→ ability（能力，才干），capable（有能力的，能干的）→ capability（能力，性能，容量），changeable（可改变的）→ changeability（可变性，易变性），但是请注意 hospitable（好客的，招待周到的）→ hospitality（好客，殷勤）。
【经典例题】Thank you so much for your generous hospitality.
【译　　文】非常感谢您的盛情款待。

hostage ['hɔstidʒ]
n. 人质

hostile ['hɔstail]
a. 敌方的，敌意的，敌对的
【固定搭配】be hostile to 对某人怀有敌意
【经典例题】I don't like her manner — she's very hostile.
【译　　文】我不喜欢她的态度——待人如仇敌。

hostility [hɔs'tiləti]
n. 敌对，敌意，对抗；抵制，反对；（*pl.*）交战，战争

hound [haund]
n. 猎犬　*vt.* 追逼，烦扰，纠缠
【名师导学】本词属于常考词汇，考生要注意相关短语：be hounded out of 从……中被赶出，hound a person on 激励某人，hound out 挑唆，煽动。
【经典例题】The police are always hounding the murderer.
【译　　文】警方一直在追捕这名凶手。

household
['haushəuld]

n. 户,家庭 *a.* 家庭的,家常的

【名师导学】辨析 household, family, home：household 是抽象的家庭,并含有家事、家务之意；family 着重强调家庭成员；home 强调的是家的概念。

【经典例题】They also did more household work and participated in more of such organized activities as soccer and ballet.

【译　文】他们同样做很多家务,且参与许多有组织的活动,像足球和芭蕾舞。

hover
['hɔvə]

vi. (鸟等)翱翔,盘旋；逗留在近旁,徘徊

【经典例题】A hawk hovers in the sky when it looks for animals to kill on the ground.

【译　文】一只鹰在空中盘旋,寻找地上的动物来猎杀。

hug
[hʌg]

vt. (热烈地)拥抱；紧抱,怀抱 *vi.* 紧紧抱在一起,互相拥抱 *n.* 紧抱,热烈拥抱

【名师导学】本词属于常考词汇,考生要注意相关短语：hug oneself for（为……而）庆幸,沾沾自喜；give sb. a big hug 紧紧抱住某人,例如：Jack hugged himself for being so lucky. 杰克庆幸自己是那么幸运。

【经典例题】He hugged his daughter closely and feared losing her again.

【译　文】他紧紧拥抱女儿,害怕再次失去她。

humble
['hʌmbl]

a. 低下的,卑贱的；恭顺的,谦卑的

【名师导学】辨析 humble, modest：两词都有"谦逊"之意。humble 强调对自己的成就不自满的品德,有时也可以指自感卑微；modest 更强调人的谦虚,无自卑、恭顺之意。

【经典例题】The doctor was humble about his work, although he cured many people.

【译　文】这位医生虽然治好了许多人的病,但他对他的工作仍很谦逊。

humidity
[hju:'miditi]

n. 湿度

【经典例题】Store the camera away from humidity and in a dust-free place.

【译　文】要把相机置于干燥、无尘的地方。

humo(u)r
['hju:mə]

n. 幽默,诙谐

【固定搭配】in a good / bad humor 情绪好（不好）；in the humor for sth. 有做某事的心情；out of humor 情绪不好

humo(u)rous
['hju:mərəs]

a. 幽默的

hunt
[hʌnt]

n. / v. 打猎,狩猎；寻找,搜索

【固定搭配】hunt down 穷追……直至捕获；搜寻……直至发现；hunt for / after 追猎；搜寻

hurl
[hə:l]

vt. 猛投,力掷；大声叫骂

【经典例题】He hurled the brick through the window to show his resentment.

【译　文】他用力把砖头从窗户扔了过去,表示自己的愤怒。

hurricane
['hʌrikən, -kein]

n. 飓风

【经典例题】The hurricane flung their motorboat upon the rocks.

【译　文】飓风把他们的摩托艇抛到岩石上了。

hypothesis
[hai'pɔθisis]

n. 假设

【名师导学】以 -sis 结尾的名词，变成复数时词尾变为 -ses，例如：thesis → theses 论题，论文；hypothesis → hypotheses 假设，臆测；analysis → analyses 分析，分解。

【经典例题】This is only a sort of scientific hypothesis which has not been proved by experiments.

【译　　文】这仅仅是一个尚未被实验证明的科学假说。

hysterical
[hi'sterikəl]

a. 情绪异常激动的，歇斯底里般的

【经典例题】The young man grew hysterical when he heard that he had been infected with AIDS.

【译　　文】这名年轻男子得知自己染上艾滋病后，开始歇斯底里起来。

ideal
[ai'diəl]

a. 理想的，称心如意的；唯心论的　*n.* 理想

identical
[ai'dentikəl]

a. 相同的；同一的

【固定搭配】be identical with / to 和……完全相同　be identical in 在……方面相同

【名师导学】辨析 be similar to, be the same as, be identical with / to：be similar to 和……相似；be the same as 和……相同；be identical with / to 和……完全相同。

【经典例题】The jobs of wildlife technicians and biologists seemed identical to him, but one day he discovered their difference.

【译　　文】在他看来，野生动物技术员和生物学家的工作似乎是一样的，但是有一天他发现了这二者之间的区别。

identification
[ai,dentifi'keiʃən]

n. 辨认，视为同一；证明，鉴定

【固定搭配】identification card = identity card 身份证

【经典例题】He used a letter of introduction as identification.

【译　　文】他用一封介绍信作为身份的证明。

identify
[ai'dentifai]

vt. 认出，鉴定；等同，打成一片

【固定搭配】identify oneself with... 参加到……中去，和……打成一片；identify...with 认为……等同于

【名师导学】辨析 identify, recognize：identify 指通过某些内在的东西辨认出某人某物；recognize 指认出曾经见过或原来认识的人或物，强调通过外表认出。

【经典例题】The basic causes are unknown, although certain conditions that may lead to cancer have been identified.

【译　　文】尽管目前已经确认了会导致癌症发生的一些条件，但根本原因还不清楚。

identity
[ai'dentiti]

n. 身份；个性，特征

【经典例题】The police are trying to find out the identity of the woman killed in the traffic accident.
【译　　文】警方正在设法查清那名在交通事故中亡的女性的身份。

ideological
[ˌaidiə'lɔdʒikl]

a. 意识形态的

ideology
[ˌaidi'ɔdʒi, id-]

n. 思想（体系），思想意识

【名师导学】后缀 -ology 表示"……学"，"……论"，"……研究"，如：biology 生物学，生物；psycology 心理学；sociology 社会学；ecology 生态学。
【经典例题】This ideology is very dangerous to our country because it includes undemocratic philosophies.
【译　　文】这种意识形态对我们国家是非常危险的，因为其中包含了非民主的观点。

idiot
['idiət]

n. 白痴，傻子，笨蛋

【经典例题】You may disagree with me as to how we ought to deal with the problem, but you shouldn't treat me as an idiot.
【译　　文】至于我们应该怎样解决这个问题，你可以和我持不同看法，但是你不应该把我当个傻瓜来看。

idle
['aidl]

a. 闲散的，闲置的；无用的，无效的 *v.* 使空闲，虚度

【固定搭配】idle away (one's time) 消磨时光
【经典例题】Now, off their work on way home, they can take a breath and be idle for a while.
【译　　文】现在，在下班回家的路上，他们可以呼吸一下新鲜空气，闲逛一下。

ignite
[ig'nait]

vt. 引燃，点火机，着火

【经典例题】His speech ignited the audience's cheer.
【译　　文】他的讲话激起了听众的喝彩。

ignorance
['ignərəns]

n. 无知，愚昧

【经典例题】Ignorance of the law is no excuse.
【译　　文】不懂法律不能成为借口。

ignorant
['ignərənt]

a. 无知的，愚昧的；不知道的

【固定搭配】be ignorant of / that... 不知道，不了解
【名师导学】辨析 ignorant, innocent：两词都有"无知的"意思。ignorant 指对某种情况"不知道的，不了解的"；innocent 指由于缺乏头脑产生的"无知的，幼稚的"。
【经典例题】A tiny insect, trying to shake a mighty tree, is ludicrously ignorant of its own weakness.
【译　　文】蚍蜉撼大树，可笑不自量。

illegal
[i'li:gəl]

a. 不合法的，非法的

【经典例题】Selling cigars without a license is illegal.
【译　　文】无执照而销售雪茄烟是违法的。

illicit
[i'lisit]

a. 违法的，违禁的，不正当的

【名师导学】近义词群：unlawful, prohibited, unauthorized, improper; adulterous, illegal, wrong

illuminate
[i'lju:mineit]

vt. 照明；阐明；说明 *vi.* 照亮；用灯装饰

【名师导学】近义词：interpret, elucidate, clarify, explain; lighten, irradiate, illumine, brighten

【经典例题】Floodlights illuminated the stadium.

【译　　文】泛光灯照亮了体育馆。

illusion
[i'luːʒən, i'ljuː-]

n. 幻觉，错觉，错误的信仰（或观念）

【名师导学】考生要注意相关短语 be under no illusion about sth. 对某事不存幻想，cherish the illusion that 错误地认为，have no illusion about 对……不存幻想。

【经典例题】The magician made us think he cut the girl into pieces, but it was merely an illusion.

【译　　文】魔术师让我们以为他把那个女孩切成了碎片，但这只是错觉。

illustrate
['iləstreit]

vt. 举例说明，图解

【经典例题】The following account by the author illustrates the difference between European and American reactions.

【译　　文】作者做出的下列解释说明了欧洲人和美国人在反应方面的区别。

imitate
['imiteit]

vt. 模仿，仿效；仿造，伪造

immense
[i'mens]

a. 巨大的，广大的

immerse
[i'məːs]

vt. 使浸没；（in）使沉浸在，使专心于

【名师导学】此词常以被动形式出现于短语中：be immersed in 沉浸于，沉溺于，专心于。

【经典例题】They were immersed in their scientific research, not knowing what happened just outside their lab.

【译　　文】他们沉浸在科学研究中，不知道实验室外面发生了什么。

immigrant
['imigrənt]

n. 移民，侨民 *a.* 移民的

【名师导学】辨析 immigrant, emigrant：immigrant 指的是来自国外的移民，指为永久居住目的而从别国到居住国的人；emigrant 指的是离开国家或地区到别国永久居住的人。

immune
[i'mjuːn]

a. 被豁免的，免除的；免疫（性）的，有免疫力的；不受影响的

【固定搭配】be immune to / against / from sth. 免受某事影响，对某事有免疫力

【名师导学】此词常与介词 against, from, to 连用，表示"免疫的、免受伤害的"，如：be immune from taxation 免于纳税，be immune from criminal prosecution 免于刑事诉讼，be immune to persuasion 不能被说服的，be immune from punishment 免受惩罚。

【经典例题】This hypothesis states that environments that are too clean may actually make the immune system develop oversensitive responses.

【译　　文】这个假设认为过于洁净的环境实际上可能会使免疫系统产生过敏反应。

immunize
['imjunaiz]

vt. 使免疫；使免除（against）

impact
['impækt]

n. 影响，作用；冲击，碰撞
【固定搭配】have an impact on sth. 对……的影响
【经典例题】Professor Taylor's talk has indicated that science has a very strong _____ on the everyday life of nonscientists as well as scientists.
A. motivation B. perspective
C. impression D. impact [D]
【译　　文】泰勒教授指出，科学不仅仅对科学家而且对普通人的日常生活都会产生强烈的影响。

impair
[im'pɛə]

v. 损害，损伤，削弱
【名师导学】近义词：spoil, injure, hurt, damage, destroy; diminish, undermine, reduce, weaken
【经典例题】Memory can be both enhanced and impaired by use of drugs.
【译　　文】使用药物可以提高也可以损伤记忆力。

impart
[im'pɑ:t]

v. 给予，传授；告知，透露

impatient
[im'peiʃənt]

a. 不耐烦的，急躁的
【固定搭配】be impatient of 对……不耐烦，不能忍受；be impatient for / to do 急切

impede
[im'pi:d]

vt. 妨碍；阻碍

imperative
[im'perətiv]

a. 必要的，紧急的；命令的 *n.* 必要的事，必须完成的事；祈使语气
【经典例题】Military orders are imperative and cannot be disobeyed.
【译　　文】军令是强制性的，必须遵守。

imperial
[im'piəriəl]

a. 帝国的，帝王的；（度量衡）英制的
【经典例题】All the single rooms are occupied. But if you like, I can check with Imperial Hotel to see if they have any.
【译　　文】所有的单间都住满了。如果您愿意，我可以和帝国旅馆联系，看他们是否还有单间。

impetus
['impitəs]

n. 促进，刺激，推动力
【名师导学】近义词：force, impulsion, spur, stimulus, incentive, purpose

implement
['implimənt]

n. (*pl.*) 工具，器具 *vt.* 实行，实施，执行

implicit
[im'plisit]

a. 含蓄的，不言明的；内含的；固有的；无疑的；无保留的

imply
[im'plai]

vt. 意指，暗示
【经典例题】These life-prolonging drugs were not prescribed to many patients who appeared to be eligible for them, implying that both generalists and specialists could do better.
【译　　文】这些延长生命的药物通常不会对那些有权使用的病人开出处方，暗示着全科大夫和专业医生都还有改进的空间。

impose
[im'pəuz]

vt. 把……强加于，加重……负担；征收（税款）

第二部分 核心意义词汇（A-K）

impress [im'pres]
vt. 印；给……以深刻印象；使铭记；*n.* 印象、印记
【经典例题】Other dermatologists are impressed by the work.
【译　文】其他皮肤病学家对这份研究印象深刻。

impression [im'preʃən]
n. 印象，感想；印记
【固定搭配】have the impression of / that 有……印象；leave a good / deep impression on sb. 给……留下很好 / 深的印象
【经典例题】He gives people the impression of having spent all his life abroad.
【译　文】他给人的感觉是好像一直在国外生活。

impressive [im'presiv]
a. 给人印象深刻的，感人的
【经典例题】However, he calls the reported risk reduction unimpressive.
【译　文】但是，他认为报道中的风险控制不怎么出色。

improve [im'pru:v]
vt. 改善，改进　*vi.* 好转，进步
【经典例题】The popular idea that classical music can improve your maths is falling from favor.
【译　文】认为古典音乐能提升数学能力的传统观念已经不再流行了。

improvement [im'pru:vmənt]
n. 改进，改良，增进；改进措施
【经典例题】No group showed any statistically significant improvement in their abilities.
【译　文】没有任何一个小组从统计数据能显示出能力的显著提升。

impulse ['impʌls]
n. 冲动，驱使
【固定搭配】on impulse 一时冲动；give an impulse to sth. 促进
【经典例题】In fact as he approached this famous statue, he only barely resisted the impulse to reach into his bag for his camera.
【译　文】实际上，当他走近这座著名雕像时，他差点忍不住从包里拿出照相机来。

inaugurate [i'nɔ:gjureit]
vt. 开始，开展；为……举行就职典礼，使正式就任；为……举行开幕式，为……举行落成仪式
【经典例题】The new president of the company will be inaugurated in January.
【译　文】公司新总裁将在1月份就任。

incentive [in'sentiv]
n. 激励前进的动力
【固定搭配】price incentive 价格刺激；tax incentive 税收鼓励；give sb. an incentive to do sth. 激发某人去干某事
【经典例题】Money is still a major incentive to most people.
【译　文】对于大多数人来说，金钱仍是主要动机。

incidence ['insidəns]
n. 发生（率）
【名师导学】注意形近词，以 -ence 结尾的名词不少，如：evidence, confidence, dependence。
【经典例题】The＿＿＿of lung cancer is particularly high among long-term heavy smokers, especially chain smokers.
A. incident　　B. accident　　C. incidence　　D. evidence　　[C]
【译　文】肺癌的发病率在长期吸烟的人群中特别高，尤其是连续吸烟人群。

219

incident
['insidənt]

n. 事件，政治事件，事变

【经典例题】Have you got a funny ____ or unusual experience that you would like to share?
A. amusement　B. incident　C. accident　D. section　　[B]
【译　　文】你有没有有意思的或者非凡的经历来分享？

incidentally
[,insi'dentəli]

ad. 附带提及地，顺便地

【名师导学】有些副词用来表示评价一件事，或说明一种状态，可以单独放在句首，除 incidentally 以外，常见的还有：fortunately 幸运的是，unfortunately 不幸地，luckily 幸运地，generally（或 generally speaking）一般说来。

【经典例题】I must go now. Incidentally, if you want that book I'll bring it next time.
【译　　文】我现在该走了。顺便提一句，如果你要那本书，我下次带来。

incite
[in'sait]

vt. 煽动，鼓动

【名师导学】近义词群：arouse, rouse, instigate, impel, stimulate, provoke, foment, excite, spur

incline
[in'klain]

v. 使倾向，使倾斜，使偏向　n. 斜坡，斜面

【派生词汇】inclination n. 偏向，倾向
【固定搭配】incline to / towards sth. 有……的倾向；be inclined to do sth. 想做某事，有……的趋势

incorporate
[in'kɔ:pəreit]

vt. 结合，合并，使加入，收编　vi. 合并，混合

【经典例题】We will incorporate your suggestion in the new plan.
【译　　文】我们将把你的建议纳入新计划。

increasingly
[in'kri:siŋli]

ad. 日益地，越来越多地

【经典例题】The international situation has been growing ____ difficult for the last few years.
A. invariably　B. presumably　C. increasingly　D. dominantly　　[C]
【译　　文】最近几年国际形势越来越严峻。

incredible
[in'kredəbl]

a. 难以置信的，不能相信的

incur
[in'kə:]

v. 招致，遭受，引起

independence
[,indi'pendəns]

n. 独立，自主，自立

independent
[,indi'pendənt]

a. 独立的，自立的，自主的

【固定搭配】be independent of 独立……之外，不受……支配
【联想记忆】depend / rely / count on 依赖；independent of 不依赖

index
['indeks]

a. 索引；指标，指数

【名师导学】index 复数形式为 indexes 或 indices。
【经典例题】If exercise is a bodily maintenance activity and an index of physiological age, the lack of sufficient exercise may either cause or hasten aging.

A. instance　　B. indicator　　C. appearance　D. option　　　　　　[B]
【译　　文】如果锻炼既能维持身体机能同时也是生理年龄指标的话，那么缺乏足够的锻炼要么会造成老化，要么会加速老化。

indicate
['indikeit]

vt. 指示，表示；暗示
【经典例题】In some non-Western cultures, even a warm, open smile does not necessarily indicate pleasure or agreement.
【译　　文】在一些非西方文化中，哪怕一个温暖、开放的微笑都未必暗示着愉悦和赞同。

indicative
[in'dikətiv]

a. 指示的；表示的；象征的；预示的　n. 陈述语气

indication
[ˌindi'keiʃən]

n. 指示，表示；暗示

indicator
['indikeitə]

n. 指示器，指示器；[计算机]指示符
【经典例题】If exercise is a bodily maintenance activity and an index of physiological age, the lack of sufficient exercise may either cause or hasten aging.
A. instance　　　　　　　　B. indicator
C. appearance　　　　　　　D. option　　　　　　　　　[B]
【译　　文】如果锻炼能够维持身体机能同时也可成为生理年龄指标，那么缺乏足够的锻炼可能会造成老化，也可能会加速老化。
【名师导学】denote, indicate 这两个动词都有"表示"之意。
denote：指用符号等表示。
indicate：指用词语或标记表达较明确的意义。
mean, imply, indicate, represent, denote, signify, suggest 这些动词均含有"表示……的意思"之意。
mean：最普通用词，指文字或符号等所表示的各种明确的或含蓄的意义。
imply：侧重用文字或符号表示的联想，暗示。
indicate：指明显的表示。
represent：指体现或代表。
denote：指某一词字面或狭义的意思，或指某些符号或迹象的特指含义。
signify：指用文字、说话或表情等表示单纯的意思。
suggest：通常指暗含地、隐晦地表达意思。

indifferent
[in'difərənt]

a. 不关心的，冷漠的

indignant
[in'dignənt]

a. 愤慨的，义愤的
【名师导学】注意和不同的介词搭配时，意义的区别：be indignant at sth. 对某事感到愤慨，be indignant with sb. 对某人表示愤愤不平。
【经典例题】The members of Parliament were indignant that the government had not consulted them.
【译　　文】议会成员对于政府没有与他们协商这件事而很愤怒。

indignation
[ˌindig'neiʃn]

n. 愤怒，义愤

indispensable
[ˌindis'pensəbl]

a. 不可缺少的

induce
[in'dju:s]
vt. 引起，感应
【名师导学】注意相关短语：induce sb. to do sth. 劝导某人做某事。
【经典例题】When he realized he had been induced to sign the contract by intrigue, he threatened to start legal proceedings to cancel the agreement.
【译　　文】当他意识到自己被诡计诱导着签了合同时，他威胁说要通过法律行动来取消合约。

inductive
[in'dʌktiv]
a. 引入的；诱导的；归纳的

indulge
[in'dʌldʒ]
v. 放任，纵容，沉溺；使（自己）纵情享受
【名师导学】本词属于常考词汇，常以该短语出现：indulge in 沉溺于，纵情享受。
【经典例题】On weekends my grandma usually indulges in a glass of wine.
【译　　文】我的祖母常在周末畅饮一杯。

inevitable
[in'evitəbl]
a. 不可避免的，必然的
【经典例题】It is inevitable that some changes will take place.
【译　　文】有些变化将要发生，不可避免。

inertia
[i'nə:ʃiə]
n. 惯性；惰性，保守
【经典例题】The reason why many badly needed reforms were never introduced is the inertia of the system.
【译　　文】许多急需的改革迟迟没有进行，都是由于制度具有惰性。

infer
[in'fə:]
vt. 推论，推断
【固定搭配】infer from sth. 从……推论，由……推知

inferior
[in'fiəriə]
a. 次的，低劣的；下级的，低等的
【固定搭配】be inferior to... 比……差，比……地位低
【联想记忆】superior to 优于；prior to 优先于，先于；junior to 比……年少；senior to 比……年长；preferable to 比……更好
【经典例题】Their products are frequently overpriced and ＿＿＿ in quality.
A. influential　　　　　　B. subordinate
C. inferior　　　　　　　D. superior　　　　　　[C]
【译　　文】他们的产品经常是价格偏高，质量又很差。

infinite
['infinit]
a. 无限的，无穷的
【经典例题】She remains confident and infinitely untroubled by our present problems.
【译　　文】面对我们现在的问题她总是能够保持自信和乐观。

infinity
[in'finiti]
n. 无限；永恒

inflation
[in'fleiʃən]
n. 通货膨胀

influence
['influəns]
n. 势力，权势　*vt./n.* 影响，感化
【固定搭配】have influence on / upon 影响
【联想记忆】have / make an impact on, have an effect on 影响
【经典例题】It also has some negative influence.
【译　　文】这也有些负面影响。

influential [ˌɪnfluˈenʃəl]	*a.* 有影响的，有势力的
infringe [ˈɪnfrɪndʒ]	*vt.* 破坏；侵犯；违犯，违反
ingenious [ɪnˈdʒiːnjəs]	*a.* 机灵的，聪明的；精巧制成的，别致的，有独创性的

ingenuity [ˌɪndʒɪˈnjuːɪti]	*n.* 智巧，创造力，精巧的设计
	【联想记忆】in 最先进的，在里面的 + gen（gene）基因 +uity（unite）联合 = 最先进的基因的联合 =ingenuity 创造力
	【经典例题】The difficult case tested the ingenuity of even the most skillful physician.
	  A. credibility B. commitment
	  C. honesty D. talent [D]
	【译　　文】即使是最熟练的医师，疑难杂症也是对其智谋的考验。
	【名师导学】近义词群：creativity, dexterity, genius, originality

ingredient [ɪnˈgriːdiənt]	*n.*（混合物的）组成部分，配料；成分，要素 【经典例题】Why does a vegetarian restaurant make its dishes resemble meat in every way except ingredients? 【译　　文】为什么素食饭店的每道菜除了配料都像是荤菜？
inhabitant [ɪnˈhæbɪtənt]	*n.* 居民，住户
inherent [ɪnˈhɪərənt]	*a.*（in）内在的，固有的，生来就有的 【名师导学】近义词：innate, inborn, inbred, indigenous to, intrinsic, internal, original, native, deep-rooted, built-in, latent. 【经典例题】He has pointed out the dangers inherent in this type of nuclear power station. 【译　　文】他已经指出这类核电站内在的危险。
inherit [ɪnˈherɪt]	*v.* 继承，遗传而得 【固定搭配】inherit...from 从……继承，遗传
inhibit [ɪnˈhɪbɪt]	*vt.* 阻止，妨碍，抑制 【经典例题】Childhood viral infections will inhibit the development of brain cells. 【译　　文】幼年时的病毒感染会抑制脑细胞的发育。
initial [ɪˈnɪʃəl]	*a.* 最初的，开头的　*n.* 首字母 【名师导学】辨析 initial, original, primary, primitive：initial 意为"最初的，开始的"，强调处于事物的起始阶段的，开头的，也可指位于开头地方的；original 意为"最早的，最先的"，强调处于事物的起始阶段的，按顺序应是首位的，也可指原始的、原件的，即非仿造的东西；primary 指在时间、顺序或发展上领先的（第一的、基本的、主要的）；primitive 指处于人类生命或事物发展的早期阶段的、原始的。 【经典例题】Though the initial idea was to just sit in the sun a bit, we were drawn toward the sidewalk. 【译　　文】尽管最初的想法是多沐浴阳光，但我们还是被吸引到人行道上。

initiate [i'niʃieit]	*vt.* 开始，创始，发动；启蒙，使入门；引入，正式介绍 【固定搭配】be initiated into 正式加入；initiate sb. into sth. 准许或介绍某人加入某团体，把某事传授给某人 【经典例题】We should initiate a new social custom. 【译　　文】我们要开创社会新风尚。
initiative [i'niʃiətiv]	*n.* 创始，首创精神；决断的能力；主动性　*a.* 起始的，初步的 【经典例题】We can't teach them how to think and to take initiative. 【译　　文】我们不能教他们如何思考，以及如何采取主动。
inject [in'dʒekt]	*vt.* 注射，注入；插进（话），引入 【名师导学】本词属于常考词汇，考生要注意相关短语：inject into 把……注入，给……增添；inject with 用……注入 【经典例题】Look at your talk and pick out a few words and sentences which you can turn about and inject with humour. 【译　　文】注意自己的言语，挑出几个你能把握的词句，注入幽默。
inland ['inlənd]	*a.* 内地的，内陆的，国内的　*ad.* 在内地，向内地 【名师导学】通常用在这样的搭配里：go inland 到内地去，live inland 住在内地，inland trade 国内贸易，inland telegraph 国内电报。注意前缀 in-，可以表示"在……里面，进入……之内"，例如：incage（*n.* 囚禁），incase（*v.* 装进箱、筒、包等容器内），input（*n. / v.* 输入）；还可以表示"否定，与……相反"，例如：incalculable（*a.* 不可计算的），inability（*n.* 无能力）。 【经典例题】I headed inland for some place of hiding. 【译　　文】我跑到内陆去找藏身之所。
innocent ['inəsnt]	*a.* 无罪的，清白的；无害的；天真的，单纯的 【固定搭配】be innocent of 无意识的，无……罪的 【联想记忆】be guilty of 有……罪
innovation [,inəu'veiʃən]	*n.* 创新，改革 【经典例题】Given this optimistic approach to technological innovation, the American worker took readily to that special kind of nonverbal thinking required in mechanical technology. 【译　　文】有了这种对技术革新的乐观态度，美国工人很快便习惯了机械技术所需要的非语言的思维方式。
input ['input]	*n.* 输入
insane [in'sein]	*a.* 蠢极的，荒唐的；（患）精神病的，精神失常的，疯狂的 【派生词汇】insanity *n.* 愚蠢，疯狂 【经典例题】I know all about your insane plan. 【译　　文】我对你的愚蠢计划了如指掌。
insight ['insait]	*n.* 洞察力，见识，深刻了解 【经典例题】The author of the book has shown his remarkably keen ＿＿＿ into human nature. 　A. perspective　B. dimension　C. insight　D. reflection　　[C] 【译　　文】此书的作者已经表现出了对人性敏锐的洞察力。

installment
[in'stɔːlmənt]

n. 分期付款；（连载）一部分，一期

【经典例题】We pay for our holidays in installment of $50 a month.
【译　　文】我们用每月付 50 美元分期付款的方式度假。

instance
['instəns]

n. 例证，实例
【固定搭配】for instance 举例说，比如

instant
['instənt]

n. 瞬间，时刻　*a.* 立即的，立刻的；紧急的，迫切的；（食品）速溶的，方便的
【固定搭配】on the instant 立即；the instant (that) 一……就（引导时间状语从句）
【经典例题】You see the lightening the instant it happens, but you hear the thunder later.
【译　　文】你可以在闪电发生的瞬间立刻看见它，但要稍后才能听到雷声。

instinct
['instiŋkt]

n. 本能，直觉；天性
【固定搭配】have an instinct for 生来爱好；by instinct 出于本能
【联想记忆】instinctive *a.* 本能的，直觉的，冲动的
【经典例题】Human behavior is mostly a product of learning, whereas the behavior of an animal depends mainly on instinct.
【译　　文】人类行为主要是后天学习的产物，而动物的行为则大都出于本能。

institute
['institjuːt]

n. 学会，研究所；学院

institution
[ˌinstiˈtjuːʃən]

n. 协会，公共机关，学校；制度，习俗

institutional
[ˌinstiˈtjuːʃənəl]

a. 设立的，规定的，制度上的

instruct
[in'strʌkt]

vt. 教，教授；指示，指令
【固定搭配】instruct sb. to do sth. 通知（或吩咐）某人做某事；instruct sb. in sth. 教导某人某事
【联想记忆】teach sb. sth. 教某人某事
【经典例题】The hotel fire officer will instruct you in how to evacuate the building if a fire breaks out.
【译　　文】酒店的消防人员将会告诉你万一着火如何逃生。

insulate
['insjuleit]

vt. 绝缘
【经典例题】Many houses in the north are warm in winter because they are insulated so that the heat is not lost.
【译　　文】北方的许多房子在冬天很暖和，因为它们都做了保温处理，使热量不会散失。

intact
[in'tækt]

a. 未经触动的，原封不动的，完整无损的

intake
['inteik]

n. 吸入，进气；（液体等）进入口；摄入，摄取；纳入（数）量
【经典例题】Choose medicine, because it is a profession that allows you to pursue many different paths, catering for the diverse personalities that constitute any medical school's intake.
【译　　文】选择医学作为职业，是因为它可以让你追求许多不同的道路，满足构成任何医学院入学需要的多元化人格。

integral
['intigrəl]
a. 组成的，完整的，构成整体所需要的

integrate
['intigreit]
vt. 使结合，使一体化
【固定搭配】integrate...with... 把……与……相结合；integrate...into 使……并入
【经典例题】Many suggestions are needed to integrate the plan.
【译　　文】需要许多建议使计划更加完整。

integrity
[in'tegriti]
n. 诚实，正直，完整
【经典例题】They have always regarded man of integrity and fairness as a reliable friend.
【译　　文】他们一直认为诚实、正直的人是可信赖的朋友。

intellect
['intilekt]
n. 理智，智力；有才智的人

intellectual
[,inti'lektʃuəl]
n. 知识分子　*a.* 智力的；显示智力的，能发挥才智的
【经典例题】More legislation is needed to protect the ＿＿ property rights of the patent.
A. integrative　　　　　B. intellectual
C. intelligent　　　　　D. intelligible　　　　　[B]
【译　　文】需要更多立法保护专利知识产权。

intelligence
[in'telidʒəns]
n. 智力；理解力；情报，消息，报道

intelligent
[in'telidʒənt]
a. 聪明的，理智的
【经典例题】He was intelligent enough to understand my questions from the gestures I made.
【译　　文】他非常聪明，能根据我的手势明白我的问题。

intelligible
[in'telidʒəbl]
a. 可以理解的，易领悟的，清晰的
【联想记忆】intelligence n. 智慧，智力，智商（intelligible=intellig+ible(able)需要智慧才能理解的）；intelligent a. 智慧的，聪明的
【经典例题】This report would be intelligible only to an expert in computing.
A. intelligent　　　　　B. comprehensive
C. competent　　　　　D. comprehensible　　　　　[D]
【译　　文】只有电脑专家才能明白这个报道。

intend
[in'tend]
vt. 想要，打算，企图
【固定搭配】intend to do sth. 打算做某事；be intended as / for 原意要，意指……
【名师导学】intend to have done 表示打算做而实际未做，有虚拟含义，此类的表达还有 plan to have done，mean to have done。

intense
[in'tens]
a. 强烈的，激烈的，热烈的

intensity
[in'tensəti]
n. 强烈；紧张；剧烈；强度；烈度
【经典例题】The attack was anticipated but its intensity came as a shock.
【译　　文】这次袭击是预料之中的，但其强度令人震惊。

intensive [in'tensiv]

a. 加强的，密集的；精工细作的

【名师导学】辨析 intense, intensive：intense 意为"激烈的，强烈的"，如 intense competition（激烈的竞争）；intensive 意为"集中的，加强的"，如 intensive reading（精读）。

【经典例题】The patient's health failed to such an extent that he was put into intensive care.

【译　　文】这名病人的病情恶化得相当严重，已对他进行了重病特别护理。

intent [in'tent]

n. 意图，目的，意向　*a.* 专心的，专注的；急切的

【固定搭配】intent on 专心的，急切的

interactive [,intər'æktiv]

a. 相互作用的，相互影响的

intercourse ['intə(:)kɔ:s]

n. 交际，交往，交流

intention [in'tenʃən]

n. 意图，意向，目的

【经典例题】She had clearly no intention of doing any work, although she was very well paid.

【译　　文】她明显不打算干任何工作，尽管她的工资待遇很不错。

interface ['intə(:),feis]

n. 界面，接口

interfere [,intə'fiə]

vi. 干涉，干预；妨碍

【固定搭配】interfere in / with 妨碍，阻碍，干扰，干涉

【经典例题】I don't want to interfere with you; proceed with your work.

【译　　文】我不想打扰你了，你继续工作吧。

interference [,intə'fiərəns]

n. 干涉，冲突

intermittent [,intə(:)'mitənt]

n. 间歇的，断断续续的

【经典例题】The weather forecast is for sun, with an intermittent shower.

【译　　文】天气预报是晴天，间歇有阵雨。

Internet ['intənet]

n. 因特网

interpret [in'tə:prit]

vt. 解释；说明；口译；翻译

【名师导学】辨析 translate, interpret：translate 指口头或笔头翻译；interpret 仅指口头翻译。

【经典例题】I interpret his answer as a refusal.

【译　　文】我把他的回答理解为拒绝。

interpretation [in,tə:pri'teiʃən]

n. 解释，阐明

interrogation [in,terə'geiʃn]

n. 询讯，审问

interrupt [,intə'rʌpt]

vt. 打断，打扰；断绝，中断

【名师导学】辨析 bankrupt, corrupt, interrupt：bankrupt 意为"破产的"；corrupt 意为"贪污的"；interrupt 意为"中断，打断"。

intersection
[ˌintə(ː)ˈsekʃn]
n. 横断；交叉；交点，交叉线

intersperse
[ˌintəˈspəːs]
vt. 散布，散置，点缀
【经典例题】Sunny periods will be interspersed with occasional showers.
A. interrupted B. blocked C. blended D. intersected [C]
【译　　文】晴日里总是不时地被点缀上几场雷阵雨。

interval
[ˈintəvəl]
n. 间隔，间歇
【固定搭配】at intervals 有时，不时，时时；at an interval of 间隔／间距（多长时间／多远）
【经典例题】Schumann wrote a great deal of music during his manic intervals.
【译　　文】舒曼在精神病发作的间歇写了大量的音乐作品。

intervene
[ˌintəˈviːn]
vi. 干预，干涉；介入
【经典例题】The first step before making any decision to ＿＿ was to determine exactly who did the killing.
A. interact B. integrate C. intervene D. intensify [C]
【译　　文】在做决定介入前，第一步要做的是确定谁杀的人。

interview
[ˈintəvjuː]
n. 接见，会见，面试 *vt.* 接见，会见
【联想记忆】preview *n.*／*vt.* 预习，预演；review *n.*／*vt.* 复习；view *n.* 风景，看法；viewpoint *n.* 观点
【经典例题】Obviously the long interviews were the more successful ones.
【译　　文】很明显，持续时间久的面试更有可能成功。

intimate
[ˈintimət]
a. 亲密的，密切的
【经典例题】Much more frequent are forms of misconduct that occur as part of the intimate relationship between a faculty member and a student.
【译　　文】更频繁的不当行为，是以师生间亲密关系的形式发生的。

intimidate
[inˈtimideit]
v. 恐吓，威胁
【固定搭配】be intimidated by 被……吓倒（该词常用在被动语态里）
【名师导学】近义词群：scare, overawe, cow, browbeat; frighten, threaten

intricate
[ˈintrikət]
a. 复杂的，错综的
【经典例题】Although the problem is intricate and complex, it can be solved very quickly with an electronic computer.
【译　　文】这道题虽然错综复杂，但用电子计算机很快就能解出。

intrinsic
[inˈtrinsik]
a. 固有的，内在的，本质的
【经典例题】The emphasis is no longer on equilibrium but on the intrinsic dynamics of urban change.
【译　　文】重点不再是城市变化的平衡性，而是城市变化的内在动力。

intuition
[ˌintjuː(ː)ˈiʃən]
n. 直觉
【经典例题】His intuition was telling him that something was wrong.
【译　　文】直觉告诉他出事了。

invalid
[inˈvælid]
a. （指法律上）无效的，作废的；无可靠根据的，站不住脚的 *n.* (the) 病弱者，残疾者
【经典例题】Your license has been invalid.
【译　　文】你的执照已经作废了。

inventory
['invəntri]

n. 存货，库存量；财产等的清单

【名师导学】后缀 -ory 可构成形容词和名词，表示"……所在，……地方"或"……性质，与……有关的"，例如：inventory 详细目录，存货清单；advisory 劝告的；crematory 与火葬有关的；monitory 训诫的。

【经典例题】Nike misjudged the strength of the aerobics shoe craze and was forced to unload huge inventories of running shoes through discount stores.

【译　文】耐克公司错误地估计了健身鞋的热销程度，于是不得不通过廉价商店来倾销大量的跑鞋存货。

invert
[in'və:t]

v. 颠倒，翻转

【经典例题】Invert the subject and predicate of a sentence.

【译　文】颠倒句子的主语和谓语。

investigate
[in'vestigeit]

v. 调查，调研

【固定搭配】investigate (into) sth. 对某事进行调查

【经典例题】What we need now is for national medical research bodies and cancer research organizations to investigate the relative risks and benefits of sunshine.

【译　文】我们现在需要的是国家的医疗机构和癌症研究组织能调查阳光的相关风险和益处。

involve
[in'vɔlv]

vt. 卷入，陷入，连累；包含，含有

【固定搭配】be involved in 陷入，使专心于；involve with 和……混在一起，和……有密切联系

【名师导学】① involve 后接动名词做宾语。② involved 做定语前置和后置含义不同，如 the people involved 所涉及的人；an involved sentence 复杂的句子。

【经典例题】There are highly professional criminals involved in car theft.

【译　文】在汽车盗窃案件中，有较多的职业窃贼。

irrespective
[,iri'spektiv]

a. 不考虑的，不顾及的

【联想记忆】respective *a.* 分别的，各自的

ironic(al)
[ai'rɔnik(əl)]

a. 讽刺的，冷嘲的

irony
['aiərəni]

n. 反话，讽刺

【经典例题】The irony of the historian's craft is that its practitioners always know that their efforts are but contributions to an unending process.

【译　文】对历史学家这一行业具讽刺意味的是，从业者总是明白，他们的努力只是对一个无穷的过程的小小奉献。

irradiate
[i'reidieit]

v. 照耀，辐射，（使）灿烂，（使）明亮

【联想记忆】ir（表示"红外辐射"的缩写）+radiate（辐射，传播，流露）=irradiate 辐射，灿烂

【经典例题】He rapidly became＿＿＿ with his own power in the team.
A．irrigated　　B．irradiated　　C．irritated　　D．initial　　[B]

【译　文】他的能力使他很快在团队中脱颖而出。

【名师导学】近义词群：illuminate, lighten, brighten

irritate
['iriteit]

v. 激怒，使恼怒

【经典例题】Please do not be irritated by his offensive remarks since he is merely trying to attract attention.

【译　　文】请不要因为他无礼的言语生气，那只是他想吸引别人的注意力罢了。

isolate
['aisəleit]

vt. 隔离，孤立

【固定搭配】be isolated from 脱离，被隔离，被孤立

【经典例题】Several villages have been isolated by the floods.

【译　　文】洪水使好几座村庄与外界隔绝了。

isolation
[,aisə'leiʃn]

n. 隔绝，孤立，绝缘

issue
['isju:]

n. 问题，论点，争端；发行，发行物　*vt.* 发行，发布

【固定搭配】at issue 在争论中；有分歧的；待裁决的

【经典例题】"The basic issue," he says, "is that adults who are responsible for issuing licenses fail to recognize how complex and skilled a task driving is."

【译　　文】他说："最基本的问题是，那些负责发驾驶执照的成人没有意识到驾驶的复杂程序和所需的技术。"

jealous
['dʒeləs]

a. 嫉妒的

【固定搭配】be jealous of 嫉妒

【名师导学】辨析 jealous, envious, envy：jealous 主要指恶意的"妒忌"；envy 和 envious 主要指"羡慕"。

【经典例题】He is jealous of his rivals.

【译　　文】他忌妒他的敌手。

jeopardize
['dʒepədaiz]

vt. 危及，损害

【经典例题】Isn't it possible that something could happen there that would jeopardize the fundamental interests?

【译　　文】难道就不会出现损害其根本利益的事情？

jog
[dʒɔg]

n. 慢跑；（尤指不正当的）轻轻碰撞

【名师导学】此词须掌握重点词组：jog sb.'s memory 使某人记起某事；jog along / on 持续而缓慢地进行。

【经典例题】He goes jogging every evening.

【译　　文】他每天晚上都进行慢跑。

journal
['dʒə:nl]

n. 日报，期刊；日志，日记

jumble
['dʒʌmbl]

vi. 掺杂，混杂 *vt.* 使混乱，搞乱 *n.* 混杂，混乱
【经典例题】Various books and papers are _____ up together on her desk.
A．jumbled　　　B．tumbled　　　C．bumbled　　　D．humbled　　　[A]
【译　　文】各种各样的书和论文杂乱地堆积在她的书桌上。

junction
['dʒʌŋkʃən]

n. 连接；会合处，交叉点
【经典例题】The morning news says a school bus collided with a train at the junction and a group of policemen were sent there immediately.
【译　　文】早间新闻说一辆校车和一辆火车在交叉路口相撞，一组警察被立刻派往现场。

jungle
['dʒʌŋgl]

n. 丛林；激烈的竞争场合 *a.* 丛林的，蛮荒的，野性的
【固定搭配】the law of the jungle 弱肉强食的原则

junior
['dʒu:njə]

a. 年少的，年幼的；后进的，下级的 *n.* 年少者，晚辈，下级
【联想记忆】freshman 一年级学生；sophomore 二年级学生；junior 三年级学生；senior 四年级学生
【固定搭配】be junior to 比……小（级别低）
【经典例题】His supervisor recommended he be promoted to the junior programmer.
【译　　文】他的上司推荐他晋升为初级程序员。

justice
['dʒʌstis]

n. 公道，公平；审判，司法
【固定搭配】bring to justice 把……交付审判，使归案受审；do justice to 公平地对待、审判

justification
[,dʒʌstifi'keiʃ(ə)n]

n. (做某事的) 正当理由，借口；齐行，整版

justify
['dʒʌstifai]

vt. 认为有理，证明……正当
【固定搭配】be justified in doing sth. 有理由做某事；justify oneself 为自己辩护
【经典例题】She worked hard at her task before she felt sure that the results would justify her long effort.
【译　　文】她一直努力工作，直到她认为她所取得的成绩足以证明她长期的努力。

keen
[ki:n]

a. 锋利的，尖锐的；敏捷的，敏锐的；热心的，渴望的
【固定搭配】be keen on (doing) sth. 喜爱；be keen about sth. 对……着迷
【经典例题】Are you keen on disco?
【译　　文】你喜欢迪斯科吗？

kidnap
['kidnæp]

vt. 诱拐，绑架

【名师导学】此词在阅读中出现较多，注意要连同与此词相关联的词一起记，如劫持、人质、赎金等。

【经典例题】Terrorists kidnapped the minister and demanded $10,000 from the government for his release.

【译　　文】恐怖分子绑架了部长，向政府索要一万美元赎金。

kneel
[ni:l]

vi. 跪，下跪

【固定搭配】kneel down 跪下

【名师导学】kneel 过去式／过去分词均为 knelt。

knob
[nɔb]

n. （门、抽屉的）球形把手，球形柄；（收音机等的）旋钮；小块

【名师导学】此词常在说明性的阅读中出现，注意其含义均与球形有关。

【经典例题】This machine has lots of knobs on it. Which one starts it?

【译　　文】这机器有许多旋钮。哪一个是启动它的？

knot
[nɔt]

n. 结；节，海里

【固定搭配】cut the knot 快刀斩乱麻

【经典例题】In the past, people usually tied a knot in a piece of string.

【译　　文】过去，人们经常在一根绳子上打结。

第三部分
核心意义词汇（L-Z）

全国医学博士英语
统考词汇巧战通关

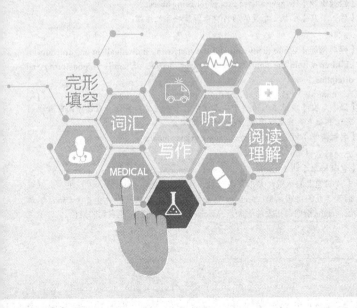

L

label
['leibl]

n. 标签，标记　*v.* 贴标签，把……称为

【固定搭配】acquire the label of... 获得……的绰号；be given the label of... 被起……的绰号

【名师导学】辨析 label, mark：label 意为"标签，标记"，通常是另外贴上或加上的；mark 意为"痕迹，记号，标记"，通常是直接写或画在某物上的。

【经典例题】By the end of 1994, 558 kinds of products had been ＿＿ green food.

A. named　　B. restricted　　C. classified　　D. labeled　　[D]

【译　　文】到 1994 年年末，已经有 558 种产品被列为绿色食品。

laboratory
[lə'bɔrətəri, 'læbərətəri]

n. 实验室，研究室

lace
[leis]

n. 网眼花边，透孔织品，花边；鞋带，系带

【固定搭配】lace up 用带子束紧

【经典例题】Please lace up your shoes.

【译　　文】请系紧你的鞋带。

lame
[leim]

a. 跛的，瘸的；站不住脚的，差劲的，蹩脚

【名师导学】注意此词的引申意义：是考查的重点，如：a lame excuse 不充分的理由。

【经典例题】He gave a lame excuse for being absent.

【译　　文】他找了个蹩脚的借口来解释缺席的原因。

lament
[lə'ment]

n. 悲叹，悔恨，恸哭　*v.* 哀悼，悔恨，悲叹

【经典例题】While many applaud the increasing individualism and freedom of children within the family, others lament the loss of family responsibility and discipline.

A. mourn　　B. delight　　C. prosecute　　D. condemn　　[A]

【译　　文】当很多人为孩子在家庭中的个人主义和自由与日俱增而鼓舞喝彩时，其他人则在哀叹家庭责任和纪律的缺失。

【名师导学】近义词 bemoan, deplore, grieve, mourn

landscape
['lændskeip]

n. 风景，景色

【名师导学】辨析 landscape, scene, scenery, sight, view：landscape 强调一大片陆地上的风景，尤指有山有水、乡间的景色；scene 意为"景色，景象"，指某一处的自然风光；scenery 更强调景色之意，从美的角度去看一些自然景色；sight 指展现在眼前的风景；view 指从人的视觉所能看到的景色。

laser
['leizə]

n. 激光

lash [læʃ]

v. (用绳索等)将(物品)系牢;鞭打,抽打,(风、雨等)猛烈打击;骂,挖苦,严厉斥责 n. 鞭打;眼睫毛;鞭梢

【名师导学】注意此词引申意义:lash out 猛烈攻击;抨击;大量捐(款)。
【经典例题】He lashed the horse across the back with a whip.
【译　文】他用鞭子抽打马背。

latitude [ˈlætitjuːd]

n. 纬度,界限;(pl.)纬度地区

【经典例题】The test of any democratic society lies not in how well it can control expression but in whether it gives freedom of thought and expression the widest possible latitude.
【译　文】任何社会的民主,不在于它对言论的控制,而在于是否给予了人们思考和表达的最广泛的自由。

laughter [ˈlɑːftə]

n. 笑,笑声

【名师导学】辨析 laugh,laughter:laugh 是可数名词,表示行为;laughter 是不可数名词,具有抽象或概括作用,意为"笑,笑声"。

launch [lɔːntʃ, lɑːntʃ]

vt. 发射;下水;开始,发起 n. 发射;下水

【固定搭配】launch an attack on / against 对……发动进攻

lawsuit [ˈlɔːsjuːt]

n. 诉讼

layman [ˈleimən]

n. 门外汉,外行

【经典例题】Where the law is concerned, I am only a layman.
【译　文】就法律知识而言,我是个门外汉。

leaflet [ˈliːflit]

n. 传单

【经典例题】He was standing at the door of the theatre handing out leaflets.
【译　文】他正站在剧院门口发传单。

lean [liːn]

vi. 倾斜,歪斜;屈身,躬身;靠,依

【经典例题】She leaned against his shoulder.
【译　文】她靠在他的肩上。

leap [liːp]

v. 跳跃,跳过

【固定搭配】by / in leaps and bounds 极其迅速地;leap to a conclusion 匆忙下结论;leap to the eye 跳入眼眶

lease [liːs]

n. 租约,契约

leather [ˈleðə]

n. 皮革,皮革制品

【联想记忆】feather n. 羽毛;fur n. 毛皮

legal [ˈliːɡəl]

a. 合法的,正当的;法律的

legend [ˈledʒənd]

n. 传说,传奇;传奇文学;传奇性人物或事件

【经典例题】He has been a legend for centuries for his heroic deeds.
【译　文】几个世纪以来,他由于自己的英勇事迹而成为传奇人物。

legislation [ˌledʒisˈleiʃən]

n. 立法,法律的制定 / 通过

legitimate
[li'dʒitimit]

a. 合情合理的；合法的，法律认可的

【名师导学】近义词：licit, legal, rightful, authorized, lawful, legal; reasonable, probable, consistent; logical , understandable; verifiable, valid, reliable, genuine

【经典例题】Protect (or safeguard) the legitimate rights and interests of women and children.

【译　　文】维护妇女和儿童合法权益。

legalization
[,li:gəlai'zeiʃn]

n. 合法化，得到法律认可

legislative
['ledʒis,leitiv]

a. 立法的，立法机关的　*n.* 立法机关

legislator
['ledʒis,leitə]

n. 立法者

leisure
['leʒə; 'li:ʒə]

n. 空闲，闲暇

【固定搭配】at leisure 有空，有闲暇时；从容不迫地，不慌不忙地

【联想记忆】measure *n.* 尺寸，措施；treasure *n.* 财富；pleasure *n.* 愉快，乐趣；exposure *n.* 暴露，揭露

【经典例题】Children's leisure time dropped from 40% of the day in 1981 to 25%.

【译　　文】孩子们的空闲时间从1981年的一天的40%减少到现在的25%。

lest
[lest]

conj. 唯恐，免得

lethal
['li:θl]

a. 致命的，毁灭性的，有效的　*n.* 基因异常，致死基因

【经典例题】It has been proved that the chemical is lethal to rats but safe for cattle.
A. fatal　　　B. reactive　　　C. unique　　　D. vital　　　　　[A]

【译　　文】经证实，这种化学药品对于鼠类是致命的，但对家禽无害。

【名师导学】deadly, fatal, mortal, lethal 这些形容词均有"致命的"之意。
deadly：指能致命或实际已致命的事物，也可指企图致死他人的人。
fatal：正式用词，强调死亡的不可避免性，多用于指伤或疾病等。
mortal：语气强，指导致死亡的直接原因。
lethal：指由于某物本身具有致命的性能。

levy
['levi]

n. / v. 税款，征税

【名师导学】此词常用的相关同义词有：tax（*n. / v.* 税，征税），tariff（关税，税率）。

【经典例题】The judge levied a $3 million fine against the factory for polluting the river.

【译　　文】由于该厂污染河流，法官对该厂征税300万美元。

liability
[,laiə'biliti]

n. 责任，义务；（*pl.*）债务，负债

【固定搭配】liability for 对……有责任；liability to do 有责任做

【名师导学】辨析 duty, liability, obligation, responsibility: duty 指按照道德、法律或良心必须要去做的事，比较强调自觉性；liability 指对某事物有责任或义务；obligation 多指履行某一特定的契约、诺言或根据社会习惯等的约束而对他人应尽的责任或义务；responsibility 指法律上和道义上应负的责任或职务上应尽的义务。

【经典例题】A few common misconceptions: Beauty is only skin-deep. One's physical assets and liabilities don't count all that much in a managerial career.
【译　　文】有一些普遍的错误看法：美丽只是表面的。在管理职业生涯中，一个人外表的美丑并不意味着全部。

liable ['laiəbl]
a. 有……倾向性，易于；有偿付责任的
【固定搭配】be liable to 易于；be liable for 对……有责任
【经典例题】A child can be born weak or liable to serious illness as a result of radiation.
【译　　文】由于辐射，孩子刚刚出生就可能很虚弱或者易于罹患严重的疾病。

liberal ['libərəl]
a. 慷慨的，大方的；丰富的，充足的；自由的，思想开明的
【固定搭配】be liberal in sth. 对事宽大；be liberal to sb. 对人宽容

liberate ['libəreit]
vt. 解放；释放

liberty ['libəti]
n. 自由；许可
【固定搭配】at liberty 自由地，不受囚禁地

license ['laisəns]
n. 执照，许可证；特许　*vt.* 准许，许可，认可
【经典例题】She is licensed to practice nursing.
【译　　文】她获准从事护理工作。

likelihood ['laiklihud]
n. 可能，可能性

linger ['liŋgə]
vi. （因不愿离开而）继续逗留，留恋徘徊；（on）继续存留，缓慢消失
【名师导学】常与 over、on 连用表示拖延；常与 on 连用表示苟延残喘。比如：The custom still lingers on in some villages. 有些村庄里还有这个风俗。
【经典例题】Mother told him not to linger on the way home.
【译　　文】妈妈告诉他不要在回家的路上逗留。

liquid ['likwid]
n. 液体　*a.* 液体的，液态的；流动的；可兑换现金的
【联想记忆】solid *n.* 固体；gas *n.* 气体

literacy ['litərəsi]
n. 识字，有文化，读写能力；教养
【名师导学】注意该词的派生词。其反义词是加前缀 il-，即 illiteracy。注意一些以 l 开头的词的反义词都是加前缀 il-，如：legal — illegal; liberal — illiberal。
【经典例题】Despite almost universal acknowledgment of the vital importance of women's literacy, education remains a dream for far too many women in far too many countries of the world.
【译　　文】尽管几乎全世界都承认妇女识字的重要性，但是在很多国家，接受教育仍然只是很多妇女的梦想。

literally ['litərəli]
ad. 确实地，毫不夸张地；照字面地，逐字地

literary ['litərəri]
a. 文学的；精通文学的，从事写作的
【联想记忆】literal *a.* 字面的，本义的；literate *a.* 有文化的，识字的。

literature ['litəritʃə]
n. 文学，文学作品；文献
【固定搭配】contemporary literature 当代文学；light literature 通俗文学

litter
['litə]

n. 废弃物，被胡乱扔掉的东西；一窝（幼崽）；（一堆）杂乱的东西，（随处）乱扔东西 *vt.* 乱扔废弃物

【经典例题】If the dangers from bacterially contaminated chicken were so great as some people believe, the streets would be littered with people lying here and there.

【译　文】如果来自被细菌污染的鸡肉的危险像一些人想象的那么严重的话，那么街道上将到处都是躺倒的人。

loaf
[ləuf]

n. 一条（面包）

locate
[ləu'keit]

vt. 找出，查出；设置在，位于 *vi.* 定居下来

【联想记忆】be situated in，lie in 位于，坐落于

【固定搭配】be located in / by / on 坐落于，位于

【名师导学】辨析 locate，place，situate，spot：locate 意为"确定……的地点或范围"；place 意为"放置，安置"；situate 意为"使位于，使处于"，多用其被动形式；spot 意为"准确地定出……的位置（主要用于军事目标的定位）"，还可表示"认出，弄污"等。

【经典例题】Early settlers located where there was water.

【译　文】早期的移民们在在有水的地方定居下来。

location
[ləu'keiʃən]

n. 位置，地点；定位，测量

lodge
[lɔdʒ]

vt. 供临时住宿 *vi.* 暂住，借宿

【固定搭配】board and lodging 食宿

【名师导学】辨析 lodging，board：lodging 仅指临时性住宿；board 指附有膳食的住宿。

log
[lɔg]

n. 原木，木料 *v.* 记录；行驶

【固定搭配】log in 登录　log out 退出

loom
[lu:m]

n. 织布机 *vi.* 阴森地逼近，隐现；即将来临

【经典例题】A dark shape loomed up ahead of us.

【译　文】一个黑乎乎的影子隐隐出现在我们面前。

lounge
[laundʒ]

n. 休息厅，休息室 *vi.*（懒洋洋地）倚，（懒散地）躺；闲逛，闲荡

【经典例题】There are more comfortable chairs in the lounge, if you find the dining room chair too hard.

【译　文】如果你觉得餐厅的椅子太硬，休息厅里有一些更舒服的椅子。

loyal
['lɔiəl]

a. 忠诚的，忠贞的

loyalty
['lɔiəlti]

n. 忠诚，忠心

【经典例题】As a demanding boss, he expected total loyalty and dedication from his employees.

【译　文】他是个苛刻的老板，要求他的雇员对他忠心耿耿、鞠躬尽瘁。

lubricate
['lu:brikeit]

vt. 润滑，加润滑油

【名师导学】注意该词的派生词，其名词有两个，去 e 加名词后缀 tion 或 or，意思不同。

【经典例题】You should lubricate the wheels of your bicycle once a month.

【译　文】你应该每个月给自行车轮子加一次润滑油。

第三部分 核心意义词汇（L-Z）

luggage ['lʌgidʒ]
n. 行李
【名师导学】luggage 和 baggage 都是不可数名词，因此"一件行李"应该说 a piece of luggage。

luminous ['lu:minəs]
a. 发光的，发亮的，光明的
【经典例题】I bought an alarm clock with a luminous dial, which can be seen clearly in the dark.
【译　　文】我买了一只带有发光钟面的闹钟，可以在黑暗中清楚地看到。

lunar ['lu:nə]
n. 月亮的

lure [luə]
n. 吸引人的东西，诱惑物　*vt.* 引诱，吸引
【名师导学】注意该词加前缀 al- 后意思基本相同，即：allure（*n.* 诱惑力，魅力；*v.* 吸引，引诱，诱惑）。
【经典例题】Many young Japanese engineers have been lured to the Middle East by the promise of high wages.
【译　　文】在高薪允诺的引诱下，许多年轻的日本工程师去了中东。

luxury ['lʌkʃəri]
n. 奢侈，奢侈品　*a.* 奢侈的
【派生词汇】luxious *a.* 奢侈的
【经典例题】He saved some money for artistic luxuries such as tinsel paintings.
【译　　文】他攒了一些钱来购买诸如金箔画之类的艺术奢侈品。

machinery [məˈʃi:nəri]
n. 机器，机械，结构
【名师导学】machine 是可数名词，表示机器；machinery 是不可数名词，表示机器的总称。

magic ['mædʒik]
n. 魔法，巫术；戏法

magistrate ['mædʒistrit, -treit]
n. 地方执政
【名师导学】注意该词常用的同义词有：judge, officer, official。
【经典例题】The magistrate ruled that the young man was innocent.
【译　　文】治安官裁定那个年轻人无罪。

magnet ['mægnit]
n. 磁铁，磁石，磁体

magnetic [mægˈnetik]
a. 磁的，有吸引力的
【经典例题】In order to be a successful diplomat you must be enthusiastic and magnetic.
　A. arrogant　　B. industrious　　C. zealous　　D. attractive　　[D]
【译　　文】想要成为一名成功的外交官，你必须热情且有魅力。

☐ **magnetism**
['mægnitizəm]
n. 磁，磁力，磁学

☐ **magnify**
['mægnifai]
vt. 放大，扩大，夸张
【经典例题】He tried to magnify the part he played in the battle.
【译　　文】他试图夸大他在那场战斗中所起的作用。

☐ **magnitude**
['mægnitju:d]
n. 巨大，重大；大小，量级
【名师导学】注意此词的动词形式也不容忽视，即 magnify，以 fy 结尾的多为动词，意思是"使……"，如：satisfy，justify 等。注意常用短语 of the first magnitude，意思是"头等重要的"。
【经典例题】The destruction an earthquake causes depends on its magnitude and duration, or the amount of shaking that occurs.
【译　　文】地震引起的破坏程度由震级和持续的时间，或者发生的次数决定。

☐ **mainstream**
['meinstri:m]
n. 主流

☐ **maintain**
[mein'tein]
vt. 维持；赡养；维修
【联想记忆】obtain *v.* 获得；retain *v.* 保持，保留；contain *v.* 包括；attain *v.* 达到；entertain *v.* 使感兴趣；招待
【经典例题】The leaders of the two countries are planning their summit meeting to maintain and develop good ties.
【译　　文】为保持并发展友好关系，两国的领导人正在策划一场峰会。

☐ **maintenance**
['meintinəns]
n. 维持，保持；维修

☐ **malignant**
[mə'lignənt]
a. 恶性的；恶意的；恶毒的
【经典例题】Cancer cells hide among healthy cells to conceal their ＿＿ proteins.
A．abundant　　B．malignant　　C．equivalent　　D．prevalent　　[B]
【译　　文】癌细胞藏匿在健康细胞中，以此掩盖它们的有害蛋白质。

☐ **malpractice**
[mæl'præktis]
n. 玩忽职守

☐ **maneuver**
[mə'nu:və]
n. 谨慎而熟练的动作；策略，花招；（*pl.*）演习 *v.*（敏捷或巧妙地）操纵，控制；用策略，耍花招
【名师导学】此词常与 into, out of 连用，意思是"操纵，设法使……"。

☐ **manifest**
['mænifest]
a. 明显的，显然的，明了的 *vt.* 表明，清楚显示；使显现，使显露
【名师导学】注意区分此词和几个常用同义词的区别：manifest 指让隐蔽的事物明白地表现出来，常接抽象名词；show 为最普通用词，表示"显示"的意思；demonstrate 指通过实例、实验来推理证明。
【经典例题】Social tensions were manifested in the recent political crisis.
【译　　文】最近的政治危机显示了社会关系的紧张。

☐ **manipulate**
[mə'nipjuleit]
vt. 操纵，利用，操作，巧妙地处理
【经典例题】In this exercise, we'll look at how we can manipulate the columns and rows in a table.
【译　　文】在此练习中，我们将了解如何处理表中的列和行。

manual ['mænjuəl]	*a.* 用手的,手工的;体力的 *n.* 手册 【经典例题】They could receive reports from students and decide what action to take by following a due process laid out in the faculty manual. 【译　　文】他们可以接收学生的报告,并根据教师手册中规定的正当程序来决定采取何种行动。
manufacture [,mænju'fæktʃə]	*vt.* 制造,加工 *n.* 制造(业);产品
manufacturer [,mænju'fæktʃərə]	*n.* 制造者,制造商;制造厂 【经典例题】In the US, car manufacturers have already had to redesign air bags so they inflate to lower pressures making them less of a danger to smaller women and children. 【译　　文】在美国,汽车制造商已经重新设计了气囊,以便在其弹出后会对体型较小的女性和孩子伤害更小。
manuscript ['mænjuskript]	*n.* 手稿,原稿 【名师导学】与该词意思相反的是 print(印刷物)。 【经典例题】The 215-page manuscript, circulated to publishers last October, sparked an outburst of interest. 【译　　文】去年10月传到出版商那里的215页手稿激发了他们浓厚的兴趣。
margin ['mɑ:dʒin]	*n.* 页边空余;边缘 【经典例题】You shouldn't have written in the margin since the book belongs to the library. 【译　　文】既然这本书是属于图书馆的,你就不应该在页边空白处写字。
marginal ['mɑ:dinl]	*a.* 边缘的,边际的
marine [mə'ri:n]	*a.* 海的,海产的,航海的,船舶的,海运的
marvellous ['mɑ:viləs]	*a.* 奇迹般的,惊人的,了不起的 【名师导学】辨析 marvellous,wonderful:marvellous 形容非凡得令人难以置信;wonderful 指因未曾见过或不寻常而令人惊奇。
masculine ['mæskjulin]	*a.* 男性的,男子的;男子气的 【名师导学】注意此词的常用同义词 manly(男子气概的);其反义词是 feminine(女性的,女人气的)。
mask [mɑ:sk]	*n.* 面具;口罩
massive ['mæsiv]	*a.* 大量的;巨大的;大而重的;结实的;非常严重的 【经典例题】It showed a massive tumor and widespread metastatic disease. 【译　　文】它显示了一个巨大的肿瘤和遍布全身的转移性疾病。
masterpiece ['mɑ:stəpi:s]	*n.* 杰作,名著
maternity [mə'tə:niti]	*n.* 母性,为母之道;产科医院 *a.* 孕妇的,产妇的,产科的

mature
[mə'tjuə]

a. 成熟，考虑周到的　*v.* （使）成熟，长成

【名师导学】辨析 mature，ripe：mature 用于人时，指生理和智力发展到了成年，用于物时，指机能发展到可以开花结果，还可指想法、意图等"经过深思熟虑的"；ripe 用于物时，指植物的果实完全成熟，可以食用，也可指时机"成熟的，适宜的"。

【经典例题】Boys mature more slowly than girls both physically and psychologically.

【译　　文】无论在生理上或心理上，男孩都比女孩成熟得慢。

maximize
['mæksməiz]

vt. 取……最大值，最佳化

maximum
['mæksiməm]

n. 最大量，最高值　*a.* 最大的，最高的

【名师导学】maximum 的复数形式为 maxima 或 maximums。

【经典例题】The level of formaldehyde（甲醛）gas in her kitchen was twice the maximum allowed by federal standard for chemical workers.

【译　　文】她家厨房的甲醛浓度是联邦政府为化工厂工人规定的最大值的两倍。

meantime
['mi:n'taim]

n. 其时，在此期间　*ad.* 同时，当时

mediate
['mi:dieit]

v. 仲裁，调停　*a.* 间接的

mediator
['mi:dieitə(r)]

n. 调停者，仲裁人

medieval
[,medi'i:vəl]

a. 中世纪的，中古（时代）的

medicare
['medikɛə(r)]

n. 医疗保险，医疗保险制度

medium
['mi:diəm]

n. 中间，适中；（*pl.* media）媒体；媒介，媒介物；传导体　*a.* 中等的，适中的

【名师导学】medium 的复数形式为 media。类似的词还有 datum — data。但应注意 premium — premiums；gymnasium — gymnasiums。

【经典例题】He is medium height.

【译　　文】他是中等身高。

melody
['melədi]

n. 曲调，旋律

【经典例题】When the melody is repeated in various forms in a longer composition, this basic tune is said to constitute its theme, or subject.

【译　　文】当旋律在一个较长的作品里以不同形式反复出现时，人们便认为这一基调构成了作品的主旋律或主题。

melt
[melt]

v. 融化，溶化，溶解

【名师导学】melt 的过去式 / 分词有两种：melted，molten。过去分词用做形容词而修饰金属时应用 molten，如 molten steel 熔化的钢（钢水）；而指融化的冰，黄油等时应用 melted，如 melted ice 融化的冰。

memorial
[mi'mɔ:riəl]

a. 纪念的，记忆的　*n.* 纪念物，纪念碑，纪念馆

第三部分　核心意义词汇（L-Z）

memorize ['meməraiz]
vt. 记住，熟记，背熟
【经典例题】He memorized the list of dates, but neglected the main facts corresponding to them.
【译　　文】他记住了那一系列日期，但却忽略了与其对应的主要事情。

menace ['menəs]
n. 具有危险性的人；威胁，威吓　*vt.* 威胁，威吓
【经典例题】A man who drives fast is a menace to other people.
【译　　文】开快车的人对其他人是个威胁。

mentor ['mentɔ:(r)]
n. 导师　*vt.* 做……的良师；指导
【经典例题】In particular, they said that faculty members should avoid neglectful teaching and mentoring.
【译　　文】他们尤其谈到教职员工应该避免不上心的教学和辅导。

mercy ['mə:si]
n. 怜悯，宽恕，仁慈
【固定搭配】at the mercy of 在……支配下

merge [mə:dʒ]
v. 合并，结合，融合
【名师导学】此词经常在经济类的阅读文章中出现。如：Two of Indonesia's top banks are planning to merge. 印度尼西亚有两家顶级银行正在计划合并。常用的介词搭配是 with 和 into，搭配意思是"融合"。
【经典例题】The board of directors decided to merge the two sections into the public relations department.
【译　　文】董事会决定将这两个科室并至公共关系部。

metabolism [me'tæbəlizəm]
n. 新陈代谢
【经典例题】Diabetes upsets the ____ of sugar, fat and protein.
A. metastasis　　　　　B. metabolism
C. malaise　　　　　　D. maintenance　　　　　[B]
【译　　文】糖尿病扰乱了糖、脂肪和蛋白质的代谢。

methodology [meθə'dɔlədʒi]
n. 方法学，方法论

metropolitan [metrə'pɔlit(ə)n]
n. / a. 大城市（的）
【经典例题】In a recent survey, questionnaires were sent to reporters in five middle size cities around the country, plus one large metropolitan area.
【译　　文】在最近的一次调查中对全国的五座中等城市及一座大都市的记者发放了调查问卷。

microphone ['maikrəfəun]
n. 麦克风，扩音器

microscope ['maikrəskəup]
n. 显微镜

migrant ['maigrənt]
n. 移居者；候鸟

migrate [mai'greit, 'maigreit]
v. 迁移，迁居；定期移栖
【经典例题】We find that some birds migrate twice a year between hot and cold countries.
【译　　文】我们发现，有些鸟每年在热带与寒带国家之间迁徙两次。

☐ **military** ['militəri]	*a.* 军事的，军队的，军用的
☐ **millimeter** ['milimi:tə(r)]	*n.* 毫米
☐ **mingle** ['miŋgl]	*vt.* 使混合，使相混 *vi.* 混合起来，相混合；相交往，相往来 【名师导学】该词常与介词 with 连用，意思是"与……混合，与……相联系"。例如：The king mingled with the people in the streets. 国王和街上的人群混在一起了。 【经典例题】If we mingle with the crowd we shall not be noticed. 【译　　文】如果我们混在人群里，就不会被人注意了。
☐ **miniature** ['minətʃə]	*n.* 缩图，缩影 *a.* 微型的，缩小的 【经典例题】The toy maker produces a miniature copy of the space station, exactly in every detail. 【译　　文】这个玩具制造商制造了一种每个细节都很逼真的空间站缩微模型。
☐ **minimal** ['miniml]	*a.* 最小的，最小限度的
☐ **minimize** ['minimaiz]	*vt.* 使减少到最少，使降到最低 【经典例题】The fire has caused great losses, but the factory tried to minimize the consequences by saying that the damage was not as serious as reported. 【译　　文】这场大火灾造成了巨大损失，但这家工厂却竭力降低对其后果的评估，说并没有报道的那么严重。
☐ **minimum** ['minimǝm]	*n.* 最小量，最低限度 *a.* 最小的，最低的 【经典例题】He said China would reduce losses incurred by SARS to the minimum. 【译　　文】他说中国会把 SARS 引起的损失降到最低程度。
☐ **ministry** ['ministri]	*n.* 部门
☐ **minus** ['mainǝs]	*a.* 负的，减的 *prep.* 减去 *n.* 减号，负号
☐ **mischief** ['mistʃif]	*n.* 调皮；危害，损害
☐ **missing** ['misiŋ]	*a.* 失去的，失踪的 【经典例题】John complained to the bookseller that there were several pages missing in the dictionary he bought. 【译　　文】约翰向书商抱怨说，他买的字典里面缺了几页。
☐ **mission** ['miʃən]	*n.* 使命，任务 【固定搭配】on a...mission 负有……使命
☐ **misunderstand** ['misʌndə'stænd]	*vt.* 误解，误会，曲解

moan [məun]	*vi.* 呻吟，呜咽；(about)抱怨，发牢骚 *vt.* 抱怨 *n.* 呻吟声，呜咽声；怨声，牢骚 【固定搭配】moan about 抱怨，发牢骚 【经典例题】Each time she moved her leg, she let out a moan. 【译　　文】每次她动一下腿，就发出一声呻吟。
mob [mɔb]	*n.* 暴民，乌合之众 *vt.* 成群围住，聚众袭击 【经典例题】When he left the hall after his speech, the party leader was mobbed by his supporters. 【译　　文】当这位政党领袖结束演讲离开大厅时，一大群支持者围住他欢呼。
mock [mɔk]	*v.* 嘲弄，嘲笑 【名师导学】近义词：deride, make fun of, taunt, ridicule 【经典例题】Although he failed in the math test, it was wrong to mock his efforts. 【译　　文】虽然他的数学考试没有考及格，但是嘲笑他的努力是不对的。
moderate ['mɔdərit]	*a.* 中等的，适度的；温和的，稳健的
modify ['mɔdifai]	*vt.* 修改，变更；缓和，减轻 【经典例题】Adverbs modify verbs and adjectives. 【译　　文】副词修饰动词和形容词。
module ['mɔdju:l]	*n.* 模数，模块；太空舱
moist [mɔist]	*a.* 湿润的，潮湿的 【经典例题】The thick steam in the bathroom had made the walls moist. 【译　　文】浴室内浓浓的水蒸气把墙壁弄潮了。
moisture ['mɔistʃə]	*n.* 潮湿，湿气，湿度
mold [məuld]	*n.* 霉，霉菌；模子，模型，铸模；(人的)性格，气质，类型 *vt.* 用模子制作，浇铸，塑造；使形成，影响……的形成，把……铸造成
molecule ['mɔlikju:l, 'məu-]	*n.* 分子 【经典例题】A molecule is made up of atoms. 【译　　文】分子由原子组成。
momentum [məu'mentəm]	*n.* 气势，冲力；动量
monetary ['mʌnitəri]	*a.* 货币的，钱的 【经典例题】China's policymakers may lack the monetary tools to engineer a soft landing. 【译　　文】制定政策的中国官员可能缺乏金融工具来安排软着陆。
monopoly [mə'nɔpəli]	*n.* 垄断，垄断专利权 【经典例题】A university education shouldn't be the monopoly of the minority whose parents are rich. 【译　　文】大学教育不应是少数富家子弟的专利。

mood [muːd]
n. 心情，情绪；语气
【固定搭配】be (not) in the mood for / to do sth. 有（没有）情绪做某事；be in good (bad) mood 情绪好（不好）
【经典例题】A mood of optimism pervaded the gathering.
【译　　文】聚会上充满乐观的气氛。

moral ['mɒrəl]
a. 道德的，道义的，有道德的　*n.* 寓意，教育意义
【经典例题】As regards the development of moral standards in the growing child, consistency is very important in parental teaching.
【译　　文】对于在成长中的孩子的道德水平的发展，家长教导的一致性是非常重要的。

morale [mə'ræl]
n. 士气，斗志

morality [mə'ræləti]
n. 道德
【经典例题】When it comes to teaching ____, many parents believe that if they love their children and treat them kindly, the kids will know how to behave.
A. mentality　　B. morality　　C. majesty　　D. majority　　[B]
【译　　文】提到道德教育，许多父母认为如果他们爱自己的孩子并和蔼地对待他们，孩子们就会知道如何正确表现。

mortal ['mɔːtl]
a. 致死的；终有一死的；人世间的

mortgage ['mɔːgidʒ]
n. 抵押；抵押单据，抵押所借的款项
【经典例题】The China Construction Bank offered mortgage loan to commercial residence house buyers.
【译　　文】中国建设银行为商品房购买者提供了按揭贷款。

motivate ['məutiveit]
vt. 作为……的动机，促动；激励
【经典例题】Examinations do not motivate a student to seek more knowledge.
【译　　文】考试不能激励学生去追求更多的知识。

motive ['məutiv]
n. 动机，目的　*a.* 发动的，运动的

mourn [mɔːn]
v. 哀悼，悲哀
【经典例题】While many applaud the increasing individualism and freedom of children within the family, others mourn the loss of family responsibility and discipline.
【译　　文】当很多人为孩子在家庭中的个人主义和自由与日俱增鼓舞喝彩时，另外一些人则在哀叹家庭责任和纪律的缺失。

mount [maunt]
vt. 登上，爬上，骑上；装配，固定，镶嵌　*n.* 支架，底座，底板；山峰
【名师导学】辨析 mount, ascend, climb：mount 指一步一步向上移动，可与抽象名词连用；ascend 指不一定很费力气地向上爬或上升，不与抽象名词连用；climb 指费劲或曲折地向上爬。

multicultural [ˌmʌltɪ'kʌltʃərəl]
a. 多种文化的；融有多种文化的

multilateral
[ˌmʌltiˈlætərəl]
a. 多边的

multinational
[ˌmʌltiˈnæʃən(ə)l]
a. 多国的，跨国公司的，多民族的

multiple
[ˈmʌltɪpl]
a. 多样的，多重的
【经典例题】As a medical team we simultaneously performed multiple procedures.
【译　　文】作为医疗团队，我们同时处理多重程序。

multiply
[ˈmʌltɪplɪ]
vt. 乘；增加；繁殖

multitude
[ˈmʌltɪtjuːd]
n. 众多，大量；人群，大众
【名师导学】注意此词的相关常用短语：a multitude / multitudes of 许多，大量。
【经典例题】A multitude of factors, both inherited and environmental, influence the development of health-related behaviors.
【译　　文】大量因素——既有遗传因素也有环境因素——影响着关于健康的行为的发展。

mundane
[mʌnˈdeɪn]
adj. 世俗的；平凡的；宇宙的；寻常的
【经典例题】Other mundane factors also affect how phones are used.
【译　　文】其他一些世俗的因素也影响电话的使用方式。

municipal
[mjuː(ː)ˈnɪsɪpəl]
a. 市政的，市立的，地方性的，地方自治的

mutual
[ˈmjuːtʃuəl]
a. 相互的；共同的
【名师导学】辨析 mutual, joint：mutual 指两者之间的相互关系，主要强调兴趣、观点、看法、感情等的共通；common 意为"共同的，共有的"，指三者或三者以上共同所有的东西；joint 主要强调两者真正地拥有某物。
【经典例题】He had taken the all-important first step to establish mutual trust.
【译　　文】为了建立相互信任关系，他迈出了最重要的第一步。

mute
[mjuːt]
a. 哑的；缄默的 *n.* 哑巴；弱音器
【名师导学】注意此词的引申含义，如例句所示。再者，注意此词的几个常用同义词：speechless, voiceless。
【经典例题】Sometimes when her friend asked her questions, she pretended to be deaf and mute.
【译　　文】有时她朋友问她问题时，她装聋作哑。

mutter
[ˈmʌtə]
v. 喃喃说出（不满、怨言等），低声嘀咕 *n.* 嘟哝，喃喃之言
【经典例题】He was muttering on the telephone so I asked him to speak more clearly.
【译　　文】他打电话声音很低，因此我让他说得清楚些。

| naked
['neikid] | *a.* 裸体的；毫无遮掩的 |

| naive
[nɑː'iːv] | *a.* 幼稚的，轻信的；天真的
【经典例题】Parents take a great interest in the naive questions raised by their children.
【译　　文】父母对孩子们提出的天真的问题很有兴趣。 |

| narrate
[næ'reit] | *v.* 叙述 |

| nasty
['næsti] | *a.* 极令人不快的；很脏的；危险的
【名师导学】和该词意思相反的是 pleasant（愉快的，可爱的）。
【经典例题】The news gave me a nasty shock.
【译　　文】这消息可把我吓死了。 |

| nationality
[ˌnæʃə'næliti] | *n.* 国籍；民族 |

| naval
['neivəl] | *a.* 海军的，军舰的
【联想记忆】navy *n.* 海军；navigation *n.* 航行
【经典例题】Germany planned to challenge Britain's naval supremacy.
【译　　文】德国计划向英国的制海权挑战。 |

| navigate
['nævigeit] | *v.* 航行；驾驶 |

| navigation
[ˌnævi'geiʃən] | *n.* 航行，航海，航空 |

| negative
['negətiv] | *a.* 否定的，消极的，反面的；负的，阴性的 |

| neglect
[ni'glekt] | *vt.* 忽视，忽略；疏忽 |

| neglectful
[ni'glektful] | *a.* 忽略的；不留心的 |

| negligible
['neglidʒəbl] | *a.* 可以忽略的，不予重视的
【经典例题】Most experts say that the new tax plan will have a negligible effect on the country's economic problems.
A. indefinite　B. indispensable　C. infinite　　D. insignificant　　　[D]
【解　　析】negligible "微不足道"，indefinite "无限期的"，indispensable "不可或缺的"，infinite "无限的"，insignificant "无足轻重的"，可知 D 为正确答案。
【译　　文】大多数专家表示，新的税收计划对该国经济问题的影响可以忽略不计。 |

第三部分 核心意义词汇（L-Z）

negotiate [ni'gəuʃieit]
v. 谈判，交涉，商议
【固定搭配】negotiate with sb. about / over / on / for sth. 与某人谈判某事

negotiable [ni'gəuʃiəbl]
a. 可谈判的，可协商的，可通行的

neighbo(u)rhood ['neibəhud]
n. 邻近，附近，周围
【固定搭配】in the neighborhood of 在……附近，大约

nerve [nə:v]
n. 神经；勇敢，胆量
【派生词汇】nervous a. 紧张的
【固定搭配】get on one's nerves 惹得某人心烦

network ['netwə:k]
n. 网络，网状系统；广播网，电视网

neutral ['nju:trəl]
a. 中立的，中性的
【经典例题】She is neutral in this argument, she does not care who wins.
【译　文】在这场辩论中她保持中立，不在乎谁赢谁输。

neutralize ['nju:trəlaiz]
v. 使中立

nightmare ['naitmeə(r)]
n. 噩梦；恐怖的经历，可怕的事件

nitrogen ['naitrədʒən]
n. 氮

nonsense ['nɔnsəns]
n. 胡说，废话
【固定搭配】speak / talk nonsense 胡说八道

nominal ['nɔminl]
a. 名义上的，有名无实的；（费用等）很少的，名称上的；名词性的
【经典例题】The old man is only the nominal head of the business.
【译　文】那老人只是这个公司的挂名总裁。

nominate ['nɔmineit]
vt. 提名，任命
【名师导学】注意此词加前缀 in-，即 innominate（a. 未名的，无名的，匿名的）。
【经典例题】To their surprise, she has been nominated as candidate for the Presidency.
【译　文】出乎他们意料的是，她被提名为总统候选人。

nominee [,nɔ:mi'ni:]
n. 被提名（任命、推荐）者

nonprofit [,nɔn'prɔfit]
a. 非营利的

norm [nɔ:m]
n. 标准，规范；平均数

normalize ['nɔ:məlaiz]
vt. 使正常化，使标准化，使规格化

notion [ˈnəʊʃən]	n. 概念，意念；想法，见解
notorious [nəʊˈtɔːriəs]	a. 臭名昭彰的，众所周知的 【名师导学】该词的常用同义词有：infamous（声名狼藉的），反义词较多：celebrated, famous, renowned, outstanding。 【经典例题】That part of the city has long been notorious for its street violence. 【译　文】这个城市的那个地区一直因为街头暴力而臭名昭著。
notwithstanding [ˌnɒtwɪθˈstændɪŋ]	prep. 虽然，尽管 ad. 尽管，还是 conj. 虽然，尽管
nourish [ˈnʌrɪʃ]	vt. 提供养分，养育；培养 【名师导学】注意和此词的派生词一起记：nourishing（a. 滋养的）；nourishment（n. 食物）。 【经典例题】By investing in education, we nourish the talents of our children. 【译　文】我们通过教育投资，培养孩子们的才能。
novel [ˈnɒvəl]	n. 小说 a. 新的，新颖的 【经典例题】The novel development, however, is often overlooked. 【译　文】然而，新的发展却往往被忽视。
nowhere [ˈnəʊhweə]	ad. 哪儿也不，什么地方都没有 【固定搭配】get nowhere 使无进展，使不能成功；nowhere near 远远不，远不及 【名师导学】nowhere 放在句首时，句子用倒装结构。 【经典例题】Help will come from the UN, but the aid will be nowhere near what's needed. 【译　文】联合国将提供援助，但这远远满足不了需要。
nuclear [ˈnjuːklɪə]	a. 原子核的；核的，核心的 【经典例题】Some scientists favor pushing asteroids off course with nuclear weapons. 【译　文】一些科学家更倾向于用核武器将行星从它们的轨道推出去。
nucleus [ˈnjuːklɪəs]	n. 核，核心；原子核 【名师导学】nucleus 复数形式为 nuclei 或 nucleuses。
nuisance [ˈnjuːsns]	n. 麻烦事，讨厌的人/事 【经典例题】Don't make a nuisance of yourself. 【译　文】别那么讨厌。
numeral [ˈnjuːmərəl]	n. 数字，数码
numerical [njuː(ː)ˈmerɪkl]	a. 数字的，用数表示的
numerous [ˈnjuːmərəs]	a. 众多的，大批的，无数的 【经典例题】This product, skillfully done and of high quality, is appreciated by numerous customers. 【译　文】该产品的制作精巧和高质量赢得了广大顾客的赞誉。
numb [nʌm]	a. 麻木的，失去知觉的；惊呆的 vt. 使麻木，使失去知觉；使目瞪口呆

nursery ['nə:səri]	*n.* 护理，养育，喂奶
nurture ['nə:tʃə]	*n.* 营养物；养育，培育，教养 *vt.* 给……营养；养育，培育，教养 【经典例题】The marketplace must nurture the idea that society must value, care for, and educate each human being. 【译　　文】市场必须培育这种思想：社会必须珍视、关心和教育每一个人。
nutrient ['nju:triənt]	*a.* 营养的，滋养的 *n.* 营养物
nutrition [nju:'triʃən]	*n.* 营养，营养学

oath ['əuθ]	*n.* 誓言，誓约；咒骂，诅咒语 【名师导学】近义词：swearword, blasphemy, curse; affirmation, vow, testimony, word, deposition, contract, pledge 【固定搭配】swear / take an oath 宣誓 【经典例题】He swore an oath to support the king. 【译　　文】他宣誓支持国王。
oblivious [ə'bliviəs]	*a.* 没注意到的，不知道的 【联想记忆】obvious 明显的 +li（谐音"离"）=oblivious 离开了明显的（东西）= 没注意到不知道的 【经典例题】She was often oblivious of the potential consequences of her action. A. unaware　　B. confident　　C. afraid　　D. convinced　　[A] 【译　　文】她总是注意不到自己行为所带来的潜在影响。
obtain [əb'tein]	*vt.* 获得，得到
obscure [əb'skjuə]	*a.* 不著名的，不重要的；费解的，晦涩的 *vt.* 使变模糊，掩盖 【经典例题】The poetry of Ezra Pound is sometimes difficult to understand because it contains so many obscure references. 【译　　文】埃兹拉·庞德的诗有时很难理解，因为它包含了很多隐晦的比喻。
obsolete ['ɔbsəli:t]	*adj.* 废弃的；老式的，已过时的；[生] 已废退的 *n.* 废词；被废弃的事物 *vt.* 淘汰；废弃 【联想记忆】old-fashioned, outdated; abandoned. 【经典例题】That is, it either requires more skill or can be done by more people around the world or is being buried and made obsolete fast. 【译　　文】也就是说，它要么需要更多的技能，要么可以被世界上更多的人完成，或者正在迅速被埋没，被淘汰。

obsession
[əbˈseʃən]

n. 痴迷；困扰

obstinate
[ˈɔbstinət]

a. 固执的，倔强的，不易屈服的；（病）难治的
【经典例题】She was so stubborn that she wouldn't change her opinions.
A. unwilling　　　　　B. talented
C. obstinate　　　　　D. determined　　　　[C]
【译　　文】她特别固执，不会改变她的想法。
【名师导学】obstinate, stubborn 这两个形容词均可表示"固执的，顽固的"之意。
obstinate：指无理地固执己见或听不进他人忠告、意见等的顽固性格。
stubborn：用于褒义指"坚定不移，执意顽强"；用于贬义指"固执己见，生性固执"。

obstruct
[əbˈstrʌkt]

vt. 阻塞，阻挡，妨碍

occasion
[əˈkeiʒən]

n. 场合；大事，节日；时机，机会
【固定搭配】on occasion 有时，偶尔；on the occasion of ... 在……的时候
【联想记忆】between times，once in a while，now and then，every once in a while，every so often 有时

occasional
[əˈkeiʒənəl]

a. 偶然的，不时

occupation
[ˌɔkjuˈpeiʃən]

n. 占领，职业
【固定搭配】by occupation 职业上
【经典例题】Some of us have made interdisciplinary study in our occupation, which is no surprise.
【译　　文】一部分人在自己的职业领域里从事跨学科研究，这不足为奇。

occupational
[ˌɔkjuˈpeiʃnəl]

a. 职业的；占领的

occupy
[ˈɔkjupai]

vt. 占，占领，占据；使忙碌，使从事
【固定搭配】occupy oneself in doing sth. / with sth. 忙着（做某事）；忙（于某事）；be occupied with / in 忙于
【联想记忆】be engaged in / with，be busy with，be absorbed in，be involved in 忙于做某事
【经典例题】You were signaled forward to occupy the seat opposite him.
【译　　文】有人暗示你向前去占他对面的座位。

occurrence
[əˈkʌrəns]

n. 发生，出现，事件

odd
[ɔd]

a. 奇数的，单的；奇怪的，古怪的；临时的，不固定的；挂零的，剩余的
【固定搭配】against (all) the odds 尽管有极大的困难，尽管极为不利；at odds (with) 与……不；与……争吵，与……不一致；odds and ends 零星杂物，琐碎物品
【名师导学】辨析 odd, queer, peculiar, strange：odd 指一反常态或出乎意料，因而引起人"诧异，稀奇，有趣"的感觉；queer 表示"古怪的，怪僻的，神经不正常的或可笑的"；peculiar 强调与众不同，强调奇异的独特性，不同寻常；strange 所指范围较广泛，凡异乎寻常或较少看到乃至新奇的东西都可称为 strange。

odds
[ɔːdz]

n. 可能性，概率
【固定搭配】against all odds 困难重重

odo(u)r
[ˈəudər]

n. 气味，名声

offend
[əˈfend]

vt. 冒犯，触犯，得罪；使不快，使恼火
【固定搭配】be offended at / by / with 因……而生气
【经典例题】I have offended him.
【译　　文】我得罪了他。

offensive
[əˈfensiv]

a. 极讨厌的，冒犯的，无礼的；进攻性的

offset
[ˈɔːfset]

n. 抵消，弥补　*vt.* 弥补，抵消

omission
[əˈmiʃn]

n. 省略，删除；遗漏，疏忽，失职

opponent
[əˈpəunənt]

n. 对手，敌手
【名师导学】辨析 opponent, match, rival：opponent 对手，指比赛、争论的对手；match 指在水平等方面与自己相当的对手、敌手；rival 指同一目标、目的的竞争者，有时可能怀有恶意或不可告人、不友好的动机。
【经典例题】We cannot look down upon our opponent, who is an experienced swimmer.
A. player　　B. competitor　　C. referee　　D. partner　　[B]
【译　　文】我们不能轻视对手，他是一名有经验的游泳选手。

oppose
[əˈpəuz]

vt. 反对，反抗
【固定搭配】be opposed to sth. / doing sth. 反对
【联想记忆】have an objection to, go against, object to 反对
【名师导学】be opposed to 后面接名词或动名词。
【经典例题】But they won't think this way; They will oppose us stubbornly.
【译　　文】可是，他们不会这样想，他们将坚决反对我们。

optical
[ˈɔptikəl]

a. 光学的，光的；视觉的，视力的

optimistic
[ˌɔptiˈmistik]

a. 乐观（主义）的
【联想记忆】pessimism *n.* 悲观（主义）；pessimist *n.* 悲观（主义）者；pessimistically *ad.* 悲观（主义）地
【经典例题】We should be optimistic because of the upward trend of the development.
【译　　文】既然事情发展是上升趋势，那我们就应该保持乐观。

optimize
[ˈɔptimaiz]

vt. 使最优化，使尽可能有效
【经典例题】In order to optimize benefit equitably across the population, physicians and services need to be ready to change and adapt to new ways of working.
【译　　文】为了在人口中平等地优化福利，医生和服务机构需要随时准备改变，适应新的工作方式。

optimum ['ɔptiməm]	*n.* 最适合条件，最佳效果，最优化 【名师导学】注意以 mum 结尾的词义都是"最……"，如：maximum（n. 最大量，最大极限；a. 最高的，最多的，最大极限的），minimum（n. 最小值，最小化；a. 最小的，最低的）。 【经典例题】If you wait for the optimum moment to act, you may never begin your project. 【译　　文】如果你一味等待最佳行动时机，那你可能永远不会着手你的计划。
option ['ɔpʃən]	*n.* 选择；供选择的事物 【固定搭配】at one's option 随意
optional ['ɔpʃenəl]	*a.* 可以任选的，非强制的 【经典例题】Is English an optional lesson, or does everyone have to learn it? 【译　　文】英语是选修课，还是每个人必修的课程？
oral ['ɔ:rəl]	*a.* 口头的，口述的 【经典例题】This drug is available for both oral and parenteral administration. 【译　　文】本药可供口服或注射用。
orbit ['ɔ:bit]	*n.* 轨道　*v.* 沿轨道运行 【经典例题】Most orbit the sun far from Earth and don't threaten us. 【译　　文】大多数的行星围绕太阳运转，它们的轨道远离地球，不会威胁到我们。
orchestra ['ɔ:kistrə, -kes-]	*n.* 交响/管弦乐队 【经典例题】The orchestra will prepare for a concert of New Year. 【译　　文】管弦乐队要为新年音乐会排练。
organ ['ɔ:gən]	*n.* 器官；机构；风琴 【经典例题】The FBI is an organ of the Justice Department. 【译　　文】联邦调查局是司法部的一个机构。
organic [ɔ:'gænik]	*a.* 有机体的，器官的
organization [,ɔ:gənai'zeiʃən]	*n.* 组织，体制；团体，机构
organize ['ɔ:gənaiz]	*vt.* 组织，组编 【经典例题】The hay field is getting organized. 【译　　文】干草地开始井然有序。
orient ['ɔ:riənt]	*vt.* 使适应；确定方向，使朝向 【固定搭配】orient to / toward 以……为方向（目标） 【经典例题】We run a commercially oriented operation. 【译　　文】我们经营一个商业性的企业。
oriental [,ɔ(:)ri'entl]	*n.* 东方人　*a.* 东方诸国的，亚洲的，东方的
orientation [,ɔ(:)rien'teiʃən]	*n.* 方向，方位，定位，倾向性 【经典例题】Educators have always been familiar with those parts of the two-year college curriculum that have a "service" or vocational orientation. 【译　　文】教育者们往往对具备服务功能或是带有职业导向的两年制大学课程很熟悉。

origin ['ɔridʒin]	*n.* 起源，由来；出身，血统 【名师导学】辨析 origin, root, source：origin 指事物的起源或者开端，着重于其发生的最早的时间或最初的地点，常表示某种历史文化现象、风俗习惯的起源，也可指人的门第或血统；root 常译为"根源、起因"，强调导致某事物最终出现的最根本的、最重要的原因，由此所产生的现象或事物常成为一种外观的产物；source 指河流或泉水的发源地，也是非物质的或无形的东西的出处或起源，常指情况或信息的来源、出处。
original [ə'ridʒənəl]	*a.* 最初的，原始的，原文的；新颖的，有独创性的
originate [ə'ridʒineit]	*vt.* 引起，发明，发起，创办 *vi.* 起源，发生 【固定搭配】originate from / in / with 产生于
ornament ['ɔ:nəmənt]	*n.* 装饰，装饰品 *vt.* 装饰 【经典例题】On Christmas Eve, she spent two hours ornamenting the room with flower chains. 【译　文】圣诞节前夜，她花了两个小时用花链装饰房间。
orthodox ['ɔ:θədɔks]	*a.* 传统的；正统的，正宗的 【经典例题】Such orthodox thinking will not lead to a new solution to the problem. 【译　文】这样传统的思维不会产生解决问题的新方法。
oscillate ['ɔsileit]	*v.* （使）振动；摇摆
outbreak ['autbreik]	*n.* （战争、情感、火山等的）爆发；（疾病、虫害等的）突然发生 【经典例题】During the acute phase of the outbreak, it is necessary to keep suspects at special risk under observation. 【译　文】在（疾病）爆发的紧急阶段，必须将面临特殊威胁的疑似病例置于监视之下。
outcome ['autkʌm]	*n.* 结果，后果，成果
outdated [aut'deitid]	*vt.* 使过时 *a.* 过时的
outer ['autə]	*a.* 外部的，外层的，外表的
outfit ['autfit]	*n.* （为特殊用途的）全套装备，全套工具，用品；全套服装，一套特别的服装 *v.* 配备 【名师导学】该词常以被动语态形式出现。 【经典例题】The expedition was outfitted with the latest scientific equipment. 【译　文】探险队装备了最先进的科学设备。
outline ['əutlain]	*n.* 轮廓，外形；大纲，概要，图略 *vt.* 概述，列提纲 【固定搭配】in outline 扼要地
outlook ['autluk]	*n.* 展望，远景；眼界，观点 【名师导学】辨析 outlook, prospect：outlook 强调以专业人士的眼光来展望预测未来，得出的结论常有准确的细节且比较可靠；prospect 一般做复数，意为"前景、前程、前途"，指能使人感兴趣、能引起情感反应的事情的前景。

☐ **output**
['autput]

n. 产量，产品，输出

【名师导学】辨析 output, production, yield: output 和 production 指工业产量；yield 多指农业产量或矿物开采量。

【经典例题】Weisberg found that Schumann's compositional output indeed swelled during his manic years.

【译　　文】韦斯伯格发现，舒曼的创作量的确在他患有狂躁症的几年间有很大的增加。

☐ **outrage**
['autreidʒ]

n. 暴行，粗暴；失礼；震怒，愤慨　*v.* 使（某人）震怒；使愤慨；违背，破坏（法律、道德）

【名师导学】近义词：indignity, abuse, affront, insult; offend, abuse, insult

☐ **outstanding**
[aut'stændiŋ]

a. 突出的，显著的

【名师导学】许多形容词是由动词加 ing 的或加 ed 构成，加 ing 表示其本身的性质，加 ed 表示使人如何。

【经典例题】Asian Americans have made outstanding contributions to the United States.

【译　　文】亚裔美国人对美国做出了杰出的贡献。

☐ **overall**
['əuvərɔ:l]

a. 全面的，综合的

【经典例题】The overall goal of the book is to help bridge the gap between research and teaching, particularly between researchers and teachers.

【译　　文】这本书的总体目标是要帮助建立研究与教学之间的桥梁，尤其是要加强研究人员与教师之间的沟通。

☐ **overcome**
[,əuvə'kʌm]

vt. 战胜，克服

【经典例题】With this gene-altering technique to overcome our immune rejection to foreign organs, scientists hope to use pig hearts for transplants in the near future.

【译　　文】转基因技术能克服我们免疫系统对植入器官的排斥，科学家们希望，在不远的将来，猪的心脏能移植给人体。

☐ **overflow**
[,əuvə'fləu] *v.*
['əuvəfləu] *n.*

v. （使）溢出，（使）泛滥；涌出　*n.* 泛滥；过剩；超出额，溢出物

【名师导学】注意该词的引申义词组 overflow with。

【经典例题】The river overflowed its banks because of the heavy rain.

【译　　文】由于大雨，河水溢出了堤岸。

☐ **overhead**
['əuvəhed]

ad. 在头顶上，在空中，在高处

☐ **overlap**
[,əuvə'læp]

v. （与……）部分重叠；（与……）部分相同　*n.* 重叠，重叠的部分

【经典例题】The two images overlap and match perfectly.

【译　　文】这两张图像重叠起来，吻合得天衣无缝。

☐ **overlook**
[,əuvə'luk]

vt. 眺望，俯瞰；忽略，漏掉，未看见；宽容，放任

☐ **oversea(s)**
[,əuvə'si:z]

ad. 在海外　*a.* 海外的

overt
[əuˈvəːt, ˈəuvəːt]

a. 公开的，不隐蔽的

【经典例题】She criticized any overt display of emotion and attempts at open rebellion against the Ruling Power.

【译　　文】凡是明显的感情流露或者公开反抗执政党的企图，她都予以批评。

overtake
[ˌəuvəˈteik]

vt. 追上，赶上，超过；突然袭击

【名师导学】过去式/分词：overtook, overtaken。

overthrow
[ˌəuvəˈθrəu]

vt. 推翻，颠覆

【经典例题】They will fight until the government is overthrown.

【译　　文】他们将战斗到政府被推翻。

overturn
[ˌəuvəˈtəːn]

v. （使）推翻，（使）颠倒

overwhelm
[ˌəuvəˈwelm]

vt. 使不知所措；征服，制服

【联想记忆】over 过，超过 + whelm 淹没，覆盖，压倒 = overwhelm 征服，不知所措

【经典例题】We are all overwhelmed with more facts and information than we can possibly absorb.

【译　　文】我们淹没在大量难以吸收的事实和信息中。

overwhelming
[ˌəuvəˈwelmiŋ]

a. 势不可挡的，压倒性的

【经典例题】Of the thousands of known volcanoes in the world, the overwhelming majority are inactive.

【译　　文】在世界上已知的数以千计的火山中，大多数是死火山。

owing
[ˈəuiŋ]

a. 欠着的，未付的；应给予的

【固定搭配】owing to 由于，因为

【联想记忆】because of, on account of, due to, as a result of, thanks to, in view of, by reason of 由于，因为

【经典例题】I must decline your invitation owing to a subsequent engagement.

【译　　文】由于有约在后，不得不谢绝您的邀请。

oxygen
[ˈɔksidʒən]

n. 氧

【经典例题】Water is made from oxygen and hydrogen.

【译　　文】水是由氧和氢构成的。

ozone
[ˈəuzəun]

n. 臭氧；（海岸等的）新鲜空气

【经典例题】The destruction of Earth's ozone layer could contribute to the general process of impoverishment by allowing ultra-violet rays to harm plants and animals.

【译　　文】地球臭氧层的破坏致使紫外线伤害动植物，这可能造成普遍的生态环境恶化。

☐ **panel** ['pænl]
n. 专门小组；面板，控制板，仪表盘

☐ **panting** ['pæntiŋ]
n. 大口喘气，（裤子）织料 *a.* 气喘的
【经典例题】For years, biologists have known that chimpanzees and even some monkeys produce a panting sound akin to human laughter.
A. rocking　　B. gasping　　C. vibrating　　D. resonating　　[B]
【译　　文】多年以来，生物学家已经知道，黑猩猩甚至有些猴子能发出类似于人类笑声的（呼气的）声音。

☐ **parade** [pə'reid]
n. 游行，检阅 *v.* 游行

☐ **paradise** ['pærədais]
n. 天堂
【经典例题】It is sheer paradise to be home again and be able to relax.
【译　　文】能再次回家放松真是太棒了！

☐ **paradox** ['pærədɔks]
n. 似乎矛盾而（可能）正确的说法；自相矛盾的人（或事情）
【经典例题】We work to make money, but it's a paradox that people who work hard and long often don't make the most money.
【译　　文】我们工作是为了挣钱，但矛盾的是，那些工作辛苦、时间又长的人并不是挣钱最多的人。

☐ **paragraph** ['pærəgrɑ:f]
n. 段，节

☐ **paralyze** ['pærəlaiz]
vt. 使瘫痪，使麻痹；使丧失作用；使惊愕，使呆若木鸡
【经典例题】The accident left him paralyzed from the waist down.
【译　　文】那场事故使他腰部以下都瘫痪了。

☐ **parameter** [pə'ræmitə]
n. 参数，参量；[常 *pl.*] 因素

☐ **parasite** ['pærəsait]
n. 寄生动物
【经典例题】Don't be a parasite, and earn your own way in life.
【译　　文】不要当寄生虫，要自食其力。

☐ **partial** ['pɑ:ʃəl]
a. 部分的，局部的；偏爱的，不公平的
【经典例题】The research project was only a partial success.
【译　　文】那个研究项目只取得了部分成功。

☐ **participate** [pɑ:'tisipeit]
vi. 参与，参加
【派生词汇】participation *n.* 参与
【固定搭配】participate in 参加，参与
【名师导学】辨析 participate in，take part in：participate in 比较正式，用于正式场合；take part in 是日常用语。
【经典例题】Americans want to participate in all kinds of activities.
【译　　文】美国人想参加各种各样的活动。

partner
['pɑ:tnə]

n. 伙伴，合伙人，舞伴；搭档，配偶

passion
['pæʃən]

n. 激情，热情，酷爱
【派生词汇】passionate *a.* 激情的，热情的
【固定搭配】have a passion for 喜爱；be passionate for 对……热衷，对……热爱
【经典例题】His skills as a player don't quite match his passion for the game.
【译　　文】他作为玩家的水平与他对这项游戏的酷爱程度不太相配。

passive
['pæsiv]

a. 被动的，消极的
【经典例题】There are about 3,000 passive smokers died of lung cancer.
【译　　文】大概有 3 000 个被动吸烟者死于肺癌。

passport
['pɑ:spɔ:t]

n. 护照

paste
[peist]

n. 糨糊　*v.* 贴，粘

pathetic
[pə'θetik]

a. 可怜的，悲惨的

pastime
['pɑ:staim]

n. 消遣，娱乐
【名师导学】近义词：diversion, recreation, amusement, sport, entertainment
【经典例题】She sacrificed her pleasure and pastime to look after the old man.
【译　　文】她牺牲了自己的消遣和娱乐时间去照料这位老人。

pasture
['pɑ:stʃə]

n. 牧草地，牧场　*vt.* 放牧
【经典例题】Nothing can be compared with the sight of the rising sun glinting on the trees and pastures.
【译　　文】冉冉升起的旭日照在树林和牧场上闪烁发光，没有什么能与这个景色相媲美。

pat
[pæt]

n. / v. 轻拍
【固定搭配】pat on the back 赞扬，鼓励
【经典例题】She patted the baby's cheek.
【译　　文】她轻轻地拍了拍婴儿的脸蛋儿。

patch
[pætʃ]

n. 小片，小块，补丁　*vt.* 补，修补
【固定搭配】patch up 解决（争吵、麻烦）等；修补，草草修理

patriot
['peitriət]

n. 爱国者

patriotic
[ˌpætri'ɔtik, ˌpeitri-]

a. 爱国的
【经典例题】At Llewellyn's funeral service, she was remembered as a patriotic American who had served her country well.
【译　　文】在卢埃林的葬礼上，她作为一个鞠躬尽瘁的有爱国心的美国人而为大家所铭记。

patriotism
['peitriətizəm]

n. 爱国精神，爱国心，爱国主义

patrol [pə'trəul]	*n.* 巡逻，巡逻队 *v.* 巡逻，巡查 【经典例题】At that moment a patrol came within sight of our observation post. 【译　　文】那时，一支巡逻队进入我们观察哨所的视野。
patron ['peitrən, 'pæ-]	*n.* 保护人，赞助人 【经典例题】This restaurant offers a discount for its regular patrons. 【译　　文】这家饭馆为老主顾提供一定的折扣。
pave [peiv]	*vt.* 铺砌，铺（路） 【固定搭配】pave the way for / to 为……铺平道路，使……容易进行 【经典例题】The agreement paves the way for a lasting peace. 【译　　文】该协议为永久的和平铺平了道路。
peak [pi:k]	*n.* 峰，山峰；尖端，突出物
peanut ['pi:nʌt]	*n.* 花生
pedestrian [pe'destriən]	*n.* 步行者，行人 【经典例题】More than one third of all pedestrian injuries are children. 【译　　文】行人受伤的事故中，三分之一以上的伤者是小孩。
peel [pi:l]	*v.* 削皮，剥皮 *n.* 果皮 【经典例题】One speaks of orange peel, banana peel, and apple peel, but of tomato skin. 【译　　文】人们说"橘子皮""香蕉皮""苹果皮"时用"peel"，但西红柿皮却用"skin"。
peer [piə]	*v.* 偷看，窥探 *n.* 同辈；伙伴
penalty ['penlti]	*n.* 处罚，罚款；受苦；报应 【固定搭配】on / upon penalty of（违者）受……处罚 【名师导学】辨析 punishment, penalty：punishment 惩罚，指一般的惩罚行动；penalty 指法律上或规则上的惩罚，如监禁或罚款等。 【经典例题】It is well known that the minimum penalty for this crime is 2 years' imprisonment. 　A. conviction　B. span　C. mercy　D. punishment　[D] 【译　　文】众所周知，这类犯罪的最轻判罚是两年监禁。
penetrate ['penitreit]	*v.* 穿透，渗入，看穿 【固定搭配】penetrate through / into 穿过，渗透 【经典例题】Electrical fields cannot penetrate the body significantly. 【译　　文】电场无法完全穿透人体。
pension ['penʃən]	*n.* 抚恤金，养老金 【固定搭配】draw one's pension 领退休金；retire on a pension 领养老金退休 【经典例题】Despite losing his job he retains his pension. 【译　　文】他虽然失去了工作，但仍然享有养老金。
per [pə:, pə]	*prep.* 每

perceive [pə'si:v]
vt. 察觉，感知；理解，领悟
【固定搭配】perceive sb. do / doing sth. 觉察到某人做某事
【经典例题】One study found that job applicants who make more eye contacts are ____ as more alert, dependable, confident and responsible.
A. referred B. perceived
C. recommended D. presumed [B]
【译　文】一项研究发现，多用目光进行交流的应聘者被认为思维更敏捷、更可靠、更自信、更有责任心。

perception [pə'sepʃən]
n. 感知能力，觉察能力；认识，观念，看法

percentage [pə'sentidʒ]
n. 百分比
【名师导学】辨析 percent, percentage：percent 表示"百分之……"，相当于"%"，其前面为一具体数字；percentage 表示"百分比"，"百分数"，其前面不能是一具体数字，可被 high, low, large 等形容词修饰。

perform [pə'fɔ:m]
vt. 做，施行，完成；表演，演出

performer [pə'fɔ:mə(r)]
n. 表演者，演奏者

performance [pə'fɔ:məns]
n. 表演，演出；执行，完成；工作情况，表现情况
【经典例题】The performance of the Mozart group improved.
【译　文】莫扎特小组的表现改善了。

perfume ['pə:fju:m]
n. 香水，香料，香气 *vt.* 使充满芳香；洒香水于
【经典例题】What does the perfume smell like?
【译　文】这种香水闻起来怎样？

periodical [ˌpiri'ɔdikl]
a. 周期的，定期的 *n.* 期刊，杂志

peril ['perəl]
n. （严重）危险；祸害；险情 *vt.* 置……于危险中；危及
【经典例题】Although science and technology have advanced tremendously over the past century, the Pandemic peril remains.
【译　文】尽管科学技术在过去一个世纪取得了巨大进步，但大流行的危险依然存在。

perish ['periʃ]
vi. 丧失，毁灭，消亡；（橡胶、皮革等）失去弹性，老化
【名师导学】近义词：die, pass away, depart
【经典例题】Thousands of people perished in the earthquake.
【译　文】成千上万的人在那场地震中丧生。

perpetual [pə'petʃuəl]
a. 永久的

perplex [pə'pleks]
vt. 使困惑，使费解，使复杂化
【经典例题】They were perplexed by her response.
【译　文】她的答复令他们困惑不解。

persecution [ˌpə:si'kju:ʃn]
n. 迫害，烦扰

persist [pə(:)'sist]	vi. 坚持 【固定搭配】persist in doing sth. 坚持 【联想记忆】persevere in, insist on 坚持
persistent [pə'sistənt]	a. 坚持的,百折不挠的;固执的 【名师导学】近义词:tenacious, steadfast, determined, resolute
perspective [pə'spektiv]	n. 前景,前途;观点,看法;透视法 【经典例题】There is no need to choose between these two perspectives in art. 【译　文】在艺术中没有必要选定一个视角。
persuasive [pə'sweisiv]	a. 能说服的;善说服的
pervasive [pə'veisiv]	a. 弥漫的;遍布的;普遍的
pessimistic [,pesi'mistik]	a. 悲观的,悲观主义的,厌世的
pest [pest]	n. 有害的生物,害虫;讨厌的人 【经典例题】Animal and vegetable pests spread with extreme rapidity. 【译　文】动植物疫害传播极快。
pesticide ['pestisaid]	n. 杀虫剂;农药
petition [pi'tiʃən]	n. 请愿,祈求,请愿书 v. 请愿,祈求 【经典例题】The townspeople sent a petition to the government asking for electric light for the town. 【译　文】市民们向政府递交请愿书,要求为该市安装电灯。
petty ['peti]	a. 不重要的,次要的;渺小的,偏狭的;地位低下的 【名师导学】近义词:small, insignificant, frivolous, trivial, unimportant; small-minded, close-minded, narrow, narrow-minded, insular
pharmacy ['fɑːməsi]	n. 药房,药剂学,配药业,制药业
phenomenon [fi'nɔminən]	n. 现象 【名师导学】phenomenon 复数形式为 phenomena。
philosopher [fi'lɔsəfə]	n. 哲学家,哲人
phrase [freiz]	n. 短语,词组,习语
physical ['fizikəl]	a. 物质的,有形的;身体的;自然科学的,物理的 【固定搭配】physical education 体育;physical strength 体力;physical constitution 体格 【经典例题】When a danger is psychological rather than physical, fear can force you to take self-protective measures. 【译　文】当出现心理危险而非身体危险时,恐惧会迫使你采取自我保护措施。

☐ **physician** [fɪˈzɪʃən]	*n.* 内科医生	
	【联想记忆】doctor 医生（一般用语）；practitioner *n.*（医生、律师等）从业者；surgeon *n.* 外科医生；dentist *n.* 牙医	
☐ **physicist** [ˈfɪzɪsɪst]	*n.* 物理学家	
☐ **physiological** [ˌfɪziəˈlɒdʒɪkl]	*a.* 生理学的，生理学上的	
	【联想记忆】physi(cal) 物理的，生理的 +o+log(y) 学科 +ical=physiological 生理学的	
	【经典例题】If exercise is a bodily maintenance activity and an index of physiological age, the lack of sufficient exercise may either cause or hasten aging. A. instance　B. indicator　C. appearance　D. option　[B]	
	【译　　文】如果锻炼既维持身体机能也是生理年龄指标的话，那么缺乏足够的锻炼要么会造成老化要么会加速老化。	
☐ **pierce** [pɪəs]	*v.* 刺穿；看穿，洞察	
☐ **pirate** [ˈpaɪərɪt]	*n.* 海盗　*v.* 侵犯版权，盗版	
☐ **piracy** [ˈpaɪərəsi]	*n.* 海盗行为，侵犯版权，盗版	
☐ **plagiarism** [ˈpleɪdʒərɪzəm]	*n.* 抄袭；剽窃；剽窃物；抄袭物	
	【经典例题】Incidents in the news tend to describe the most serious violations of scientific standards, such as plagiarism for fabricating data.	
	【译　　文】上了新闻的不当行为往往描述最严重的学术违规行为，例如伪造数据的剽窃行为。	
☐ **plague** [pleɪg]	*n.* 瘟疫；麻烦，苦恼，灾祸　*vt.* 折磨，使苦恼	
☐ **plastic** [ˈplæstɪk, plɑːstɪk]	*a.* 塑料的，塑性的；可塑的　*n.* (*pl.*) 塑料	
☐ **plausible** [ˈplɔːzəbl]	*a.* 似乎合理的；似乎可能的，似是而非的	
	【经典例题】One team from Bristol announced that it had evidence to back a controversial but plausible theory which would explain how power lines might cause cancer.	
	【译　　文】来自布里斯托尔的一个团队对外宣布，该团队已经有证据支持一个充满争议但似乎合理的理论，该理论能够对电线可能引发癌症做出解释。	
☐ **plea** [pliː]	*n.* 恳求，请求；辩解，借口	
☐ **plead** [pliːd]	*v.* 请求，恳求	
	【名师导学】近义词：implore, solicit, appeal, beg; defend, advocate, allege, prosecute, argue, debate	
	【经典例题】Your youth and simplicity plead for you in this instance.	
	【译　　文】在这种情况下你的年轻和单纯成为有力的辩护。	

pledge
[pledʒ]

n. 誓约，保证 *vt.* 发誓，保证
【固定搭配】keep / break a pledge 信守 / 违背诺言；pledge to do / that 保证做
【联想记忆】commit oneself to do 答应做；engage oneself to do 保证做；undertake to do 承诺做
【经典例题】Take this ring as a pledge of our friendship.
【译　　文】把这个戒指作为我们友谊的信物。

plentiful
['plentiful]

a. 丰富的，富裕的

plot
[plɔt]

n. 一块地；计策，阴谋；情节 *v.* 策划

plug
[plʌg]

n. 塞子，插头 *v.* 堵，插
【固定搭配】plug in 给……接通电源，连接

plunge
[plʌndʒ]

vt. 跳入，（使）投入，（使）陷入；猛冲 *n.* 投入
【固定搭配】plunge into 冲入，投入；take the plunge（经过踌躇）决定冒险一试，采取决定性步骤
【联想记忆】dive / sink / throw into 投入
【经典例题】He made a headlong plunge into the river.
【译　　文】他一头栽进河里。

plus
[plʌs]

prep. 加 *a.* 正的，加的 *n.* 加号，正号
【联想记忆】add *v.* 加；subtract *v.* 减；multiply *v.* 乘；divide *v.* 除

poke
[pəuk]

vt. 戳，捅；用……戳（或捅），戳向；伸出，穿出 *vi.* 伸出，突出 *n.* 戳，捅
【固定搭配】poke one's nose into 探问，干预
【经典例题】Don't go poking your nose into other people's business!
【译　　文】少管闲事！

poise
[pɔiz]

v. 使均衡，保持平衡；使……保持某种姿态 *n.* 平衡，均衡；举止，态度

poison
['pɔizn]

n. 毒物，毒药 *v.* 放毒，毒害

poisonous
['pɔiznəs]

a. 有毒的；恶毒的

polar
['pəulə]

a. 两极的；极地的
【联想记忆】pole *n.* 极
【经典例题】Love and hatred are polar feelings.
【译　　文】爱与恨是完全相反的感情。

policy
['pɔlisi]

n. 政策，方针

polish
['pɔliʃ]

v. 磨光，擦亮；使优美，润色 *n.* 光泽，光滑；优美，品质；擦光剂，上光蜡
【经典例题】He took off his glasses and gave a polish to them.
【译　　文】他摘下眼镜擦了擦。

political
[pə'litikəl]

a. 政治的

poll [pəul]
n. 投票，投票数，民意测验 *v.* 投票，进行民意测验

pollutant [pə'lu:tənt]
n. 污染物质

pollute [pə'lu:t, -'lju:t]
vt. 污染，玷污
【经典例题】You are one of the guilty people who are helping to pollute the planet.
【译　　文】你是污染这个星球的罪人之一。

pollution [pə'lu:ʃən, -'lju:-]
n. 污染

ponder ['pɔndə]
v. 沉思，考虑
【名师导学】近义词：meditate, deliberate, consider, reflect

pop [pɔp]
n. 流行音乐 *v.* 突然出现，发生 *a.* 流行的，通俗的

populate ['pɔpjuleit]
v. 使人民居住，移民
【派生词汇】population *n.* 人口；populous *a.* 人口稠密的

pore [pɔ:, pɔə]
n. 毛孔 *vi.* 钻研；注视；细心思索
【固定搭配】pore over 仔细阅读
【经典例题】She was poring over an old map of the area.
【译　　文】她正在仔细查阅该地区的旧地图。

portal ['pɔ:tl]
n. 壮观的大门；豪华的入口；门户网站；入口站点
【经典例题】The site acts as a portal for thousands of online dealers.
【译　　文】该站点为数千名网络交易者的门户网站。

porter ['pɔ:tə]
n. 搬运工人

portion ['pɔ:ʃən]
n. 部分，份
【名师导学】"a portion of + 复数名词"做句子主语时，谓语用单数。
【经典例题】Two portions of the total market were targeted.
【译　　文】瞄准了全部市场的两个领域。

portrait ['pɔ:trit]
n. 肖像，画像

portray [pɔ:'trei]
vt. 描写，描绘；扮演，饰演

pose [pəuz]
v. 摆好姿势；提出（问题）*n.* 姿势

positive ['pɔzətiv]
a. 确定的，肯定的；正面的，积极的；正的，阳性的
【固定搭配】be positive about / of / that 确信；对……有自信
【经典例题】We still don't have a positive answer as to how he died.
【译　　文】他究竟是如何死的，我们还没有得出明确的答案。

possess
[pə'zes]

vt. 占有，拥有

【固定搭配】be possessed of 拥有；be possessed by / with 被……所迷住，被……所缠住

【名师导学】辨析 possess，own：possess 意为"占有，拥有"，既可指对某物有所有权或支配权，也指拥有才能、特点、品质等；own 意为"拥有，支配"，表示合法或天生地拥有某物，不能有抽象意义。

posture
['pɔstʃə]

n. 姿态，态度；看法，态度 *vi.* 摆出（不自然的）姿势，装模作样

【经典例题】She went on a diet to maintain good posture.

【译　　文】她节食以保持良好的体态。

potential
[pə'tenʃ(ə)l]

a. 潜在的，可能的 *n.* 潜力，潜能

【经典例题】It's much to be regretted that he died so young, his potential unfulfilled.

【译　　文】他才华未展，英年早逝，十分令人惋惜。

poverty
['pɔvəti]

n. 贫穷，贫困

【根源词汇】poor *a.* 贫穷的，可怜的

【固定搭配】poverty of / in 缺乏，不足

【经典例题】The Athens County poverty rate still remains at more than 30 percent — twice the national average.

【译　　文】雅典郡的贫困率仍然保持在30%以上，是全国平均水平的两倍。

practitioner
[præk'tiʃənə]

n. 开业医生；律师

pray
[prei]

v. 祈祷，祈求；请求，恳求

【固定搭配】pray for 为……祈祷；pray sb. to do sth. 恳求某人做某事

【联想记忆】ask for，beg for，request for，appeal for 请求

prayer
[prɛə]

n. 祈祷，祷告，祷文

preach
[pri:tʃ]

v. 传教，布道；劝诫，宣扬

【经典例题】The minister preached a sermon on the parable of the lost sheep.

【译　　文】牧师讲道时用了亡羊的比喻。

precaution
[pri'kɔ:ʃən]

n. 预防，留心，警戒 *vt.* 预告，警告

【经典例题】Our first priority is to take every precaution to protect our citizens at home and around the world from further attacks.

【译　　文】我们的首要任务是采取每一个预防措施，以保证我们的国民不论是在国内还是在世界上的其他地方都不再受到袭击。

precede
[pri(:)'si:d]

vt. 先于，在……（之）前；比……更重要

【经典例题】A further stimulus to invention came from the "premium" system, which preceded our patent system and for years ran parallel with it.

【译　　文】推动发明的另一种刺激因素来自"奖赏"制度，它产生于专利制度之前，并与之并存了多年。

precedent
['presidənt]

n. 先例

preceding
[pri(:)'si:diŋ]

a. 在前的，在先的

precise
[pri'sais]

a. 精确的，准确的

precision
[pri'siʒn]

n. 精确；精密度

preclude
[pri'klu:d]

v. 排除；阻止；妨碍

predecessor
['pri:disesə]

n. 前辈，前任

【名师导学】该词在考题中会比其近义词 ancestor 出现的频率高，注意一些词的同义异形。

【经典例题】Judging by the past, we can expect that a new species will arise out of man, surpassing his achievements as he has surpassed those of his predecessor.

【译　　文】由过去来判断，我们可以展望，一个新的物种将从人类中出现，就像人类超过祖先的成就一样，新物种也将超过人类的成就。

predict
[pri'dikt]

v. 预言，预测

【经典例题】With the constant change of the conditions, the outcome is not always predictable.

【译　　文】随着情况的持续变化，结果并不总是可以预测的。

prediction
[pri'dikʃn]

n. 预言，预报

predispose
[ˌpri:di'spəuz]

v. （使）易罹患，（使）预先偏向于

【联想记忆】pre 提前，预先 +dispose 处理，处置，安排 =predispose 预先处置，使……偏向于

【经典例题】His weak chest ＿＿＿ him to winter illness.
A. predicts　　B. preoccupies　C. prevails　　D. predisposes　　[D]

predominant
[pri'dɔminənt]

a. 卓越的；支配的；主要的；突出的；有影响的

【联想记忆】pre 主要的 +dominant 显著的，支配的 =predominant 主要的，突出的

【经典例题】In front of the platform, the students were talking with the professor over the quizzes of their ＿＿＿ subject.
A. compulsory　　　　　　B. compulsive
C. alternative　　　　　　D. predominant　　[A]

【解　析】compulsory 被强制的，必修的；compulsive 强制的；alternative 选择性的；predominate 卓越的；支配的。所以答案为 A。

【译　　文】学生们在讲台前跟教授谈论他们必修课的考试。

【名师导学】dominant, predominant, sovereign 这些形容词均含有"占优势的，支配其他的"之意。
dominant 强调权威。
predominant 侧重指影响与新近的优势。
sovereign 侧重指其他事物都从属于或低于它的地位。

preface
['prefis]

n. 序言，引言，前言

pregnancy ['pregnənsi]	*n.* 怀孕，怀孕期
pregnant ['pregnənt]	*a.* 怀孕的
prejudice ['predʒudis]	*n.* 偏见，成见
preliminary [pri'liminəri]	*a.* 预备的，初步的
premature [priːmə'tʃur]	*a.* 未成熟的，早熟的
premier ['premjə, -miə]	*n.* 首相，总理
premise ['premis]	*n.* 前提，根据 【经典例题】Advice to investors was based on the premise that interest rates would continue to fall. 【译　文】给予投资者们的建议是以利率将继续下降这一点为前提的。
premium ['primjəm]	*n.* 奖赏，奖金／品，佣金；（利息，工资等以外的）酬金；额外的费用 【固定搭配】put / place a premium on sth. 高度评价，重视；pay a premium for 付……佣金；at a premium 奇缺的，难得的
preoccupy [pri(ː)'ɔkjupai]	*v.* 使全神贯注，迷住
prescribe [pri'skraib]	*vt.* 开处方，开药；规定，指示 【经典例题】The doctor prescribed his patient a receipt. 【译　文】医生给病人开了一张药方。
prescription [pri'skripʃən]	*n.* 药方，处方 【经典例题】If you want this painkiller, you'll have to ask the doctor for a prescription. 【译　文】如果你想要这种止疼药，你就必须请医生开处方。
presence ['prezns]	*n.* 出席，在场；存在 【固定搭配】in the presence of sb. 当着某人的面，有某人在场；presence of mind 镇定自若
presentation [,prezen'teiʃən]	*n.* 介绍，陈述；表现形式
presently ['prezəntli]	*ad.* 不久，一会儿，目前，现在 【经典例题】Dinner will be ready ____, but we still have time for a drink. A. finally　B. currently　C. presently　D. lately　[C] 【译　文】宴会马上就开始了，但是我们还是有时间喝一杯。
preserve [pri'zəːv]	*vt.* 保护，保存；保藏，腌渍；维持，保持 【固定搭配】preserve...from 保护……免于 【经典例题】I tried to preserve family harmony. 【译　文】我努力维持家庭和睦。

preside
[prɪˈzaɪd]

v. 主持

prestige
[preˈstiːʒ, -ˈtiːdʒ]

n. 声望，威望，威信

pressure
[ˈpreʃə(r)]

n. 压力，紧张；强制；压强

【固定搭配】under the pressure of 在……强迫下，在……压力下
【名师导学】辨析 pressure，stress：pressure 指液体产生的压力，在这种压力下，各方面的受力是同样的，也指某事物所产生的压力、影响力；stress 指一定的困难或精神上、肉体上的痛苦所带来的压力，也指作用在物体上的力。

presume
[prɪˈzjuːm]

vt. 假定，假设，姑且认为 *vi.* 揣测
【经典例题】Twelve passengers are missing, presumed dead.
【译　　文】12 名乘客失踪，估计已死亡。

presumably
[prɪˈzjuːməbli]

ad. 推测上，大概

presumption
[prɪˈzʌmpʃn]

n. 假定

pretext
[ˈpriːtekst]

n. 借口，托词 *v.* 借口
【经典例题】He left immediately on the pretext that he had to catch a train.
A. claim　　B. clue　　C. excuse　　D. talent　　[C]
【译　　文】他借口赶火车，立即离开了。

prevail
[prɪˈveɪl]

vi. 取胜，占优势；流行，盛行
【固定搭配】prevail over / against 战胜，压倒；prevail in / among 流行，普遍存在；prevail on / upon sb. to do sth. 劝说某人做某事
【经典例题】Nothing is so uncertain as the fashion market where one style ＿＿＿＿ over another before being replaced.
A. dominates　　B. manipulates　　C. overwhelms　　D. prevails　　[D]
【译　　文】任何事情都是不确定的，就像在时装市场中，一种样式在被取代前，和其他样式相比都占优势地位。

prevalent
[ˈprevələnt]

a. 流行的，普遍的
【名师导学】近义词：widespread, accepted, common, prevailing
【经典例题】Diabetes is one of the most ＿＿＿＿ and potentially dangerous diseases in the world.
A. crucial　　B. virulent　　C. colossal　　D. prevalent　　[D]
【译　　文】糖尿病是世界上最普遍的、具有潜在危险的疾病之一。

preview
[ˈpriːvjuː]

n. 事先查看，[计]预览 *vt.* 事先查看，预展，预演

previous
[ˈpriːvjəs]

a. 先，前，以前的
【固定搭配】be previous to 在……之前
【名师导学】辨析 preceding, previous, prior：preceding 指"此前的"，多用于指文章中某一处之前；previous 多指时间发生在前的；prior 比 previous 多一层"优先"的意思。

prey [prei]

n. 被捕食的动物，捕获物；受害者　*v.* (on) 捕食；折磨，使烦恼
【名师导学】该词是常考词，要特别注意以下词组：fall prey to 成为……的牺牲品，深受……之害；prey on 捕食。还要注意该词与 pray（祈祷）的区别。
【经典例题】She fell an easy prey to his charm.
【译　　文】她一下子就被他迷住了。

prime [praim]

a. 主要的，基本的；极好的，第一流的　*n.* 全盛时期；青壮年时期

primitive ['primitiv]

a. 原始的，早期的；简单的，粗糙的
【经典例题】Farmers began primitive genetic engineering at the dawn of agriculture.
【译　　文】农民们在农业的初期就开始了早期的基因工程。

principal ['prinsəp(ə)l]

a. 主要的，最重要的，首要的　*n.* 负责人，校长；资本，本金
【经典例题】Smith has one principal rule for all teaching instructions.
【译　　文】史密斯对所有的授课程序有一个主要的原则。

principle ['prinsəpl]

n. 原则，原理；主义，信念
【固定搭配】in principle 原则上，大体上；on principle 根据原则

prior ['praiə]

a. 在前的；优先的
【固定搭配】prior to 在……之前
【联想记忆】priority *n.* 优先权，优先考虑；superiority *n.* 优势，优越性；seniority *n.* 年长，资深
【经典例题】The competitor must make this decision prior to seeing either the time or the score from the initial attempt.
【译　　文】选手必须在看到初次比赛的时间与分数前做出决定。

private ['praivit]

a. 私人的，私有的，私立的；私下的，秘密的
【固定搭配】in private 私下地
【经典例题】Mr. Morgan can be very sad　　　, though in public he is extremely cheerful.
A. by himself　　B. in person　　C. in private　　D. as individual　　[C]
【译　　文】虽然摩根先生在公开场合表现得十分愉悦，但是私底下他还是非常伤心的。

privilege ['privilidʒ]

n. 特权，优惠，特许　*vt.* 给予优惠，给予特权
【经典例题】Parking in this street is the privilege of the residents.
【译　　文】在这条街上停车是此处居民特有的权利。

probe [prəub]

n. 探针，探测器　*vt.* 穿刺；探察，查究，调查
【固定搭配】probe into 调查，探索
【名师导学】考试中经常考查这个用法：probe into sth. 探究，调查。

procedure [prə'si:dʒə]

n. 程序

proceed [prə'si:d]

vi. 继续进行
【固定搭配】proceed to do sth. 继续做（另一件事）；proceed with sth. 继续进行
【联想记忆】go on to do sth., go on doing sth., continue sth. / to do sth., keep on doing sth., keep on with sth. 继续做
【经典例题】Once your PIN has been reset, you may proceed to create a new PIN.
【译　　文】一旦您的 PIN 被重新设置，您就可以继续创建新的 PIN。

process
['prəuses]

n. 过程，历程；工序，工艺 *vt.* 加工，处理
【固定搭配】in the process of 在……过程中
【经典例题】Achieving a high degree of proficiency in English as a foreign language is not a mysterious process without scientific basis.
【译　　文】在英语学习中获得较高造诣并不是一个没有任何科学基础的神秘过程。

proclaim
[prə'kleim]

vt. 宣布，声明；表明
【名师导学】近义词：declare, announce, give out, blazon

productive
[prə'dʌktiv]

a. 多产的，（土地）肥沃的；有收获的，很多成果的
【名师导学】近义词：rich, fruitful, prolific, fertile
【经典例题】They work hard, but their efforts are not very productive.
【译　　文】他们很努力，但他们的努力缺乏成效。

productivity
[,prɔdʌk'tiviti]

n. 生产力，生产能力
【经典例题】Raise labor productivity, land productivity and utilization rate of the resources.
【译　　文】提高劳动生产率、土地生产力和资源利用率。

proficiency
[prə'fiʃənsi]

n. 精通，熟练，精练
【固定搭配】proficiency in (doing sth.) 精通
【经典例题】The tutor tells the undergraduates that one can acquire proficiency in a foreign language through more practice.
【译　　文】导师告诉这些大学生，要熟练掌握一门外语需要更多的练习。

profile
['prəufail]

n. （面部或头部的）侧面（像）；传略，人物简介；轮廓，形象；姿态，引人注目的状态 *vt.* 为……描绘（轮廓等），写……的传略（或概括）
【经典例题】But these high-profile infractions occur relatively rarely.
【译　　文】但是这些高调的违法行为相对少见。

profound
[prə'faund]

a. 深奥的，渊博的；由衷的；深远的，深刻的
【名师导学】近义词：intelligent, learned, scholarly, abstruse, sage, serious, sagacious, penetrating, discerning, knowing, wise, reflective, knowledgeable, intellectual, enlightened, thorough, informed
【经典例题】The new research has profound implications for the environmental summit in Rio de Janeiro.
【译　　文】这项新研究对里约热内卢的环境峰会具有深远的意义。

prohibit
[prə'hibit]

vt. 禁止，阻止
【经典例题】Good manners prohibit me from so rude an answer.
【译　　文】礼貌不允许我作如此粗鲁的回答。

project
[prə'dʒekt] *v.*
['prɔdʒekt] *n.*

n. 计划，方案；工程，项目 *vt.* 设计，规划；投射；放映；使突出

prolong
[prə'lɔŋ]

vt. 延长，拉长，拖延
【经典例题】The operation could prolong his life by two or three years.
【译　　文】这次手术可使他多活两三年。

prominent
['prɔminənt]

a. 凸起的；显著的，杰出的
【经典例题】A new theory is the most prominent feature of the book.
【译　　文】一个新的理论是这本书最突出的特性。

promising ['prɔmisiŋ]

a. 有希望的,有前途的
【联想记忆】promise *n.* 诺言 *v.* 承诺
【名师导学】注意 promise 的现在分词形式的词义之一是形容词。
【经典例题】The weather report wasn't very promising.
【译　　文】天气预报不太乐观。

promote [prə'məut]

vt. 提升,晋升;促进,增进,助长
【经典例题】They have greatly promoted American culture, and improved the living standards of the whole American people.
【译　　文】他们极大促进了美国文化的发展,提高了所有美国人的生活水平。
【经典例题】The government is trying to do something to＿＿＿better understanding between the two countries.
A. raise　　B. promote　　C. heighten　　D. increase　　[B]
【译　　文】政府正试图促进两国间的相互理解和认识。

promotion [prə'məuʃən]

n. 升级,晋级;宣传,推广

prompt [prɔmpt]

a. 敏捷的,迅速的,即刻的　*vt.* 促使,推动
【固定搭配】be prompt in sth. / doing sth. 在……方面敏捷的
【经典例题】Fuel scarcities and price increase prompt automobile designers to scale down the largest models and to develop completely new lines of small cars and trucks.
【译　　文】燃料匮乏和价格上扬促使汽车设计人员开始减少大型车的设计,开始转向发展小型轿车和小型卡车的新产品线。

prone [prəun]

a. 易于……的,有……倾向的;俯卧的
【固定搭配】be prone to sth. / to do sth. 易于……的
【经典例题】Doctors are interested in using lasers as a surgical tool in operations on people who are prone to heart attack.
【译　　文】医生倾向于用激光作为外科工具给那些易患心脏病的人做手术。

proof [pru:f]

n. 证据,证明

prop [prɔp]

n. 支柱,顶杠,支持;支持物,支持者　*vt.* 支撑,支持;依靠,靠立

propaganda [ˌprɔpə'gændə]

n. 宣传
【经典例题】There has been a good deal of propaganda about the dangers of smoking.
【译　　文】关于吸烟的害处,人们已做了大量的宣传。

propagate ['prɔpəgeit]

vt. 繁殖,传播,传送
【经典例题】That old scientist did a lot in propagating scientific knowledge.
【译　　文】那位老科学家在传播科学知识方面做了许多事情。

property ['prɔpəti]

n. 财产,所有物;性质,特性
【固定搭配】movable / personal property 动产; real property 不动产

prophet ['prɔfit]

n. 先知,预言者;预言书
【经典例题】I'm afraid I'm no weather prophet.
【译　　文】我可不会预测天气。

proportion [prə'pɔːʃən]
n. 部分，份额；比例，比重；均衡，相称
【固定搭配】in proportion to 与……成比例 out of proportion to 与……不成比例
【经典例题】Gradually raise the proportion of the tertiary industry in the national economy.
【译　文】逐步提高第三产业在国民经济中的比重。

proposal [prə'pəuzəl]
n. 提议，建议；求婚
【名师导学】在 proposal 跟的同位语从句和表语从句中，谓语用虚拟语气。
【名师导学】辨析 proposal, suggest：proposal 意为"提议，忠告"，指正式或通过一定程序或途径而提出的建议；suggest 意为"建议"，指所提建议不一定正确，仅供对方参考。

propose [prə'pəuz]
vt. 提议，建议；求婚
【固定搭配】propose doing 建议做某事；propose to do 打算做某事；propose to sb. 向某人求婚
【名师导学】propose 所带的宾语从句中谓语用虚拟语气。

proposition [ˌprɔpə'ziʃən]
n. 提议，建议；主张，观点；命题
【联想记忆】propose v. 建议，打算

prose [prəuz]
n. 散文
【经典例题】He delivered a long prose full of platitudes.
【译　文】他发表了一篇充满陈词滥调的散文。

prosecute ['prɔsikjuːt]
vt. 实行，从事；告发，起诉 vi. 告发，起诉，做检察官
【固定搭配】prosecute sb.（for sth.\ doing sth.）因某事检举、告发某人
【经典例题】He was prosecuted for exceeding the speed limit.
【译　文】他因超速行驶而被起诉。

prospect ['prɔspekt]
n. 展望，前景
【固定搭配】in prospect 期望中的，展望中的
【经典例题】I see little prospect of an improvement in his condition.
【译　文】我看他的情况没有什么改进的希望。

prospective [prə'spektiv]
a. 预期的

prosperity [prɔ'speriti]
n. 繁荣，兴旺

prosperous ['prɔspərəs]
a. 繁荣的，兴旺的

protein ['prəutiːn]
n. 蛋白质

protest ['prə'test] v. ['prəutest] n.
v. / n. 抗议，反对
【固定搭配】protest against / at / about sth. 反对，抗议
【联想记忆】oppose to，object to，go against，have an objection to 抗议；反对
【经典例题】Tens of thousands of demonstrators hit the streets yesterday in protest against the proposed anti-subversion law.
【译　文】数以万计市民昨日上街游行，抗议政府就基本法立法。

prototype [ˈprəutətaip]	n. 原型
provoke [prəˈvəuk]	vt. 挑动，激发，招惹 【固定搭配】provoke sb. to do，provoke sb. into doing 激起某人做某事 【经典例题】The attitude of Japanese government provoked widespread criticism. 【译　文】日本政府的态度激起了广泛的批评。
prudent [ˈpru:dnt]	a. 谨慎的，有远见的，精打细算的 【经典例题】The bacterial infection is curable with judicious use of antibiotics. 　A. impudent　　　　　　B. imprudent 　C. purulent　　　　　　D. prudent　　　　　　　[D] 【译　文】如谨慎使用抗生素，细菌感染可以治愈。
psychiatrist [saiˈkaiətrist]	n. 精神病医师，精神病学家 【联想记忆】psych（用精神分析治疗，使做好心理准备）+ia(I am)+tr(try)+ist 人＝试图用精神分析治疗病人的人＝psychiatrist 精神病学家，精神病医师 【经典例题】"The material on immigrant health shocked me when we first reviewed it." says panel member Arthus M. Kleinman, a psychiatrist and anthropologist at Harvard Medical School in Boston. 【译　文】"当我们第一次审阅移民健康的资料时，我感到十分震惊。"审阅委员会的成员亚瑟 M. 克莱曼说。他是波士顿哈佛医学院的精神病学家和人类学家。 【名师导学】psychic 通灵的人；psychiatry 精神病学；psycho 精神病患者；psychology 心理学；psychologist 心理学家
publication [ˌpʌbliˈkeiʃən]	n. 公布；出版；出版物
publicity [pʌbˈlisiti]	n. 众所周知，闻名；宣传，广告
publicize [ˈpʌblisaiz]	v. 宣扬；引人注意；广为宣传；推销
publish [ˈpʌbliʃ]	vt. 公布，发表；出版
pulse [pʌls]	n. 脉搏，脉冲
pump [pʌmp]	n. 泵　vt. 打气，泵送
punch [pʌntʃ]	vt. 冲压，穿孔　n. 冲压机，穿孔机
punctual [ˈpʌŋktjuəl]	n. 准时的，正点的 【经典例题】Not being punctual is his greatest shortcoming. 【译　文】不守时间是他最大的缺点。
purchase [ˈpə:tʃəs]	n. 购买；购买的东西　vt. 购买

pursue [pə'sjuː]

vt. 追逐，追击；从事，进行

【经典例题】Dozens of scientific groups all over the world have been ____ the goal of a practical and economic way to use sunlight to split water molecules.
A. pursuing　　B. chasing　　C. reaching　　D. winning　　[A]
【译　文】全世界许多的科学团队都在追求运用可行又经济的方法使太阳能来分离水分子。
【经典例题】He was free to pursue his own life in his own way.
【译　文】他有自由以自己的方式过自己的生活。

qualification [ˌkwɔlifi'keiʃən]

n. 资格，条件；限制，限定

qualify ['kwɔlifai]

vt. 取得资格，使合格，使胜任
【固定搭配】qualify as 有条件成为
【经典例题】He does not qualify as a teacher of English for his poor pronunciation.
【译　文】他不适合当一名英语教师，因为他的发音很差。

quarterly ['kwɔːtəli]

a. / ad. 季度的/地　*n.* 季刊
【联想记忆】quarter *n.* 四分之一
【经典例题】I receive quarterly bank statements.
【译　文】我每个季度收到一份银行结账单。

queue [kjuː]

n. 行列，长队　*vi.* 排长队
【固定搭配】jump the / a queue 插队

quench [kwentʃ]

vt. 止（渴），扑灭（火焰）
【经典例题】It is hard to quench people's thirst for truth.
【译　文】人们追求真理的渴望是很难扑灭的。

quest [kwest]

v. / n. 探索，寻找，追求
【名师导学】近义词：cast about, hunt, look, search, seek., pursuit
【经典例题】He left home in quest of adventure.
【译　文】他离家去探险了。

question(n)aire [ˌkwestiə'nɛə, -tʃə-]

n. 问卷，调查表
【联想记忆】question 问题
【经典例题】The purpose of the survey was to discover the views of the students on a number of matters of personal concern. The survey was conducted by means of a questionnaire given to the students to complete.
【译　文】调查的目的是，了解学生在一系列个人关心的问题上的观点。调查以发给学生问卷的方式完成。

quiver ['kwivə]
n. / vi. 颤抖，发抖，抖动
【经典例题】A quiver of his lips showed that he was about to cry.
【译　　文】他嘴唇一阵颤动，表明他要哭了。

quiz [kwiz]
n. 小型考试，测验，问答比赛

quota ['kwəutə]
n. 定额，限额，配额
【经典例题】No boat is allowed to catch more than its quota of fish.
【译　　文】任何船都不允许捕获超过配额的鱼。

quotation [kwəu'teiʃən]
n. 引语，语录

quote [kwəut]
vt. 引用，援引
【经典例题】He quotes the *Bible*.
【译　　文】他引用《圣经》的话。

racial ['reiʃəl]
a. 人种的，种族的
【经典例题】There is no racial discrimination to be felt in this city.
【译　　文】在这座城市里感觉不到种族歧视。

racism ['reisizəm]
n. 种族主义；种族歧视（意识）

racket ['rækit]
n. 球拍；敲诈
【经典例题】The police investigating the fraud suspected him of being in the racket.
【译　　文】调查这一诈骗案的警方怀疑他涉嫌参与诈骗活动。

radar ['reidə]
n. 雷达

radical ['rædikəl]
a. 基本的，重要的；激进的，极端的
【经典例题】Radical psychoanalyst Wilhelm Reich believed that many of us inhibit or deny impulses, feelings, traumas, and stresses by tightening our muscles and creating a kind of body armor.
【译　　文】激进的精神分析学家威廉·赖希认为，我们许多人通过收缩肌肉和创造一种身体防御来抑制或拒绝冲动、感情、创伤和压力。

radioactive [,reidiəu'æktiv]
a. 放射性的
【经典例题】Radium and uranium are radioactive elements.
【译　　文】镭和铀是放射性元素。

radiologist [,reidi'ɔlədʒist]
n. 放射专家
【联想记忆】radiological *adj.* 放射的，放射学的

radius ['reidiəs]
n. 半径
【经典例题】Police searched all the woods within a radius of six miles.
【译　文】警方在树林半径六英里范围内进行了搜索。

rag [ræg]
n. 破布，碎布
【固定搭配】be in rags 衣衫褴褛

rage [reidʒ]
n. 愤怒
【固定搭配】be in a rage / fall into a rage 勃然大怒

raid [reid]
n. / v. 袭击，突击；搜查，搜捕；抢劫

rally ['ræli]
v. 集合，重整；恢复（元气），振作（精神）　*n.* 群众集会；汽车拉力赛

random ['rændəm]
a. 随机的；任意的，随便的　*n.* 偶然的（或随便的）行动（或过程）
【固定搭配】at random 随便的，任意的
【经典例题】When a psychologist does a general experiment about the human mind, he selects people at random and asks them questions.
【译　文】当一位心理学家做一项关于人类心理的普遍实验时，他通常随机选择一些人来问一些问题。

rape [reip]
n. 强奸；劫取　*vt.* 强奸；洗劫
【经典例题】Her rape had a profound psychological effect on her.
【译　文】她被强奸这件事给她心理上造成了严重的创伤。

rare [rɛə]
a. 稀有的，难得的，珍奇的；稀薄的，稀疏的
【名师导学】辨析 rare，scarce：rare 指罕见的、稀奇的物品；scarce 指寻常物的短缺。
【经典例题】It is a rare treasure of historical records.
【译　文】这是罕见的史料宝藏。

rarely ['rɛəli]
ad. 稀少，很少，难得
【经典例题】San Francisco is usually cool in the summer, but Los Angeles　　　.
A. is rarely　　B. is scarcely　　C. hardly is　　D. rarely is　　[D]
【译　文】在夏天，旧金山通常很凉爽，但是在洛杉矶就极少这样了。

rash [ræʃ]
a. 轻率的，鲁莽的
【联想记忆】rush *v.* 冲
【经典例题】I'm not very happy about our rash decision.
【译　文】我不很赞成我们的草率决定。

rate [reit]
n. 速率，比率；等级；价格，费　*vt.* 评级，评价
【固定搭配】at any rate 无论如何，至少
【联想记忆】in any circumstances，under any condition，ad any cost，in any case, by all means 无论如何
【名师导学】辨析 rate，ratio：rate 意为"速率，速度"，一般用词，既可指速度又可指比率，如 survival rate（成活率）；ratio 意为"比率，比例"，指两个同类数互相比较，其中一个数是另一个数的几倍或几分之几，如 4:3。

rating ['reitiŋ]
n. 评价，估计，评分；等级，规格
【经典例题】Blue Funk's new hit has had good ratings in the charts.
【译　文】布鲁·芬克的新唱片在流行音乐排行榜上名列前茅。

ratio [ˈreiʃiəu]	*n.* 比率，比
rational [ˈræʃənl]	*a.* 理性的，合理的 【名师导学】辨析 rational，reasonable：rational 强调有思考、推理的能力；reasonable 指公平合理，暗示行为或要求等不过火。 【经典例题】It's usually the case that people seldom behave in a _____ way when in a furious state. A. stable　　B. rational　　C. legal　　D. credible　　[B] 【译　文】通常人们在暴怒的情况下很少能表现得有理性。
raw [rɔː]	*a.* 生的，未煮熟的；未加工过的
realistic [riəˈlistik]	*a.* 现实的，现实主义的；逼真的
reality [riː(ː)ˈæliti]	*n.* 现实，实际；真实 【固定搭配】in reality 实际上，事实上
realism [ˈriːəlizəm]	*n.* 现实主义
realization [ˌriːəlaiˈzeiʃən]	*n.* 实现
realm [relm]	*n.* 王国，国度；领域，范围
reap [riːp]	*v.* 收割，收获 【经典例题】Anyone clever enough to modify this information for his own purposes can reap substantial rewards. 【译　文】任何一个足够聪明的人为了个人目的修改这项资料，就能从中获取丰厚的酬劳。
rear [riə]	*n.* 后部，尾部　*a.* 后方的，背后的　*vt.* 饲养；抚养 【固定搭配】at the rear of 在……的后部
reasonable [ˈriːznəbl]	*a.* 合理的，讲理的；公道的 【经典例题】This statement is a reasonable conclusion looking at world politics and economics. 【译　文】看看世界的政治与经济就可以说这是个合理的断言。
reassure [ˌriːəˈʃuə]	*vt.* 使安心 【经典例题】They tried to reassure her, but she still felt anxious. 【译　文】他们设法让她安心，可她还是焦虑不安。
rebel [riˈbel]	*vi.* 反抗，反叛，起义　*n.* 叛逆者，起义者
rebellion [riˈbeljən]	*n.* 谋反，叛乱，反抗，不服从
rebound [riˈbaund]	*n.* 回弹　*v.* 回弹

recede
[ri'si:d]

vi. 退，退去；向后倾斜，缩进

【名师导学】近义词：fall / draw back, shrink, withdraw, retreat; abate, decline, decrease

【经典例题】We reached the open sea and the coast receded into the distance.

【译　文】我们驶抵公海，海岸似乎退到了远方。

receipt
[ri'si:t]

n. 收据，收条；收到，接到

【固定搭配】on receipt of 收到……后

reception
[ri'sepʃən]

n. 接见，接待，招待会；接受，接收，接收效果

【固定搭配】hold a reception 举行招待会

recession
[ri'seʃən]

n. 退回，后退；（经济）衰退，不景气

【经典例题】I used to make a small profit on my travel allowances, but since the recession I haven't been able to.

【译　文】我以前会在旅行津贴上赚点小利润，但是自从经济衰退以后就不能了。

recipe
['resipi]

n. 食谱；方法，窍门

【经典例题】When you write a recipe, you need to explain what ingredients will be needed and how they will be used.

【译　文】写食谱时，你需要说明所需的配料以及加工方法。

recipient
[ri'sipiənt]

n. 接受者，接收者

【经典例题】This kind of support, like all government support, requires decisions about the appropriate recipients of the fund.

【译　文】这种类型的支持，像所有政府的支持一样，需要对资金的合适接受人选做出决定。

reciprocal
[ri'siprəkəl]

a. 相互的，互惠的

【经典例题】The two countries will assign counter-drug officials to their respective embassies on a reciprocal basis.

【译　文】这两个国家将在互惠的基础上，委派缉毒官员到他们各自的大使馆。

recite
[ri'sait]

v. 背诵，朗诵

【经典例题】He can recite that poem from memory.

【译　文】他能凭记忆背诵那首诗。

reckless
['reklis]

a. 粗心大意的，鲁莽的

【名师导学】近义词：thoughtless, heedless, breakneck, wild

【经典例题】He showed a reckless disregard for his own safety.

【译　文】他对个人安危全然不顾。

reckon
['rekən]

v. 数，计算；想，料想

【固定搭配】reckon...as 把……看作；reckon on 指望，依靠

【经典例题】The movement of the moon conveniently provided the unit of month, which was ＿＿＿＿ from one new moon to the next.

A. measured　　B. reckoned　　C. judged　　D. assessed　　[B]

【译　文】月亮的运动很方便地提供了"月"这个单位，我们可以把它看作从一个新的月亮到下一个新的月亮出现之间的时间。

reclaim
[riˈkleim]
vt. 要求归还,收回;开垦

recognition
[ˌrekəgˈniʃən]
n. 认出,承认
【固定搭配】grant recognition 给予承认

recognize
[ˈrekəgnaiz]
vt. 认出,识别;承认

recommend
[ˌrekəˈmend]
vt. 劝告,建议;介绍,推荐
【固定搭配】recommend sb. to do sth. 推荐某人(做)某事
【经典例题】Although my sister and her husband have eight children, they do not recommend other couples to have families of this size.
【译　　文】尽管我姐姐姐夫有8个孩子,他们并不建议别的夫妇也生这么多子女。

recommendation
[ˌrekəmenˈdeiʃən]
n. 劝告,建议;推荐;最高纪录,最佳成绩;履历,历史

reconcile
[ˈrekənsail]
vt. 使协调;使和谐;(to)使顺从(于),使甘心(于)
【名师导学】注意与 compromise, harmonize, assort 等词的区别运用:compromise with sb. on sth. 妥协;harmonize with 协调;assort with 相称,协调。常用短语:reconcile to / with sb. 与某人和解,reconcile oneself to sth. / doing sth. 安于,听从。其中 to 为介词,后接动名词。
【经典例题】Since the couple could not reconcile their differences, they decided to get a divorce.
【译　　文】由于不能调和彼此的分歧,这对夫妻决定离婚。

recount
[riˈkaunt]
v. 叙述

recovery
[riˈkʌvəri]
n. 复原,痊愈;收回,复得

recreation
[ˌrekriˈeiʃ(ə)n]
n. 娱乐,消遣

recruit
[riˈkruːt]
v. 征募新兵,吸收新成员;补充　*n.* 新兵,新成员

rectangular
[rekˈtæŋgjulə]
n. 长方形的,矩形的
【联想记忆】triangular 三角形的,三人间的;quinquangular 五角形的
【经典例题】The national flags in some countries are not rectangular.
【译　　文】有些国家的国旗并不是长方形的。

rectify
[ˈrektifai]
vt. 纠正,修复
【名师导学】注意 rectify 转化成名词时 y 变成 i 加 cation,在英语中多以 y 结尾的动词以同样的方法变成名词如有:purify, clarify, unify, personify 等。
【经典例题】Of course, to rectify the economic order, we must straighten out the price system.
【译　　文】当然,要真正建立市场秩序,不理顺价格是不行的。

recur
[ri'kə:r]

v. 再发生,重现,反复出现

recyclable
[ri:'saikləbl]

a. 能再循环的,可回收的

recycle
['ri:'saikl]

vt. 使再循环,反复利用

【经典例题】The environment on our planet is a closed system. Nature recycles its resources. Water, for example, evaporates and rises as visible drops to form clouds.
【译　　文】我们星球的环境是个封闭的系统。大自然循环使用它的资源。例如,水蒸发,上升成为可见的水滴而形成云。

redundant
[ri'dʌndənt]

a. 被裁减的,多余的;不需要的

reel
[ri:l]

n. 卷筒,线轴　*v.* 卷,绕

【名师导学】reel 常与 off 搭配,意思是"(很快)背出所记忆的信息"。
【经典例题】When she heard the bad news, the streets reeled before her eyes.
【译　　文】她听到坏消息时,感到街道在她眼前打旋。

reference
['refrəns]

n. 提及,涉及;参考,查阅;参考文献,参考书目;介绍人/信,证明人/信

【固定搭配】in / with reference to 关于;have / bear some / no reference to 与……有关/无关
【经典例题】During the time we have done business you have been a very reliable customer, and if your suppliers approach us for a reference, we shall be very happy to support your request for credit facilities.
【译　　文】在我们双方进行交易期间,贵公司一直是可靠的买主,如贵公司的供货商同我们联系了解你公司的资信情况,我们将乐于支持贵公司对赊购做法的要求。

refine
[ri'fain]

vt. 精炼,精制,提纯;改善,改进

【经典例题】Technological advances over the past few decades mean that such investigations now can be refined.
【译　　文】过去数十年的技术发展意味着如今这样的调查可以得到改进。

reflect
[ri'flekt]

vt. 反射;反映,表现　*vi.* 反射,映出;思考,仔细考虑

【固定搭配】reflect on / upon 仔细考虑

reflection
[ri'flekʃən]

n. 映像,倒影,反射;沉思,熟虑

【经典例题】Many novels that attempt to mirror the world are really reflections of the reality that they represent.
【译　　文】许多意图呈现现实世界的小说都做到了对事实的如实反映。

reform
[ri'fɔ:m]

vt. 革,改良;改造;重新组成　*n.* 改革,改良;改过,自新

【固定搭配】advocate a reform 倡导改革;carry out a reform 执行改革;initiate a reform 着手改革

refrain
[ri'frein]

vi. 抑制,克制　*n.* (诗歌的)叠句,副歌

【名师导学】熟记固定搭配 refrain from doing sth.
【经典例题】He could not refrain from tears at the sight of it.
【译　　文】他一见那情景就不禁潸然泪下。

refresh [riˈfreʃ]

vt. 提神，振作，（使）清新

【名师导学】辨析 refresh, renew, restore：refresh 指提供某种必要的条件以恢复活力、生机、雄心或权力；renew 表示使已旧或已丧失力气、活力等物变新；restore 指某人借助他人的力量使某物回到原来的状态或使某物失而复得。

【经典例题】Get your car in top condition and refresh your driving experience.

【译　　文】让爱车处于最佳状态，会让您获得更加顺畅的驾驶感受。

refuge [ˈrefjuːdʒ]

n. 避难（处），藏身（处）

【固定搭配】take refuge in 躲避在……；靠……逃避

【名师导学】辨析 refuge, shelter：refuge 指躲避危险或灾难的地方；shelter 指暂时的保护，以避免暴露在自然环境中。

refugee [ˌrefju(ː)ˈdʒiː]

n. 难民，逃亡者

refund [riˈfʌnd]

v. 归还，偿还　*n.* 归还（额），偿还（额）

【名师导学】作为名词时常与动词 obtain, make, demand 等词连用；与其他词搭配如：full refund 全部退还；tax refund 退税。

【经典例题】If the shoes don't wear well, the shop will refund your money.

【译　　文】如果鞋子不合适，商店会给你退钱。

refute [riˈfjuːt]

v. 驳斥，驳倒

【经典例题】Their claims to damages have not been convincingly refuted.

【译　　文】他们要求赔偿的主张还没有被令人信服地驳倒。

regime [reiˈʒiːm]

n. 政府，政权；政治制度

【经典例题】People hoped that things would change for the better under the new regime.

【译　　文】人们希望在新政权下，一切都会变得更好。

regiment [ˈredʒimənt]

n. （军队）团；*vt.* 把……编组成团，把……组织化；统一制定，把……规格化

【固定搭配】review a regiment 检阅兵团；serve with regiment 服役于兵团

【经典例题】As Jack hated army life, he decided to desert his regiment.

【译　　文】因为杰克厌恶军队生活，所以他决心背弃自己所在的那个团。

region [ˈriːdʒən]

n. 地区，区域；范围

【固定搭配】in the region of 在……左右，接近

【经典例题】The bacteria which make the food go bad prefer to live in the watery regions of the mixture.

【译　　文】能使食物变坏的细菌更喜欢在混合物的水样区域生存。

register [ˈredʒistə]

vt./n. 登记，注册，挂号　*n.* 登记，注册；登记簿，注册簿　*vi.* 登记，注册

【经典例题】A company which issues corporate bonds shall keep a corporate bonds register.

【译　　文】发行公司债券的公司应当保存公司债券存根簿。

regulate [ˈregjuleit]

vt. 管理，控制；调整，调节，校准

【经典例题】The speed of the machine may be automatically regulated to pace the packing operation by an inner microcomputer.

【译　　文】机器的速度可通过内部的微型电脑自动调节得同包装速度一致。

regulation
[ˌreɡjuˈleiʃən]

n. 管理，控制；规章，规则

【固定搭配】adopt new regulations 采取新规定；break / violate a regulation 违反规定；obey / observe regulations 遵守规定

rehearsal
[riˈhəːsəl]

n. 预演，排练

【经典例题】They think of putting your play in rehearsal at once.

【译　　文】他们想立刻对你们的戏进行排练。

rehearse
[riˈhəːs]

v. 排练，练习，演习，背诵

reinforce
[ˌriːinˈfɔːs]

vt. 增援，加强

【经典例题】The same factors push wages and prices up together, the one reinforcing the other.

【译　　文】相同的因素促使工资和物价同时上涨，彼此促进。

rein
[rein]

n. 缰绳　v. 严格控制，加强管理；用缰绳勒马

【固定搭配】hold / take over the reins 掌握、支配……的权利

reject
[riˈdʒekt]

vt. 拒绝，谢绝，驳回；舍弃，排斥，退掉

【经典例题】The university rejects a forth of all applicants.

【译　　文】这所大学拒绝了1/4的申请者。

rejoice
[riˈdʒɔis]

vi. 欣喜，高兴，庆祝，欢乐　vt. 使欣喜，使高兴

【名师导学】rejoice 一般与介词 at / over 搭配，意思是"对……感到欣喜"。

【经典例题】The whole family are rejoicing at their unexpected good fortune.

【译　　文】全家人都在为意外的好运气而感到高兴。

relate
[riˈleit]

vi. 联系，关联　vt. 叙述，讲述

【固定搭配】be related to 与……有关系

related
[riˈleitid]

a. 叙述的，讲述的；有关系的

relationship
[riˈleiʃənʃip]

n. 关系，联系

relay
[ˈriːlei]

vt. 中继，转播；接力

【名师导学】relay 当表示"转发，播放"等意思时，其过去式和过去分词均为 relayed；当表示"重新放置"的意思时，过去式和过去分词均为 relaid。

【经典例题】The World Cup football game will be relayed and broadcasted live through satellite tonight.

【译　　文】今晚世界杯足球赛将通过卫星进行实况转播。

release
[riˈliːs]

vt. 释放，放出；发布，发行；放开，松开

【经典例题】As a defense against air-pollution damage, many plants and animals＿＿a substance to absorb harmful chemicals.

A. relieve　　B. release　　C. dismiss　　D. discard　　[B]

【译　　文】作为防止空气污染的屏障，许多的树木和动物都会释放一种能够吸收有害化学成分的物质。

relevant [ˈrelivənt]	*a.* (to) 相关的，切题的；适当的，中肯的 【经典例题】He failed to supply the facts relevant＿＿＿ the case in question. 　A. for　　　B. with　　　C. to　　　D. of　　　[C] 【译　文】他不能够提供与该案例相关的事实依据。
reliable [riˈlaiəbl]	*a.* 可靠的 【经典例题】The only reliable penicillin was that made by the Allies. 【译　文】唯一可靠的盘尼西林是盟军制造的。
reliance [riˈlaiəns]	*n.* 依靠，信赖；依靠的人/物 【名师导学】reliance 是动词 rely 的名词形式，常与介词 on 连用。例如：You can place full reliance on her honesty. 对她的诚实你尽可放心。 【经典例题】He has failed me so many times that I no longer place any reliance on what he promises. 【译　文】他多次让我失望，我再也不能信赖他的承诺了。
relief [riˈli:f]	*n.* 缓解，消除；救济，援救 【经典例题】I felt great relief when I heard I had passed the examination. 【译　文】听到已经通过考试的消息后，我感到轻松多了。
relieve [riˈli:v]	*vt.* 缓解，消除，减轻 【固定搭配】relieve...of 解除（痛苦、磨难、诱惑等）
religion [riˈlidʒən]	*n.* 宗教，信仰 【经典例题】Citizens enjoy the freedom to believe in religion and freedom not to believe in religion and to propagate atheism. 【译　文】公民有信仰宗教和不信仰宗教、宣传无神论的自由。
religious [riˈlidʒəs]	*a.* 宗教的，信教的，虔诚的
reluctant [riˈlʌktənt]	*a.* 不情愿的，勉强的 【名师导学】be reluctant to do sth.，不情愿做某事。这是一个含有否定含义却没有否定前缀或后缀的单词。它的近义词为 unwilling。 【经典例题】Footballers are often reluctant, for superstitious reasons, to discard their old boots. 【译　文】出于迷信的原因，足球运动员往往不愿意扔掉他们的旧靴子。
rely [riˈlai]	*vi.* 依靠，信赖，依仗 【固定搭配】rely on / upon 依靠；信赖 【经典例题】The poor used to rely on government aid. 【译　文】穷人过去都依靠政府的援助。
remarkable [riˈmɑ:kəbl]	*a.* 值得注意的；显著的，异常的，非凡的 【经典例题】A newspaper is even more remarkable for the way one reads it. 【译　文】报纸对于读者来说，阅读的方式是更值得注意的。
remedy [ˈremidi]	*n.* 药品；治疗措施，补救办法　*vt.* 纠正，补救；医疗，治疗 【固定搭配】beyond remedy 无法补救的，无可救药的；prescribe a remedy 开药方；work out a remedy 想出补救办法 【经典例题】The remedy is worse than the disease. 【译　文】治不得法，越治越糟。

第三部分 核心意义词汇（L-Z）

reminiscence [ˌremiˈnisəns]
n. 回忆，怀旧；缅怀往事；记忆力，回想力

remnant [ˈremnənt]
n. 残余部分，剩余部分，零料

remorse [riˈmɔːs]
n. 懊悔，悔恨
【经典例题】The nurse was filled with remorse of not believing her.
A. anguish B. regret C. apology D. grief [B]
【译　文】没有相信她，护士非常后悔。

remote [riˈməut]
a. 遥远的，偏僻的；疏远的，远缘的
【经典例题】The elementary schools in this area have begun teaching English, but it is difficult for those schools in remote, rural areas to hire qualified English teachers.
【译　文】该地区的小学已经开始教授英语，但对于偏僻的农村地区来说，找到有水平的教师是很困难的。

renaissance [rəˈneisəns]
n. （欧洲14~16世纪的）文艺复兴（时期）；（文学艺术等的）复兴，再生
【名师导学】请注意 renaissance 一些短语，如：Renaissance humanism（欧洲）文艺复兴时期的人文主义（运动）；Renaissance man 多才多艺的人。
【经典例题】The book ranges historically as far back as the Florence of the Renaissance.
【译　文】这部书一直回溯到文艺复兴时期佛罗伦萨的历史。

render [ˈrendə]
vt. 致使，使成为；给予，提供；翻译；提出，呈递
【经典例题】Firms decide what goods to produce or what services to render in order to satisfy that demand.
【译　文】公司生产何种产品以及提供何种服务均是为了满足需求。

renew [riˈnjuː]
v. 重新开始，继续；使更新，更换
【固定搭配】renew a contract 续约

renowned [riˈnaund]
a. 著名的，有声望的

rent [rent]
n. 租金 *vt.* 租，租赁 *vi.* 出租

repay [ri(ː)ˈpei]
v. 付还，偿还
【固定搭配】repay sb. by / with / for sth. 通过／以……方式／为……而偿还某人
【经典例题】There is no way I can repay the kindness that you and your family have shown me.
【译　文】我无法报答你和你的家人对我的一片深情厚谊。

repeat [riˈpiːt]
vt. 重复，重说，重做；背，背诵 *n.* 重复

repeatedly [riˈpiːtidli]
ad. 重复地；再三地

repel
[ri'pel]

vt. 使厌恶；击退，驱逐；排斥

【经典例题】This kind of material can repel heat and moisture.
【译　　文】这种材料能够防热防潮。

repetition
[ˌrepi'tiʃən]

n. 重复，反复；背诵

【经典例题】If the work of remedying of any defect or damage may affect the performance of the works, the engineer may require the repetition of any of the tests described in the contract.
【译　　文】如果任何缺陷或损害的修补工作可能影响到工程运行时，那么工程师就可要求重新进行合同中列明的任何检验。

replace
[ri(:)'pleis]

vt. 放回；替换，取代

【固定搭配】replace...with... 以……代替……
【名师导学】辨析 replace, substitute：replace 指取代、替换陈旧的、用坏的或遗失的东西，用法是 replace A with B（用 B 代替 A）；substitute 指用一件东西替换另一件东西，用法是 substitute B for A（用 B 代替 A）。
【经典例题】The new city, Brasilia, replaced Rio de Janeiro as the capital of Brazil in 1960.
【译　　文】巴西利亚这座新城市于 1960 年取代了里约热内卢成为巴西的首都。

replacement
[ri'pleismənt]

n. 取代，替换，交换；替代品，代用品

represent
[ˌrepri'zent]

vt. 表示，阐明，说明；描写，表现，象征；代理，代表

【固定搭配】represent...as 把……描述成
【经典例题】They elected him to represent them.
【译　　文】他们选他当代表。

representative
[ˌrepri'zentətiv]

n. 代表，代理人　*a.* 典型的，有代表性的

【固定搭配】be representative of 有代表性的，典型的

repression
[ri'preʃn]

n. 镇压，压制；克制

repressive
[ri'presiv]

a. 压抑的，压制的

reproach
[ri'prəutʃ]

n. / vt. 责备，批评

【名师导学】reproach 的同义词有：blame, scold, accuse, criticize 等。另外注意短语 reproach sb. for sth. 为某事训斥某人。
【经典例题】Don't reproach him with laziness; he has done his utmost.
【译　　文】不要责备他懒惰；他已尽了最大努力。

reproduce
[ˌri:prə'dju:s]

v. 繁殖，生殖；复制，仿造

reputation
[ˌrepju(:)'teiʃən]

n. 名声，声望

【固定搭配】have a reputation for 因……而出名；gain / acquire / establish a reputation 博得名声
【经典例题】And if a company wants to use a technology with a bad reputation, it is the firm's responsibility to educate the consumer about why it is beneficial.
【译　　文】如果一个公司想使用口碑不好的技术，那么让消费者认识到这项技术的益处便是这个公司的责任了。

第三部分 核心意义词汇（L-Z）

requirement
[ri'kwaiəmənt]

n. 需求，要求
【固定搭配】to meet / satisfy one's requirement 满足某人的要求
【名师导学】require 的各种形式出现在句中，那么句中与其相关的名词性从句谓语部分使用虚拟语气。
【经典例题】One of the requirements for a fire is that the material ＿＿＿＿ to its burning temperature.
A. is heated　　　　　　　　B. will be heated
C. be heated　　　　　　　　D. would be heated　　　　[C]
【译　　文】燃火的要求之一就是被点的材料必须加热到它的燃点。

requisite
['rekwizit]

a. 必要的，需要的　*n.* 必需品
【经典例题】I worked to develop the requisite skill for managerial skills.
A. perfect　　　　　　　　　B. exquisite
C. unique　　　　　　　　　D. necessary　　　　　　　　[D]
【译　　文】我努力提高必要的管理技能。

rescue
['reskju:]

vt. / n. 援救，营救
【固定搭配】come / go to sb.'s rescue 来 / 去救某人
【名师导学】辨析 rescue，save：rescue 指"营救，援救"，从危险、祸患中迅速有效地把人解救出来，也指抢救东西不至损坏；save 指"挽救，救出"，指援救某人或某物使其脱离危险或灾难，使其生存或保存下来。
【经典例题】Police and helicopter rescue crews were at the scene within minutes.
【译　　文】警方和直升机救援队伍于数分钟内赶抵现场。

resemblance
[ri'zembləns]

n. 相似，相像

resemble
[ri'zembl]

vt. 像，类似

resent
[ri'zent]

vt. 愤恨，憎恶，怨恨
【名师导学】熟记该词常用句型：resent doing sth. 表示愤恨做某事。并注意 resent 的名词形式是在其末尾加 ment。
【经典例题】I resent being told to wash my face when visitors are present.
【译　　文】我恨有客人来时让我洗脸。

reservation
[,rezə'veiʃən]

n. 预定，预订；保留
【固定搭配】make a reservation for 预订
【经典例题】When he tried to make a reservation , he found that the hotel that he wanted was completely filled because of a convention.
【译　　文】当他试图预订时，却发现那个饭店由于某个会议已经客满了。

reserve
[ri'zə:v]

vt. 储备；保留；预订　*n.* 储备品，储备金，储备；保留地；节制，谨慎
【固定搭配】without reserve 毫无保留地
【经典例题】We'd like to reserve a table for five for dinner this evening.
【译　　文】我想预订一个今晚的 5 人饭桌。

reshuffle
[,ri:'ʃʌfl]

v. 改组；重新洗牌　*n.* 改组

residence
['rezidəns]

n. 住宅，住处
【经典例题】That big house is the president's official residence.
【译　　文】那个大房子是总统的官邸。

reside [ri'zaid]	*vi.* 居住（in） 【固定搭配】reside in 居住；属于，在于，取决于；reside with sb. 与某人在一起居住
resident ['rezidənt]	*n.* 居民，常住者 *a.* 居住的，住校的，住院的
resign [ri'zain]	*vt.* 辞去，辞职，放弃 *vi.* 辞职
resignation [,rezig'neiʃən]	*n.* 辞职，辞职书
resist [ri'zist]	*vt.* 抵抗，反抗；忍住，抵制 【经典例题】We must raise the Party's capacity to resist corruption. 【译　文】我们必须提高党的拒腐能力。
resistance [ri'zistəns]	*n.* 抵抗，反抗；抵抗力，阻力；电阻 【固定搭配】resistance to 对……有阻力
resistant [ri'zistənt]	*a.* 抵抗的，反抗的 【固定搭配】be resistant to 对……有抵抗力的 【经典例题】The researchers are already working with food companies keen to see if their products can be made resistant to bacterial attack through alterations to the food's structure. 【译　文】研究人员已经和食品公司联合起来，希望他们的产品能通过改变食品的结构来抵抗细菌的侵袭。
resolution [,rezə'lu:ʃən]	*n.* 决心，坚决；决定，决议（案） 【固定搭配】make / come to a resolution to do 做出决议，下决心做
resolve [ri'zɔlv]	*vt.* 解决（问题等）；决定，下决心；决议；分解 *n.* 决心，决议 【固定搭配】be resolved to 决心做 【经典例题】Only friends who could discuss and resolve their differences openly are true friends. 【译　文】只有能说不同意见的朋友才是最好的朋友。
resonance ['rezənəns]	*n.* 共鸣；洪亮；共振
resort [ri'zɔ:t]	*vi.* 诉诸，凭借 resort to 诉诸，求助于 *n.* 度假胜地
resource [ri'sɔ:s]	*n.* 资源，财力；谋略；应付办法
respective [ris'pektiv]	*a.* 各自的，各个的 【联想记忆】respectable *a.* 值得尊敬的；respectful *a.* 尊敬别人的；respected *a.* 受尊敬的
respectively [ri'spektivli]	*ad.* 各自，独自，个别地，分别地 【经典例题】Retail sales volume in local urban and rural areas rose 57.8 percent and 46.8 percent,_____, over February 1995. A. individually　　　　　　B. accordingly C. correspondingly　　　　D. respectively　　　　[D] 【译　文】1995年2月，当地城市和农村的零售销售量分别增长了57.8%和46.8%。

respond [ri'spɔnd]

vi. 作答，答复；响应，起反应
【固定搭配】respond to 回答，响应；（药物）有效
【经典例题】Slowly he began to respond to the ward staff around him who hung over the side of his crib.
【译　　文】慢慢地，他开始对徘徊在摇篮周围的看护人员有了回应。

respondent [ri'spɔndənt]

n. 应答者，响应者

response [ris'pɔns]

n. 回音，回答；反应，响应
【固定搭配】in response to 回答，响应
【经典例题】The tax cuts produced a favorable response from the public.
【译　　文】税额削减受到了公众的欢迎。

responsibility [ri,spɔnsəbiliti]

n. 责任；职责
【固定搭配】do sth. on one's responsibility 自觉地尽职尽责；accept / assume / take on responsibility for... 为……负责

responsible [ri'spɔnsəbl]

a. 应负责任的，有责任的；可靠的，认真的，尽责的；责任重大的，重要的
【固定搭配】be responsible for 为……负责
【经典例题】It does not alter the fact that he was the man ＿＿＿＿ for the death of the little girl.
A．accounting　　　　　　B．guilty
C．responsible　　　　　　D．obliged　　　　　　　　[C]
【译　　文】什么都不能改变他应该对这个小女孩的死亡负责的事实。

responsive [ri'spɔnsiv]

n. （常与 to 连用）反应的；表示回答的；易反应的

restless ['restlis]

a. 不安的，坐立不安的

restore [ri'stɔ:]

vt. 归还，放回；修复，恢复

restrain [ri'strein]

v. 管制，阻止，约束（自己）

restraint [ri'streint]

n. 约束力；管理措施；控制

restrict [ri'strikt]

vt. 限制，约束
【固定搭配】restrict...to... 把……限制在……范围之内
【经典例题】A graduated license requires that a teenager first prove himself capable of driving in the presence of an adult, followed by a period of driving with night or passenger restrictions, before graduating to full driving privileges.
【译　　文】在取得完全的驾驶资格前，青少年必须先取得临时驾照，证明他能在成人的陪同下驾驶，然后要有一段时间的夜间行驶或载客行驶的经历。

retort [ri'tɔ:t]

n. / v. 反驳，反击
【固定搭配】retort against sb. 反驳某人

retrieval [ri'tri:vəl]	*n.* 取回，寻回
retrieve [ri'tri:v]	*vt.* 重新得到，取回；挽回，补救；检索 【名师导学】近义词：regain, bring back, reclaim, recover 【经典例题】The dog was intelligent and quickly learned to retrieve the game killed by the hunter. 【译　　文】那条狗很聪明，很快就学会了取回猎人杀死的猎物。
retrospect ['retrəuspekt]	*n.* 回顾 *v.* 回顾，反思（过去） 【名师导学】考生要注意相关短语：retrospect to 追溯到；retrospective exhibition 回顾展。 【经典例题】There are some things that you only become totally conscious of in retrospect. 【译　　文】有些事情的含义只有在事后回想时才能完全意识到。
resume [ri'zju:m]	*vt.* 恢复；重新开始 【经典例题】Resume his teaching post at City University. 【译　　文】恢复他在城市大学的教职。
resume [rezju:mei]	*n.* 简历
retail ['ri:teil]	*n.* 零售 *a.* 零售的 *v.* 零售 【固定搭配】sell by/at retail 零售
retain [ri'tein]	*vt.* 保持，保留 【经典例题】Several studies have reported that people can retain conscious or subconscious memories of things that happened while they were being operated on. 【译　　文】几项研究都认为，人们在动手术期间对过程中发生的事情会保留有意识或者潜意识的记忆。
retire [ri'taiə]	*vi.* 退下，离开；退休，引退；隐退
retreat [ri'tri:t]	*vi.* 撤退，退却 【经典例题】A person who has been a beacon of vision and idealism retreats into despair or cynicism. 【译　　文】一个曾是远见卓识和理想主义代表的人沦落到绝望或是尖酸刻薄之境。
retrospective [ˌretrə'spektiv]	*a.* 回顾的，回想的；溯及既往的
reunification [ˌri:ju:nifi'keiʃən]	*n.* 再统一，重新团结
reunion [ri:'ju:njən]	*n.* 团圆，重逢，聚会
reveal [ri'vi:l]	*vt.* 揭示，揭露，展现；告诉，泄露 【经典例题】I hate people who reveal the end of a film that you haven't seen before. 【译　　文】我讨厌那些在你还没看完电影之前提前说出结局的人。

revelation
[ˌreviˈleiʃən]

n. 揭示，透露，启示；被揭示的真相，新发现

【经典例题】"Spilling the beans" means confessing or making a startling revelation.

【译　　文】"洒了豆子"意思是坦白交代或者透露惊人的真相。

revenge
[riˈvendʒ]

vt. / n. 报复，复仇

【名师导学】该词常用的动词短语有：revenge for 为……报复；revenge oneself on for 因某事向某人报仇。名词短语：in revenge for 以报复……；take revenge on sb. 对某人报复。

【经典例题】Out of sheer revenge, he did his best to blacken her character and ruin her reputation.

【译　　文】纯粹出于报复，他挖空心思诋毁她的人品，败坏她的名誉。

revenue
[ˈrevinjuː]

n. 收入，税收

【固定搭配】collect revenue 收税；raise revenue 增加收入

【经典例题】Local government＿＿＿＿ could be obtained through a local income tax and / or a local sales tax.

A．budget　　　B．expense　　　C．finance　　　D．revenue　　　[D]

【译　　文】当地政府的收入可以通过当地的收入所得税和营业税获得。

reverse
[riˈvəːs]

v. 颠倒，翻转，后退　*n. / a.* 反面（的），颠倒（的），相反（的）

【经典例题】Several international events in the early 1990s seem likely to reverse, or at least weaken, the trends that emerged in the 1980s.

【译　　文】在20世纪90年代初期的少数国际事件似乎会扭转20世纪80年代出现的那个趋势，至少是减弱。

reversible
[riˈvəːsəbl]

a. 可翻转的，可逆的

【联想记忆】reverse *v.* 倒转，颠倒

【名师导学】opposite, contrary, adverse, reverse, converse 这些形容词均含"相反的，对立的"之意。

opposite：指位置、方向、行动或想法等完全相反。

contrary：一般指与某种主张、看法或行为等正好相反，隐含否定一方并不意味着肯定另一方的意味。

adverse：通常指危害利益的、无生命的势力或条件等，侧重分歧。

reverse：指朝相反方向的或反面（背面）的。

converse：指在方向、行动或意见上相反的。

revert
[riˈvəːt]

v. 回复；恢复；（财产、权力等）归还，归属（to）

revise
[riˈvaiz]

vt. 修订，修正

revive
[riˈvaiv]

v. （使）复活；（使）复兴

【经典例题】These flowers will revive in water.

【译　　文】这些花在水中会复活。

revolt
[riˈvəult]

v. / n. 反抗，起义

【固定搭配】revolt against 反叛

【名师导学】辨析 revolt, rebellion：revolt 指不再效忠，拒绝接受目前的状况和控制；rebellion 指公开的武装反抗，以要挟或推翻政府为目的。

revolutionary
[ˌrevəˈluːʃənəri]
a. 革命的，革新的 *n.* 革命者

revolve
[riˈvɔlv]
v. 旋转，转动
【固定搭配】revolve around 以……为中心；revolve round / about 围绕……而旋转，环绕
【经典例题】In the first year or so of web business, most of the action has revolved around efforts to tap the consumer market.
【译　　文】在网上交易的第一年左右，大部分业务活动都是围绕着努力开发消费者市场来进行的。

reward
[riˈwɔːd]
n. 酬谢，报酬，奖金 *vt.* 酬谢，报答，报酬
【固定搭配】in reward for 作为回报

rhythm
[ˈriðəm, ˈriθəm]
n. 节奏，韵律；有规律的循环运动

rid
[rid]
vt. 使摆脱，使去掉
【固定搭配】get rid of 摆脱，除去

ridge
[ridʒ]
n. 岭，山脉；屋脊；鼻梁
【经典例题】The waves had pushed the sand into little ridges.
【译　　文】海浪推动沙子形成了小小的沙垄。

ridiculous
[riˈdikjuləs]
a. 荒谬，可笑
【经典例题】I think it ridiculous to lend them so much money.
【译　　文】我认为借这么多钱给他们是荒唐可笑的。

rigid
[ˈridʒid]
a. 坚硬的，刚性的，严格的

rigorous
[ˈrigərəs]
a. 严格的
【经典例题】They set up a rigorous training schedule for the new comers.
【译　　文】他们为新手制订了严格的训练计划。

riot
[ˈraiət]
n. / v. 骚乱，闹事
【固定搭配】raise a riot 引起暴动

rip
[rip]
v. 撕裂，扯开
【名师导学】rip 的动词以下短语容易记混，需格外注意：rip into 猛攻，穿进，刺入；rip off 撕掉；rip out 狠狠地发出；rip up 把……撕成碎片。
【经典例题】After she read the letter, she ripped it up.
【译　　文】看完信后，她把信撕成了碎片。

ripe
[raip]
a. 熟的，成熟的，时机成熟的

risk
[risk]
n. 风险 *vt.* 冒风险
【固定搭配】at / face / take / run the risk of... 冒……风险

ritual
[ˈritjuəl]
a. 宗教仪式的，典礼的 *n.* 仪式，典礼；例行公事，习惯
【经典例题】She went through her usual ritual of making sure all the doors were locked before she went to bed.
【译　　文】她上床之前按惯例检查一下是不是所有的门都锁上了。

rival ['raivəl]

vt. 竞争，与……抗衡 *a.* 竞争的 *n.* 竞争对手

【经典例题】Although the two players are _____ in the tennis court, they are really good friends.
A. partners B. enemies
C. rivals D. companions [C]

【译　文】虽然这两个运动员在网球比赛场上是对手，但他们实际上是很好的朋友。

【经典例题】Of all the flowers in the garden few can rival the lily.

【译　文】在花园的所有花卉中，能与百合媲美的很少。

rivalry ['raivlri]

n. 竞争，竞赛；敌对，对立

roar [rɔ:]

vi. 吼，咆哮，轰鸣

【经典例题】The roar of airplane engines announced a coming air raid.

【译　文】飞机发动机的轰鸣声预示着空袭即将到来。

rob [rɔb]

vt. 抢劫，盗取

【固定搭配】rob sb. of sth. 掠夺某人某物，使某人丧失某物

robust [rəu'bʌst]

a. 强健的，耐用的，富有活力的

romance ['rəumæns]

n. 恋情，浪漫史；传奇性，浪漫情调；爱情故事，冒险故事

【经典例题】There is an air of romance traveling in the Inner Mongolia grassland.

【译　文】在内蒙古大草原旅游，颇有浪漫气氛。

romantic [rə'mæntik]

a. 浪漫的，传奇的；不切实际的，好幻想的

rot [rɔt]

v. / n. 腐烂，腐朽

【固定搭配】rot away 烂掉，变虚弱

rotary ['rəutəri]

a. 旋转的

【经典例题】She sprained her ankle when trying to perform a rotary motion.

【译　文】当她试图完成一个旋转的动作时，扭伤了脚踝。

rotate [rəu'teit]

v. (使) 旋转

【名师导学】辨析 rotate, revolve, swirl, twirl: rotate 指围绕某物体自己的轴心的旋转运动，即自转运动；revolve 指围绕某一中心所做的圆周运动，即公转运动；swirl 指水、空气等使某物旋转而动，打着漩涡；twirl 常指用手操作某物而产生的一系列复杂的旋转运动。

【经典例题】You can rotate the wheel with your hand.

【译　文】你可以用手转动轮子。

rouse [rauz]

vt. 激起，使振奋；唤起，唤醒

route [ru:t]

n. 路线，航线

【经典例题】If you know exactly what you want, the best route to a job is to get specialized training.

【译　文】如果你确切知道你想要的，那么找工作最好的方法就是接受专业的训练。

routine
[ruːˈtiːn]

a. 常规的，例行的 *n.* 常规，例行公事
【固定搭配】break the routine 打破常规；follow the routine 墨守成规
【经典例题】Children and old people do not like having their daily _____ upset.
A. habit B. routine C. practice D. custom [B]
【译　　文】孩子和老人都不喜欢他们的日常生活被打乱。

rub
[rʌb]

v. 摩擦，擦 *n.* 摩，擦；障碍
【固定搭配】rub out 擦掉，拭去

rude
[ruːd]

a. 粗鲁，不礼貌；粗糙，粗陋 *n.* 小地毯
【经典例题】I was always taught that it was _____ to interrupt.
A. rude B. coarse C. rough D. crude [A]
【译　　文】我经常被教导说，打断别人是不礼貌的。

rumo(u)r
[ˈruːmə]

n. 谣言，谣传，传闻
【固定搭配】circulate / spread a rumor 散布谣言

rupture
[ˈrʌptʃə]

n. （体内组织等的）破裂，断裂，绝交
v. （体内组织等的）破裂，断裂，绝交

rural
[ˈruər(ə)l]

a. 农村的
【经典例题】He pointed out that the living standard of urban and _____ people continued to improve.
A. remote B. municipal C. rural D. provincial [C]
【译　　文】他指出，城市和农村地区的人们的生活水平还在继续提高。

sabotage
[ˈsæbətɑːʒ]

n. 阴谋破坏，破坏活动 *vt.* 对……采取破坏行动，妨害，破坏
【固定搭配】safeguard sb. / sth. from / against sth. 保护……以免……
【经典例题】The police investigating the traffic accident have not ruled out _____.
A. salvage B. safeguard
C. sabotage D. sacrifice [C]
【译　　文】对交通事故进行调查的警察没有排除恶意行为的可能性。

sacred
[ˈseikrid]

a. 神圣的，宗教的；严肃的，郑重的
【名师导学】近义词：pure, pious, saintly, divine, holy; consecrated, ordained, sanctioned
【固定搭配】be sacred from 免除，不受
【经典例题】It is the sacred duty of every citizen to safeguard their motherland.
【译　　文】保卫祖国是每个公民神圣的义务。

sacrifice
[ˈsækrifais]

n. 牺牲，牺牲品；祭品，供品 *v.* 牺牲，献祭
【固定搭配】at the sacrifice of 牺牲；sacrifice one's life for sth. / to do sth. 为……牺牲生命

第三部分 核心意义词汇（L-Z）

safeguard ['seif,gɑ:d]
v. 保护，保障，捍卫 *n.* 安全设施，保护措施

salary ['sæləri]
n. 薪金，薪水
【固定搭配】boost / increase / raise salaries 加薪

salute [sə'lu:t, -'lju:t]
vt. / vi. 招呼，敬礼 *n.* 招呼，敬礼
【经典例题】He took off his hat to salute her.
【译　　文】他向她脱帽致敬。

salvation [sæl'veiʃən]
n. 拯救，救助
【固定搭配】attain salvation 得到救赎；work out one's own salvation 自寻出路
【经典例题】In some religious groups, wealth was a symbol of salvation and high morals, and fatness a sign of wealth and well-being.
【译　　文】在一些宗教团体中，财富是济世善和崇高道德的象征，而肥胖则是财富与幸福的标志。

sanction ['sæŋkʃən]
n. 认可，许可，批准；支持，赞成；制裁，处罚

sarcasm ['sɑ:kæzəm]
n. 讥讽；嘲笑；挖苦

satisfactory [,sætis'fæktəri]
a. 令人满意的
【名师导学】辨析 satisfactory, satisfying, satisfied：satisfactory 意为"令人满意的，符合要求的"，因为可以满足某种愿望或合乎某种要求而令人满意，常指事物本身所特有的特性，含有主动意味，该词在句子中常做定语和表语；satisfying 表示事物"令人满意的"，具有较强的主动性，通常做定语；satisfied 表示"感到满意的"，指人达到某种希望时感到满足和愉快，含有被动意味。
【经典例题】The plan is almost satisfactory in every way.
【译　　文】这个计划从各方面来看几近完美。

saturate ['sætʃəreit]
vt. 使湿透，浸透；使充满，使饱和
【名师导学】与 saturate 连用的介词是 with。
【经典例题】During the heavy fog, the air was saturated with moisture.
【译　　文】大雾期间，空气中充满水气。

savage ['sævidʒ]
a. 残暴的，凶猛的，粗鲁的；未开化的，野蛮的 *n.* 野蛮人，粗鲁的人 *vt.*（狗等）乱咬；猛烈抨击
【经典例题】Darwin had a phrase to describe those ignorant of evolution: they "look at an organic being as a savage looks at a ship, as at something wholly beyond his comprehension."
【译　　文】达尔文有一句话描述那些对进化一无所知的人，他们"看有机的生命如同野人看船那样，在看超出他们理解能力的东西"。

scale [skeil]
n. 规模，标度，刻度（*pl.*）天平，天平盘；标尺，比例尺；音阶
【固定搭配】on a large scale 大规模地
【经典例题】It may be possible for large-scale change to occur without leaders with magnetic personalities, but the pace of change would be slow.
【译　　文】缺乏独特个人魅力的领导者也有可能推动大规模的变化，但变化的进度可能会慢一些。

295

scan [skæn]

n. / v. 浏览；扫描

【名师导学】辨析 scan，skim，skip：scan 特指搜寻特定信息，目的性较强，可引申为"审视，仔细打量"；skim 指为了寻找文章主题，获得总体印象，往往含有"粗略地看一看"之意；skip 意为"略读，跳过"，指跳过不重要的或无关的部分。

【经典例题】He scanned *Time* magazine while waiting at the doctor's office.

【译　　文】在医生的诊所候诊的时候，他翻阅了《时代》杂志。

scandal ['skændl]

n. 丑闻

【经典例题】There was a great scandal when we found out that the doctor had been sent to prison for stealing.

【译　　文】我们发现这位医生因偷盗而被送进监狱，真是个大丑闻。

scar [skɑ:r]

n. 伤疤，（精神上的）创伤；煞风景之处

v. 在……上结疤，给……留下精神创伤；损害……的外观

scatter ['skætə]

vi. 撒，驱散，散开；散布，散播　*vt.* 分散，消散

【名师导学】辨析 scatter, disperse, spread：scatter 指由于外力使人或物杂乱地向不同的方向散开或散播；disperse 指有目的地、安全地解散或彻底散开，范围较前者广；spread 指在表层分散，也可指疾病、谣言的传播。

【经典例题】I hate to scold, but you mustn't scatter your things all over the place.

【译　　文】我不想训斥你，但你不该总把东西到处乱丢。

scent [sent]

n. 气味，香气；香水

【固定搭配】be scented with 充满香气

【经典例题】The Japanese scientists have found that scents enhance efficiency and reduce stress among office workers.

【译　　文】日本科学家们发现香味能够提高工作人员的办公效率并减少紧张感。

scheme [ski:m]

n. 计划，方案；阴谋，诡计　*v.* 计划，图谋

scope [skəup]

n. 范围，视野；余地，机会

【固定搭配】scope for sth. / to do sth.（做……的）机会；within / outside the scope of 在……范围之内 / 外

【经典例题】In my opinion, you can widen the ＿＿＿ of these improvement through your active participation.

A. dimension　B. volume　C. magnitude　D. scope　[D]

【译　　文】我认为，你能够通过积极参与来延伸进步的范围。

scorn [skɔ:n]

n. 轻蔑，鄙视　*vt.* 轻蔑，鄙视；拒绝，不屑（做）

【名师导学】将 scorn 和其同义词一起记：scoff, despise, contempt, disdain 等。

【经典例题】She realizes that his eyes hold neither pity, nor scorn.

【译　　文】她意识到他的目光里既无怜悯，也无轻蔑。

scramble ['skræmbl]

vi. / n. 攀登，爬行；争夺，抢夺　*vt.* 扰乱，搞乱

【固定搭配】scramble for 争夺，勉强拼凑

【经典例题】The players were scrambling for the possession of the ball.

【译　　文】选手们为了控制球，在争抢着。

scrap [skræp]
n. 小片，碎片 *vt.* 废弃
【名师导学】scrap 做动词时其过去式和过去分词为 scrapped。
【经典例题】Water birds, for example, can choke on plastic bottle rains and get cut by scrap metal.
【译　　文】例如，水鸟可能窒息死在铺天盖地的"塑料瓶雨"中或者被废弃金属片割伤。

scrape [skreip]
v. / n. 擦，刮

scratch [skrætʃ]
v. 搔，抓，扒；勾销，删除 *n.* 搔，抓，抓痕
【固定搭配】scratch a living 勉强维持生活
【经典例题】The scratch on your hand will soon be well.
【译　　文】你手上的划伤不久就会好。

screen [skri:n]
vt. 掩蔽，庇护；选拔，淘汰 *n.* 屏风；屏幕

script [skript]
n. 手稿，打字原稿；笔迹

scrub [skrʌb]
vt. 用力擦洗 *vi.* 用力擦洗，把……擦净；取消（计划等） *n.* 矮树丛，灌木丛
【经典例题】Scrub your back with this long-handled brush.
【译　　文】用这把长柄刷擦洗你的后背。

scrutiny ['skru:təni]
n. 细看，仔细检查；仔细研究

sculpture ['skʌlptʃə]
n. 雕刻，雕塑
【经典例题】He is sculpturing a running horse out of the tree root.
【译　　文】他正在把树根雕刻成一匹奔驰的马。

seal [si:l]
n. 封口，封蜡，封条；印戳；海豹 *vt.* 封，密封

seam [si:m]
n. 缝，接缝
【经典例题】Big seams appeared on the dried-up riverbed.
【译　　文】干涸的河床上现出大的裂缝。

secondary ['sekəndəri]
a. 第二的，中级的；次要的，次等的

section ['sekʃən]
n. 章节；部分；地区；截面，剖视图
【经典例题】One section of the class was reading and the other section was writing.
【译　　文】班上的一部分人在看书，另一部分人在写东西。

sector ['sektə]
n. 扇形，部门

secure [si'kjuə]
a. 安心的；可靠的 *vt.* 得到，获得；防护，保卫
【固定搭配】secure sth. from / against 保护（免于……的危险）
【经典例题】Your SMTP mail server could not start a secure connection.
【译　　文】SMTP 邮件服务器无法启动安全链接。

security [siˈkjuəriti]	n. 安全（pl.）治安防卫；证券，债券
segment [ˈsegmənt]	n. 片，部分，断片，段
segregate [ˈsegrigeit]	v. 隔离并区别对待（不同种族、宗教或性别的人）；（使）隔离
segregation [ˌsegriˈgeiʃən]	n. 种族隔离；隔离
select [siˈlekt]	vt. 选择，挑选 a. 精选的，选择的 【经典例题】I was selected for the team. 【译　文】我被选入这个队。
selection [siˈlekʃən]	n. 选择，挑选；被挑选出来的人，精选品 【固定搭配】make one's own selection 自己选择
selfish [ˈselfiʃ]	a. 自私的，利己的
semester [siˈmestə]	n. 学期
seminar [ˌsemiˈnɑː]	n. （专家）研讨会；（大学）研究班 【经典例题】China will, in cooperation with the US and Singapore, hold an ARF seminar on non-proliferation in 2006. 【译　文】中国将与美国、新加坡于2006年共同承办东盟地区论坛防扩散研讨会。
sensation [senˈseiʃən]	n. 感觉，知觉；激动，轰动一时的东西 【经典例题】It appealed to both refined and popular tastes and caused a great social sensation in the 1960s. 【译　文】它取得了雅俗共赏的艺术效果，并在20世纪60年代引起强烈的社会反响。
sensational [senˈseiʃənəl]	a. 轰动性的；耸人听闻的；极好的
sensible [ˈsensəbl]	a. 明理的，明智的 【经典例题】Surely, it would be sensible to get a second opinion before taking any further action. 【译　文】当然，在进一步采取行动之前改变看法是明智的。
sensitive [ˈsensitiv]	a. 敏感的；灵敏的
sensual [ˈsenʃuəl]	a. 肉体（上）的；感官的；肉欲的
sentiment [ˈsentimənt]	n. 伤感；感情，情绪 【经典例题】There is strong sentiment on the question of unemployment. 【译　文】公众对于失业问题的情感反应非常强烈。

sequence
['si:kwəns]

n. 连续，继续；序列，数列；先后，次序，顺序

【固定搭配】in sequence 依次，逐一

【名师导学】辨析 sequence，series，succession：sequence 指先后衔接次序，字母顺序，强调事情发生的先后逻辑顺序；series 指一连串相同的东西彼此间有共同的关系，有独立的个性，但又构成一个整体；succession 指时间上或次序上相连续的事物，强调一个接一个没有间断。

【经典例题】What each person does is to put together, out of the pages of that day's paper, his own selection and sequence, his own newspaper.

【译　　文】每个人所做的是将其从报纸中拿出来，再组合到一起。用他自己的选择和顺序，做成他自己的报纸。

【联想记忆】sequent *adj.* 接连而来的

serial
['siəriəl]

n. 连续剧，连载故事　*a.* 连续的，顺序排列的

【名师导学】注意区别 serial 和 series。series 连续，系列，丛书，级数。

【经典例题】His masterpiece at first appeared as a serial novel on the newspaper.

【译　　文】他的杰作最初以连载小说的形式出现在报纸上。

series
['siəri:z]

n. 一系列，一连串；序列；丛书

【固定搭配】a series of 一系列，一连串

session
['seʃən]

n. 会期；一届会议；（某种活动）一场，一段时间

setback
['setbæk]

n. 退步；挫折，挫败

【名师导学】与 setback 搭配使用的主要动词有 have，meet with receive 以及 suffer 等。

【经典例题】Since that time there has never been any setback in production.

【译　　文】从那时候起，生产就一直没有任何阻碍。

setting
['setiŋ]

n. 安装，放置；周围，环境

settlement
['setlmənt]

n. 调停，解决；居留地，住宅区；清偿，结算

【固定搭配】come to / make / reach a settlement 达成和解

severe
[si'viə]

a. 严厉，严格；严重，凛冽；严峻，艰难

【名师导学】辨析 severe，strict，stern：severe 指法律、惩罚、言行等方面严格；strict 指对规则不仅自己严格遵守，而且对别人也毫不放松；stern 指利用权力使人服从，毫不讲情面，不为哀求和眼泪所动。

【经典例题】Severe punishment will be imposed on various tourist- concerning irregularities such as illegal operation in travel services.

【译　　文】严厉查处非法经营旅游业务、销售假冒伪劣旅游商品。

shabby
['ʃæbi]

a. 破烂的；衣衫褴褛的；卑鄙的，不公正的

【经典例题】She is nonetheless beautiful for her shabby clothing.

【译　　文】即使她衣衫褴褛，却仍然美丽。

shaft
[ʃɑ:ft]

n. 柄，杆；（光的）束，光线；轴；竖井

【经典例题】The Washington Monument is a hollow shaft without a break in its surface except for the tiny entrance.

【译　　文】华盛顿纪念塔是一个空心的柱子，除了一个小入口之外，表面没有一处裂痕。

☐ **shallow** ['ʃæləu]	*a.* 浅的；浅薄的，肤浅的 *n.* (*pl.*) 浅滩，浅处
☐ **shatter** ['ʃætə]	*vt.* 使粉碎，砸碎；使破灭，使震惊 *vi.* 碎裂 【名师导学】近义词：break, fracture, shiver, smash; bankrupt, break down, cross up, demolish, destroy, finish, ruin, sink, smash, spoil 【经典例题】The shells became so thin that they shattered before the babies hatched. 【译　文】蛋壳太薄了，在幼鸟孵出之前它们就破碎了。
☐ **shed** [ʃed]	*vt.* 脱落，脱去；流出，流下；发出，散发
☐ **sheer** [ʃiə]	*a.* 纯粹的，绝对的，全然的 【经典例题】Out of ____ revenge, he did his worst to blacken her character and ruin her reputation. A. perfect　　B. total　　　C. sheer　　　D. integral　　[C] 【译　文】除了纯粹的报复，他还尽可能地诽谤她的人格并损毁她的名誉。
☐ **shelter** ['ʃeltə]	*n.* 隐蔽处，掩蔽部 *v./n.* 掩蔽，庇护 【固定搭配】under the shelter of 在……掩蔽下；find / take shelter from 躲避……
☐ **shield** [ʃi:ld]	*n.* 盾，屏障 *vt.* 防护，保护
☐ **shift** [ʃift]	*v./n.* 转移，移动，转变 【固定搭配】be on the night / day shift 上夜班 / 白班；shift sth. from...to... 把……从……转移到 【经典例题】Shift the economic growth mode from an extensive one to an intensive one. 【译　文】把走外延增长的经济模式转变到走内含增长的模式。
☐ **shipment** ['ʃipmənt]	*n.* 装货，运输；装载的货物，装货量 【经典例题】Our firm specializes in the shipment of goods abroad. 【译　文】我们公司专注于出国货物装运。
☐ **shiver** ['ʃivə]	*vi./n.* 颤抖，哆嗦 【经典例题】He shivered as he heard the strange noise in the night. 【译　文】当他在夜晚听见这奇怪的声音时，吓得直发抖。
☐ **shortcoming** ['ʃɔ:t,kʌmiŋ]	*n.* 短处，缺点
☐ **shortly** ['ʃɔ:tli]	*ad.* 立刻，马上
☐ **shove** [ʃʌv]	*vt.* 乱推，挤；乱塞，随意放 *vi.* 用力推，挤 *n.* 猛推 【固定搭配】shove around 推来推去；shove in 推进；shove off 开船，离开；shove sth. under the carpet 掩盖某事 【经典例题】Help me shove this furniture aside. 【译　文】帮我把这件家具推到一边去。
☐ **shrewd** [ʃru:d]	*a.* 精明的；有眼光的，判断得准的

第三部分 核心意义词汇（L-Z）

shrink [ʃriŋk]
vi. 起皱，收缩；退缩，畏缩
【经典例题】In our highly technological society, the number of jobs for unskilled workers is shrinking.
【译　　文】在我们高度科技化的社会里，非技术工作的岗位将会紧缩。

sightseeing [ˈsaitsiːiŋ]
n. 观光，游览
【固定搭配】go sightseeing 观光

signify [ˈsignifai]
vt. 表示……的意思，意味，预示
【名师导学】注意习惯用语：signify one's consent with a nod 点头同意。
【经典例题】A fever usually signifies that there is something wrong with the body.
【译　　文】发烧通常说明身体有病。

silicon [ˈsilikən]
n. 硅
【名师导学】在科技类的阅读文章中常出现的术语有：silicon chip 硅片；silicon cell 硅电池。

simulate [ˈsimjuleit]
vt. 模仿，模拟；假装，冒充
【经典例题】We used to use this trick in the army to simulate illness.
【译　　文】我们在军队服役时常用这一伎俩装病。

simultaneous [simlˈteinjəs]
a. 同步的，同时发生（或进行）的

simultaneously [siməlˈteiniəsli]
ad. 同时发生地，同时做出地，同时地
【联想记忆】simu (same)+l+tane(time)+ous（形容词后缀）+ly（副词后缀）= 同时地
【经典例题】Reading a book and listening to music simultaneously seems to be on problem for them. (2005)
A. intermittently　　　B. constantly
C. concurrently　　　D. continuously
【译　　文】对于他们来说，边看书边听音乐是个难题。
【名师导学】近义词群：all together 同时，at the same time 同时，coincident 同时发生的，concurrently 同时地，in chorus 一齐，instantaneously 即刻地，meantime 与此同时，synchronous 同时的。

sincere [sinˈsiə]
a. 真诚的；诚挚的
【经典例题】We have just learned of your success, sincere congratulations and best wishes for the future.
【译　　文】我们刚刚获悉你成功的消息，谨向你表示衷心的祝贺，并祝愿你日后更加飞黄腾达。

situated [ˈsitjueitid]
a. 位于，坐落于
【固定搭配】be situated at / in / on 位于
【经典例题】The housing development must be situated near public transportation.
【译　　文】住房开发必须位于靠近公共交通的地方。

skeleton [ˈskelitən]
n. 骨骼，骨架
【名师导学】熟记 skeleton in the cupboard / closet（一个被隐藏了多年的秘密或令人不快的事情）。
【经典例题】I have written the skeleton of my report, but I have to fill in the details.
【译　　文】我已经写了报告的框架，但我还必须填补细节。

skeptical
['skeptikəl]

a. 表示怀疑的

【名师导学】和它的近义词一起记忆：doubtable, suspicious。

【经典例题】Ignorant people were skeptical of Columbus' theory that the earth is round.

【译　　文】那时，无知的人对于哥伦布的地球是圆形的理论表示怀疑。

sketch
[sketʃ]

n. 素描，速写；略图，梗概，大意 *vt.* 速写，写生；概述，简述

【固定搭配】sketch out 画出轮廓；概述

【经典例题】A＿＿＿ of the long report by the budget committee was submitted to the mayor for approval.

A. shorthand　　B. scheme　　C. schedule　　D. sketch　　[D]

【译　　文】预算委员会做的长篇报告的概要已经呈递给市长等待批复。

skil(l)ful
['skilful]

a. 灵巧的，娴熟的

【固定搭配】be skillful in / at 擅长做

【名师导学】辨析 skilled, skillful：skilled 意为"熟练的，需要技能的"，既可修饰人，也可修饰物；skillful 意为"熟练的"，用以修饰人。

skilled
[skild]

a. 有技能的，熟练的；需要技能的

【固定搭配】be skilled in / at 擅长做

skim
[skim]

vt. 略读，快读；撇，撇去

【固定搭配】skim over 掠过；skim through 翻阅

skip
[skip]

v. 轻快地跳，蹦蹦跳跳；跳过，错过；不参加

【名师导学】注意短语 skip over 有两个意义相差很大的意思：skip over 略过，遗漏；短期旅行。

【经典例题】She likes to skip rope as a warm-up.

【译　　文】她喜欢以跳绳来热身。

skull
[skʌl]

n. 头骨，颅骨

【固定搭配】get it into your thick skull 理解，明白；skull protector 安全帽

【经典例题】Archeologists recently discovered a complete skull of anthropoid (ape).

【译　　文】考古学家最近发现了一个完整的类人猿头盖骨。

slack
[slæk]

a. 淡季的，不景气的；萧条 *n.* (*pl.*) 便装裤，运动裤

【经典例题】There's a certain amount of slack in the car industry at the moment.

【译　　文】眼下汽车工业不太景气。

slap
[slæp]

vt. / n. 拍，掌击

【固定搭配】slap sb. in the face 打某人耳光

slash
[slæʃ]

v. 猛砍，挥斩，切开，打过去；贬斥，严厉批评；（雨）猛烈拍打 *n.* 猛砍，砍击；（衣服的）开叉

【固定搭配】slash at 猛击；slash with 用……砍削

【经典例题】The consumer welcomes a slash in meat price.

【译　　文】消费者欢迎肉食品价格的削减。

slaughter
['slɔːtə]

n. 屠杀，杀戮；屠宰

【名师导学】表示杀的词还有：butcher 屠宰，屠杀；massacre 残杀，集体屠杀；carnage（尤指在战场上的）残杀，大屠杀，流血；assassinate 暗杀，行刺。

【经典例题】I could not stand to watch them slaughter the cattle.

【译　　文】看到他们在屠杀那头牛，我受不了。

slender ['slendə]

a. 细长的，苗条；微小的，微薄的
【联想记忆】slenderly *ad.* 细长地，苗条；slenderness *n.* 苗条
【名师导学】辨析 slender, slim, thin, lean：slender 多用于女性，强调高而细，匀称而优美；slim 指瘦而健康之意；thin 可指一般的瘦，也可指不健康的瘦；lean 指自然而健康的瘦。
【经典例题】You have a beautifully slender figure.
【译　　文】你的体形十分苗条。

slide [slaid]

vi. / n. 滑，滑动　*n.* 幻灯片
【固定搭配】slide into 陷入
【名师导学】辨析 slide, slip, glide：slide 指物体在与其他物体的接触面上滑行或滑落；slip 指由于失误而不自主地滑动；glide 指在空中或水中无声地、较长时间地滑动、滑翔。
【经典例题】The drawers slide in and out easily.
【译　　文】这些抽屉很容易推进和拉出。

slight [slait]

a. 轻微的，细微的；纤细的，瘦弱的
【固定搭配】not in the slightest 一点也不，毫不

slim [slim]

a. 苗条的；微小的，不充实的

slip [slip]

vi. 滑，滑倒；溜走；犯错误　*n.* 疏忽，笔误，口误
【固定搭配】make a slip of tongue 失言
【经典例题】Along the long way of changing, you may occasionally slip and fall. You have to learn to face failures, for the road to success is full of ups and downs.
【译　　文】在不断变化的路途中，你偶尔可能会滑倒，会跌倒，你必须学会面对失败，因为成功的路上充满了起起落落。

slogan ['sləugən]

n. 口号，标语
【名师导学】注意短语：under a slogan of... 在……口号下

slope [sləup]

n. 坡，斜坡；倾斜；斜度
【经典例题】He ran up the slope to the top of the hill.
【译　　文】他爬上斜坡，到了山顶。
【固定搭配】slope off （为了逃避或躲避工作）偷偷溜走

slump [slʌmp]

v. 突然倒下，跌落；（物价、景气、名气等）暴跌，萧条，骤然低落　*n.* 暴跌，萧条；消沉，萎靡
【名师导学】在做名词时常与形容词 bad, worst, severe, great 等搭配使用。
【经典例题】When some markets slump, there are always other markets remaining buoyant.
【译　　文】当某些市场疲软时，总还有另一些市场坚挺。

smash [smæʃ]

vt. / n. 打碎，粉碎
【固定搭配】smash up 撞毁，毁坏
【经典例题】We are determined to smash terrorism.
【译　　文】我们一定要消灭恐怖主义。
【经典例题】A window in the kitchen was ____; there was rubbish everywhere, and the curtains and carpets had been stolen.
A. scattered　　B. scraped　　C. scratched　　D. smashed　　[D]
【译　　文】厨房的窗户被打碎了。到处都是垃圾，窗帘和地毯也都被偷了。

smog [smɔg]	*n.* 烟雾
smuggle [ˈsmʌgl]	*v. / n.* 走私 【名师导学】本词属于常考词汇，考生要注意相关短语：smuggle in 偷运进来；smuggle out 私运出去；smuggle through 走私运出。 【经典例题】As many as 200,000 cars are smuggled out of the country every year. 【译　文】每年有多达 20 万辆汽车被走私出国。
snap [snæp]	*v.* 突然折断；拍快照；猛咬，厉声说 【固定搭配】snap out of 使迅速从……中恢复过来；snap up 抢购；争相拿取 【经典例题】The rope snapped and the boy fell off. 【译　文】绳子突然断了，男孩子摔了下来。
snatch [snætʃ]	*vt. / n.* 攫取，抢夺 【固定搭配】snack bar 快餐柜，小吃店　snack food 点心，小吃　go snacks 平分，均摊 【经典例题】There isn't time for a proper meal so we'll get a snack at the coffee stall. 【译　文】因为没时间吃顿像样的饭，所以我们将在一家咖啡厅弄点小吃。
sneak [sniːk]	*v.* 偷偷地走；偷拿；偷偷地做　*n.* 打小报告者　*a.* 突然的，出其不意的
sneaker [ˈsniːkə(r)]	*n.* 鬼鬼祟祟的人，卑鄙者；运动鞋
sniff [snif]	*v.*（嗅嗅地）以鼻吸气，用力吸入；嗅，闻　*n.* 吸气（声）；嗅，闻 【固定搭配】sniff at 嗅，闻；不喜欢，（傲慢地）拒绝；sniff out 发现，寻找 【经典例题】The dog sniffed suspiciously at the stranger. 【译　文】狗怀疑地嗅那位陌生人。
sob [sɔb]	*v. / n.* 哭泣，呜咽 【经典例题】She shut herself in her bedroom and sobbed her heart out. 【译　文】她把自己关在卧室里，哭得死去活来。
sober [ˈsəubə]	*a.* 未醉的；冷静的；素净的　*v.*（使）变得冷静
so-called	*a.* 所谓的，号称的
social [ˈsəuʃəl]	*a.* 社会的；社交的，交际的 【经典例题】Social studies is the study of how man lives in societies. 【译　文】社科课程研究的是人们怎样在社会中生活。
socialize [ˈsəuʃəlaiz]	*vt.* 使社会（主义）化
sociologist [ˌsəusiˈɔlədʒist]	*n.* 社会学者，社会学家
sociology [ˌsəusiˈɔlədʒi]	*n.* 社会学

☐ **software** ['sɔftwɛə]	*n.* 软件，计算方法
☐ **solar** ['səulə]	*a.* 太阳的，日光的 【固定搭配】solar system 太阳系
☐ **sole** [səul]	*a.* 单独的，唯一的
☐ **solemn** ['sɔləm]	*a.* 冷峻的；庄严的，隆重的
☐ **solicitor** [sə'lisitə]	*n.* 法务官；事务律师 【名师导学】注意区别使用同义词：attorney＜美＞律师；barrister（在英国有资格出席高等法庭并辩护的）律师，法律顾问；lawyer 律师；counsellor 顾问，律师。
☐ **solidarity** [ˌsɔli'dæriti]	*n.* 团结 【经典例题】National and international solidarity is indispensable if victory is to be achieved. 【译　文】如果要获得胜利，国内与国际的团结一致是必不可少的。
☐ **solitary** ['sɔlətri]	*a.* 独自的，喜欢独处的，孤单的 *n.* 隐士，独居者 【经典例题】Someone who isในัง＿＿＿confinement is kept alone in a room in prison. A. precise　　B. solitary　　C. remote　　D. confidential　　[B] 【译　文】单独监禁的意思是被单独关在监狱的单间里。
☐ **solo** ['səuləu]	*n.* 独唱，独奏 *a.* 独自的，单独的 *ad.* 独自 【经典例题】She was left solo to await the returning hunters. 【译　文】她独自留下等候归来的猎人。
☐ **soluble** ['sɔljubl]	*a.* 可溶的；可以解决的 【名师导学】soluble 的反义词是 insoluble。 【经典例题】Common salt is soluble in water. 【译　文】普通的盐在水里是可溶的。
☐ **solution** [sə'lu:ʃən]	*n.* 解答，解决办法；溶解，溶液。 【固定搭配】arrive at / come to / reach a solution of / for / to a problem 找到解决……问题的办法 【经典例题】The solution to the problem was apparent to all. 【译　文】问题的解决方法是显而易见的。
☐ **solve** [sɔlv]	*vt.* 解答，解决 【固定搭配】solve a problem / puzzle / riddle 解决问题 / 解谜 / 解答谜语
☐ **sophisticated** [sə'fistikeitid]	*a.* 先进的，复杂的；精密的；老于世故的 【经典例题】The British in particular are becoming more sophisticated and creative. 【译　文】特别是英国人正在变得更加的成熟和有创造力。 【经典例题】The courses aim to give graduated an up-to-date grasp of their subject and＿＿＿laboratory skills. A. superficial　　　　B. subjective C. structural　　　　D. sophisticated　　[D] 【译　文】这门课程的目标是使毕业生能够掌握当前最新的专业技能和最尖端的试验技能。

sorrow ['sɔrəu]	n. 悲哀，悲伤 【固定搭配】to one's sorrow 令人遗憾（伤心）的是；feel sorrow 感到悲伤 【经典例题】My father still carried the sorrow and pain of my mother's death twenty years ago. 【译　　文】我父亲对于20年前我母亲的去世仍感到十分悲痛。
sour ['sauə]	a. 酸的，酸腐的；脾气坏的，刻薄的
source [sɔ:s]	n. 源，源泉；来源，根源
sovereign ['sɔvrin]	n. 君主，元首　a. 有主权的；完全独立的；掌握全部权利的
spacious ['speiʃəs]	a. 宽广的，宽敞的
span [spæn]	n. 跨距，跨度；一段时间 【固定搭配】for a long / short span of time 长（短）时间内；the span of life 寿命
sparkle ['spɑ:kl]	v. 发火花，闪耀 【名师导学】近义词：glitter, glisten, twinkle, shine 【经典例题】Her jewellery sparkled in the candlelight. 【译　　文】烛光下，她的首饰光彩熠熠。
specialist ['speʃəlist]	n. 专家 【固定搭配】a specialist in / on……方面的专家
specialization [,speʃəlai'zeiʃn]	n. 特殊化，专门化
specialize ['speʃəlaiz]	vi. 专攻，专门研究 【固定搭配】specialize in 专攻
specially ['speʃəli]	ad. 特别地，特地；格外地
specialty ['speʃəlti]	n. 特性，性质；专门研究，专业，专长；特产，特有的产品 【经典例题】Seafood is a specialty on the island. 【译　　文】海味是该岛的特产。
species ['spi:ʃiz]	n. （物）种，种类
specific [spi'sifik]	n. 特效药；细节　a. 详细而精确的，明确的；特殊的，特效的；（生物）种的
specification [,spesifi'keiʃən]	n. (pl.) 规格，规范；明确说明；（产品等的）说明书 【名师导学】specification 多以其复数形式出现。 【经典例题】The specifications for the new classroom to be built next year are now ready. 【译　　文】明年将建的新教室的规格标准现在准备好了。

specifically [spi'sifikəli]	ad. 特定，明确
specify ['spesifai]	vt. 指定，详细说明
specimen ['spesimin, -mən]	n. 样本，标本 【固定搭配】collect specimens 采集标本
spectacle ['spektəkl]	n. (pl.) 眼镜　n. 场面，景象；奇观，壮观 【经典例题】To keep a conversation flowing smoothly, it is better for the participants not to wear dark spectacles. 【译　　文】为了保持会话流畅地进行，参与者最好不要戴深色眼镜。
spectacular [spek'tækjulə]	a. 壮观的
spectator [spek'teitə, 'spekteitə]	n. 观众，旁观者 【名师导学】注意 spectator 同 audience 区别，前者尤其指体育比赛的观众，后者则可指不同类型的观众。 【经典例题】The spectators are filled with fury before those absurd contests. 【译　　文】观众们面对这些荒谬的比赛怒火满腔。
spectrum ['spektrəm]	n. 光谱，频谱；领域，范围 【名师导学】spectrum 的复数形式是 spectra。 【经典例题】There is discrimination in a wide spectrum of fields of employment. 【译　　文】很多行业聘请雇员时都有歧视情况。
speculate ['spekju,leit]	vi. 思索，推测；投机 【固定搭配】speculate about / on / over 推测；speculate in 投机 【经典例题】We are living in the here and can only speculate about the hereafter. 【译　　文】我们生活在现在，只能预测未来。
speculative ['spekjulətiv, -leit-]	a. 推测的；投机性的；揣摩的
spelling ['speliŋ]	n. 拼法，拼写
sphere [sfiə]	n. 球，球体，范围，领域 【固定搭配】enlarge / widen one's sphere of knowledge 扩大知识范围 【联想记忆】globe n. 球体，地球，地球仪；bulb n. 灯泡；ball n. 球状物；cylinder n. 圆柱体；sphere n. 球体；triangle n. 三角形；square n. 正方形；diamond n. 菱形；circle n. 圆形；column n. 圆柱形；cube n. 立方体；disc n. 圆盘
spill [spil]	v. (使) 溢出来 【经典例题】One is not supposed to cry over spilled milk. 【译　　文】对着已经洒了的牛奶哭是无济于事的。
spin [spin]	v. / n. 旋转，自转　vi. 纺，纺纱；结网，吐丝

spinal
['spainl]
a. 脊柱的；有关脊柱的

spiral
['spaiərəl]
a. 螺旋的 *n.* 螺旋（线），螺旋式的上升（或下降）*vi.* 盘旋上升（或下降）；（物价等）不断急剧地上升（或下降）
【经典例题】A spiral staircase takes less space than a regular one.
【译　　文】螺旋形的楼梯比起普通楼梯占较少的空间。

spiritual
['spiritjuəl]
a. 精神（上）的，心灵的

spit
[spit]
vi. 吐；唾，吐痰 *n.* 唾液
【固定搭配】spit in one's face 侮辱某人
【经典例题】Please do not spit; do not litter.
【译　　文】请不要随地吐痰，乱扔杂物。

spite
[spait]
n. 恶意，怨恨
【固定搭配】in spite of 尽管，不顾

splash
[splæʃ]
v. 溅，泼 *n.* 溅泼声；溅出的水；（光色等的）斑点
【固定搭配】splash down 溅落，（宇宙飞船等）着陆；splash into 溅入，滴入；make a splash 引起关注
【经典例题】The children were splashing water on each other in the swimming pool.
【译　　文】孩子们正在游泳池中相互泼水嬉戏。

split
[split]
v. 劈开，裂开 *a.* 分裂的 *n.* 裂缝，裂口；分化，分裂
【固定搭配】split up（使）分裂，（使）关系破裂
【联想记忆】divide into 把……分成；separate...from 把 ... 分开；burst into 爆发出；break into 破门而入；split *v.* 劈开；divide *v.* 分开；cut *v.* 切开；chop *v.* 砍开
【经典例题】My daughter is heartbroken because she has just split up with her boyfriend, but she'll soon get over it.
【译　　文】我女儿的心碎了，因为她刚同男朋友分手，不过她会很快摆脱出来的。

spoil
[spɔil]
vt. 搞糟，损坏；宠坏，溺爱 *vi.* 食物变坏
【经典例题】Children who are over-protected by their parents may become＿＿＿＿.
A. hurt　　B. damaged　　C. spoiled　　D. harmed　　[C]
【译　　文】始终在父母羽翼之下的孩子会被宠坏的。

sponsor
['spɔnsə]
n. 发起人，主办者；资助者 *vt.* 发起，主办
【经典例题】He sponsored all sorts of questions.
【译　　文】他提出了各种问题。

spontaneous
[spɔn'teinjəs, -niəs]
n. 自发的，自然产生的
【经典例题】Hearing the joke, we burst into spontaneous laughter.
【译　　文】听到笑话，我们不由自主地大笑起来。

spot
[spɔt]
n. 地点，场所；点，斑点，污点
【固定搭配】on the spot 当场，在现场
【经典例题】There is no proof that he was on the crime spot.
【译　　文】没有证据证明他当时在犯罪现场。

spotlight ['spɔtlait]
n. 照明灯，车头灯
【经典例题】Throughout his political career he has always been in the_____.
A. twilight　B. spotlight　C. streetlight　D. torchlight　[B]
【译　文】在整个政治生涯中，他总是成为焦点。

spouse [spauz]
n. 配偶
【经典例题】Mr. Smith is Mrs. Smith's spouse, and she is his spouse.
【译　文】史密斯先生是史密斯太太的配偶，而她也是他的配偶。

spray [sprei]
vt. 喷，喷射，喷雾 *n.* 浪花，水沫；喷雾
【经典例题】The seed was sprayed over the ground in huge qualities by aeroplane.
【译　文】飞机把这些草籽大量地喷洒在地面上。

sprinkle ['spriŋkl]
v. 撒，洒；把……撒（或洒）在……上 *n.* 少量，少数

spur [spə:]
n. 刺激，刺激物
【固定搭配】on the spur of the moment 一时冲动之下，当即，当场
【经典例题】A business tax cut is needed to spur industrial investment.
【译　文】需要用减少商业税的办法刺激工业投资。

squad [skwɔd]
n. 班，分队；部队，小队
【经典例题】The men were divided into squads to perform different tasks.
【译　文】人们被分成小组去执行不同的任务。

squeeze [skwi:z]
vt. 压榨，挤

stabilize ['steibilaiz]
vt. 使安定，使稳固

stab [stæb]
v. 刺，戳
【固定搭配】stab in the back 出卖，攻击（朋友）
【经典例题】The killer stabbed his victim with a carving knife.
【译　文】杀人犯用一把雕刻刀捅了受害者。

stable ['steibl]
a. 安定的，稳定的
【经典例题】People guess that the price of oil should remain stable for the rest of the year.
【译　文】人们估计在今年剩下的日子里油价会保持稳定。

staff [stɑ:f]
n. 工作人员，全体职员；参谋，参谋部 *vt.* 配备工作人员

stagger ['stægə]
vi. 摇晃，蹒跚 *vt.* 使吃惊；使错开，使交错
【经典例题】The school was so crowded they had to stagger the classes.
【译　文】这所学校的学生人数太多，他们只得错开时间上课。

stain [stein]
n. 污染，污点 *vt.* 沾染，污染
【经典例题】Please be careful when you are drinking coffee in case you_____the new carpet.
A. crash　B. pollute　C. spot　D. stain　[D]
【译　文】当你喝咖啡的时候要小心别把新的地毯弄脏了。

☐ **stainless** [steinlis]
a. 纯洁的，无瑕疵的；不生锈的

☐ **stake** [steik]
n. 桩，标桩；赌注
【固定搭配】at stake 在危险中，利害攸关
【联想记忆】be in danger 在危险中；be in trouble, be in difficulty 在困境中
【经典例题】The stake had been sharpened to a vicious-looking point.
【译　　文】木桩削得尖得吓人。

☐ **stale** [steil]
a. 陈腐的，不新鲜的
【经典例题】There are pieces of stale bread on the ground which she threw away.
【译　　文】地上到处都是她扔的坏面包。

☐ **stall** [stɔ:l]
n. 货摊；畜舍
【经典例题】At the public market different things are sold in different stalls under one big roof.
【译　　文】在公共市场，不同的物品由同一大屋顶下的不同货摊出售。

☐ **standby** [stændbai]
n. 备用设备，备用品
【固定搭配】on standby 待命，随时准备

☐ **standoff** ['stændɔf, -ɔ:f]
n. 僵持

☐ **standpoint** ['stændpɔint]
n. 立场，观点
【固定搭配】maintain / alter one's standpoint 坚持 / 改变立场

☐ **staple** ['steipl]
n. 钉书钉，U形钉；主食；主要产品 *vt.* 用钉书钉钉
【经典例题】The weather is the staple subject of conversation in England.
【译　　文】在英国，天气是人们会话的主要话题。

☐ **startle** [stɑ:tl]
v. 使惊吓，使吓一跳，使大吃一惊
【经典例题】When he finally emerged from the cave after thirty days, John was startlingly pale.
A. amazingly　B. astonishingly　C. uniquely　　D. dramatically　　　[A]
【译　　文】30天后，当他最终从山洞里出现的时候，约翰非常震惊。

☐ **starve** [stɑ:v]
vt. 使饿死 *vi.* 饿得要死
【固定搭配】starve for 渴望，急需

☐ **statement** ['steitmənt]
n. 陈述，声明
【固定搭配】confirm a statement 证实某一说法

☐ **static** ['stætik]
a. 静力的，静态的

☐ **stationery** ['steiʃ(ə)nəri]
n. (总称) 文具

☐ **statistic** [stə'tistik]
n. 统计数值

☐ **statue** ['stætju:]
n. 塑像，雕像
【联想记忆】portrait *n.* 肖像；photo *n.* 照片；picture *n.* 画片，图片；illustration *n.* 插图；sketch *n.* 素描；portrait *n.* 肖像；perspective *n.* 透明画法，透视图；figure *n.* 画像，肖像，塑像；image *n.* 肖像，影像；landscape *n.* 风景（画）；(oil) painting *n.* 油画，绘画；drawing *n.* 图画

status ['steitəs]

n. 地位，身份；情形，状况

【经典例题】China believes that nuclear-weapon states should respect the status of nuclear-weapon-free zones and assume corresponding obligations.

【译　　文】中国认为，核武器国家应尊重无核武器区的地位并承担相应的义务。

steady ['stedi]

a. 稳定的，不变的；稳固的，平稳的；坚定的，扎实的 *v.* (使)稳定

steep [sti:p]

a. 险峻的，陡峭的 *vt.* 浸，泡

steer [stiə]

vt. 驾驶，掌舵

【经典例题】He managed to steer the discussion away from the subject of money.

【译　　文】他设法把讨论内容从钱的话题上岔开了。

stem [stem]

n. 茎，干 *vt.* 堵住，挡住 *vi.* 起源于，由……造成

【固定搭配】stem from 起源于

【联想记忆】leaf *n.* 叶；root *n.* 根；branch *n.* 枝；shoot *n.* 苗 spring from, come from, originate from, derive from, result from 起源于，由……造成

stereo ['steəriəu]

a. 立体声的

【经典例题】It seems that the progress of man includes a rising volume of noise. In every home a stereo or television will fill the rooms with sound.

【译　　文】似乎人类的进步总是伴随着噪声音量的扩大。在每个家庭，立体音响或电视都能用声音把每间屋子填满。

stereotype ['steəriəutaip]

n. 陈规，老套，固定模式（或形象） *vt.* 对……形成固定看法

【经典例题】It is a stereotype, but nobody lines up to protest this.

【译　　文】这确实是刻板印象，但没有人会排队去抗议它。

sterilize [sterilaiz]

vt. 使不育，杀菌，使贫瘠

【经典例题】All instruments that come into contact with the patient must be ＿＿＿＿ before being used by others.

A. sterilized　　　　　　B. labeled
C. quarantined　　　　　D. retained　　　　　　　　[A]

【译　　文】所有与此病人接触的器械在别人使用前必须消毒。

stern [stə:n]

a. 严厉，苛刻

【名师导学】近义词：demanding, exacting, hard, harsh, rigid, severe, strict, tough, unyielding

【固定搭配】be stern to 对……严厉；be strict with sb. 对某人严格要求；be hard on sb. 对某人过分严厉

【经典例题】We have a very stern headmaster.

【译　　文】我们有位非常严厉的校长。

stiff [stif]

a. 硬，僵直；生硬，死板

stimulate
['stimjuleit]

vt. 刺激，激励，使兴奋

【固定搭配】stimulate sb. into / to sth. 鼓励某人做

【经典例题】An important property of a scientific theory is its ability to _____ further research and further thinking about a particular topic.
A. stimulate　　B. renovate　　C. arouse　　D. advocate　　[A]

【译　　文】一个科学理论的最重要的特性在于它能够推进某个特定主题的进一步研究和思考。

stimulus
['stimjuləs]

n. 刺激物

【名师导学】stimulus 后通常与介词 to 搭配。

【经典例题】During the first two months of a baby's life, the stimulus that produces a smile is a pair of eyes.

【译　　文】婴儿出生的头两个月，刺激他微笑的是别人的眼睛。

sting
[stiŋ]

n. 叮，刺痛，刺激

stipulate
['stipjuleit]

v. 规定，保证

【经典例题】These rules could stipulate that professors must return substantive feedback on drafts within 15 days.

【译　　文】这些规定要求教授们必须在 15 天内对初稿做出实质性反馈。

stir
[stə:]

vt. 动，移动；搅拌，搅动；激动，轰动 *vi.* 微动，活动 *n.* 微动，动静；搅动；轰动

【固定搭配】stir up 惹起，煽动

stitch
[stitʃ]

n. 针脚，（编织的）一针，针法 *v.* 缝补，缝合；做成

storage
['stɔridʒ]

n. 贮藏，保管；存储器

straightforward
[streit'fɔ:wəd]

a. 正直的，坦率的；简明的，易懂的

【经典例题】It's quite straightforward to get here.

【译　　文】来这儿相当容易。

strain
[strein]

n. 紧张，过劳；张力 *vt.* 拉紧，伸张；拉伤，扭伤

【固定搭配】ease / relieve the strain 缓和紧张；impose / lay / place / put (a) strain on 使紧张

【联想记忆】twist *n.* 扭伤；strain *n.* 拉伤；hurt *n.*（肉体、感情上的）创伤；injure *vt.*（因偶然事故、名誉）受伤，伤害；wound *n.* 负（刀枪）伤；harm *n.* 损伤，伤害

strand
[strænd]

vt. 使（船等）触礁，搁浅；使处于困境；扔下，抛开（某人）

【经典例题】I was stranded in the strange town without money or friends.

【译　　文】我被困在那个陌生的镇上，举目无友，身无分文。

strap
[stræp]

n. 皮带；皮条 *vt.* 用带缚住，用带捆扎

strategy
['strætidʒi]

n. 战略；策略

【固定搭配】adopt / apply / pursue a strategy 采取策略

【经典例题】Meanwhile, we will also carry out the open strategy of Going Global and encourage qualified companies with competence to make overseas investment.

【译　　文】同时，我们还要实施"走出去"开放战略，鼓励有条件有实力的企业到境外投资办厂。

straw
[strɔ:]

n. 稻草，麦秆；吸管

【固定搭配】catch / clutch / grasp at a straw 捞救命稻草，依靠完全靠不住的东西

stray
[strei]

vi. 走失，迷路；分心；离题　*a.* 迷路的，走失的；孤立的，零星的　*n.* 走失的家畜

【名师导学】此词经常与 ramble, roam, wander 放在一起辨析。stray 强调偏离正确路线；ramble 指漫游、逍遥自在地漫步，用于比喻时表说话离题；roam 着重于相当大的区域里自由移动；wander 指漫无目的地徘徊。

【经典例题】When on safari in Africa I used to sleep with my rifle close to hand because lions would sometimes stray into the camp looking for food.

【译　　文】在非洲狩猎远征时，我都是把步枪放在身边睡觉，因为狮子有时会闯进帐篷寻找食物。

stream
[stri:m]

n. 河；流　*vi.* 流出

【固定搭配】in streams 川流不息

【联想记忆】stream *n.* 小河，溪流；river 河流，江河；spring *n.* 泉，源泉；fountain *n.* 喷泉；rapid *n.* 急流；waterfall *n.* 瀑布；overflow *v.* 溢出；spill *v.* 溢出；discharge *v.* 流出；shed *v.* 流出（眼泪，光、热）；stream *v.* 涌出；drip *v.* 滴下，滴出；flow *v.* 流动；pour *v.* 注，倾泻；run *v.* 流淌

streamline
['stri:mlain]

vt. 使成流线型；使简化，使有效率；使现代化

【名师导学】该词在翻译句子里使用很广，应该多加注意，并记住相关的单词如：efficiency *n.* 效率，效能，功能；simplify *v.* 简化，使简明。

【经典例题】We must streamline our production procedures.

【译　　文】我们必须精简生产程序以提高效率。

strenuous
['strenjuəs]

a. 奋发的，费力的，狂热的

stretch
[stretʃ]

v. / n. 拉长，延伸　*n.* 连续的一段时间；一大片

【固定搭配】at full stretch 倾注全力；stretch oneself 伸懒腰

【名师导学】辨析 stretch, extend, prolong, expand：stretch 意为"拉伸"，extend 意为"长度的延展"，prolong 意为"时间的延长"，expand 意为"范围的扩大"。

【经典例题】Having finished morning work, the clerks stood up behind the desks, ____ themselves.

A. stretching　　B. extending　　C. prolonging　　D. expanding　　[A]

【译　　文】忙完了早上的工作，店员们站在桌子后，伸展他们的身体。

stride
[straid]

vi. 大踏步走　*n.* 大步，步法，步态，进步，进展

string [striŋ]
n. 一串，一行，一列；弦，线，绳
【固定搭配】a string of 一串

strip [strip]
n. 窄条，长带 *vt.* 剥，剥去……衣服
【固定搭配】strip of 剥取，夺取
【联想记忆】deprive sb. of 剥夺某人的；rob sb. of sth. 抢夺某人某物

strive [straiv]
vi. 努力，奋斗，力求
【名师导学】本词的重点是"strive for / after sth."的意义与用法。
【经典例题】Newspaper editors all strive to be first with a story.
【译　　文】报纸编辑都力争率先报道。

stroke [strəuk]
n. 击，敲；报时的钟声；（网球等）一击，（划船等）一划，（绘画等）一笔，一次努力；打击 *vt.* 抚摸
【固定搭配】at a stroke 一举，一下子

stroll [strəul]
vi. / n. 散步，闲逛
【名师导学】与本词同义的重要词语还有：range, wander, amble, ramble。
【经典例题】He strolls in and out as he pleases.
【译　　文】他随意地出来进去，到处闲逛。

structure ['strʌktʃə]
n. 结构，构造；建筑物

stuff [stʌf]
n. 物品，物质；个人所有物；材料，原料；东西 *vt.* 填满，塞满
【固定搭配】be stuffed with 被……填满
【联想记忆】be filled / crowded / packed with 被填满
【经典例题】Do I stuff too much laundry in the washer?
【译　　文】我是不是塞进太多的衣服到洗衣机里头了呢？

sturdy ['stə:di]
a. 强壮的，结实的；坚固的；坚定的，坚强的
【名师导学】近义词：firm, secure, solid, sound, stable, strong, substantial, sure, unshakable. See continue; athletic, muscular, robust
【经典例题】He is a sturdy child.
【译　　文】他是一个结实的孩子。

stubborn ['stʌbən]
a. 顽固的，倔强的，固执的；棘手的
【名师导学】该词属于常考词汇，应注意形容某人非常固执时，经常可以用到 stubborn 的固定搭配 stubborn as a mule 或 stubborn as a stone。同时可以注意一下它的反义词 flexible（灵活的）。
近义词：obstinate, unreasonable, unyielding, headstrong, resolute
【经典例题】She was so stubborn that she wouldn't change her opinions.
【译　　文】她特别固执，绝不会改变她的想法。

stumble ['stʌmbl]
vi. 蹒跚（而行）；结结巴巴地说
【名师导学】表示"被某物绊倒"时，该词往往与 over 搭配。
【经典例题】It is where prices and markets do not operate properly that this benign trend begins to stumble, and the genuine problem arises.
【译　　文】在那些价格和市场手段不能正常运转的地方，这种良好的趋势就失灵了，于是真正的问题就产生了。

stun [stʌn]
vt. 打昏，使昏迷；使震惊，使惊叹
【名师导学】该词常常考到"使某人感到震惊"的意思，特别是在阅读中出现的概率更高。
【经典例题】The punch stunned me for a moment.
【译　　文】那一拳把我打昏了一阵。

style [stail]
n. 风格，文体；时尚，时髦；种类，类型
【固定搭配】in style 流行的；out of style 不再流行的
【联想记忆】in fashion 合时尚，时髦；out of fashion 过时

subdivide [ˈsʌbdivaid]
v. 再分；细分

submarine [ˈsʌbməriːn]
a. 水底的，海底的 *n.* 潜水艇；海底生物
【名师导学】sub- 是在名词或形容词前的前缀，表示"在……之下""低于……""不完全的""次要部分的"。sub 单独还可以做动词"替补"的意思。

submerge [səbˈməːdʒ]
vt. 使浸水，使陷入 *vi.* 潜入水中
【经典例题】The flood submerged the town.
【译　　文】洪水淹没了整个城市。

submissive [səbˈmisiv]
a. 服从的，顺从的，柔顺的
【经典例题】Children were expected to be obedient and contribute to the well-being of the family.
A．smart　　　　　　　B．efficient
C．painstaking　　　　 D．submissive　　　　　　　　[D]
【译　　文】孩子们应该服从长辈，并为家庭的幸福做贡献。

submit [səbˈmit]
v. 屈服，服从；呈送，提交
【固定搭配】submit oneself / sth. to 服从；呈送；submit sb. to 使某人服从；submit sth. to 把……交给
【名师导学】辨析 submit, yield：submit 强调放弃抗拒，屈服于某一势力、权力或意志；yield 指在压力、武力或恳求下让步。
【经典例题】I was able to submit my paper before the bell rang.
【译　　文】在铃响之前我及时交出了答卷。

subordinate [səˈbɔːdinit]
a. 次要的，下级的；附属的，从属的 *vt.* 使服从（或从属）于
【固定搭配】subordinate to 次要的，附属的
【经典例题】Just because I'm subordinate to him, my boss thinks he can order me around without showing me any respect.
【译　　文】就因为我归他领导，我的老板就以为他可以毫不尊重地使唤我。

subscribe [səbˈskraib]
vi. 订阅，订购（书籍等）；同意，赞成 *vt.* 捐助，赞助
【固定搭配】subscribe to (sth.) 订阅，订购（杂志等）

subsequent [ˈsʌbsikwənt]
a. 随后的，后来的
【联想记忆】frequent *a.* 频繁的；consequent *a.* 作为结果的；sequent *a.* 连续的
【经典例题】Original documents must be sent by registered airmail, and duplicate by subsequent airmail.
【译　　文】单据的正本须用挂号航空邮寄，副本随后用航空邮寄。

subsidiary [səb'sidjəri]
a. 辅助的，次要的，附属的
【经典例题】GMAC is a wholly owned subsidiary of General Motors established in 1919.
【译　　文】通用汽车金融服务公司是通用集团（GM）全资子公司，于 1919 年建立。

subsidy ['sʌbsidi]
n. 津贴，补贴
【名师导学】注意与该词同义的重要词还有：allowance, sponsorship。
【经典例题】By the end of the war, in August 1945, more than 100,100 children were being cared for in day-care centers receiving Federal subsidy.
【译　　文】至 1945 年 8 月战争结束之前，超过十万儿童在联邦补贴的看护幼儿中心受到照顾。

substance ['sʌbstəns]
n. 物质；实质，本质；要旨，大意
【固定搭配】in substance 大体上是，从本质上说
【经典例题】Water consists of various chemical substances.
【译　　文】水由各种不同的化学物质构成。

substitute ['sʌbstitju:t]
n. 代用品，代替者　*vt.* 代，代替
【固定搭配】substitute...for 替代；取代，代替

subtle ['sʌtl]
a. 微妙的，细微的；敏锐的；精巧的，精密的
【经典例题】There is a subtle difference in meaning between the words "surroundings" and "environment".
【译　　文】surroundings 和 environment 这两个词的词义有细微的区别。

subtract [səb'trækt]
vt. 减，减去
【经典例题】He could add and subtract, but hadn't learned to divide.
【译　　文】他会做加减法，但还没有学会除法。

succession [sək'seʃən]
n. 连续，系列；继任，继承
【固定搭配】in succession 一连，一个接一个

successive [sək'sesiv]
a. 连续的，接连的
【联想记忆】succeeding *a.* 后来的；successful *a.* 成功的

successor [sək'sesə]
n. 继承人
【名师导学】注意以下同义词：heir（继承人），substitute（代用品，代替人）。同时还要注意此词一般与介词 "to" 搭配。
【经典例题】This car is the successor to our popular hatchback model.
【译　　文】这种汽车是我厂著名的带上掀式斜背小轿车的换代产品。

sue [sju:, su:]
vi. 控告，起诉；要求，请求　*vt.* 控告，起诉
【经典例题】If you don't complete the work, I will sue you, for money to compensate for my loss.
【译　　文】如果你不把工作做完，我就控告你，要你付损害赔偿金。

sufficient [sə'fiʃənt]
a. 足够的，充分的
【固定搭配】be sufficient for 足够 be sufficient in 在……方面充足
【联想记忆】be adequate to 足够；be rich in... 在……方面富有；be abundant in... 在……方面充足
【经典例题】Sufficient data have been collected for the building project.
【译　　文】为这项建筑工程收集的资料已经很充分了。

suffocate
['sʌfəkeit]

v. 窒息；（使）窒息而死；（把……）闷死；让人感觉闷热；憋气
【经典例题】The baby will suffocate if the blanket is over his face.
【译　　文】毯子如果盖在小宝宝脸上，他可能会窒息。

suffocation
[ˌsʌfə'keiʃən]

n. 窒息；窒息炼狱；窒息乐队；梗塞；绞杀
【经典例题】To reduce the chance of suffocation, pillows should not be placed in the cradle of the kid.
A. breathing　　B. choking　　C. sweating　　D. swallowing　　[B]
【译　　文】为了减少孩子窒息的概率，枕头不应该放在孩子的摇篮里。

suggest
[sə'dʒest]

vt. 建议，提出；使想起，暗示

suggestion
[sə'dʒestʃən]

n. 建议，提议；暗示，示意
【固定搭配】make / offer / put forward a suggestion 提出建议
【经典例题】The suggestion that the mayor＿＿＿the prizes was accepted by everyone.
A. would present　　　　　B. ought to present
C. present　　　　　　　　D. presents　　　　　　　　　　　[C]
【译　　文】由市长发奖牌的建议得到所有人的认可。

suicide
['sjuisaid]

n. 自杀
【固定搭配】commit suicide 自杀

suite
[swi:t]

n. 一套（家具）；套房；随从人员
【名师导学】注意不要跟 suit（一套外衣）一词相混。

sum
[sʌm]

n. 总数，总和；金额　v. 总结，概括；估量，估计
【固定搭配】sum up 总结，概括

summarize
['sʌməraiz]

vt. 概括，总结

summary
['sʌməri]

n. 摘要，概要
【固定搭配】in summary 概括起来
【经典例题】This historic decision was based on a summary of the experiences of 24 years after the founding of the Party.
【译　　文】这是总结建党24年经验做出的历史性决策。

summit
['sʌmit]

n. 顶，最高点；巅峰，高峰；最高级会议

summon
['sʌmən]

vt. 传唤；召集
【经典例题】They had to summon a second conference and change the previous decision.
【译　　文】他们不得不召集第二次会议，改变之前的决定。

super
['sju:pə]

a. 极好的，超级的

superb
[sju:'pə:b]

a. 极好的

superficial
[sju:pə'fiʃəl]

a. 表面的；肤浅的，浅薄的

superior [ˌsjuːˈpiəriə]
n. 长者；高手；上级 a. 较高的；上级的；上好的，出众的；高傲的
【固定搭配】be superior to 优越于，地位高于
【经典例题】This watch is ____ to all the other watches on the market.
A. superior   B. advantageous   C. super   D. beneficial   [A]
【译　　文】这个表比市场上其他的表都要优良。

superiority [sjuːpiəriˈɔrəti]
n. 优越（性），优势
【联想记忆】形容词 superior

supersonic [ˈsjuːpəsɔnik]
a. 超声的
【经典例题】A supersonic airplane is flying in the sky.
【译　　文】天空中翱翔着一架超音速飞机。

supervise [ˈsjuːpəvaiz]
v. 管理，监督，指导，监视
【名师导学】近义词：oversee, conduct, control, manage
【经典例题】If you don't supervise the children properly, Mr. Chiver, they'll just run riot.
【译　　文】奇弗先生，如果你不严格地管教孩子，他们将胡作非为。

supervisor [ˈsjuːpəvaizə]
n. 监督人，管理人，检查员，督学，主管人

supplement [ˈsʌplimənt]
n. 补充（物）；增刊，副刊，附录 vt. 增补，补充

supplementary [ˌsʌpliˈmentri]
a. 增补的，补充的

suppress [səˈpres]
vt. 镇压，压制；抑制，查禁
【经典例题】Although there are occasional outbreaks of gunfire, we can report that the rebellion has in the main been suppressed.
【译　　文】虽然这儿不时会出现一些炮火声，但是我们可以报道说叛乱已基本平息。

surge [səːdʒ]
v. / n. 汹涌，澎湃；涌现；蜂拥
【名师导学】该词原意指"大海的翻腾"，但是考试中常常考到的是它的引申意思。
【经典例题】The gates opened and the crowd surged forward.
【译　　文】大门打开了，人群向前涌去。

surgical [ˈsəːdʒikəl]
a. 外科（医术）的；外科用的，外科手术的

surpass [səːˈpɑːs]
vt. 超过，优于，多于；超过……的界限，非……所能办到（或理解）
【名师导学】与本词同义的重要词汇还有：exceed, excel, transcend。
【经典例题】Computers match people in some roles, and when fast decisions are needed in a crisis, they often surpass them.
【译　　文】计算机在某些角色中能与人相媲美，当危急关头需快速做出决定时，计算机往往比人强。

supreme [sjuːˈpriːm]
a. 最高的；极度的，重要的

surgery
['sə:dʒəri]

n. 外科，外科手术

surplus
['sə:pləs]

n. 过剩，剩余物；盈余，顺差 *a.* 多余的，过剩的

surrender
[sə'rendə]

vi. 投降；屈服，让步 *vt.* 交出，放弃
【固定搭配】surrender oneself to... 向……投降，沉迷在……之中
【经典例题】We will not surrender without a struggle.
【译　　文】我们绝不会不战而降。

surround
[sə'raund]

vt. 围绕，包围

surroundings
[sə'raundiŋz]

n. (*pl.*) 周围的事物，环境

survey
['sə:vei]

n. 俯瞰，眺望；测量，勘察；全面审查，调查
【固定搭配】conduct / do / make a survey of 对……进行调查
【经典例题】According to a survey, which was based on the response of over 188,000 students, today's traditional-age college freshmen are "more materialistic and less altruistic" than at any time in the 17 years of the poll.
【译　　文】根据一项调查，当今的大学新生比任何时候都重视物质享受，更加自私。这是根据过去 17 年对同龄人进行的民意测验，在 18.8 万份反馈的基础上得出的结论。

survival
[sə'vaivəl]

n. 幸存(者)，生存

survive
[sə'vaiv]

vi. 幸免于，幸存 *vt.* 从……逃出
【经典例题】There's little chance that mankind would survive a nuclear war.
【译　　文】人类从核战争中幸存的概率很小。

susceptible
[sə'septəbl]

a. 易受影响的，过敏的，能经受的，容许的
【经典例题】And Schallert believes that a brain injury makes neighboring cells unusually susceptible to the neurotransmitter's toxic effects.
【译　　文】夏勒特相信脑部受伤会使得临近的细胞对于神经递素的毒害异乎寻常地容易被侵害。
【名师导学】liable, susceptible, vulnerable, subject, apt, prone 这组形容词都含"易于……的，有……倾向"的意思。
　liable 普通用词，指易产生不利的后果，如，危险、风险、伤害等。可接介词 to 或不定式 to do sth.。
susceptible 较 liable 正式，多用于正式文体英语，接介词 to。
vulnerable 侧重指易受到伤害、危险或影响等，接介词 to，常用做表语或定语。
subject 与介词 to 连用也可表示"易于……的"意思，但侧重于"容易遭受"某些不幸的事情。subject 基本意思是"受支配，受制于，从属于"。
apt 常指固有的或习惯性的倾向，常接动词不定式，表示"易于……，倾向于……"，一般是人做主语，物做主语多表示自然的倾向性。
prone 常指有某种弱点、错误或不良行为的倾向，接介词 to 或动词不定式。

suspect
[səs'pekt] v.
['sʌspekt] n.

vt. 猜想，怀疑 n. 可疑分子，嫌疑犯 a. 可疑的
【固定搭配】suspect sb. of sth. 疑心某人干某事
【经典例题】We suspect that diet is related to most types of cancer but we don't have definite proof.
【译　　文】我们怀疑饮食和多种癌症有关，但是我们没有确切的证据。

suspension
[səs'penʃən]

n. 悬吊，悬浮；暂停，中止
【经典例题】She appealed against her suspension.
【译　　文】她对被停职一事提出了上诉。

suspend
[səs'pend]

vt. 悬，挂，吊；暂停，中止

suspicion
[səs'piʃən]

n. 怀疑，猜疑
【固定搭配】arouse sb.'s suspicion 引起某人的怀疑；be under suspicion 受怀疑；with suspicion 怀疑地
【经典例题】There are suspicions that he may not be able to play at all.
【译　　文】他是否参演还是值得怀疑的。

suspicious
[səs'piʃəs]

a. 可疑的，多疑的，疑心的
【固定搭配】be suspicious about / of 有疑心的，表示怀疑的
【经典例题】The police are suspicious of his words because he already has a record.
【译　　文】警察怀疑他的话，因为他有前科。

sustain
[sə'stein]

vt. 支撑，撑住；经受，忍耐
【经典例题】Seana sustained only on pain medications .
【译　　文】西娜只能靠疼痛治疗维持着。

sustainable
[sə'steinəbl]

a. 可以忍受的，足可支撑的，养得起的

swallow
['swɔləu]

v. 吞，咽；轻信；忍受，抑制，食言 n. 燕子
【经典例题】Their homes will be swallowed up by the hungry sea.
【译　　文】他们的房屋将被汹涌的大海淹没。

swamp
[swɔmp]

n. 沼泽 vt. 淹没，浸没；难倒，压倒
【经典例题】The two kids loved the story of the ugly ogre who leaves his swamp and goes out into the world in search of adventure.
【译　　文】这两个小孩很喜欢这个关于一只丑陋的怪物离开沼泽到世界各地冒险的故事。

swap
[swɔp]

v. 交换 n. 交换
【联想记忆】swap 强调的是"互换"，而 change 多指"变换，换"的意思。exchange 意为"交换，调换，兑换；交流，交易"。

sway
[swei]

n. 摇摆，影响力，支配 vt. 摇动

swear
[swɛə]

vi. 宣誓，发誓；咒骂，骂人
【固定搭配】swear at 骂（某人）；swear in（常用被动语态）使宣誓就职
【经典例题】Don't swear, for I dislike swearing.
【译　　文】别骂人，我不喜欢骂人。

□ sweat [swet]	n. 汗 v. 出汗
□ swell [swel]	vi. 膨胀，增大，隆起 【固定搭配】swell with anger 满腔怒火
□ swift [swift]	a. 快的，迅速的
□ swing [swiŋ]	vi. 摇摆，摇荡；回转，转向 n. 秋千 【固定搭配】in full swing 正在全力进行中
□ symbol ['simbəl]	n. 象征，符号，标志
□ symmetry ['simitri]	n. 对称（性）；匀称，整齐 【名师导学】注意该词形容性（symmetric）的反义词的特殊变化：asymmetric。
□ symmetrical [si'metrikl]	a. 对称的，均匀的
□ sympathetic [,simpə'θetik]	a. 同情的，共鸣的 【固定搭配】be sympathetic to... 对……表示同情 【联想记忆】sympathize with sb., show sympathy towards sb., feel / express sympathy for / with sb., have sympathy for sb. 同情
□ sympathize ['simpəθaiz]	vi. 同情，怜悯；同感，共鸣
□ sympathy ['simpəθi]	n. 同情，同情心；赞同，同感 【固定搭配】feel / have sympathy for 同情某人
□ symphony ['simfəni]	n. 交响乐，交响曲；（色彩等的）和谐，协调 【名师导学】该词通常跟 orchestra 一词同时出现，表示"交响乐团"。
□ symposium [sim'pəuziəm, -'pɔ-]	n. 讨论会，专题报告会；专题论文集
□ symptom ['simptəm]	n. 症状，征候 【固定搭配】have / show the symptoms of a cold 显出感冒的症状
□ syndrome ['sindrəum]	n. 综合征；并存特性；常见的共存情况 【名师导学】注意该词不要跟 symptom 混淆。symptom 只是指生病的症状而已。 【经典例题】Unemployment, inflation, and low wages are all parts of the same economic syndrome. 【译　　文】失业、通货膨胀以及低工资都是在同一经济状况下的现象。
□ synthesis ['sinθəsis]	n. 综合，合成
□ synthetic [sin'θetik]	a. 合成的，人工的；综合的 n. 人工制品（尤指化学合成物） 【经典例题】The store now offers 531 varieties of synthetic fabrics, all Chinese-made. 【译　　文】这个店现在出售 531 种合成纤维，全部都是中国生产的。

tablet
['tæblit]
n. 片，药片；匾额，门牌

taboo
[tə'buː]
n. 禁忌；忌讳，戒律

tackle
['tækl]
vt. 解决，处理
【经典例题】The local government leaders are making every effort to tackle the problem of poverty.
【译　　文】当地政府领导正在努力解决贫困问题。

tactful
['tæktful]
a. 机智的；老练的，圆滑的
【经典例题】The doctor tried to find a tactful way of telling her the truth.
A. delicate　　　　　　B. communicative
C. skillful　　　　　　D. considerate　　　　　　[D]
【译　　文】医生尽量用得体的方式告诉她真相。

tag
[tæg]
n. 标签，货签

talent
['tælənt]
n. 天资；才能；人才
【固定搭配】have a talent for 对……有天赋　cultivate / develop one's talent 培养自己的才能
【经典例题】They also say that the need for talented, skilled Americans means we have to expand the pool of potential employees.
【译　　文】他们也指出对有才华的、技术熟练的美国人的需求，这意味着我们要挖掘员工的潜力。

tame
[teim]
n. 驯养　*a.* 驯服的，易驾驭的
【联想记忆】train *n.* 培训，训练；cultivate *n.* 培养；discipline *n.* 训导，训练；domesticate *n.* 驯养；harness *n.* 治理
【经典例题】It took him several months to ＿＿ the wild horse.
A. tend　　B. cultivate　　C. breed　　D. tame　　[D]
【译　　文】驯服那匹野马花了他好几个月的时间。

tangle
['tæŋgl]
v. (使)纠缠，(使)乱作一团　*n.* 乱糟糟的一堆，混乱；复杂的问题（或形势），困惑
【经典例题】Her hair got all tangled up in the barbed wire fence.
【译　　文】她的头发让刺钢丝篱笆给挂住了。

target
['tɑːgit]
n. 靶子，目标
【固定搭配】hit / miss the target 射中 / 未射中靶子
【经典例题】The Government has set the target for full implementation of whole-day primary schooling for 2007-2008.
【译　　文】政府已定下目标，将于2007～2008学年全面推行全日制小学。

☐ tariff ['tærif]	*n.* 关税，关税表
☐ tax [tæks]	*vt.* 征税 *n.* 税款 【固定搭配】escape taxes 逃税；collect taxes 征税 【联想记忆】tax-free 免税；taxpayer *n.* 纳税人
☐ tease [ti:z]	*vt.* 戏弄，取笑，挑逗，撩拨 *n.*（爱）戏弄他人者
☐ technology [tek'nɔlədʒi]	*n.* 工业技术，应用科学
☐ tedious ['ti:diəs]	*a.* 沉闷的，冗长乏味的 【经典例题】In particular, different cases have to be distinguished, or these will make works tedious. 【译　文】应特别指出，不同的案例必须区分开，否则会使工作变得乏味。
☐ telecommunication [,telikə,mju:ni'keiʃn]	*n.* 通信，电信
☐ telescope ['teliskəup]	*n.* 望远镜
☐ temperament ['temprəmənt]	*n.* 气质，性格 【经典例题】Whether a person likes a routine office job or not depends largely on temperament. 　A. disposition　　　　　　B. qualification 　C. temptation　　　　　　D. endorsement　　　　[A] 【译　文】一个人是否喜欢程式化的办公室工作很大程度上取决于性格。
☐ temporal ['tempərəl]	*a.* 暂时的，短暂的；世俗的，现世的
☐ tempt [tempt]	*vt.* 引诱，勾引；吸引，引起……的兴趣 【名师导学】近义词：lure, entice, fascinate, seduce, appeal to, induce, intrigue, incite, provoke, allure, charm, captivate, stimulate, move, motivate, rouse 【经典例题】Your offer does not tempt me at all, and nothing can tempt me to leave my present position. 【译　文】你的建议一点也打动不了我的心，什么东西都不能诱使我离开现在的职位。
☐ temptation [temp'teiʃən]	*n.* 引诱，诱惑；迷人之物，诱惑物 【经典例题】It is not easy for us to resist temptation. 【译　文】对于我们来说，抵制诱惑是不太容易的。
☐ tenaciously [tə'neiʃəsli]	*ad.* 坚韧不拔地，执着地 【经典例题】She kept to her point tenaciously, and would not give way. 　A. persistently　　　　　　B. constantly 　C. perpetually　　　　　　D. vigorously　　　　　[A] 【译　文】她执着地坚持自己的观点，决不妥协。

tend
[tend]

vt. 照料，护理　*vi.* 趋向，趋于

【经典例题】Most candidates make promises during a campaign to win voters' support. But after they get elected, they tend to forget most of things they promise to achieve.

【译　　文】大多数候选人在竞选过程中都做出各种保证，以赢得选民支持，但等他们当选后，他们往往忘记去兑现大部分的诺言了。

tendency
['tendənsi]

n. 趋向，趋势

【固定搭配】have a tendency to do 有做……的倾向

【名师导学】辨析 tendency, trend：tendency 指自然因素决定的趋势、倾向；trend 指在外界压力下事物发展的趋势、大的潮流，强调外界压力，人的作用。

【经典例题】Their profits have grown rapidly in recent years, and this upward ＿＿＿＿ is expected to continue.

A. trend　　B. increase　　C. tendency　　D. movement　　[C]

【译　　文】他们的利润最近几年增长很快，而且这种上升的趋势有望继续。

tender
['tendə]

a. 嫩的，柔软的；温柔，温厚的；脆弱的，纤细的

【经典例题】My leg was very tender after the injection.

【译　　文】接受注射后我的腿发软。

tense
[tens]

a. 拉紧的，绷紧的；紧张的

【经典例题】The air is so tense here. I feel like I cannot even cough.

【译　　文】这里气氛太紧张，我觉得好像连咳嗽都不行。

tenure
['tenjə(r)]

n. 终身职位

【名师导学】记忆技巧：ten 拿住 +ure 表示结果→拿住→占有权　tenure application 终身教职申请

terminal
['tə:minl]

a. 末端的，终点的；学期的，期末的；晚期的，致死的　*n.* 末端；总站；计算机终端

【固定搭配】terminal cancer 癌症晚期；terminal heart disease 心脏病晚期

【经典例题】His mom has a terminal illness.

【译　　文】他母亲的病已进入晚期。

terminate
['tə:mineit]

v. 停止，（使）终止

termination
[,tə:mi'neiʃn]

n. 结局，结束；终止

terrace
['terəs]

n. 梯田；平台，阳台

testify
['testifai]

v. 证实，作证；证明，表明

【名师导学】近义词：affirm, give evidence, swear, attest, witness, certify, warrant, depose

【经典例题】Two witnesses will testify against her and three will testify on her behalf.

【译　　文】两位证人将作不利于她的证明，三位证人将作有利于她的证明。

testimony
['testiməni]

n. 证言，证明

【经典例题】This is nearly 16 times the number of business graduates in 1960, a testimony to the widespread assumption that the MBA is vital for young men and women who want to run business someday.

【译　　文】这几乎是1960年商科毕业生的16倍，从而证实了人们的普遍假设，即MBA对那些想在将来某一天开公司的青年男女来说非常关键。

terrific
[tə'rifik]

a. 极好的，非常的，极度的

【名师导学】该词经常用在口语里，表示"极好的。"与此意思相近的词还有：wonderful, excellent, marvelous, amazing, brilliant。

【经典例题】We had a terrific time at the party.

【译　　文】我们在聚会中度过了一段极好的时光。

terrify
['terifai]

v. 使恐怖，使惊吓

【名师导学】注意该词的形容词形式是terrified而不是terrific。同时terrified后边常常与介词of/at搭配。

territory
['teritəri]

n. 领土，地区；领域，范围

【经典例题】Wild animals will not allow other animals to enter their territory.

【译　　文】野生动物不许其他动物进入它们的领地。

terror
['terə]

n. 恐怖，恐怖的人/事

【固定搭配】quiver in terror 怕得发抖

【经典例题】A rabid dog became the terror of the neighborhood.

【译　　文】一条狂暴的狗让邻居们觉得很恐怖。

textile
['tekstail]

a. / n. 纺织品（的）

【经典例题】China's woollen textile industry is forging ahead to meet the needs of the country.

【译　　文】中国的毛纺工业正迅速发展以适应国家的需要。

texture
['tekstʃə]

n. 质地；（材料等的）结构

【名师导学】注意把该词与textile区别开。textile指的是"织物；纺织物"，而texture的意思则要加抽象一点，表示"质地，手感"等深层意义。

【经典例题】Their outward appearance seems rather appealing because they come in variety of styles, textures, and colors.

【译　　文】因为它们有多种类型、质地和颜色，所以它们的外表看上去十分诱人。

theft
[θeft]

n. 偷窃（行为）

【名师导学】注意与该词意义相近的词并注意它们之间的区别：robbery（抢劫案），burglary（盗劫案），hijacking（劫持人质案）。

【经典例题】If the current trends continue, experts predict annual vehicle thefts could exceed two million by the end of the decade.

【译　　文】照现在这个趋势发展下去，专家们预测十年后，每年的汽车失窃案会超过200万件。

theme
[θi:m]

n. 主题，话题

【名师导学】此单词经常在阅读题的题干中出现，如：what is theme (topic) of the passage? 文章的主题是什么？
【名师导学】辨析 theme, topic：theme 意为"主题"，指音乐或文学作品所表现出的思想；topic 意为"话题"，一般作为演讲或谈话的主题。
【经典例题】Stamp collecting was the theme of his talk.
【译　　文】集邮是他谈话的主题。

theory
[ˈθiəri]

n. 理论；学说；意见
【固定搭配】in theory 理论上

therapy
[ˈθerəpi]

n. 治疗，疗法
【名师导学】辨析 therapy，treatment，cure，heal：therapy "疗法"，尤指不用药物或手术的矫正疗法；treatment "医疗方法"，指用药物或手术进行的治疗；cure "治愈"；heal "治疗外伤"。

therapeutic
[ˌθerəˈpju:tik]

a. 治疗的　*n.* 治疗剂

thermal
[ˈθə:məl]

a. 热的，热量的；温泉的
【名师导学】该词属于阅读理解中，特别是科技文章里的高频词汇。
【经典例题】One of the more severe thermal food processes is referred to as commercial sterilization.
【译　　文】商业灭菌是较严格的食品热处理过程之一。

thermometer
[θəˈmɔmitə(r)]

n. 温度计

thesis
[ˈθi:sis]

n. 论题，论文
【名师导学】该词的复数形式比较特殊，为"theses"。与本词同义的重要词还有：dissertation，essay。
【经典例题】He is busy writing thesis which is the requirement to graduate and gain diploma.
【译　　文】他正忙于写论文，这是毕业和取得文凭所要求的。

thorn
[θɔ:n]

n. 刺，荆棘；带刺小灌木
【经典例题】The thorns on the roses scratched her hands.
【译　　文】玫瑰上的刺把她的手划了。

thoughtful
[ˈθɔ:tful]

a. 深思的，沉思的；体贴的，关心的

threshold
[ˈθreʃhəuld]

n. 门槛，门口；入门，开端，起始点
【名师导学】该词往往考查其引申意思"入门，开始，开端"，与其意思相近的同义词还有：sill，entrance，prelude。
【经典例题】Teaching students of threshold level is hard but the effort is very rewarding.
【译　　文】教尚未入门的学生是一件很辛苦的工作，但这种努力是值得的。

thrift
[θrift]

n. 节俭，节约

thrill [θril]
n. 令人激动的事 *v.* 使激动，使兴奋；使毛骨悚然
【名师导学】该词属于英语考试中的常考词汇，尤其是该词的形容词形式"thrilling"和"thrilled"，其用法跟"excite"的用法一样。

thrive [θraiv]
vi. 兴旺，繁荣
【联想记忆】flourish *n.* / *v.* 繁茂；prosper *v.* 繁荣；boom *n.* / *v.* 兴旺
【经典例题】She seems to thrive on hard work.
【译　　文】她看起来是靠艰苦的工作而发迹的。
【经典例题】The timber rattlesnake is now on the endangered species list, and is extinct in two eastern states in which it once＿＿＿.
A. thrived　　B. swelled　　C. prospered　　D. flourished　[A]
【译　　文】这种森林响尾蛇现在已经属于濒危物种，而且在东部曾经常见的两个州也已经灭绝了。

thrombus ['θrɔmbəs]
n. [医] 血栓
【经典例题】The thrombus forms in a blood vessel or within the heart and obstructs the circulation. (2006)
A. clot　　B. mass　　C. node　　D. knot　[A]
【译　　文】血栓形成于血管或心脏当中，堵塞血液流通。

throne [θrəun]
n. 宝座，王位，王权
【名师导学】该词在意为"王位，王权"时，一般以"the throne"的形式出现。用来表示"继位"的搭配可以用：come to / ascend / mount the throne。
【经典例题】This throne symbolized the supreme power of the feudal society.
【译　　文】这个宝座是封建皇权的象征。

thrust [θrʌst]
n. 插，戳，刺，猛推 *vt.* 插入，猛推
【经典例题】She thrust herself through the crowd.
【译　　文】她挤过了人群。

tick [tik]
n. 滴答声，钩号 *v.* 滴答响，打钩
【经典例题】While we waited the taxi's meter kept ticking away.
【译　　文】我们等候时，出租车里的计程表一直在滴答地响着。

tide [taid]
n. 潮，潮汐
【经典例题】It is the tide of the times, an inevitability of history.
【译　　文】这是时代的潮流，历史的必然。

tidy ['taidi]
vt. 整理，收拾 *a.* 整洁；整齐
【固定搭配】tidy up 使整洁
【经典例题】They went into the house and found that it is extremely tidy.
【译　　文】他们进入房子，发现房子真整洁。

tilt [tilt]
v. （使）倾斜，（使）倾倒 *n.* 倾斜，倾ράντ
【经典例题】Popular opinion has tilted in favor of the Socialists.
【译　　文】公众舆论已倒向社会党人一边。

timber ['timbə]
n. 木材，木料；森林；梁
【联想记忆】lumber *n.* 木材，木料；log *n.* 原木，圆木；board *n.* 木板
【经典例题】The main products of the district are wool, cotton and timber.
【译　　文】这个地区的主要产品是羊毛、棉花和木材。

timid
['timid]
a. 羞怯的，胆小的
【经典例题】You are as timid as a rabbit.
【译　　文】你胆小如兔。

tire
['taiə]
v. 使疲倦，疲劳；使厌倦（与 of 连用）*n.* 轮胎

tiresome
['taiəsəm]
a. 令人厌倦的，讨厌的

tissue
['tisju:]
n. 织物，薄纸；（机体）组织
【经典例题】What he said is a tissue of lies.
【译　　文】他所说的是一整套谎话。

title
['taitl]
n. 书名，题目；头衔，称号
【固定搭配】bestow / confer a title on sb. 授予某人头衔

toast
[təust]
n. 烤面包，吐司；祝酒词 *v.* 烤（面包片等）；提议为……祝酒
【经典例题】This bread toasts well.
【译　　文】这个面包烤得不错。

token
['təukən]
n.（用作某种特殊用途的，替代货币的）筹码；信物，标志，纪念品；代价券，礼券 *a.* 象征性的，装样子的
【固定搭配】by the same token 相应地，基于同一理由的　in token of something 作为某事的证据
【经典例题】Here's a little token of my appreciation for all that you have done for me over the years.
【译　　文】这是我一点小小的心意，感谢您这么多年来为我所付出的一切。

tolerate
['tɔləreit]
vt. 忍受，容忍，容许
【经典例题】Some old people don't like pop songs because they can't＿＿＿so much noise.
A．resist　　　　　　　　B．sustain
C．tolerate　　　　　　　D．undergo　　　　　　　[C]
【译　　文】一些老人不喜欢流行歌曲是因为他们受不了那么嘈杂的声音。

toll
[təul]
n. 通行费；牺牲，损失；死伤人数
【固定搭配】take a heavy toll / take its toll (of sth.) 造成重大损失
【经典例题】Cars account for half the oil consumed in the U.S. They take a similar toll of resource in other industrial nations and in the cities of the developing world.
【译　　文】汽车消耗了美国的一半石油。他们在其他工业国和发展中国家城市中差不多也消耗了同样份额的石油资源。

tone
[təun]
n. 音，音调，声调；腔调，语气；色调；气氛，调子
【固定搭配】tone in... 与……和谐；与……相配

topic
['tɔpik]

n. 题目；论题，话题
【固定搭配】bring up a topic 提出话题

torment
['tɔ:ment] n. v.

n. 苦痛，拷问 v. 使苦痛，拷问
【经典例题】Nobody can stand for long <u>agony</u> of a severe toothache.
A. sufferance　　　　　　B. suppuration
C. plague　　　　　　　　D. torment　　　　　　[D]
【译　　文】没有人能够忍受强烈的牙痛带来的煎熬。
【名师导学】agony, anguish, torment, torture, grief, misery, distress, sorrow 这些名词均有"苦恼，痛苦"之意。
agony：侧重指精神或身体痛苦的剧烈程度。
anguish：指精神方面令人难以忍受的极度痛苦；用于身体时，多指局部或暂时的痛苦。
torment：强调烦恼或痛苦的长期性。
torture：语气比 torment 强，指在精神或肉体上受到的折磨所产生的痛苦。
grief：指由某种特殊处境或原因造成的强烈的感情上的苦恼与悲痛。
misery：着重痛苦的可悲状态，多含不幸、可怜或悲哀的意味。
distress：多指因思想上的压力紧张、恐惧、忧虑等所引起的精神上的痛苦，也可指某种灾难带来的痛苦。
sorrow：语气比 grief 弱，指因不幸、损失或失望等所产生的悲伤。

torture
['tɔ:tʃə]

n. / vt. 拷问，拷打；折磨，痛苦
【固定搭配】put sb. to torture 拷问某人
【名师导学】辨析 torture，torment：torture 指身体上或肉体上所受的撕裂般的巨大痛苦；torment 在现代英语中多用来指精神上的强烈痛苦或不安，也可表示由于连续性伤害所引起的肉体上的重复性剧痛。
【经典例题】He would rather die than surrender under the enemy's cruel torture.
【译　　文】在敌人的酷刑之下，他宁死不屈。

toss
[tɔs]

vt. 向上扔，向上掷；摇摆，颠簸 n. 扔，投，抛；摇动
【固定搭配】toss oneself in bed 辗转反侧
【经典例题】I tossed the book aside and got up.
【译　　文】我把书丢在一边，站了起来。

tough
[tʌf]

a. 坚韧的，难嚼烂的；结实的，能吃苦耐劳的；艰巨的，困难的，严厉的
【固定搭配】be / get tough with sb. 对某人强硬

tow
[təu]

v. / n. 拖引，牵引
【经典例题】If you park your car here the police may tow it away.
【译　　文】你要是把汽车停在这里，警察就会把它拖走。

toxic
['tɔksik]

a. 有毒的，因中毒引起的
【名师导学】下列同义词值得关注：poisonous, venomous。
【经典例题】The chemical was found to be toxic to human health.
【译　　文】这种化学品已证实对人类健康有害。

trace [treis]

n. 痕迹，踪迹 *vt.* 跟踪，查找

【固定搭配】trace back to 追溯到

【名师导学】辨析 trace，track，trail：trace 意为"痕迹，踪迹，遗迹"，指在其他物体上留下的明显痕迹；track 意为"（人、动物、车等）踪迹，足迹"，常指由人或动物经常往返而自然踩出的路；trail 意为"（人或动物留下的）足迹"，还可表示人或动物留下的其他痕迹，如气味，尘土等。

【经典例题】Much of Chinese mythology is lost, and what is not lost is scattered and difficult to trace.

【译　　文】中国神话散失很多，仅存的文献又很分散，难以寻查。

trademark ['treidmɑ:k]

n. 商标

tradition [trə'diʃən]

n. 传统，惯例

tragedy ['trædʒidi]

n. 悲剧；惨事，灾难

trail [treil]

n. 痕迹，足迹 *vt.* 跟踪，追踪

trait [treit]

n. 特征，特点，特性

tranquil ['træŋkwil]

a. 宁静的，平静的

【经典例题】It is not easy to remain tranquil when events suddenly change your life.
A. cautious　　B. motionless　　C. calm　　D. alert　　[B]

【译　　文】当重大事件突然改变你的生活的时候，你很难保持平静。

transaction [træn'zækʃən]

n. 交易，事务，处理事务

【固定搭配】conduct transaction 进行交易

【名师导学】注意该词可以有复数形式，transactions 还可以表示"报告会，讨论会"。前缀 tran- 有"穿越，超"的意思。例如：translation（翻译），transcribe（誊抄），transparent（透明的）。

【经典例题】As they bought and sold assets, they had trouble remembering that each transaction could impact their monthly cash flow.

【译　　文】当他们买卖资产时，总是难以记住每笔交易都会对他们的每月现金流量产生影响。

transcend [træn'send]

vt. 超出，超越（经验、理性、信念等）范围

【名师导学】近义词：exceed, overreach, overrun, overstep, surpass, excess

transcribe [træn'skraib]

vt. 抄写；誊写

transfer
['trænsfə:] *v.*
['trænsfə:] *n.*

vt. 迁移，调动；换车；转让，过户 *n.* 迁移，调动；换车；转让，过户

【固定搭配】transfer sth. from...to 转移，调任，换乘

【名师导学】transfer, transmit, transport：transfer 意为"转移"，指从一处到另一处；transmit 意为"传送"，指通过媒介或设备传导、输送；

transport 意为"运输",指用火车、轮船等交通工具运送人或货物。
【经典例题】Transfer research results into commodities according to market rules.
【译　文】将研究成果按市场规律转换成商品。

transform
[træns'fɔ:m]

vt. 转换,变形;变化,变压
【联想记忆】change...into, turn...into 由……变成
【名师导学】在词汇题中以词义辨析为主,而只要能辨认前缀 trans- 后的词义,就不难辨析词义,而阅读中则以变化的形式出现。
【经典例题】The photochemical reactions transform the light into electrical impulses.
【译　文】光化学反应使光变为电脉冲。

transient
['trænziənt]

a. 短暂的,转瞬即逝的,临时的,暂住的
【联想记忆】tran"转移,移动"+si(l)ent"安静的"=transient 转瞬即逝的,短暂的,临时的
【经典例题】Certain drugs can cause transient side effects, such as sleepiness.
　A. permanent　　　　　　B. residual
　C. irreversible　　　　　　D. fleeting
【译　文】某些药会带来短暂的副作用,例如嗜睡。
【名师导学】temporary, momentary, transient 这些形容词均含"短暂的,瞬息的"之意。
temporary:普通用词,其反义是 permanent。指持续有限的可计时间,着重暂时的存在、应用或效应。
momentary:指瞬间即逝的,也表明时间很短。
transient:指停留或延续的时间很短。

transit
['trænsit]

n. 通行,运输
【经典例题】We observed the transit of Venus across the sun last night.
【译　文】我们昨晚观测到了金星凌日。

transition
[træn'ziʒən, -'siʃən]

n. 转变,变迁,过渡(时期)
【名师导学】近义词：shift, passage, flux, passing, development, transformation, turn
【经典例题】The transition from childhood to adulthood is always a critical time for everybody.
【译　文】从童年到成年的过渡对每个人来说都是一个关键的时期。

transistor
[træn'zistə]

n. 晶体管(收音机)

translate
['trænsleit]

v. 翻译,变成
【固定搭配】translate into 变成,转变

translation
[træns'leiʃən]

n. 翻译

transmit
[trænz'mit]

vt. 传送,传输,传达,传导,发射 *vi.* 发射,信号,发报
【固定搭配】transmit a match live 实况转播比赛
【经典例题】Some diseases are transmited by certain water animals.
【译　文】一些疾病是通过某种水栖动物传播的。

transparent
[træns'pɛərənt]

a. 透明的，显然的；易懂的

transplant
[træns'plɑːnt] *vt.*
['trænsplɑːnt] *n.*

vt. 移栽，移种（植物等）；移植（器官）；使迁移，使移居 *n.*（器官的）移植

【名师导学】注意该词的名词形式同样也可以做定语。

【经典例题】When any non-human organ is transplanted into a person, the body immediately recognizes it as foreign.

【译　　文】当任何非人类的器官移植到人体内，身体很快便能识别出它是异物。

transport
[træns'pɔːt] *vt.*
['trænspɔːt] *n.*

vt. / n. 运输，运送

【经典例题】Additional social stresses may also occur because of the population explosion or problems arising from mass migration movements — themselves made relatively easy nowadays by modern means of transport.

【译　　文】由于人口猛增或大量人口流动（现在交通运输工具使大量人口流动得相对容易）所引起的各种社会问题也会对社会造成新的压力。

transportation
[ˌtrænspɔːˈteɪʃən]

n. 运输，运输系统

trap
[træp]

n. 陷阱，圈套　*vt.* 诱捕，使中圈套

【固定搭配】fall into a trap 陷入圈套

【经典例题】I just want your boys to have a chance to avoid the trap.

【译　　文】我只希望你的孩子们有机会避开陷阱。

trash
[træʃ]

n. 垃圾，废物

trauma
['trɔːmə]

n. 外伤；精神创伤

traverse
['trævə(ː)s]

vt. 横渡，横越

【经典例题】The road traverses a wild and mountainous region.

【译　　文】这条公路穿过荒芜的山区。

treaty
['triːti]

n. 条约；协定

【经典例题】Under the treaty, inspection are required to see if any country is secretly developing nuclear weapons.

【译　　文】基于此条约，如果任何一个国家在秘密地发展核武器，那么就需要对其进行调查。

trend
[trend]

n. 倾向，趋势

【经典例题】The development of the trend toward multi-polarity contributes to world peace, stability and prosperity.

【译　　文】多极化趋势的发展有利于世界的和平、稳定和繁荣。

trial
['traɪəl]

n. 试验；审判

【固定搭配】on trial 受审

triangle
['traɪæŋgl]

n. 三角，三角形

【经典例题】Her earrings were in the shape of triangles.

【译　　文】她的耳环是三角形的。

tribute ['tribju:t]	*n.* 颂词，称赞；（表示敬意的）礼物，贡品
trifle ['traifl]	*n.* 少量，少许；小事，琐事；无价值的东西 *v.* 怠慢；小看 【名师导学】该词做动词用时常与 with 搭配，表示"轻视"或"随便对待某人或某事"。 【经典例题】He spends all his time on crosswords and other trifles. 【译　　文】他把所有的时间都用在做填词游戏和其他无聊的活动上。
trigger ['trigə]	*n.* 扳机 *vt.* 引起，激发起 【名师导学】与该词意思相近的词还有：provoke，stimulate。
trim [trim]	*vt. / n.* 整理，修剪，装饰 【固定搭配】trim down 削减；trim off 减掉
triumph ['traiəmf]	*n.* 胜利，成功 *vi.* 得胜，战胜 【固定搭配】triumph over 获胜 【联想记忆】win sb. over 把某人争取过来 【名师导学】辨析 triumph，conquest，victory：triumph 指辉煌的胜利、征服、大成功；conquest 指把战败的一方的人或国家置于完全的控制之中；victory 指战争、比赛、竞赛等所有各类斗争的胜利。 【经典例题】This year has seen one signal triumph for them in the election. 【译　　文】今年是他们在选举中取得重大胜利的一年。
trivial ['triviəl]	*a.* 琐碎的，不重要的
tropical ['trɔpikl]	*a.* 热带的 【经典例题】Bananas are tropical fruit. 【译　　文】香蕉是热带水果。
tuck [tʌk]	*vt.* 折起，卷起；把……塞进 【名师导学】该词意为"藏入"时常与介词 away 搭配，表示"将某物存起来或藏起来"。 【经典例题】For now, the subject of their research is little more than a stack of gleaming chips tucked away in a laboratory drawer. 【译　　文】目前，他们的研究对象仅仅是藏在实验室抽屉里的一堆发光的芯片。
tuition [tju:'iʃən]	*n.* 学费
tumble ['tʌmbl]	*vi.* 摔倒，跌倒；滚落；翻筋斗 *vt.* 使摔倒；弄乱 *n.* 翻滚；混乱 【经典例题】He slipped and tumbled down the stairs. 【译　　文】他脚一滑滚下了楼梯。
tune [tju:n]	*n.* 调子，曲调；和谐，协调 *vt.* 为……调音；调整，调节 【固定搭配】in tune with 与……和谐 / 协调；tune in (to sth.) 收看，收听 【经典例题】There's many a good tune played on an old fiddle. 【译　　文】[谚]提琴虽老，仍可奏出好的曲子。/ 老当益壮。

turbulent ['tə:bjulənt]
a. 狂暴的；混乱的，动乱的
【名师导学】近义词：stormy, tempestuous, tumultuous; rough, rugged, ugly, violent, wild
【经典例题】The lane is a safe haven for those struggling in the turbulent sea of humans to enjoy a sense of security.
【译　文】巷，是汹汹人海中的一道避风塘，给人带来安全感。

turmoil ['tə:mɔil]
n. 混乱；焦虑
【经典例题】Many of us are taught from an early age that the grown-up response to pain, weakness, or emotional＿＿＿ is to ignore it, to tough it out.
A. turmoil　　B. rebellion　　C. temptation　　D. relaxation　　[A]
【译　文】我们很多人从很小就被教导，对待痛苦、脆弱和情绪波动的成熟反应，就是无视它，忍受它。turmoil "混乱，焦虑"，rebellion "背叛"，temptation "诱惑"，relaxation "放松"。句子中 pain, weakness 和 emotional＿＿＿ 是并列结构且语义走向相似，即三者都是人类的脆弱和不利情况，因此选择 A 最合适。

turnout ['tə:naut]
n. 结果；产量；生产；出动；到会人数

turnover ['tə:n,əuvə]
n. 营业额，成交量；人员调整，人员更替率

tutor ['tju:tə]
n. 家庭教师，指导教师　*v.* 指导

twin [twin]
n. 孪生儿　*a.* 孪生的，成双的

twist [twist]
v./n. 搓，捻；拧，扭　*n.* 扭弯，扭转　*v.* 歪曲，曲解
【固定搭配】twist sb.'s arm 扭某人的胳膊；强迫做某事
【经典例题】To twist the law in order to obtain bribes.
【译　文】贪赃枉法。

ulcer ['ʌlsə]
n. 溃疡，腐烂物

ultimate ['ʌltimit]
a. 最后的，最终的　*n.* 终极，顶点
【经典例题】The union leaders declared that the ultimate aim of their struggle was to increase pay and improve working conditions for the workers.
【译　文】工会领导人宣称他们斗争的最终目的是要增加工人工资和改善工作条件。

ultraviolet [ˌʌltrəˈvaiəlit]	*a.* 紫外线的 *n.* 紫外线辐射 【名师导学】词缀 ultra 有"极端、过分或超出某一限度、范围"的意思。
unanimous [ju(ː)ˈnæniməs]	*a.* 全体一致的，一致同意的 【经典例题】Over the last 30 years, social scientists have conducted more than 1,000 studies of how we react to beautiful and not-so-beautiful people. The virtually unanimous conclusions: looks do matter, more than most of us realize. 【译　　文】在过去的三十年中，社会科学家针对我们对美丽和不是很美丽的人们所做出的反应，做了一千多次试验。几乎一致的结论是：外表确实重要，而且比我们大多数人认识到的还要重要。
unbutton [ʌnˈbʌtən]	*vt.* 解开……的纽扣；打开，松开
underestimate [ˌʌndərˈestimeit]	*vt.* 对……估计不足，低估 *n.* 估计不足，低估
undergo [ˌʌndəˈgəu]	*vt.* 经历，遭受 【固定搭配】undergo hardships / changes 经历苦难 / 变化 【名师导学】在英文中有许多以 under- 这个前缀开头的单词，多指"在……之下"。 【经典例题】Security programs should undergo actuarial review. 【译　　文】对保障方案进行精算评估。
undergraduate [ˌʌndəˈgrædʒuət]	*n.* 大学生，大学肄业生 【联想记忆】undergraduate *n.* 本科生；postgraduate *n.* 研究生；Ph. student *n.* 博士生
underground [ˈʌndəgraund]	*a.* 地下的，秘密的 *n.* 地铁 *ad.* 在地下，秘密地
underlie [ˌʌndəˈlai]	*vt.* 位于……之下，成为……的基础
underline [ˌʌndəˈlain]	*vt.* 在……之下划线；强调，着重
underlying [ˌʌndəˈlaiiŋ]	*a.* 含蓄的，潜在的
undermine [ˌʌndəˈmain]	*v.* 挖掘；侵蚀……基础；逐渐伤害（健康） 【名师导学】近义词：impair, ruin, threaten, weaken 【经典例题】Although the key to a good college is a high-quality faculty, the Carnegie study found that most college do very little to encourage good teaching. In fact, they do much to undermine it. 【译　　文】虽然好大学的关键是高质量的教师队伍，但卡内基研究发现大部分大学在鼓励好的教学方面做得很少。事实上，他们在暗中伤害教学方面却做得很多。
underneath [ˌʌndəˈniːθ]	*prep.* 在……下面 *ad.* 在下面，在底层；在里面
underscore [ˌʌndəˈskɔːr]	*vt.* 在……下划线；强调

understanding [ˌʌndəˈstændɪŋ]	*n.* 理解，理解力；谅解 *a.* 能体谅人的，宽容
undertake [ˌʌndəˈteɪk]	*vt.* 接收，承担；约定，保证；着手，从事 【联想记忆】undertaking *n.* 事业，企业；承诺，保证；殡仪业 【固定搭配】undertake to do / that 答应做；undertake an attack 发动进攻；undertake a great effort 做出巨大努力
underway [ˌʌndəˈweɪ]	*a.* 在航的；在旅途中的；正在进行使用或工作中的
undo [ʌnˈduː]	*v.* 解开，松开；取消
undoubtedly [ʌnˈdaʊtɪdli]	*ad.* 毋庸置疑地，的确
uneasy [ʌnˈiːzi]	*a.* 不安的，忧虑的 【名师导学】见 nervous。
unemployment [ˌʌnɪmˈplɔɪmənt]	*n.* 失业，失业人数 【名师导学】与该词的形容词 unemployed 意思相近的词还有：jobless，sacked 等。
unexpected [ˌʌnɪksˈpektɪd]	*a.* 想不到的，意外的
unfortunately [ʌnˈfɔːtʃənətli]	*ad.* 恐怕，不幸的是
unify [ˈjuːnɪfaɪ]	*vt.* 统一，使一致 【名师导学】后缀 -fy 构成的动词多是及物动词，为"使成为；使……划一"的意思。注意 -fy 与辅音结尾的词基之间，往往添加连接字母"i"或"e"。例如：beautify（美化），classify（把……分等级，把……分类），solidify（使坚固化）等。 【经典例题】We must unify the printing with the rest of the book. 【译　　文】我们必须使该书在印刷方面与其他方面相一致。
unilateral [ˌjuːnɪˈlætrəl]	*a.* 单方面的；单边的
union [ˈjuːnjən]	*n.* 联合，结合，组合；协会，工会，联盟
unique [juːˈniːk]	*a.* 唯一的，独一无二的 【固定搭配】be unique to... 对……独一无二的 【经典例题】Speech is the unique ability possessed only by human beings. 【译　　文】讲演是人类独有的能力。
unity [ˈjuːnɪti]	*n.* 统一，整体；一致，团结，协调
universal [ˌjuːnɪˈvɜːsəl]	*a.* 宇宙的，全世界的；普通的，一般的；通用的，万能的 【经典例题】Personal computers are of universal interest; everyone is learning how to use them. 【译　　文】大家都对个人电脑感兴趣，每个人都在学习怎样使用它们。

universe ['juːnivəːs]	*n.* 宇宙，万物
unlike [ˌʌn'laik]	*a.* 不同的，不相似的 *prep.* 不像，和……不同
unsanitary [ʌn'sænətri]	*a.* 不卫生的，有碍健康的，不健康的 【经典例题】The ＿＿＿ conditions and places are likely to cause diseases. A. unsanitary　　　　B. insidious C. insane　　　　　　D. inefficacious　　　　　　[A] 【译　文】不卫生的条件和地方容易导致疾病。
update [ˌʌp'deit] *v.* ['ʌpdeit] *n.*	*v.* 更新，使最新　*n.* 最新资料，最新版 【名师导学】该词在用于"向某人提供最新消息"的时候，常常用到搭配 update sb. (on sth.)，表示"向某人提供最新信息"。 【经典例题】I updated the committee on our progress. 【译　文】我向委员会报告了我们的进展情况。
upgrade ['ʌpgreid]	*vt.* 提升，使升级　*n.* 向上的斜坡 【名师导学】注意该词的反义词 downgrade 表示"降级"。 【经典例题】She was upgraded to the post of sales director. 【译　文】她已提升为销售部主任。
uphold [ʌp'həuld]	*vt.* 支撑，赞成，鼓励，坚持 【名师导学】近义词：confirm, sustain, back up, support 【经典例题】We have a duty to uphold the law. 【译　文】维护法律是我们的责任。
upper ['ʌpə]	*a.* 上，上部的；较高的 【经典例题】A full moon was beginning to rise and peered redly through the upper edges of fog. 【译　文】一轮满月开始升起，带着红色的光芒在雾气上方朦胧出现。
upright ['ʌprait]	*a.* 直立的，竖立的；正直的，诚实的
upset [ʌp'set]	*vt.* 弄翻，打翻；扰乱，打乱；使不安　*vi.* 颠覆
up-to-date [ˌʌptə'deit]	*a.* 时兴的，新式的，跟上时代的
urge [əːdʒ]	*v. / n.* 强烈希望，竭力主张；鼓励，促进 【固定搭配】urge sth. on 竭力推荐某事 【名师导学】在 urge that... 从句中谓语动词用原形表示虚拟。 【经典例题】The urge to survive drove them on. 【译　文】求生的欲望促使他们继续努力。
urgent ['əːdʒənt]	*a.* 紧迫的；催促的 【经典例题】Since the matter was extremely ＿＿＿, we dealt with it immediately. A. tough　　B. tense　　C. urgent　　D. instant　　[C] 【译　文】既然事情比较紧急，我们就马上处理吧。

☐ **utility** [juːˈtiliti]	*n.* 效用，实用；公用事业 【经典例题】The abstract shall state briefly the main technical points of the invention or utility model. 【译　文】摘要应当简要说明发明或者实用模型的技术要点。
☐ **utilization** [ˌjuːtilaiˈzeiʃn]	*n.* 利用，使用，应用
☐ **utilize** [ˈjuːtilaiz]	*vt.* 利用，使用
☐ **utmost** [ˈʌtməust]	*a.* 最远的 *n.* 极限
☐ **utter** [ˈʌtə]	*a.* 完全的，彻底的，绝对的 *vt.* 说，发出（声音）；说出，说明，表达 【固定搭配】utter one's thoughts / feelings 说出自己的想法/感觉 【经典例题】What he is doing is utter stupidity! 【译　文】他正在做的是完全愚蠢的事！

V

☐ **vacancy** [ˈveikənsi]	*n.* 空，空白；空缺；空闲，清闲，空虚
☐ **vacant** [ˈveikənt]	*a.* 空的；（职位）空缺的；茫然的 【经典例题】Are there any rooms vacant in this hotel? 【译　文】这家旅馆有空房吗？
☐ **vaccinate** [ˈvæksineit]	*v.*（给……）接种（疫苗）；（给……）打预防针 【固定搭配】vaccinate sb. against 给某人接种疫苗以防止
☐ **vacuum** [ˈvækjuəm]	*n.* 真空；真空吸尘器 【经典例题】Her death left a vacuum in his life. 【译　文】她的去世给他的生活留下一片真空。
☐ **vain** [vein]	*a.* 无用的；无结果的；徒劳的 【名师导学】近义词：proud, arrogant, haughty; trivial, unimportant, frivolous, petty, insignificant, idle, empty, hollow
☐ **valid** [ˈvælid]	*a.* 有根据的，正确的；有效的 【经典例题】However logical and valid the argument may be, they only skim the surface of the issue. 【译　文】不管这些争论多么有逻辑性和正确，他们只看到了问题的表面。
☐ **validate** [ˈvælideit]	*vt.* 使有效，使生效，确认，证实，验证

vanish ['vænɪʃ]

vi. 消失，消散；消逝，灭绝
【固定搭配】vanish away 消失（away，表示向相反的方向离开）
【经典例题】As a rule, where the broom does not reach the dust will not vanish of itself.
【译　　文】通常，扫帚不到，灰尘不会自己跑掉。

variable ['vɛərɪəbl]

n. 变量 *a.* 易变的；可变的，可调节的

variation [,vɛərɪ'eɪʃən]

n. 变化，变动；变种，变异

vary ['vɛərɪ]

vt. 变化，改变
【派生词汇】various *a.* 各种各样的；variety *n.* 多样化，变化
【固定搭配】vary with... 随……变化；vary from...to... 由……到……情况不同
【名师导学】在词汇和阅读题中多是以 vary 的词形变化形式出现。
【经典例题】The hopes, goals, fears and desires ＿＿＿ widely between men and women, between the rich and the poor.
A. alter　　B. transfer　　C. shift　　D. vary　　[D]
【译　　文】无论男女，无论贫富，每个人的希望、目标、忧虑和愿望都大不相同。

vehicle ['vi:ɪkl]

n. 车辆，交通工具
【经典例题】Cars and trucks are vehicles.
【译　　文】小汽车和大卡车都是交通工具。

veil [veɪl]

n. 面纱，纱帐，幕
【经典例题】We'll draw a veil over your recent bad behaviour, but I must warn you that if this happens again you will be punished.
【译　　文】对你最近的不良行为，我们先不追究了，但我得警告你，要是你再犯，就要受处罚了。

velocity [vɪ'lɒsɪtɪ]

n. 速度，速率

ventilate ['ventɪleɪt]

vt. (使)通风；把……公开，公开讨论
【经典例题】My office is well-ventilated.
【译　　文】我的办公室通风良好。

venture ['ventʃə]

n. / vi. 冒险，拼，闯 *v.* 敢于，大胆表示 *n.* 冒险（事业）
【固定搭配】at a venture 胡乱地，随便地
【名师导学】辨析 venture, adventure, risk：venture 指冒生命危险或经济风险；adventure 指使人心振奋、寻求刺激性的冒险；risk 指不顾个人安危、主动承担风险的事。

venue ['venju]

n. 犯罪地点；审判地；集合地点，会议地点，比赛地点；管辖地

verbal ['və:bəl]

a. 言辞的，有关语言的，在语言上的；口头的，口头上的；逐字的，按照字面的
【经典例题】The desire for security can be satisfied through verbal reassurance and promise of steady employment.
【译　　文】通过口头安慰和许诺稳定职业，可以满足对安全感的要求。

verdict ['və:dikt]
n. (陪审团的)判/裁决；定论，判断，意见
【名师导学】注意该词在固定搭配 return a verdict 中表示"做出判决"。
【经典例题】Concerns were raised that witnesses might be encouraged to exaggerate their stories in court to ensure guilty verdict.
【译　文】为了确保做出有罪判决，证人可能被怂恿在法庭上夸大事实。这件事已引起广泛关注。

verge [və:dʒ]
n. 边，边缘　*vi.* 接近，濒临

verify ['verifai]
vt. 证实，证明；查清，核实
【经典例题】There are often discouraging predictions that have not been proved verified by actual events.
【译　文】经常会有未经过事实证明的令人泄气的预测。

versatile ['və:sətail]
a. 多才多艺的，有多种技能的；有多种用途的，多功能的，万用的
【经典例题】She is very＿＿＿, and will be able to perform all required tasks well.
A. productive　　　　B. flexible
C. sophisticated　　　D. versatile　　　　　　　　　　[D]
【译　文】她多才多艺，能出色完成所有交办的任务。

verse [və:s]
n. 诗句，诗
【经典例题】Most of the scene is written in verse, but some is in prose.
【译　文】这场戏大部分内容是用韵文写成的，但也有一些是散文形式的。

version ['və:ʃən]
n. 形式，式样；看法，说法；版本，译本，改写本　*prep.*（诉讼、竞赛等中）……对……；与……相对（比）
【经典例题】Asteroids are bigger versions of the meteoroids that race across the night sky.
【译　文】行星是划过夜空的流星的更大一些的形式。

vertical ['və:tikəl]
a. 垂直的，竖的
【经典例题】On the vertical exterior surface of the outer ring, 3,800 solar cells are mounted on panels to convert the sun's energy to electrical power.
【译　文】在外环空间的垂直外部表面上，有3800个太阳能电池被镶嵌在嵌板上，将太阳能转化为电力。

vessel ['vesl]
n. 容器，器皿；船舶；管，导管，血管
【联想记忆】steamship *n.* 蒸汽船；liner *n.* 客轮；ferry *n.* 摆渡；tanker *n.* 油轮

veteran ['vetərən]
n. 老兵，老手　*a.* 老练的

veto ['vi:təu]
n. 否决权　*vt.* 使用否决权　*vi.* 反对，不赞成；否决，禁止
【经典例题】Japan used its veto to block the resolution.
【译　文】日本使用了它的否决权反对该项决议。

via ['vaiə, 'vi:ə]
prep. 经，经由，通过
【经典例题】I went to Pittsburgh via Philadelphia.
【译　文】我经过费城到匹兹堡。

☐ **vibrate** [vaɪˈbreɪt]	*v.* (使)振动,(使)摇摆	
	【经典例题】The diaphragm vibrates, thus setting the air around it in motion.	
	【译　　文】膜片振动使得周围的空气也动了起来。	
☐ **vice** [vaɪs]	*n.* 罪恶;恶习;缺点,毛病	
	【固定搭配】vice versa 反之亦然	
☐ **vicinity** [vɪˈsɪnɪtɪ]	*n.* 周围地区,临近地区	
	【固定搭配】in the vicinity of 在……附近	
	【经典例题】Everyone knows that if he shouts in the vicinity of a wall or a mountainside, an echo will come back.	
	【译　　文】人人都知道,如果一个人在墙壁或山边附近大喊一声,回声就会传回来。	
☐ **vicious** [ˈvɪʃəs]	*a.* 恶毒的,恶意的;危险的,险恶的	
	【名师导学】近义词：wicked, evil, cruel, sinful; bad, debased, base, impious, profligate, demoralized, faulty, vile, foul, impure, lewd, indecent	
	【经典例题】I need experience to get a job but without a job I can't get experience. It's a vicious circle.	
	【译　　文】我得有经验才能找到工作,可是没有工作我就无法获得经验。这真是个恶性循环。	
☐ **video** [ˈvɪdɪəʊ]	*a.* 电视的,视频的;录像的　*n.* 电视,视频;录像	
	【经典例题】It's not just video games and movies; children see a lot of murder and crime on the local news.	
	【译　　文】不仅从电视游戏和电影,在当地的新闻中孩子也能见到许多的谋杀和犯罪。	
☐ **vigorous** [ˈvɪɡərəs]	*a.* 精力充沛的	
	【经典例题】He is successful as a doctor because of his vigorous personality. He seems to have unlimited energy.	
	【译　　文】因为精力充沛的个性,所以他是一位成功的医生。他似乎有无限的力量。	
☐ **violate** [ˈvaɪəleɪt]	*vt.* 违犯,违背,违例	
	【派生词汇】violation *n.* 违背	
	【固定搭配】violate the regulation / agreement 违反规定 / 合约	
	【经典例题】The actress violated the terms of her contract and was prosecuted by the producer.	
	【译　　文】这位女演员违反了她合同上的条款,被制片人起诉了。	
☐ **violence** [ˈvaɪələns]	*n.* 强暴,暴力;暴行;猛烈,激烈	
	【固定搭配】resort to violence 诉诸暴力	
☐ **violent** [ˈvaɪələnt]	*a.* 猛烈的,强烈的,剧烈的;强暴的,由暴力引起的	
☐ **virtual** [ˈvɜːtjʊəl, -tʃʊəl]	*a.* 虚的,虚拟的;实际上的	

virtually
['və:tjuəli']

ad. 实际上，几乎

virtue
['və:tju:]

n. 美德；优点
【固定搭配】by / in virtue of 借助，经由
【联想记忆】by means of 借助；by way of 借助，经由；as a result of, by reason of 经由
【经典例题】The manager spoke highly of such virtues as loyalty, courage and truthfulness shown by his employees.
【译　　文】经理对员工们所表现出的诸如忠诚、勇气和诚实这类的美德给予了高度的评价。

virtuous
['vət∫uəs]

n. 善良的，有道德的；贞洁的；有效力的

virus
['vaiərəs]

n. 病毒
【经典例题】This is the pernicious virus of racism.
【译　　文】这是种族主义的毒害。

visa
['vi:zə]

n. 签证
【固定搭配】apply for a visa 申请签证；extend a visa 延长签证；issue a visa 发给签证；deny sb. a visa 拒绝给某人签证

vital
['vaitl]

a. 极其重要的，致命的；生命的；有生机的
【固定搭配】be vital to 对……极其重要
【名师导学】It's vital that 从句谓语动词用原形表示虚拟形式。
【经典例题】The young people are the most active and vital force in society.
【译　　文】青年是整个社会中最积极、最有生气的一部分力量。

vivid
['vivid]

a. 鲜艳的；生动的，栩栩如生的
【经典例题】Many children turn their attention from printed texts to the less challenging, more vivid moving pictures.
【译　　文】许多孩子将他们的注意力从绘有彩图的课文转到了难度较小，却更加生动的动画片上了。

vocabulary
[və'kæbjuləri]

n. 词汇（量 / 表）
【经典例题】His English vocabulary is limited, but his Chinese vocabulary is large.
【译　　文】他英文的词汇量有限，但他中文的词汇量却很丰富。

vocal
['vəukl]

a. 喜欢畅所欲言的，直言不讳的；嗓音的，发声的 *n.*（常用复数）声乐节目

void
[vɔid]

a. 无效的；没有，缺乏的 *n.* 空虚感，寂寞感；真空，空白
vt. 使无效

volt
[vəult, vɔlt]

n. 伏特
【联想记忆】transformer *n.* 变压器；voltage *n.* 电压；volt *n.* 伏特；watt *n.* 瓦，瓦特；current *n.* 电流

voluntary
['vɔləntəri; -teri]

a. 自愿的
【经典例题】There is a voluntary conveyance of property.
【译　　文】这是一桩自愿的财产转让。

vote
[vəut]

n. 选票，选票数　*n. / v.* 选举，表决
【固定搭配】vote for / against 投票支持 / 反对
【经典例题】I have to admire the ladies who fifty years ago worked so hard to get women the right to vote.
【译　　文】我必须钦佩以前那些女士们，他们在五十年前就努力为妇女争取选举权。

vulgar
['vʌlgə(r)]

a. 粗野的，下流的；庸俗的，粗俗的
【名师导学】近义词：coarse, crude, crass, unrefined, uncouth, indelicate, boorish, uncultivated, gross, low, common, tasteless, inelegant

vulnerable
['vʌlnərəb(ə)l]

a. 易受攻击的，有弱点的；易受伤害的，脆弱的
【名师导学】该词的考查点主要在 vulnerable to（易受伤害的，易受打击的）的用法，其中 to 为介词，后面需接名词或名词短语。
【经典例题】Some researchers feel that certain people have nervous systems particularly vulnerable to hot, dry winds. They are what we call weather-sensitive people.
【译　　文】一些研究人员认为有些人的神经系统特别容易受到干燥的热风的影响，这些人就是我们称为"对天气敏感的人"。

wage
[weidʒ]

n. 工资，报酬

warrant
['wɔrənt]

n. 证明，保证；授权，许可证；付（收）款凭单
【固定搭配】warrant for sth. / doing sth. 正当理由，根据
【经典例题】The total amount of your order last year was moderate, which does not warrant an agency appointment.
【译　　文】你方去年的订货总量不大，这无法证明你方可以胜任我们的代理。

warranty
['wɔrənti]

n. 保证书，担保

wary
['wɛəri]

a. 谨慎的，机警的，小心的

watertight ['wɔ:tətait]	a. 不透水的，不漏水的；无懈可击的
weary ['wiəri]	a. 疲倦的；令人厌烦的 vt. 使疲倦，使厌烦 【名师导学】该词的考查点在于该词意为"令人厌烦"时，经常出现在"weary of sth."的搭配中。 【经典例题】Today there are many charitable organizations which specialize in helping the weary travelers. 【译　　文】如今成立了许多专门从事救助疲惫旅行者的慈善组织。
weave [wi:v]	v. 编织 【经典例题】How long does it take to weave five yards of cloth? 【译　　文】织五码布需要多长时间呢？
wedge [wedʒ]	n. 楔，楔形 v. 楔牢，楔住，挤进 【经典例题】Put a wedge under the door so that it will stay open. 【译　　文】在门底下塞一块楔子，让门保持开着。
weird [wiəd]	a. 怪诞的，离奇的 【名师导学】与本词同义的词语还有：bizarre, uncanny, strange, eccentric. 【经典例题】Weird shrieks were heard in the darkness. 【译　　文】黑暗中传来离奇的叫声。
weld [weld]	vt. 焊接，锻接；熔接，焊缝 【经典例题】These alloys weld at different heats. 【译　　文】这些合金可在不同的温度熔接。
welfare ['welfɛə]	n. 福利
well-being [wel'bi:iŋ]	n. 幸福；舒适
well-off [wel'ɔ:f]	a. 顺利的，走运的；手头宽裕的，繁荣昌盛的
whirl [(h)wə:l]	vi. 旋转，急转；发晕，（感觉等）变混乱 n. 旋转，急转；混乱，接连不断的活动 【经典例题】Leaves whirled in the wind. 【译　　文】落叶在风中旋转。
widespread ['waidspred]	a. 普遍的，分布/散布广的 【经典例题】SARS is not a widespread disease. 【译　　文】SARS 并不是一种广泛传播的疾病。
wise [waiz]	a. 智慧的，聪明的
wisdom ['wizdəm]	n. 智慧，明智；名言，格言；古训

wit [wit]	*n.* 机智；(*pl.*) 智力，才智；(*pl.*) 健全的头脑 【经典例题】It is surely not beyond the wit of the government to solve this simple problem. A. intention　　　　B. endowment C. intelligence　　　D. enlightenment　　　　[C] 【译　文】对于政府来说，解决这一简单的问题毫不费力。
withdraw [wið'drɔ:]	*vt.* 收回；撤回，撤取　*vi.* 撤退，退出 【固定搭配】withdraw...from... 将……从……撤回；withdraw from 退出 【经典例题】If after education he or she still shows no change, the Party branch shall persuade him or her to withdraw from the Party. 【译　文】经教育仍无转变的，应当劝其退党。
wither ['wiðə]	*v.*（使）枯萎
withhold [wið'həuld]	*vt.* 扣留，保留；抑制，制止 【联想记忆】with "有" +hold "持有，拥有，保存" =withhold 【经典例题】If a drug can save lives, we shouldn't withhold it without good reason. 【译　文】如果一种药物可以拯救生命，那么我们不该毫无理由抑制它。 【名师导学】keep, retain, reserve, preserve, conserve, withhold 这些动词均有"保持，保存"之意。 keep：最常用词，指长时间牢固地保持或保存。 retain：指继续保持。 reserve：正式用词，指为了将来的用途或其他用途而保存、保留。 preserve：主要指为防止损害、变质等而保存。 conserve：一般指保存自然资源，保全人的精力、力量等。 withhold：指扣住不放，暗示有阻碍。
withstand [wið'stænd]	*vt.* 抵抗，经受住 【经典例题】The new beach house on Sullivan's Island should be able to withstand a Category 3 hurricane with peak winds of 179 to 209 kilometers per hour. 【译　文】在沙利文岛的海边房屋应该能够抵挡第三类的飓风，这种飓风的最大风速为每小时179到209公里。
witness ['witnis]	*n.* 目击者，见证人　*vt.* 目击；证明 【固定搭配】bear witness to... 为……作证，做……的证人 【联想记忆】judge *n.* 法官；lawyer *n.* 律师；court *n.* 法院；accuse *n.* 指控 【经典例题】She is the witness to the accident. 【译　文】她是事故的目击者。
worldwide ['wə:ld,waid]	*a.* 世界范围的，遍及全球的 【联想记忆】nationwide *a.* 全国范围的
worship ['wə:ʃip]	*n.* 礼拜；礼拜仪式　*v.* 崇拜，敬仰 【联想记忆】church *n.* 教堂；pray *n.* 祈祷；god *n.* 神，上帝；Christianity *n.* 基督教；heaven *n.* 天堂

wrap [ræp]	*vt.* 卷，包，缠绕 *n.* 披肩 【固定搭配】wrap sth. in... 用……将某物包起来；be wrapped in... 用……包裹好；穿着……；wrap up 包好
wreck [rek]	*n.* 失事，遇难；沉船，残骸 *vt.* （船等）失事，遇难 【经典例题】The strong storm did a lot of damage to the coastal villages; several fishing boats were wrecked and many houses collapsed. 【译　文】猛烈的暴风雨破坏了海边的许多村庄，一些渔船沉没，许多房屋倒塌。
wrench [rentʃ]	*vt.* 猛拧，猛扭，挣脱，使扭伤 *n.*（离别等的）痛苦，难受，猛拉，扳手
wretched [ˈretʃid]	*a.* 不幸的，可怜的；卑鄙的，无耻的
wrinkle [ˈriŋkl]	*n.* 皱纹 *v.*（使）起皱纹 【名师导学】注意跟该词拼写相近的词：twinkle（闪耀），winkle（设法弄到），shrink（收缩，缩水）。 【经典例题】Smile is a wrinkle that should not be removed. 【译　文】微笑是一种不应消除的皱纹。

X-ray [ˈeksrei]	*n.* X 射线，X 光

yawn [jɔ:n]	*vi.* 打呵欠 *n.* 呵欠 【固定搭配】yawn out 打着哈欠说出 【经典例题】A yawn is a silent shout. 【译　文】呵欠是无声的叫喊。
yearly [ˈjə:li]	*a.* 每年的，一年一度的

yell
[jel]

n. / vi. 叫喊，尖叫

【名师导学】与本词同义的词语还有：scream, yelp, howl, cry, shout. 同时注意与该词搭配的介词为"at"。

【经典例题】She yelled at him about his constant drunkenness.

【译　文】她大嚷大叫说他总是烂醉如泥。

yield
[ji:ld]

vt. 生产，出产；让步，屈服　*vi.* 屈服，服从　*n.* 产量，收获量

【固定搭配】yield to 向……让步；increase the yield 增加产量

【联想记忆】submit *n.* 屈服；obey *n.* 服从；compromise *n.* 妥协；surrender *n.* 投降

【经典例题】They were short of sticks to make frames for the climbing vines, without which the yield would be halved.

【译　文】他们缺少搭葡萄架的杆儿，没有它们葡萄产量就会减少一半。

【经典例题】We love peace, yet we are not the kind of people to yield ____ military threat.

A. up　　　　B. to　　　　C. in　　　　D. at　　　　　　[B]

【译　文】我们热爱和平，但我们绝不会屈服于军事威胁。

Z

zigzag
[zigzg]

n. 之字形　*a. /ad.* 之字形的（地）　*v.* 曲折地进行

zone
[zəun]

n. 地带，区域

【经典例题】Which time zone is your city located in?

【译　文】你们的城市位于哪个时区？

第四部分
低频词汇

全国医学博士英语
统考词汇巧战通关

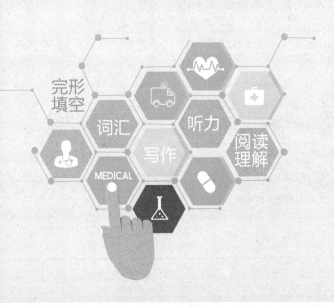

A

abate [ə'beɪt]	v. 减轻，减退 【经典例题】This topic appears to abate. 【译　文】这个话题的热度似乎降低了。
abide [ə'baɪd]	vt. 坚持；忍受 【固定搭配】abide by 服从；履行；遵守
abortion [ə'bɔːʃən]	n. 流产，夭折
abound [ə'baʊnd]	vi. 大量存在；有许多 【固定搭配】abound in / with 富于；充满，多
abstain [əb'steɪn]	vi.（投票时）弃权；戒；戒除；离开；回避
absurd [əb'sɜːd]	a. 荒谬的 【名师导学】absurd, foolish, silly 与 ridiculous 均含有"不合情理的，荒唐的，可笑的，愚蠢的"之意。absurd 强调"不符合人情或常识的"；foolish 强调"缺乏智慧和判断力的"；silly 强调"单纯的，糊涂的，低能的"；ridiculous 意为"荒谬的，令人发笑的"，常有"鄙视"之意。
accent ['æksənt] n. [æk'sent] v.	n. 口音，腔调；重音，重音符号 vt. 重读
acclaim [ə'kleɪm]	vt. 宣称；称誉某人/事物（为……）；给予高度评价 n.（尤指对艺术成就的）称誉，高度评价
accumulate [ə'kjuːmjəleɪt]	vt. 积累，积聚
acid ['æsɪd]	n. 酸 a. 酸的
acupuncture ['ækjupʌŋktʃə]	n. 针灸，针刺法
adjacent [ə'dʒeɪsənt]	a. 接近的，附近的，毗连的，相邻的
adjoin [ə'dʒɔɪn]	vt. 邻接，毗连

aerial ['ɛəriəl]	*a.* 空中的,航空的 *n.* 天线
aerospace ['ɛərəuspeis]	*a.* 航天的;太空的 *n.* 宇宙空间,航空
affix [ə'fiks]	*vt.* 使……附于;署名;粘贴 *n.* 附加物;附件,词缀
aisle [ail]	*n.* 通道,走廊
album ['ælbəm]	*n.* 相片册,邮票簿
alley ['æli]	*n.* 小巷子
aloft [ə'lɔft]	*ad.* 在高处,在上面,在空中
aluminum [ə'lju:minəm]	*n.* 铝 【联想记忆】copper *n.* 铜制品;bronze *n.* 青铜
amass [ə'mæs]	*vt.* 积累,积聚;收集
amateur ['æmətə(:)]	*a.* 业余的 *n.* 业余爱好者
ambassador [æm'bæsədə]	*n.* 大使,专使
ammunition [,æmju'niʃən]	*n.* 弹药,军火;武器,军事装备
amplitude ['æmplitju:d]	*n.* (声波、无线电波等的)振幅
antenna [æn'tenə]	*n.* 天线;触角,触须
antique [æn'ti:k]	*a.* 古代的,古式的;旧式的 *n.* 古董,古物
antiseptic [,ænti'septik]	*a.* 防腐的,抗菌的 *n.* 防腐剂;抗菌剂
arch [ɑ:tʃ]	*n.* 拱门,弓形结构

arch [ɑːtʃ]	n. 共性结构
archaeology [ˌɑːkiˈɔlədʒi]	n. 考古学
architect [ˈɑːkitekt]	n. 建筑师
architecture [ˈɑːkitektʃə]	n. 建筑
archives [ˈɑːkaivz]	n. 档案
arena [əˈriːnə]	n. 竞技场，角斗场；舞台，场地
artillery [ɑːˈtiləri]	n. 火炮，大炮；炮兵
ashore [əˈʃɔː]	ad. 在岸上，在陆地
aspirin [ˈæspərin]	n. 阿司匹林
astronomy [əˈstrɔnəmi]	n. 天文学
asylum [əˈsailəm]	n. 避难所，庇护所，避难
atlas [ˈætləs]	n. 地图，地图集
atmosphere [ˈætməsfiə]	n. 空气；大气，大气层；气氛
atmospheric [ˌætməsˈferik]	a. 大气的，空气的
audit [ˈɔːdit]	v. 审计，查账
auditorium [ˌɔːdiˈtɔːriəm]	n. 观众席，听众席；礼堂，会堂
authentic [ɔːˈθentik]	a. 真实的，真正的；可靠的，可信的
auxiliary [ɔːgˈziljəri]	a. 辅助的，备用的

☐ **aviation** [ˌeiviˈeiʃən]	*n.* 航空，航空学 【固定搭配】civil aviation 民用航空
☐ **awesome** [ˈɔːsəm]	*a.* 令人惊叹的；令人敬畏的；很好的
☐ **axis** [ˈæksis]	*n.* 轴

☐ **bachelor** [ˈbætʃələ]	*n.* 学士；单身汉
☐ **badge** [bædʒ]	*n.* 徽章，证章；标记，标志；象征
☐ **baffle** [bæfl]	*vt.* 使困惑，为难，使挫折
☐ **ballot** [ˈbælət]	*n.* （无记名投票）选举，选票
☐ **bandwidth** [ˈbændwidθ]	*n.* 带宽；频宽
☐ **bang** [bæŋ]	*v.* 猛敲，猛撞，猛地关上；砰地把（门、盖）关上；发出砰的响声
☐ **bankrupt** [ˈbæŋkrʌpt]	*a.* 破产的 *vt.* 使破产 *n.* 破产者
☐ **banner** [ˈbænə]	*n.* 旗帜，横幅
☐ **barometer** [bəˈrɔmitə]	*n.* 气压计
☐ **beckon** [ˈbekən]	*vt.* 示意，召唤；吸引，诱惑
☐ **besiege** [biˈsiːdʒ]	*vt.* 围攻，围困

beware [bi'wɛə]	v. 谨慎，当心
Bible ['baibl]	n. 圣经
bid [bid]	v. 出价，投标 n. 出价，投标
binder ['baində]	n. 包扎者，绑缚者；装订工
biochemistry [,baiəu'kemistri]	n. 生物化学
biography [bai'ɔgrəfi]	n. 传记
biomedical [,baiəu'medikl]	a. 生物医学的
bionics [bai'ɔniks]	n. 仿生学
biotechnology [,baiəutek'nɔlədʒi]	n. 生物技术
birthright [bə:rθrait]	n. 与生俱来的权利；基本人权
bishop ['biʃəp]	n. 主教；（国际象棋中的）象；热果子酒
blade [bleid]	n. 刀刃，刀片；叶片；翼
blank [blæŋk]	n. 空白；空白表格 a. 空白的，空着的；茫然的，无表情的
bleach [bli:tʃ]	v. 漂白 n. 漂白剂
bloodshed ['blʌdʃed]	n. 流血事件
bloody ['blʌdi]	a. 流着血的，有血的；血腥的，残忍的
blush [blʌʃ]	vi. 脸红；羞愧；尴尬 n. 脸红；红色，红光
boast [bəust]	vi.（of, about）夸耀，说大话 vt. 吹嘘；以有……而自豪；自夸 n. 自吹自擂夸耀，夸口

bond [bɔnd]	n. 契约；公债，债券；联结，联系
bonus ['bəunəs]	n. 奖金；津贴；红包
booklet ['buklit]	n. 小册子
boom [bu:m]	v. 轰鸣；繁荣，迅速发展 n. 隆隆声；繁荣，激增
booth [bu:ð]	n. 货摊；小间，亭子
botanical [bə'tænikl]	a. 植物学的，植物的
brace [breis]	n. 支架，托架 vt. 使做准备；加强，加固
bracket ['brækit]	n. 括号；组级；托架 v. 把……置于括号内
brass [brɑ:s]	n. 黄铜；(pl.) 黄铜制品
breadth [bredθ]	n. 宽度，(布的) 幅宽，(船) 幅
breakage ['breikidʒ]	n. 破坏，裂口，破损处
brew [bru:]	v. 酿造；调制；煎（药）
brewery ['bru:əri]	n. 啤酒厂，酿酒厂
bride [braid]	n. 新娘
brilliant ['briljənt]	a. 辉煌的，灿烂的；杰出的，有才华的
brink [briŋk]	n. （河、海、峭壁等的）边，界，岸
brisk [brisk]	a. 快的，敏捷的；忙碌的
broadband ['brɔ:dbænd]	n. 宽带

☐ **brochure** [brəuˈʃuə]	*n.* 小册子
☐ **bronze** [brɔnz]	*n.* 青铜 *a.* 青铜色的
☐ **Buddhism** [ˈbudizəm]	*n.* 佛教
☐ **bypass** [ˈbaipɑ:s]	*n.* 旁路；小道 *vt.* 绕过；忽视，回避
☐ **bystander** [ˈbaistændə]	*n.* 旁观者；局外人

C

☐ **calcium** [ˈkælsiəm]	*n.* 钙
☐ **cancer** [ˈkænsə]	*n.* 癌
☐ **cane** [kein]	*n.* 手杖，细长的茎，藤条 *vt.* 以杖击，以藤编制
☐ **canvas**	*n.* 帆布，画布，油画
☐ **capacitance** [kəˈpæsitəns]	*n.* 电容
☐ **capacitor** [kəˈpæsitə]	*n.* 电容器
☐ **cape** [keip]	*n.* 斗篷，披肩；地角，岬角
☐ **capitalism** [ˈkæpitəlizəm]	*n.* 资本主义
☐ **capsule** [ˈkæpsju:l]	*n.* 胶囊；太空舱
☐ **caravan** [ˈkærəvæn]	*n.* 大篷车；活动房屋

第四部分 低频词汇

carbon ['kɑ:bən]	n. 碳
carefree ['kɛrfri:]	a. 无忧无虑的；无牵挂的；无责任的
cargo ['kɑ:gəu]	n. 货物
caring ['kering]	a. 关心人的，人道的，有同情心的
caring ['kɛəriŋ]	a. 关心人的，人道的，有同情心的
cart [kɑ:t]	n. 大车，手推车 vt. 用车装载
casino [kə'si:nəu]	n. 夜总会，俱乐部，娱乐场
catalogue ['kætəlɔg]	n. 目录 vt. 将……编入目录；记载
cathedral [kə'θi:drəl]	n. 大教堂
Catholic ['kæθəlik]	n. 天主教徒 a. 天主教的
cavity ['kæviti]	n. 洞，空穴，凹处
Celsius ['selsiəs]	a. 摄氏的
censorship ['sensəʃip]	n. 审查，检查；审查制度
centimeter ['sentimi:tə(r)]	n. 厘米
ceramic [si'ræmik]	a. 陶瓷的 n. 陶瓷器
chamber ['tʃeimbə]	n. 室；议院
chancellor ['tʃɑ:nsələ]	n. 大臣；首席法官；校长
channel ['tʃænl]	n. 海峡；水道，沟渠，渠道；频道

☐ chart [tʃɑːt]	n. 图，图表
☐ charter ['tʃɑːtə]	n. 宪章，特许状 vt. 特许设立，发执照给……；包租（船，车等）
☐ chase [tʃeis]	v./n. 追逐，追赶；追捕
☐ chew [tʃuː]	v. 咀嚼
☐ chill [tʃil]	n. 凉气，寒气；寒战，风寒 vt. 使变冷，使冷冻，使感到冷
☐ chilly ['tʃili]	a. 寒冷的
☐ chip [tʃip]	n. 缺口；碎片；炸薯条；集成电路片
☐ chloride ['klɔːraid]	n. 氯化物
☐ chlorine ['klɔːriːn]	n. 氯（气）
☐ choke [tʃəuk]	v. 窒息，阻塞，抑制
☐ chop [tʃɔp]	v. 砍，劈；剁碎 n. 砍，劈，剁；排骨
☐ chore [tʃɔː]	n. 日常事务；例行工作；令人厌烦的任务
☐ Christian ['kristjən]	a. 基督的；基督教的
☐ chronicle ['krɔnikl]	n. 年代记，编年史；记录 【联想记忆】chronic 慢性的，长期的；chronicle=chronic+article "长期的文章"/"慢慢记录的文献"=年代记，编年史
☐ chunk [tʃʌŋk]	n. 大块，矮胖的人或物
☐ circuit ['səːkit]	n. 电路，线路
☐ circular ['səːkjulə]	a. 圆形的；环形的

☐ **cite** [saɪt]	vt. 举（例），引证，引用
☐ **civic** ['sɪvɪk]	a. 城市的；市民的，公民的
☐ **civic** ['sɪvɪk]	a. 城市的；市民的，公民的
☐ **clan** [klæn]	n. 克兰（苏格兰高地人的氏族、部族）部落，氏族，宗族，党派
☐ **clap** [klæp]	n. 鼓掌，拍手 v. 鼓掌
☐ **clash** [klæʃ]	v. 打斗，冲突；发出铿锵声，猛烈地碰撞；（意见）冲突，（色彩等）不一致 n. 打斗，冲突；争论；铿锵声；不一致
☐ **clasp** [klɑːsp]	vt. 握紧；扣住，扣紧；抱紧 n. 搭扣，扣环；紧握，紧抱
☐ **clause** [klɔːz]	n. 子句，从句；（章程、条约等的）条，项；条款
☐ **cliff** [klɪf]	n. 悬崖
☐ **clockwise** ['klɔːkwaɪz]	a. / ad. 顺时针方向转动的（地），正转的（地）
☐ **coach** [kəʊtʃ]	n. 长途客车，长途汽车；教练，私人教师 v. 训练，辅导，指示
☐ **colonel** ['kɜːnl]	n. 上校
☐ **colony** ['kɔləni]	n. 殖民地；聚居地
☐ **comet** ['kɔmɪt]	n. 彗星
☐ **compartment** [kəm'pɑːtmənt]	n. 间隔，（列车车厢的）隔间
☐ **compass** ['kʌmpəs]	n. 指南针
☐ **condom** ['kɔndəm]	n. 避孕套

cone [kəun]	n. 圆锥体；圆锥形东西
Confucian [kən'fju:ʃən]	a. 孔子的；儒家的
Confucianism [kən'fju:ʃənizm]	n. 孔子学说，儒家学说，儒教
congress ['kɔŋgres]	n. 代表大会；国会，议会
constituent [kən'stitjuənt]	n. 选民，选区居民；成分，组成要素 【名师导学】考生要注意常用的相关同义词：component（成分），element（要素，元素，成分）。
cord [kɔ:d]	n. 细绳，弦
cordless ['kɔ:dlis]	a. 无绳的，不用电线的
cork [kɔ:k]	n. 软木，软木塞
cosmetic [kɔz'metik]	n. 化妆品 a. 化妆用的
coupon ['ku:pɔn]	n. 息票；赠券
creditor ['kreditə]	n. 债权人，贷方
creek [kri:k]	n. 小湾，小溪
crown [kraun]	n. 王冠；荣誉 vt. 为……加冕
crowning ['krauniŋ]	a. 至高无上的；登峰造极的
cruise [kru:z]	v./n. 巡航，巡游
crumble ['krʌmbl]	vt. 弄碎，粉碎
crush [krʌʃ]	v. 压碎，榨；压服，压垮 n. 拥挤的人群，热恋，迷恋

☐ **crust** [krʌst]	*n.* 面包皮，干面包片；外壳，硬壳
☐ **crystal** ['kristl]	*n.* 水晶，晶体 *a.* 水晶的，晶体的；透明的
☐ **cubic** ['kju:bik]	*a.* 立体的，立方的；三次的
☐ **curfew** ['kə:fju:]	*n.* 宵禁时间；戒严时间；宵禁令
☐ **curse** [kə:s]	*n. / v.* 诅咒，咒骂
☐ **curve** [kə:v]	*v.* 弄弯，使成曲线 *n.* 曲线，弯曲
☐ **cushion** ['kuʃən]	*n.* 垫子，坐垫 【名师导学】辨析 cushion, mat, pad：cushion 指用柔软的物质做的坐垫、软垫；mat 指用稻草、纤维等做成的铺在地上的席子、垫子；pad 指用软的东西做成的衬垫。
☐ **cybernetics** [ˌsaibə:'netiks]	*n.* 控制论
☐ **cylinder** ['silində]	*n.* 圆柱体，滚筒；气缸

☐ **deadline** ['dedlain]	*n.* 最后期限，截止日期
☐ **debris** ['debri:]	*n.* 残骸，碎片；残渣，垃圾
☐ **decimal** ['desiməl]	*a.* 小数的，十进制的
☐ **deck** [dek]	*n.* 甲板
☐ **den** [den]	*n.* 兽穴，兽窝；进行私人活动的场所

derail [diˈreil]	vt. 使（火车等）出轨
detergent [diˈtə:dʒənt]	a. 使清洁的 n. 清洁剂；去垢剂
detoxify [ˌdi:ˈtɔksifai]	v. 解毒，除去……毒物，去除……的放射性沾染
dew [dju:]	n. 露水
diagram [ˈdaiəgræm]	n. 简图；图解，图表
dial [ˈdaiəl]	n. 表盘；刻度盘，调节盘 v. 拨号，打电话
diesel [ˈdi:zəl]	n. 柴油机，内燃机
dip [dip]	n. / vt. 浸；蘸
dispense [diˈspens]	vt. 分发，分配
dissertation [ˌdisə(:)ˈteiʃən]	n. 专题论文，学位论文
ditch [ditʃ]	n. 沟，渠
dive [daiv]	n. / vi. 跳水，潜水；俯冲，扑
dock [dɔk]	n. 船坞，码头
dodge [dɔdʒ]	v. 躲闪，躲避，搪塞 n. 躲闪
dogged [ˈdɔgid]	a. 顽固的；顽强的
dogma [ˈdɔgmə]	n. 教条，教义；信条
dome [dəum]	n. 圆屋顶
dough [dəu]	n. 生面团；钱，现款

dryer ['draɪə]	n. 干衣机，干燥剂
duke [djuːk]	n. 公爵
dye [daɪ]	n. 颜料，染料 vt. 染，染色
dynamite ['daɪnəmaɪt]	n. 黄色炸药；引起轰动的人（或事物）
dynasty ['daɪnəsti]	n. 王朝，朝代

Easter ['iːstə]	n. 复活节
ebb [eb]	n. 退潮，落潮 vi. 退潮，落潮；减少，衰落
ectopic [ek'tɔpik]	a. 异位的
electoral [ɪ'lektərəl]	a. 选举的；选举人的
embargo [em'bɑːgəu]	vt. 禁止（船舶进入港口或贸易） n. 封港令；禁止贸易令；禁令
embed [ɪm'bed]	vt. 把……嵌入；使深留脑中
embryo ['embriəu]	n. 胚胎
encyclop(a)edia [ɪn,saɪklə'piːdɪə]	n. 百科全书
envious ['enviəs]	a. 羡慕的；忌妒的
epoch ['iːpɔk]	n. 新纪元，时代，时期

escort ['eskɔ:t]	n. 护卫（队），陪同（人员） v. 护卫，护送，陪同
essay ['esei, 'esi]	n. 散文，随笔，短文

fabric ['fæbrik]	n. 织物，纺织品；结构，组织
fabulous ['fæbjuləs]	a. 寓言中的，神话般的；难以置信的
facet ['fæsit]	n.（多面体的）面，方面
famine ['fæmin]	n. 饥荒
fantastic [fæn'tæstik]	a. 极好的；很大的；空想的；奇异的，古怪的
fascist ['fæʃist]	n. 法西斯主义者 a. 法西斯主义的
feat [fi:t]	n. 技艺，功绩，武艺；壮举；技艺表演
ferry ['feri]	n. 渡轮，摆渡船
fertilizer ['fə:tilaizə]	n. 化肥，肥料
festival ['festəvəl]	n. 节日，喜庆日
fiber ['faibə]	n. 纤维，纤维素
fiction ['fikʃən]	n. 小说，虚构的故事；虚构，杜撰，捏造

☐ **filter** ['filtə]	*n.* 过滤器,滤波器 *vt.* 过滤
☐ **fitting** ['fitiŋ]	*a.* 适合的,相称的,适合的 *n.* 试穿,试衣;装配,装置
☐ **flame** [fleim]	*n.* 火焰,火苗;热情,激情
☐ **flank** [flæŋk]	*n.* 侧面,腰窝 *vt.* 在……的侧面
☐ **flap** [flæp]	*n.* 飘动,摆动;(翅膀的)拍打;激动 *v.* (使)拍打,鼓翼而飞,飘动
☐ **flee** [fli:]	*v.* 逃走,逃出;消失,(时间)飞逝
☐ **fleet** [fli:t]	*n.* 舰队,船队,机群
☐ **flip** [flip]	*n.* 轻抛,空翻 *vt.* 掷,弹,轻击 *vi.* 用指轻弹,翻动书页(或纸张) *a.* 无礼的,冒失的,轻率的
☐ **flush** [flʌʃ]	*n.* 红晕;冲刷(便桶) *v.* (脸)发红;冲洗,冲掉 *a.* 丰足的,完全齐平的
☐ **flutter** ['flʌtə]	*n.* 紧张,激动;鼓翼 *v.* (鸟等)鼓翼;飘动;(心脏等)怦怦乱跳
☐ **foil** [fɔil]	*n.* 箔,金属薄片;烘托,衬托 *vt.* 阻止,挫败
☐ **folklore** ['fəuklɔ:(r)]	*n.* 民间传统;民俗;民间传说
☐ **footstep** ['futstep]	*n.* 脚步声;足迹
☐ **fort** [fɔ:t]	*n.* 要塞;堡垒
☐ **furnace** ['fə:nis]	*n.* 火炉,熔炉
☐ **furthermore** [fə:ðə'mɔ:(r)]	*ad.* 而且,此外
☐ **fusion** ['fju:ʒən]	*n.* 熔化,熔解,熔合,熔接

G

gadget ['gædʒit]	*n.* 小器具,小配件,小玩意
gallon ['gælən]	*n.* 加仑 【联想记忆】ounce *n.* 盎司;pint *n.* 品脱;quart *n.* 夸脱;liter *n.* 公升
garment ['gɑ:mənt]	*n.* 衣服,(*pl.*)服装 【名师导学】辨析:dress, clothing, garment, clothes。dress 指正式场合穿着的衣服;clothing 指衣服的总称,单数形式;garment 常指一件穿在外面的衣服;clothes 指衣服的总称,复数形式,但不能与数词连用。
glossary ['glɔsəri]	*n.* 词汇表
gorge [gɔ:dʒ]	*n.* 峡谷,山谷
grab [græb]	*n./v.* 强夺,攫取,抓取
gram(me) [græm]	*n.* 克
grammar ['græmə]	*n.* 语法;语法书
grave [greiv]	*n.* 坟,坟墓 *a.* 严肃的,庄重的
gravity ['græviti]	*n.* 重力,引力;严肃,庄严
graze [greiz]	*v.* 喂草;吃草;放牧
grill [gril]	*n.* (烤肉用的)烤架,铁篦子
grim [grim]	*a.* 冷酷无情的,严厉的;讨厌的,野蛮的
groove [gru:v]	*n.* 槽,沟;常规,老一套 *v.* 开槽于
gymnastics [dʒim'næstiks]	*n.* 体育;体操

☐ **hail** [heil]	n. 冰雹；一阵 v. 赞扬……为；招手；下雹；跟……打招呼
☐ **hardware** ['hɑ:dwɛə]	n. 五金器具；硬件
☐ **heading** ['hediŋ]	n. 标题
☐ **healthcare** ['helθkɛə,]	n. 医疗保健，健康护理
☐ **hedge** [hedʒ]	n. 树篱，障碍物 v. 用树篱围住
☐ **henceforth** [hens'fɔ:θ]	ad. 从此以后，从今以后
☐ **herd** [hə:d]	n. 兽群，牧群；人群
☐ **hitherto** [,hiðə'tu:]	ad. 到目前为止，迄今
☐ **hive** [haiv]	n. 蜂箱，蜂房 v.（使）入蜂箱，群居
☐ **hoarse** [hɔ:s]	a.（嗓子）嘶哑的；沙哑的
☐ **hoist** [hɔist]	n. 起重机；吊车，（残疾人用）升降机 v. 升起，举起，吊起
☐ **holy** ['həuli]	a. 神圣的；圣洁的
☐ **homosexual** [,həuməˈsekʃuəl]	a. 同性恋的 n. 同性恋者
☐ **hono(u)rable** ['ɔnərəbl]	a. 诚实的，正直的；光荣的，荣誉的；值得尊敬的；品格高尚的
☐ **honorary** ['ɔnərəri]	a. 荣誉的，名誉的

hose [həuz]	n. 长筒袜，软管，水龙带 v. 用软管浇水（与 down 连用）
hostage [ˈhɔstidʒ]	n. 人质
housewife [ˈhauswaif]	n. 家庭主妇
housing [ˈhauziŋ]	n. 住房；住房供给
howl [haul]	n. 嚎叫，哀号，咆哮 v. 吠，嚎叫，咆哮
huddle [ˈhʌdl]	n. 杂乱的一堆人（或物品、建筑），拥挤 v.（因寒冷或害怕）挤在一起；蜷缩，缩成一团；草率从事
hut [hʌt]	n. 小屋，茅舍

ideological [ˌaidiəˈlɔdʒikl]	a. 意识形态上的
idiom [ˈidiəm]	n. 惯用语，成语，习语
impromptu [imˈprɔmptjuː]	ad. / a. 即席地（的），临时地（的），事先无准备地（的）
indoor(s) [ˈindɔː(z)]	ad. / a. 在室内（的），在户内（的）
inflict [inˈflikt]	v. 把……强加给，使遭受，使承担
injure [ˈindʒə]	vt. 伤害，损害，损伤
inlet [ˈinlet]	n. 进口，入口；水湾，小湾
input [ˈinput]	n. 输入

install [in'stɔ:l]	vt. 安装,设置
installation [,instə'leiʃən]	n. 安装,设置
instantaneous [,instən'teinjəs]	a. 即刻的,瞬间的
insurgency [in'sə:dʒənsi]	n. 叛乱,暴动
insurgent [in'sə:dʒənt]	a. 起义的,造反的,暴动的,叛乱的
interim ['intərim]	n. 过渡时期,中间时期,暂时 a. 暂时的,临时的;期中的
interior [in'tiəriə]	a. 内部的,里面的;内地的 n. 内部,内陆,内地,内政
intermediary [,intə'mi:diəri]	a. 中间的;中途的;媒介的
intermediate [,intə'mi:djət]	a. 中间的,居中的 n. 中间体,媒介物
intoxicate [in'tɔksikeit]	vt. 使陶醉,使喝醉
isle [ail]	n. 岛
italic [i'tælik]	a. [印] 斜体的,斜体字的

jerk [dʒə:rk]	n. 急推,急拉;蠢人,傻瓜 v. 使猝然一动,猛拉,猛扯
jetlag ['dʒətlæg]	n. 时差
judicial [dʒu(:)'diʃəl]	a. 司法的,法庭的,审判的;明断的,公正的

□ **judicious** [dʒuˈdiʃəs]	*a.* 明智的，明断的，审慎的
□ **jury** [ˈdʒuəri]	*n.* 陪审团

□ **kilowatt** [ˈkiləwɔt]	*n.* [物]千瓦（功率单位）
□ **knuckle** [ˈnʌkl]	*n.* 指节 *vi.*（down）开始努力工作；（under）屈服，认输

□ **lad** [læd]	*n.* 少年，青年男子
□ **landmark** [ˈlændmɑːrk]	*n.*（航海）陆标，地界标；里程碑
□ **landmine** [ˈlændmain]	*n.* 地雷
□ **lane** [lein]	*n.* 小路，小巷；行车道
□ **laundry** [ˈlɔːndri]	*n.* 洗衣房，洗衣店；要洗的衣服
□ **lavatory** [ˈlævətəri]	*n.* 厕所，盥洗室
□ **learned** [ˈləːnid]	*a.* 有学问的，博学的；学术性的
□ **lease** [liːs]	*n.* 租约，契约

lens [lenz]	n. 透镜,镜头
lesbian ['lezbiən]	n. 女同性恋者
lever ['li:və, 'levə]	n. 杠杆;控制杆,推杆
liaison [li'eizən]	n. 联络;(语音)连音
lick [lik]	n. / vt. 舔
lieutenant [lef'tenənt]	n. 陆军中尉,海军上尉;副职官员
lightning ['laitniŋ]	n. 闪电 a. 闪电般的,飞快的
lightweight ['laitweit]	n. 轻量级选手;不能胜任者
limp [limp]	vi. 蹒跚,一瘸一拐地走 a. 软弱的,柔软的,无力的
linear ['liniə]	a. 线的,直线的,线状的;长度的
linen ['linin]	n. 亚麻布,亚麻制品
liner ['lainə]	n. 邮轮,班机
liter ['li:tə]	n. 升
literally ['litərəli]	ad. 照字面地,逐字地;确实地,毫不夸张地
loaf [ləuf]	n. 一条(面包)
lobby ['lɔbi]	n. 门厅,前厅,大厅
locomotive [,ləukə'məutiv]	n. 机车,火车头 a. 运动的,移动的;运载的
locust ['ləukəst]	n. 蝗虫,蚱蜢

lofty ['lɔ:fti]	*a.* 高高的,崇高的,高傲的	
longitude ['lɔndʒitju:d]	*n.* 经度	
loop [lu:p]	*n.* 圈,环,环状物;回路,循环	
lottery ['lɔtəri]	*n.* 彩票或奖券的发行,抽彩给奖法,乐透彩	
lump [lʌmp]	*n.* 团,块 *v.* (使)成团,(使)成块	
luncheon ['lʌntʃən]	*n.* 午宴,正式的午餐	

mainstream ['meinstri:m]	*n.* 主流
malicious [mə'liʃəs]	*a.* 怀有恶意的,恶毒的
mall [mɔ:l]	*n.* (由许多商店组成的)购物中心
managerial [,mænə'dʒiəriəl]	*a.* 管理的
mansion ['mænʃən]	*n.* 大厦,官邸
marble ['mɑ:bl]	*n.* 大理石
marine [mə'ri:n]	*a.* 海的,海产的,航海的,船舶的,海运的
martyr ['mɑ:tə]	*n.* 烈士;殉教者

mask [mɑ:sk]	n. 面具；口罩
masterful ['mɑ:stəfəl]	a. 专横的
mastermind ['mɑ:stəmaind]	v. 策划
maximize ['mæksmaiz]	vt. 取……最大值；充分利用
meadow ['medəu]	n. 草地，牧场
meantime ['mi:n,taim]	n. 其时，在此期间 ad. 同时，当时
mercury ['mə:kjuri]	n. 水银（柱），汞；(the Mercury) 水星
metric ['metrik]	a. 公制的，米制的 n. 度量标准
midwife ['midwaif]	n. 助产士，接生员，产婆
militant ['militənt]	a. 好战的；好用暴力的；富于战斗性的
mill [mil]	n. 磨坊
minimal ['miniməl]	a. 最小的，最小限度的
mint [mint]	n. 薄荷，薄荷糖
minus ['mainəs]	a. 负的 prep. 减去 n. 减号，负号
mischief ['mistʃif]	n. 调皮；恶意伤害，损害
misery ['mizəri]	n. 痛苦，苦恼，悲惨

☐ **missile** ['misail]	n. 导弹；发射物
☐ **mo(u)ld** [məuld]	n. 模子，铸型 vt. 浇铸，塑造
☐ **modem** ['məudəm]	n. 调制解调器
☐ **moderator** ['mɔdəreitə]	n. 仲裁者，调停者；缓和剂
☐ **mold** [məuld]	n. 模子，模型，铸模；(人的)性格，气质，类型；霉，霉菌 vt. (用模具)浇铸，塑造；使形成，影响……的形成，把……塑造成
☐ **momentum** [məu'mentəm]	n. 气势，冲力；动量
☐ **monarchy** ['mɔnəki]	n. 君主立宪制，君主政体；君主国
☐ **morale** [mə'rɑːl]	n. 士气，斗志
☐ **mortal** ['mɔːtl]	a. 致死的；终有一死的；至死方休的
☐ **moss** [mɔs]	n. 苔藓，青苔
☐ **motel** [məu'tel]	n. 汽车旅馆

☐ **naked** ['neikid]	a. 裸体的；毫无遮掩的
☐ **nap** [næp]	n. 午睡
☐ **naturally** ['nætʃərəli]	ad. 当然，自然地；天然地，天生地

negative ['negətiv]	*a.* 否定的，消极的，反面的；负的，阴性的
neglect [ni'glekt]	*vt.* 疏于照顾；忽视，忽略；疏忽
neglectful [ni'glektful]	*a.* 忽略的；不留心的
network ['netwə:k]	*n.* 网络，网状系统；广播网，电视网
neutralize ['nju:trəlaiz]	*v.* 使中立
nickel ['nikl]	*n.* 镍，镍币 *vt.* 镀镍于
nickname ['nikneim]	*n.* 绰号，昵称 *vt.* 给……取绰号
nightmare ['naitmɛə(r)]	*n.* 噩梦；恐怖的经历，可怕的事件
nil [nil]	*n.* 无，零
nitrogen ['naitrədʒən]	*n.* 氮
noble ['nəubl]	*a.* 高尚的，贵族的，高贵的 *n.* 贵族
norm [nɔ:m]	*n.* 标准，规范；平均数
normalize ['nɔ:məlaiz]	*vt.* 使正常化，使标准化，使规格化
notation [nəu'teiʃən]	*n.* 符号
notion ['nəuʃən]	*n.* 观念，信念；想法，理解
notwithstanding [,nɔtwiθ'stændiŋ]	*prep.* 虽然，尽管 *ad.* 尽管，还是 *conj.* 虽然，尽管
nylon ['nailɔn]	*n.* 尼龙

oak [əuk]	n. 栎树，橡树，橡木 a. 橡木制的
obscene [əbˈsiːn]	a. 淫秽的，猥亵的
occurrence [əˈkʌrəns]	n. 发生的事情；发生，出现
odo(u)r [ˈəudər]	n. 气味，臭味
offset [ˈɔːfset]	n. 抵消，弥补；补偿 vt. 弥补，抵消；补偿
oily [ˈɔili]	a. 油的，油滑的
olive [ˈɔliv]	n. 橄榄树，橄榄叶；橄榄色
omission [əuˈmiʃən]	n. 省略，删除；遗漏；疏忽，失职
onset [ˈɔnset]	n. 攻击，进攻；有力的开始；某事的开始[发作]（尤指不好的事情）
opening [ˈəupniŋ]	a. 开始的，开幕的 n. 洞，孔，通道；开，开始，开端；空地；（职务的）空缺
opinionated [əˈpinjəneitid]	a. 固执己见的，武断的
opium [ˈəupjəm]	n. 鸦片
opt [ɔpt]	v. 选择
optic [ˈɔptik]	a. 眼的，视觉的；光学上的
oracle [ˈɔrəkl]	n. 神谕，预言；传神谕者

ore [ɔː(r)]	n. 矿石,矿砂
ouch [autʃ]	int. 哎唷 n.(皮带等的)扣环;胸针,饰针
ounce [auns]	n. 盎司,少量
oust [aust]	vt. 剥夺,取代,驱逐
outcome ['autkʌm]	n. 结果,后果,成果
outdated [aut'deitid]	a. 过时的;陈旧的
outer ['autə]	a. 外部的,外层的,外表的
outflow ['autfləu]	n. 外流,流出量
outlet ['autlet]	n. 出路;表现机会,专营店,批发商店;出口,排水口
outpost ['autpəust]	n. 前哨,边区村落
outreach ['autriːtʃ]	v. 超越,伸出;超出……的范围
outset ['autset]	n. 开端,开始
overhead ['əuvəhed]	ad. 在头顶上,在空中,在高处
overturn [,əuvə'təːn]	v.(使)推翻,(使)颠倒
oxide ['ɔksaid]	n. 氧化物

P

- **pamphlet** ['pæmflət] — n. 小册子
- **panel** ['pænl] — n. 专门小组；面板，控制板，仪表盘
- **panic** ['pænik] — n. 惊慌，恐慌 a. 恐慌的，惊慌的
- **parachute** ['pærəʃu:t] — n. 降落伞 v. 跳伞
- **parade** [pə'reid] — n. 游行，检阅 v. 游行
- **paragraph** ['pærəgrɑ:f] — n. 段，节
- **parcel** ['pɑ:sl] — n. 包裹，邮包 vt. 打包
- **parliament** ['pɑ:ləmənt] — n. 国会，议会
- **parliamentary** [,pɑ:lə'mentəri] — a. 议会的
- **particle** ['pɑ:tikl] — n. 粒子，微粒
- **partition** [pɑ:'tiʃən] — n. 分割，划分，瓜分，分开
- **pastry** ['peistri] — n. 面粉糕饼，馅饼皮
- **peculiarity** [pi,kju:li'æriti] — n. 特性，怪癖
- **pendulum** ['pendjələm] — n. 钟摆

☐ **petrochemical** [ˌpetrəʊˈkemɪkəl]	*a.* 石油化学的；岩石化学的	
☐ **petrol** [ˈpetrəl]	*n.* 汽油	
☐ **petroleum** [pɪˈtrəʊlɪəm]	*n.* 石油	
☐ **pilgrim** [ˈpɪlgrɪm]	*n.* 圣地朝拜者，朝圣	
☐ **pillar** [ˈpɪlə]	*n.* 柱子，栋梁	
☐ **pint** [paɪnt]	*n.* 品脱	
☐ **pioneer** [ˌpaɪəˈnɪə]	*n.* 先驱，倡导者，先锋	
☐ **piracy** [ˈpaɪərəsi]	*n.* 海上抢劫，侵犯版权，盗版	
☐ **pistol** [ˈpɪstl]	*n.* 手枪	
☐ **piston** [ˈpɪstən]	*n.* 活塞	
☐ **planetary** [ˈplænət(ə)ri]	*n.* 行星的	
☐ **plank** [plæŋk]	*n.* 板条；要点、核心	
☐ **plantation** [plænˈteɪʃən]	*n.* 种植园，大农场	
☐ **plaster** [ˈplɑːstə(r)]	*n.* 灰浆，石膏	
☐ **plateau** [ˈplætəʊ, plæˈtəʊ]	*n.* 高地，高原	
☐ **plight** [plaɪt]	*n.* 情况，状态，困境	
☐ **plural** [ˈplʊərəl]	*a.* 复数的	

polytechnic [ˌpɔliˈteknik]	a. 多种工艺的 n. 理工学院
pony [ˈpəuni]	n. 矮马，小马
Pope [pəup]	n. 天主教教皇
porch [pɔːtʃ]	n. 门廊，走廊
powder [ˈpaudə]	n. 粉末，药粉；火药
priest [priːst]	n. 传教士
proverb [ˈprɔvə(ː)b]	n. 谚语，格言
provocative [prəˈvɔkətiv]	a. 煽动的；[衣服、动作、图片等]挑逗性的
proximity [prɔkˈsimiti]	n. 接近、靠近、临近、亲近(to)
punch [pʌntʃ]	n. 冲压机，冲床；打孔机 vt. 冲孔，打孔
punctuate [ˈpʌŋktjueit]	v. 加标点(于)；强调，加强；不时打断
puppet [ˈpʌpit]	n. 木偶，傀儡

quake [kweik]	n. 地震 v. 颤抖、哆嗦
qualitative [ˈkwɔlitətiv]	a. 性质上的；定性的
quantify [ˈkwɔntifai]	vt. 确定数量，量化

☐ **quantitative** ['kwɔntitətiv]	*a.* 数量（上）的，定量的	
☐ **quart** [kwɔːt, kwɔːrt]	*n.* 夸脱（容量单位）	
☐ **quarter** ['kwɔːtə]	*n.* 四分之一；一刻钟；季度	
☐ **quilt** [kwilt]	*n.* 被子，棉被	

☐ **rack** [ræk]	*n.* 行李架	
☐ **radium** ['reidjəm]	*n.* [化] 镭	
☐ **ranger** ['reindʒə]	*n.* 森林守护员	
☐ **razor** ['reizə]	*n.* 剃刀	
☐ **reboot** [,riː'buːt]	*v.* 重新启动	
☐ **reed** [riːd]	*n.* 芦苇；芦笛，牧笛	
☐ **refinery** [ri'fainəri]	*n.* 精炼厂	
☐ **reign** [rein]	*n.* 君主统治时期，任期 *v.* 当政，统治	
☐ **relish** ['reliʃ]	*n.* 美味；味道；风味 *vt.* 爱好；喜欢	
☐ **repertoire** ['repətwɑː]	*n.* （剧团、演员等的）全部可表演节目，（某人的）全部才能	
☐ **republican** [ri'pʌblikən]	*a.* 共和国的；共和政体的 *n.* （美国）共和党党员	

☐ **reservoir** [ˈrezəvwɑː]	n. 水库；蓄水池
☐ **rifle** [ˈraɪfl]	n. 步枪
☐ **ribbon** [ˈrɪbən]	n. 带，缎带，丝带
☐ **roach** [rəʊtʃ]	n. 蟑螂
☐ **roast** [rəʊst]	v. 烤，炙，烘
☐ **royal** [ˈrɔɪəl]	a. 王室的；皇家的
☐ **rust** [rʌst]	v. 生锈

☐ **screw** [skruː]	n. 螺钉，螺 vt. 拧，拧紧；用螺丝固定
☐ **secular** [ˈsekjulə]	a. 不受宗教约束的，非宗教的；现世的，世俗的
☐ **semiconductor** [ˌsemɪkənˈdʌktə]	n. 半导体
☐ **senate** [ˈsenɪt]	n. 参议院
☐ **senator** [ˈsenətə]	n. 参议员
☐ **shrewd** [ʃruːd]	a. 精明的；有眼光的，判断得准的
☐ **shrub** [ʃrʌb]	n. 灌木丛
☐ **shrug** [ʃrʌg]	v./n. 耸肩

shutter ['ʃʌtə]	n. 遮蔽物；百叶窗，窗板；照相机快门
shuttle ['ʃʌtl]	n. 太空船，航天飞机
siege [si:dʒ]	n. 包围
sieve [siv]	n. 滤器，筛子 v. 滤；筛
sigh [sai]	vi. 叹气，叹息 n. 叹息声
signpost ['sainpəust]	n. 路标，路牌
sin [sin]	n. 罪孽 vi. 犯罪
singular ['siŋgjulə]	a. 单数的；突出的
sip [sip]	v. 小口喝，抿 n. 一小口（饮料）
siren ['saiərin]	n. 警笛
site [sait]	n. 地点，场所
sizable ['saizəbl]	a. 相当大的，大的
skyline ['skailain]	n. 地平线，以天空为背景映出轮廓
skyscraper ['skaiskreipə(r)]	n. 摩天大楼
slam [slæm]	v. 砰地关上，砰地放下
slang [slæŋ]	n. 俚语
sleeve [sli:v]	n. 袖子
slice [slais]	n. 片，薄片 v. 切片

slipper ['slipə]	n. 拖鞋
slippery ['slipəri]	a. 滑的，滑溜的；狡猾的
slot [slɔt]	n. 窄缝；(列表或名单中的)位置；投币机 v. 投放；塞进；插入
slum [slʌm]	n. 贫民窟
snack [snæk]	n. 快餐，小吃
snapshot ['snæpʃɔt]	n. 快照，快相
soak [səuk]	v. 浸湿，浸透
soar [sɔː, sɔə]	vi. 急升，猛增；高飞，翱翔
socket ['sɔkit]	n. 孔，插座
sour ['sauə]	a. 酸的，酸腐的；脾气坏的，刻薄的
source [sɔːs]	n. 源，源泉；来源，根源
sovereign ['sɔvrin]	n. 君主，元首 a. 有主权的；完全独立的；掌握全部权力的
sow [səu]	v. 播种
spacecraft ['speiskrɑːft]	n. 宇宙飞船
spacious ['speiʃəs]	a. 宽广的，宽敞的
spade [speid]	n. 铲子，铁锹
species ['spiːʃiz]	n. (物)种，种类
specific [spi'sifik]	n. 特效药；细节 a. 具体的，明确的；特殊的，特效的

specifically [spi'sifikəli]	ad. 明确地；特意；具体来说
specify ['spesifai]	vt. 指定；详细说明
spectacular [spek'tækjulə]	a. 壮观的
spelling ['speliŋ]	n. 拼法，拼写
spice [spais]	n. 香料
spinal ['spainl]	a. 脊柱的；有关脊柱的
stack [stæk]	n. 一叠，一堆；许多 v.（使）放成整齐的一叠，使成叠地放在……
stalk [stɔ:k]	n.（植物的）茎、杆 v. 偷偷接近（猎物或人）；（非法）跟踪；趾高气扬地走
sticky ['stiki]	a. 有黏性的；黏的
sting [stiŋ]	n. 叮，刺痛，刺激
stitch [stitʃ]	n. 针脚，（编织的）一针，针法 v. 缝补，缝合；做成
stout [staut]	a. 肥胖的，粗壮的；勇敢的；坚固的
strap [stræp]	n. 皮带；皮条 vt. 用带缚住，用带捆扎
streak [stri:k]	n. 条纹，条痕；个性特征；一阵子，一连 vi. 飞跑，疾驶 vt. 在……上加条纹
stump [stʌmp]	n. 树桩；残根，残余部分 vt. 把……难住，使为难，在……作巡回演说 vi. 脚步重重地走
suck [sʌk]	v. 吸，吮
suffice [sə'fais]	vi. 足够 (for)

☐ **sway** [swei]	*n.* 摇摆；影响力；支配 *vt.* 摇动
☐ **sweat** [swet]	*n.* 汗 *v.* 出汗
☐ **swift** [swift]	*a.* 快的，迅速的
☐ **symbol** ['simbəl]	*n.* 象征，符号，标志
☐ **symposium** [sim'pəuziəm]	*n.* 讨论会，专题报告会；专题论文集
☐ **synthesis** ['sinθəsis]	*n.* 综合，合成

☐ **tack** [tæk]	*n.* 平头钉，大头针，行动方向，方针 *vt.* 用平头钉钉，附加，增补
☐ **tan** [tæn]	*vt.* 使晒成棕褐色，硝制（皮革）*vi.* 晒成棕褐色 *n.* 棕褐色，棕黄色；晒成棕褐色，晒黑
☐ **tanker** ['tæŋkə]	*n.* 油轮
☐ **tentative** ['tentətiv]	*a.* 试探（性）的，实验（性）的
☐ **terrain** ['terein]	*n.* 地形，地势
☐ **thermos** ['θə:mɔs]	*n.* 热水瓶，暖瓶
☐ **thrombus** ['θrɔmbəs]	*n.* [医] 血栓 【经典例句】The thrombus forms in a blood vessel or within the heart and obstructs the circulation. A. clot　　　　　　　　　B. mass C. node　　　　　　　　　D. knot　　　　　　[A] 【译　　文】血栓形成于血管或心脏当中，堵塞血液流通。

thunder ['θʌndə]	n. 雷，轰隆响 vi. 打雷，轰隆响
tile [tail]	n. 瓦，瓷砖 vt. 铺瓦于，贴瓷砖于
torch [tɔ:tʃ]	n. 火把
tract [trækt]	n. 一片，一片土地；传单，小册子
transcontinental [,trænzkɔnti'nentəl]	a. 横贯大陆的
tribe [traib]	n. 部落，宗族
tribunal [tri'bjun(ə)l]/ [trai'bju:n(ə)l]	n. 法官席，审判员席，(特等)法庭
tribute ['tribju:t]	n. 颂词，称赞；(表示敬意的)礼物，贡品
trillion ['triljən]	n. 兆，万亿
triple ['tripl]	a. 三部分的，三方的，三倍的，三重的 v. (使)增至三倍
troop [tru:p]	n. (一)队，(一)群；(pl.)部队，军队
truly ['tru:li]	ad. 正确地，事实上；真诚地
trumpet ['trʌmpit]	n. 喇叭，小号
trunk [trʌŋk]	n. 树干，躯干；大箱子，(汽车后部)行李厢
tube [tju:b]	n. 管，软管；电子管，显像管
tuberculosis [tju,bə:kju'ləusis]	n. 结核病；肺结核
tug [tʌg]	v. 用力拖(或拉) n. 拖船，猛拉，牵引

☐ **turbine** ['tə:bain]	*n.* 汽轮机，涡轮机
☐ **turbulence** ['tə:bjuləns]	*n.* 骚动；动乱，暴乱；湍流

U

☐ **uranium** [juˈreiniəm]	*n.* 铀
☐ **utopia** [juːˈtəupiə]	*n.* 乌托邦；理想的完美境界；空想的社会改良计划

V

☐ **valve** [vælv]	*n.* 阀，阀门；电子管，真空管
☐ **vanilla** [vəˈnilə]	*n.* 香草精，香子兰精 *adj.* 香草味的
☐ **vapour** ['veipə]	*n.* 蒸气，雾气
☐ **vector** ['vektə(r)]	*n.* 矢量；向量；（传染疾病的）媒介，载体；（航空器的）航线
☐ **vent** [vent]	*n.* 通风口，排放口，（衣服底部的）开衩 *vt.* 表达，发泄（情感等）
☐ **vinegar** ['vinigə]	*n.* 醋
☐ **virgin** ['və:dʒin]	*n.* 处女 *a.* 贞洁的，纯洁的；未开发的
☐ **volt** [vəult, vɔlt]	*n.* 伏特（电压单位）

☐ **wag(g)on** ['wægən]	*n.* 运货马车，运货车
☐ **wage** [weidʒ]	*n.* 工资，报酬
☐ **wary** ['wɛəri]	*a.* 谨慎的，机警的，小心的
☐ **wasteland** ['weistlænd]	*n.* 荒地，不毛之地
☐ **watt** [wɔt]	*n.* 瓦特
☐ **wax** [wæks]	*n.* 蜡，蜂蜡 *vt.* 打蜡
☐ **webcast** ['webkɑːst]	*n.* 网络广播
☐ **whilst** [wailst]	*conj.* 当……时候；虽然，尽管
☐ **whip** [(h)wip]	*n.* 鞭子 *vt.* 鞭打，抽打；搅拌（奶油、蛋等）
☐ **whistle** ['(h)wisl]	*v.* 吹口哨，鸣笛 *n.* 口哨声，汽笛声；哨子，汽笛
☐ **wicked** ['wikid]	*a.* 邪恶的，恶劣的；淘气的，顽皮的；危险的 *n.* 恶人，邪恶的人
☐ **workshop** ['wəːkʃɔp]	*n.* 车间，工场；研讨会，讲习班
☐ **wrench** [rentʃ]	*vt.* 猛拧，猛扭，挣脱，使扭伤 *n.*（离别等的）痛苦，难受；猛拉；扳手

Y

☐ **yacht** [jɔt]	*n.* 游艇
☐ **Yankee** [ˈjæŋki]	*n.* 美国佬；(美国人中的) 北方佬
☐ **yoga** [ˈjəugə]	*n.* 瑜伽

Z

☐ **zinc** [ziŋk]	*n.* 锌

第五部分
医学专用词汇

全国医学博士英语
统考词汇巧战通关

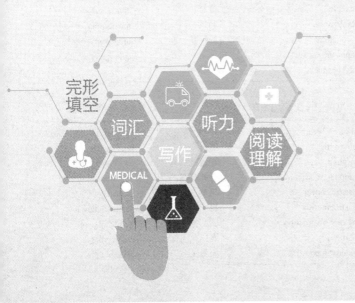

一、医学考博专业基础词汇大全

1.1 内科常用词汇

1.1.1 心血管系统 the Cardiovascular system

急性心肌梗死	acute myocardial infarction (AMI)	先天性心脏病	congenital heart disease
高血压性心血管疾病	hypertensive cardiovascular disease	心电图	electrocardiogram (ECG)
动脉硬化	arteriosclerosis	血管瘤	hemangioma
高血压	hypertension	血管扩张	vasodilatation
低血压	hypotension	肥大	hypertrophy
腺炎	adenitis 这个不常用，常用的是 lymphadenitis，淋巴结炎	静脉曲张	varicose veins
白细胞减少	leukocytopenia	白细胞	leukocyte

1.1.2 血液及淋巴系统 The Hemic and Lymphatic System

急性淋巴细胞白血病	acute lymphogenous leukemia	脾肿大	splenomegaly
系统性红斑性狼疮	systemic lupus erythematosus	贫血	anemia
无菌的	aseptic	败血症	septicemia
止血	hemostasis	输血	transfusion

1.1.3 呼吸系统 The Respiratory System

肺栓塞	pulmonary embolism	黏膜	mucosa
呼气	exhale	窒息	apnea
呼吸急促	tachypnea	肺炎	pneumonia
支气管炎	bronchitis	肺积脓	lung empyema
失语症	aphasia	失声	aphonia
语言障碍	dysphasia		

1.1.4 消化系统 The Digestive System

呼吸短促	short of breath	吞咽困难	dysphagia
齿龈炎	gingivitis	咽炎	pharyngitis
喉炎	laryngitis	食道镜检查	esophagoscopy
食道狭窄	esophagus stricture	腹腔穿刺术	abdominocentesis
胃癌	gastric cancer	胃炎	gastritis
胃肠炎	gastroenteritis	胃出血	gastrorrhagia
幽门阻塞	pyloric obstruction	十二指肠溃疡	duodenal ulcer
腹膜炎	peritonitis	肠出血	enterorrhagia
肠破裂	enterorrhexis	阑尾炎	appendicitis

（续）

结肠癌	colon cancer	直肠镜检查	proctoscopy
直肠癌	rectal cancer	肛门瘘管	anal fistula
排泄	excretion	外痔	external hemorrhoid
内痔	internal hemorrhoid	肝炎	hepatitis
肝脏肿大	hepatomegaly	胆结石	gall stone
胆石症	cholelithiasis	肝硬化	liver cirrhosis
腹水	ascites		

1.1.5 内分泌系统 The Endocrine System

高血糖	glycemia	甲状腺肿	goiter
糖尿病	diabetes mellitus	尿崩症	diabetes insipidus
汗臭症	bromidrosis	垂体肿瘤	pituitary tumor

1.1.6 神经系统 The Nervous System

脑动脉硬化	cerebral arteriosclerosis	脑出血	cerebral hemorrhage
脑水肿	cerebral edema	脑性麻痹	cerebral palsy
脑血栓	cerebral thrombosis	脑神经炎	cranial neuritis
颅内出血	intracranial hemorrhage	脑炎	encephalitis
肌电图	electromyography	神经炎	neuritis
癫痫	epilepsy	三叉神经痛	trigeminal neuralgia
佝偻症	rachitis	脊柱侧弯	rachio scoliiosis
脊椎炎	spondylitis	四肢麻痹	quadriplegia
下半身瘫痪	paraplegia	即刻意识丧失	immediately loss of consciousness
睁眼反应	eye opening response	舞蹈症	chorea
语言反应	verbal response	运动反应	motor response
角膜反射	corneal reflex	膝反射	plantar reflex
坐骨神经痛	sciatica	肌萎缩	muscle atrophy
偏头痛	migraine	帕金森症	Parkinson's disease
脑水肿	brain swelling	脑震荡	brain concussion
脑缺氧症	brain anoxia	脑死亡	brain death

1.1.7 肌肉骨骼系统 The Musculoskeletal System

前十字韧带	anterior cruciate ligament	退行性关节炎	degenerated joint disease
关节硬化	arthrosclerosis	骨盆骨折	pelvic fracture
锁骨骨折	clavicle fracture	转移性肿瘤病灶	matastatic lesion
骨质疏松症	osteoporosis	截肢	amputation
骨移植	bone graft	大拇指外翻	hallux valgus
假体置换	prosthesis replacement	运动范围	range of motion
内翻	varus	软骨软化症	chondromalacia
类风湿性关节炎	rheumatoid arthritis		

1.1.8 泌尿及男性生殖系统 The Urinary and Male Reproductive System

膀胱炎	cystitis	包皮环割术	circumcision
膀胱镜检查	cystoscopy	肾水肿	hydronephrosis
肾结石	renal stone	急性肾衰竭	acute renal failure
隐睾症	cryptorchidism	精子生成	spermatogenesis
良性前列腺肥大	benign prostatic hypertrophy	输尿管狭窄	ureteral stenosis
排尿困难	dysuria	血尿	hematuria
尿毒症	uremia	尿路感染	urinary tract infection
输精管结扎	vasoligation	阳痿	impotence

1.1.9 特殊感觉器官 The Organs of Special Senses

听力计	audiometer	耳炎	otitis
耳漏	otorrhea	中耳炎	tympanitis
鼓膜穿破术	tympanotomy	鼻炎	nasitis
鼻咽癌	nasopharyngeal carcinoma	鼻溢	rhinorrhea
眼科医师	ophthalmologist	眼内异物	intraocular foreign body
眼内压	intraocular pressure	双眼	oculus uterque
左眼	oculus sinister	右眼	oculus dexter
眼外肌	extraocular muscle	复视	diplopia
近视	myopia	眼睑下垂	blepharoptosis
角膜炎	corneitis	瞳孔大小不等	pupil size anisocoria
视网膜固定术	retinopexy	视网膜剥落	retinal detachment
视野	visual field	声带结节	vocal nodular
白内障	cataract	青光眼	glaucoma
皮肤科医师	dermatologist	皮炎	dermatitis

1.1.10 综合性词汇

避孕的	contraceptive	禁忌证	contraindication
生物学	biology	剧吐	hyperemesis
剧渴	polydipsia	同性的	homosexual
异性的	heterosexual	注射	inject
脂肪瘤	lipoma	脂肪样的	lipoid
脂肪过多症	lipomatosis	畸形	malformation
不适	malaise	坏死	necrosis
夜尿症	nocturia	多尿	polyuria
麻醉药	narcotics	增殖	hyperplasia
发育不良	dysplasia	消化不良	dyspepsia
预后	prognosis	解热剂	antipyretic
恐水症	hydrophobia	畏光	photophobia
抗生素	antibiotic	症状	syndrome
水疗法	hydrotherapy	穿孔	perforation
叩诊	percussion	脏器痛	visceralgia

1.2 妇产科常用词汇

生殖的	genital	妇科	gynecology
月经	menstruation	绝经	menopause
闭经	amenorrhea	经血过多	menorrhagia
痛经	dysmenorrhea	初潮	menarche
子宫颈癌	cervical cancer	子宫颈糜烂	cervical erosion
子宫颈炎	cervicitis	会阴	perineum
卵巢	ovary	子宫内膜异位	endometriosis
卵巢囊肿	ovarian cyst	排卵	ovulation
阴道炎	vaginitis	阴道镜检法	colposcopy
乳腺囊肿	galactocele	乳房X光摄影术	mammography
不孕症	infertility	体外受精	in vitro fertilization
羊膜	amnion	羊水穿刺术	amniocentesis
羊水栓塞	amniotic fluid embolism	羊水过多	hydramnion
产前的	antenatal	分娩前	antepartum
绒毛膜绒毛取样	chorionic villi sampling	头盆不称	cephalo-pelvic disproportion
人工授精	artificial insemination	胎头入盆	engagement
雌激素	estrogen	初乳	colostrum
黄体	corpus luteum	终止妊娠	termination of pregnancy
胎吸助产	vacuum extraction delivery	性病	venereal disease
输卵管结扎	tubal ligation	腹腔镜	laparoscope
胚胎	embryo	异位妊娠	ectopic gestation
初产妇	primipara	胎姿势	attitude of fetus
胎死腹中	dead fetus in uterus	经产妇	multipara
产次（相对于孕次 gravidity）	parity	前置胎盘	placenta previa
产后	postpartum	产后出血	postpartum hemorrhage
妊娠毒血症；子痫前期	toxemia of pregnancy	青春期	adolescence
基础体温	basal body temperature	剖腹产	cesarean section
预产期	expected date of confinement	输卵管	fallopian tube
产钳	forceps	葡萄胎	hydatidiform mole
阵痛	labor pain	无痛分娩	painless labor
胎头变形	molding	正常自然产	normal spontaneous delivery
子宫颈涂片检查	papanicolaou smear	胎膜早破	premature rupture of membrane
孕激素	progesterone	死产	stillbirth
缝合	suture	残物	stump
激素撤退后出血	withdrawal bleeding		

1.3 小儿科常用词汇

呼吸暂停	apnea	动静脉畸形	arteriovenous malformation
支气管气喘	bronchial asthma	红斑	erythema
支气管炎	bronchitis	尿道下裂	hypospadia
头皮血肿	cephalohematoma	脑积水	hydrocephalus
脱水	dehydration	多指（趾）畸形	polydactylia
阴囊积水	hydrocele	败血症	sepsis
脓皮病	pyoderma	脑炎	encephalitis
扁桃腺炎	tonsillitis	恶性的	malignant
肠胃炎	gastroenteritis	先天性畸形	congenital malformation
坏死性小肠结肠炎	necrotizing enterocolitis	腭裂	cleft palate
新生儿窒息	neonatal asphyxia	龋齿	dental caries
腹泻	diarrhea	荨麻疹	hives urticaria
颜面神经麻痹	facial nerve paralysis	疫苗	vaccine
斜颈	torticollis	兔唇	cleft lip
保温箱	incubator	马蹄内翻足	club foot
水痘	chicken pox	登革热	dengue fever
白喉	diphtheria	先天性梅毒	congenital syphilis
湿疹	eczema	巨婴	giant baby
风疹	German measles / rubella	乙型肝炎	hepatitis
手足口病	hand-foot-mouth disease	黄疸	jaundice
呼吸骤停	respiratory arrest	腮腺炎	mumps
呕吐	vomiting	幼儿急疹	roseola infantum
再生障碍性贫血	aplastic anemia		

1.4 精神科常用词汇

智力障碍	mental retardation	自闭症	autism
痴呆症	dement	酒瘾	alcoholism
阿尔茨海默症	Alzheimer's dementia	物质中毒	substances intoxication
酒精中毒	alcohol intoxication	安非他命中毒	amphetamine intoxication
精神分裂	schizophrenia	妄想性病患	delusional disorder
恐惧症	phobia	重症抑郁	major depressive disorder
强迫症	obsessive-compulsive disorder	恋童癖	pedophilia
暴露狂	exhibitionism	异装癖	transvestic fetishism
性别认同异常	gender identity disorders	心因性厌食症	anorexia nervosa
心因性暴食症	bulimia nervosa	感情迟钝	blunted affect
傻笑	silly laughter	冷漠	apathy
易怒的	irritable	忧郁	depression
感情淡漠	flat affect	物理约束	physical restraint
怪异行为	queer behavior	感情矛盾	ambivalence
怪异行为	bizarre behavior	自杀企图	suicide attempt
少话	hypo talkative	不语	mutistic

(续)

活动减退	hypoactivity	多话	hyper talkative
语言重复症	verbigeration	活动过多	hyperactivity
违拗行为	negativism	强迫行为	compulsive behavior
破坏行为	destructive behavior	木僵	catalepsy
言语贫乏	poverty of speech	言语急迫	pressured speech
思考连接松散	loosening of association	思考中断	thought blocking
不合逻辑思考	illogical thinking	思想退缩	thought withdrawal
语无伦次	incoherent	妄想	delusion
答非所问	irrelevant	恐高症	acrophobia
被害妄想	delusion of persecution	性欲	sexual drive
惧痛症	algophobia	幻觉	hallucination
错觉	illusion	失去定向力	disorientation
听幻觉	auditory hallucination	虚谈症	confabulation
记忆丧失症	amnesia	判断力	judgement
定向力	orientation	自由联想	free association
失真感	derealization	原我	id
自我	ego	自我界限	ego boundary
超我	superego	原欲	libido
梦的解析	dream analysis	内在冲突	internal conflict
代罪羔羊	scapegoat	无意识	unconsciousness
意识	consciousness	移情	transference
前意识	preconsciousness	脱离现实	derealization
人格解体	depersonalization	神经病	psychosis
神经精神病	neurosis	现实原则	reality principle
享乐原则	pleasure principle	潜在因素	predisposing factors
道德原则	moral principle	防卫机制	defense mechanism
诱发因素	precipitating factors	转化作用	conversion
补偿作用	compensation	转移作用	displacement
否认作用	denial	幻想作用	fantasy
解离作用	dissociation	内射作用	introjection
认同作用	identification	合理化作用	rationalization
外射作用	projection	退化作用	degression
反向作用	reaction formation	压抑作用	suppression
潜抑作用	repression	升华作用	sublimation
归还作用	restitution	象征作用	symbolism
取代作用	substitution	歪曲作用	distortion
抵消作用	undoing	认知行为疗法	cognitive behavioral therapy
隔离作用	isolation	阻抗	resistance
同理心	empathy	自我了解	self-awareness
试探行为	testing out behavior	增强原则	reinforcement
分离焦虑	separation anxiety	对抗	confrontation
情绪宣泄	catharsis	约束	restraint
倾听	listen	药物性约束	chemical restraint

1.5 各科常用缩写

		A			
AAD	against- advice discharge	自行离院	A	abdomen	腹部
ADL	activities of daily life	日常生活活动	A/G	albumin / globulin ration	白蛋白 / 球白比例
AK	above knee	膝上			

		B			
BE	below elbow	肘下	BH	body height	身高
b.i.d	twice a day	一日两次	Bil	bilateral	两侧的
BK	below knee	膝下	BM	bowel movement	肠蠕动
BMR	basal metabolic rate	基础代谢率	BPH	benign prostatic hypertrophy	良性前列腺肥大
BTI	biliary tract infection	胆道感染	BUS	blood, urine, stool	血液，小便，大便
BW	body weight	体重			

		C			
Ca.	Carcinoma	癌	CBC	complete blood count	全血球计数
CBD	common bile duct	胆总管	CH	cerebral hemorrhage	脑出血
Chest P-A	chest posterior-anterior	前后胸部	CO	cardiac output	心输出量
CPR	cardiopulmonary resuscitation	心肺复苏术	CPS	chronic paranasal sinusitis	慢性鼻窦炎
C/T	chemotherapy	化疗	CT	cerebral thrombosis	脑栓塞
CT scan	computerized axial tomography scan	电脑断层检查	CVA	cerebral vascular accident	脑血管意外
CVP	central venous pressure	中心静脉压			

		D			
DC	discontinue	停止	D&C	dilatation and curettage	清宫术（宫颈扩张＋吸除）
DM	diabetes mellitus	糖尿病	DPT	diphtheria, pertussis, tetanus	白喉，百日咳，破伤风
DU	duodenal ulcer	十二指肠溃疡			

		E			
ECG	electrocardiogram	心电图	EEG	electroencephalogram	脑电波图
ENT	ear, nose, throat	耳鼻喉			

		F			
FH	family history	家族史	FHS	fetal heart sounds	胎心音
FOU	fever of unknown	不明原因发烧	Fr	fracture	骨折

G

GB	gall bladder	胆囊	GI tract	gastric intestinal tract	胃肠道
GSR	general surgical routine	一般外科常规	gtt.	Drops	滴（静脉滴注的拉丁文缩写）
GU	genitourinary	生殖泌尿的	GYN	gynecology	妇科学

H

Hb	hemoglobin	血色素	HICH	hypertensive intracerebral hemorrhage	高血压性脑内出血
h.s.	at bedtime	睡前	HT	hypertension	高血压
Ht.	(Hct.) Hematocrit	血球压积	Hx	history	病例

I

ICP	intermittent catheterization program	间歇性导尿	ICU	intensive care unit	加护病房
ICT	intracerebral tumor	脑内肿瘤	I & D	incision and drainage	切开及引流
IICP	increased intracranial pressure	胪内压升高	Imp.	impression	临床印象
IM	intramuscular	肌肉内的	I & O	intake and output	出入量
IV	intravenous	静脉内的	IVKO	intravenous keep open	静脉点滴维持通畅

J

Jej.	jejunum	空肠	Jt.	joint	关节

K

Kn.	knee	膝	KUB	kidney, ureter, bladder	肾、输尿管及膀胱

L

LFT	liver function test	肝功能试验	LLQ	left lower quadrant	左下腹
LMP	last menstrual period	末次月经			

MBD	may be discharged	可出院	MN	midnight	午夜

N

NKA	non known allergy	不明原因的过敏	NP	nothing particular	并无特别的
NPC	nasopharyngeal carcinoma	鼻咽癌	NPO	nothing by mouth	禁食

O

OA	osteoarthritis	骨性关节炎	OB	occult blood	潜血
OBS	obstetrics	产科	OP	operation	手术
OPD	outpatient department	门诊	Ortho.	orthopaedic	骨科的
OS	oculus sinister	左眼主视	OT	occupational therapy	职能治疗
OU	both eyes	双眼			

P

p.c.	after meals	饭后	PCT	penicillin test	青霉素皮试
PE	physical examination	体格检查	PI	present illness	现病史
p.o.	by mouth	由口	PPU	perforated peptic ulcer	穿孔性消化溃疡
PT	physical therapy	物理治疗	PTA	prior to admission	入院前
PTN	parenteral total nutrition	肠道外营养			

Q

Q	every	每一	q.d.	every day	每日
q.h	every hour	每小时	q.i.d.	four times a day	每日四次
q.m.	every morning	每日早晨	q.n.	every night	每日晚间

R

RA	rheumatoid arthritis	类风湿性关节炎	RBC	red blood cell	红细胞
RN	registered nurse	注册护士	R/O	rule out	排除
RR	recovery room	恢复室	R/T	radio-therapy	放射治疗
RUQ	right upper quadrant	右上腹	Rx	take	完成如下医嘱
	medication	用药		treatment	治疗

S

Sc.	subcutaneous	皮下的	SOB	short of breath	呼吸短促
SP.g.r.	specific gravity	比重	S/P	status/ post operation	手术后
s-s	half	一半	St	(stat) immediately	立刻
Staph.	staphylococcus	葡萄球菌			

T

t.i.d.	three times a day	每日三次	TPR	temperature, pulse, respirations	体温、脉搏、呼吸
TURP	transurethral resection of prostate	经尿道切除前列腺			

U

URI	upper respiratory infection	上呼吸道感染

W

WBC	white blood cell	白细胞	white blood cell count	白细胞计数

Y

Y/O	year old	年龄

Z

zero		零

1.6 解剖式内外科常用词汇

心血管系统	the cardiovascular system	阑尾	appendix
血管	vessels	空肠回肠	ileum
心脏	heart	大肠	large intestine
静脉	vein	肛门	anus
血液	blood	胃	stomach
红细胞	red blood cell	肺脏	lungs
血小板	platelet	毛细血管	capillaries
主支气管	bronchial tube	动脉	artery
咽	pharynx	凝血	blood clot
气管	trachea	血液及淋巴系统	the hemic and lymphatic system
小支气管	bronchioles	白细胞	white blood cell
胸	chest	呼吸系统	the respiratory system
消化系统	the digestive system	肺泡	alveolus
牙齿	teeth	喉	larynx
胆管	bile duct	肺	lung
胸膜	pleura	虹膜	iris
气	air	内直肌	internal rectus muscle
唇	lips	泪小管	lacrimal canaliculi
舌	tongue	泪腺管	excretory lacrimal duct
胆囊	gall bladder	耳蜗	cochlea
十二指肠空肠	duodenum jejunum	耳壳	helix
小肠	small intestine	外耳道	external auditory canal
直肠	rectum	锤骨	malleus
胰	pancreas	齿龈	gingiva
食道	esophagus	前磨牙	premolars
咽	pharynx	内分泌系统	the endocrine system
腺体	glands	肾上腺	adrenals
垂体	pituitary	甲状腺和甲状旁腺	thyroid and parathyroids
乳房	breasts	卵巢	ovaries
神经系统	the nervous system	脑	brain
脊髓	spinal cord	脊椎	vertebra
颅腔	cranium	脑膜	meninges
神经	nerves	肌肉骨骼系统	the musculoskeletal system
头骨	skull	锁骨	clavicle
胸骨	sternum	肋骨	ribs
关节	joints	韧带	ligaments
肌腱	tendons	软骨	cartilage
泌尿及男性生殖系统	the urinary and male reproductive system	皮质	cortex
尿道	urethra	输尿管	ureters
肾脏	kidney	肾盂	renal pelvis
输精管	vas deferens	膀胱	urinary bladder

(续)

前列腺	prostate gland	阴囊	scrotum
睾丸	testicle	阴茎	penis
特殊感觉器官	the organs of special senses	听神经	acoustic nerve
耳朵	ear	听觉的	hearing
耳咽管	tube	耳鼓膜	eardrum
欧式管	eustachian	鼻腔	nasal cavities
鼻	nose	眼睑	eyelid
晶状体	lens	角膜	cornea
泪管	tear duct	结膜	conjunctiva
脉络膜	choroid layer	视网膜	retina
巩膜	sclera	视神经	optic nerve
妇产科	obstetrics & gynecology	输卵管	fallopian tube
卵巢	ovary	子宫	uterus
阴道	vagina	外阴	vulva
大脑	cerebrum	胼胝体	corpus callosum
视丘	thalamus	小脑	cerebellum
间脑	diencephalon	大脑脚	cerebral peduncles
漏斗	infundibulum	垂体	hypophysis
中脑	midbrain	脑桥	pons
延髓	medulla	脑干	brain stem
瞳孔	pupil	悬韧带	suspensory ligaments
睫状突	ciliary process	网膜静脉	retinal veins
网膜动脉	retinal arteries	视神经	optic nerve
前眼房	anterior chamber	后眼房	posterior chamber
玻璃体	vitreous body	尖牙	canines
泪孔	lacrimal puncta	中切牙	incisors
泪腺	lacrimal gland	上唇	upper lip
眉毛	eyebrow	齿槽突	alveolar
耳咽管	eustachian tube	颚扁桃腺	palatine tonsil
鼓膜	tympanic membrane	口腔前庭	vestibule of mouth
半规管	semicircular canals	上唇系带	upper lip frenulum
前庭耳蜗神经	vestibulocochlear nerve	硬腭	hard palate
磨牙	molars	舌下阜	sublingual caruncle

1.7 癌症相关单词

胃癌	gastric cancer	胰脏癌	pancreatic cancer
结肠癌	colon cancer	直肠癌	rectal cancer
前列腺癌	prostate cancer	鼻咽癌	nasopharyngeal carcinoma
子宫颈癌	cervical cancer	肺癌	lung cancer

(续)

食道癌	esophageal cancer	膀胱癌	bladder cancer
喉癌	laryngeal caner	卵巢癌	ovarian cancer
肝癌	liver cancer	皮肤癌	skin cancer
乳癌	breast cancer	白血病	leukemia
骨癌	bone cancer	脑瘤	brain tumor
淋巴瘤	lymphoma		

1.8 医院内常见单词

医院	hospital	护理学校	nursing school = nursing home
慢性疾病或恢复期的患者疗养的私立小医院	private convalescence hospital	内科	department of medicine = department of internal medicine
住院医师	resident in medicine	内科主任	chief of medicine (medical man)
实习生	internist = intern	访问医生	extern
医学院学生（通常大三或大四学生）	junior and senior students	护理学生	student nurse
轮转阶段的学生	clinical clerk	注册护士	registered nurse (R.N.)
护理学校毕业的护士	graduate nurse	护士长	head nurse
督导护士	supervisor	从业医生	practicing physician = physician in practice = practitioner
刷手护士	scrub nurse	可走动不必卧床的病人	ambulant
麻醉药	narcotic / anaesthetic	装病的人（malinger 装病）	malingerer
住院的可走动的患者	ambulatory patient	诊疗错误	malpractice
瘫痪患者	paretic	病房	ward
急诊室	emergency room	恢复室	recovery room
护理站	station	患者，病人	patient
护士	nurse	医生	doctor
内科医生	internist	外科医生	surgeon
牙科医生	dentist	妇科医生	gynecologist
眼科医生	oculist	骨科医生	orthopedist
小儿科医生	pediatrician	精神病医生	psychiatrist
实习医生	intern	诊疗台	examination table

403

(续)

体温计	clinical thermometer	听诊器	stethoscope
反光镜	reflector	X光检查	X-ray checkup
X光片	X-ray photograph	手术	operation
手术刀	scalpel	针筒	syringe
注射针	hypodermic needle	注射	injection
冰袋	ice bag	固定镊	fixation forceps
药品	medicine, drug	绷带	bandage
脱脂棉	absorbent cotton	纱布	gauze
口罩	mask	轮椅	wheel chair
救护车	ambulance	担架	stretcher
病历表	chart	处方	prescription
血压	blood pressure	血型	blood type
人工呼吸	artificial respiration	药丸	pill
胶囊	capsule	软膏	ointment
碘酒	iodine tincture	镇静剂	sedative
重症病房	intensive care unit (ICU)	心肺复苏术	cardiopulmonary resuscitation (CPR)
点滴	intravenous drip	化疗	chemotherapy
计算机断层扫描	computerized topography (CT)	核磁共振	magnetic resonance imaging (MRI)
骨折	fracture	石膏	gypsum

1.9 诊断用具

听诊器	stethoscope	血压计	Sphygmomanometer (blood pressure cuff)
体温计	thermometer	检眼镜	ophthalmoscope
耳镜	otoscope	喉镜	laryngeal mirror
手电	flashlight	压舌板	tongue depressor (tongue blade)
叩诊锤	hammer (percussion / reflex hammer)	音叉	tuning fork
卷尺	tape measure	尺	scale (ruler)
放大镜	loupe (magnifying glass; hand lens)	橡胶手套	rubber gloves
指套	finger cot	阴道窥器	vaginal speculum

(续)

二、医学考博专用词汇大全

2.1 【常见科室篇】

2.1.1 常见科室

department of dermatology	皮肤科	department of infectious diseases	传染病科
department of pathology	病理科	department of psychiatry	精神科
department of orthopaedic surgery	矫形外科	department of cardiac surgery	心脏外科
department of cerebral surgery	脑外科	department of thoracic surgery	胸外科
pharmacy dispensary	药房	nutrition department	营养部
diet-preparation department	配膳室	therapeutic department	治疗室
operating room/Theater	手术室	blood-bank	血站
supply-room	供应室	disinfection-room	消毒室
dressing room	换药室	mortuary	太平间
record room	病案室	department of plastic surgery	矫形外科
department of physiotherapy	理疗科	electrotherapy room	电疗科
heliotherapy room	光疗科	wax-therapy room	蜡疗科
hydrotherapy room	水疗科	central laboratory	中心实验室
clinical laboratory	临床实验室	bacteriological laboratory	细菌实验室
biochemical laboratory	生化实验室	serological laboratory	血清实验室
X-ray room	X 光室	doctor's office	医生办公室
nurse's office	护士办公室		

2.1.2 科室人员

director of the hospital	院长	physician	内科医师
chief physician	主任医师	associate chief physician	副主任医师
attending doctor	主治医师	resident doctor	住院医师
intern doctor	实习医师	general practitioner	全科医师
specialist	专科医师	head of the nursing department	护理部主任
Head nurse	护士长	Student nurse	实习护士
E.N.T.doctor	耳鼻喉科医师		

2.2 【西医篇】

2.2.1 医院部门及科室名称

2.2.1.1 医学学科

医学	Medicine	基础医学	Basic Medicine
人体解剖与组织胚胎学	Human Anatomy, Histology and Embryology	免疫学	Immunology
病原生物学	Pathogenic Organisms	病理学与病理生理学	Pathology and Pathophysiology
法医学	Forensic Medicine	放射医学	Radiation Medicine
航空航天与航海医学	Aerospace and Nautical medicine	临床医学	Clinical Medicine
内科学（含心血管病学、血液病学、呼吸系病学、消化系病学、内分泌与代谢病学、肾脏病学、风湿病学、传染病学）	Internal medicine (including Cardiology, Hematology, Respiratory, Gastroenterology, Endocrinology and Metabolism, Nephrology, Rheuma-tology, Infectious Diseases)	儿科学	Pediatrics
老年医学	Geriatrics	神经病学	Neurology
精神病与精神卫生学	Psychiatry and Mental Health	皮肤病与性病学	Dermatology and Venereology
影像医学与核医学	Imaging and Nuclear Medicine	临床检验诊断学	Clinical Laboratory Diagnostics
护理学	Nursing	外科学（含普通外科学、骨外科学、泌尿外科学、胸心血管外科学、神经外科学、整形外科学、烧伤外科学、野战外科学）	Surgery (General Surgery, Orthopedics, Urology, Cardiothoracic Surgery, Neurosurgery, Plastic Surgery, Burn Surgery, Field Surgery)
妇产科学	Obstetrics and Gynecology	眼科学	Ophthalmic Specialty
耳鼻咽喉科学	Otolaryngology	肿瘤学	Oncology
康复医学与理疗学	Rehabilitation Medicine Physical Therapy	运动医学	Sports Medicine
麻醉学	Anesthesiology	急诊医学	Emergency Medicine
口腔医学	Stomatology	口腔基础医学	Basic Science of Stomatology
口腔临床医学	Clinical Science of Stomatology	公共卫生与预防医学	Public Health and Preventive Medicine
流行病与卫生统计学	Epidemiology and Health Statistics	劳动卫生与环境卫生学	Occupational and Environmental Health
营养与食品卫生学	Nutrition and Food Hygiene	儿少卫生与妇幼保健学	Maternal, Child and Adolescent Health
卫生毒理学	Hygiene Toxicology	军事预防医学	Military Preventive Medicine

（续）

中医学	Chinese Medicine	中医基础理论	Basic Theories of Chinese Medicine
中医临床基础	Clinical Foundation of Chinese Medicine	中医医史文献	History and Literature of Chinese Medicine
方剂学	Formulas of Chinese Medicine	中医诊断学	Diagnostics of Chinese Medicine
中医内科学	Chinese Internal Medicine	中医外科学	Surgery of Chinese Medicine
中医骨伤科学	Orthopedics of Chinese Medicine	中医妇科学	Gynecology of Chinese Medicine
中医儿科学	Pediatrics of Chinese Medicine	中医五官科学	Ophthalmology and Otolaryngology of Chinese Medicine
针灸推拿学	Acupuncture and Moxibustion and Tuina of Chinese medicine	民族医学	Ethnomedicine
中西医结合医学	Chinese and Western Integrative Medicine	中西医结合基础医学	Basic Discipline of Chinese and Western Integrative
中西医结合临床医学	Clinical Discipline of Chinese and Western Integrative Medicine	药学	Pharmaceutical Science
药物化学	Medicinal Chemistry	药剂学	Pharmaceutics
生药学	Pharmacognosy	药物分析学	Pharmaceutical Analysis
微生物与生化药学	Microbial and Biochemical Pharmacy	药理学	Pharmacology
中药学	Science of Chinese Pharmacology		

2.2.1.2 医院部门

out-patient department	门诊部	In-patient department	住院部
Nursing department	护理部	Admission office	住院处
Discharge office	出院处	Registration office	挂号处
Reception room, waiting room	候诊室	Consultation room	诊察室
Isolation room	隔离室	Delivery room	分娩室
Emergency room	急诊室	Ward	病房室
Department of internal medicine	内科	Department of surgery	外科
Department of pediatrics	儿科	Department of obstetrics and gynecology	妇科
Department of neurology	神经科	Department of ophthalmology	眼科
E.N.T.department	耳鼻喉科	Department of stomatology	口腔科
Department of urology	泌尿科	Department of orthopedic	骨科
Department of traumatology	创伤科	Department of endocrinology	内分泌科
Department of anesthesiology	麻醉科		

2.2.2 医务人员名称

Ophthalmologist	眼科医师	Dentist	牙科医师
Orthopedist	骨科医师	Dermatologist	皮肤科医师
urologist surgeon	泌尿外科医师	neurosurgeon	神经外科医师
plastic surgeon	矫形外科医师	anaesthetist	麻醉科医师
Doctor for tuberculosis	结核科医师	Physiotherapist	理疗科
Doctor for infectious diseases	传染病科	Dietician	营养科医师
Pediatrician	儿科医师	Obstetrician	产科医师
Midwife	助产师	Gynecologist	妇科医师
Radiologist	放射科医师	Epidemiologist	流行病医师
Pharmacist	药剂医师	Assistant pharmacist	药剂医士
Laboratory technician	化验员	Assistant nurse	卫生员
Cleaner	清洁员	Controller	总务科长
Registrar	挂号员	Sanitation worker	消毒员

2.2.3 常用临床医学术语

diseases	疾病	acute diseases	急性病
advanced diseases	病沉重期，晚期疾病	chronic diseases	慢性病
communicable diseases	传染病	complicating diseases	并发病
congenital diseases	先天性疾病	acquired diseases	后天性疾病
low-residue diet	低渣饮食	nourishing diet	滋补饮食
obesity diet	肥胖病饮食	prenatal diet	孕期饮食
regimen diet	规定食谱	smooth (soft) diet	细软饮食
shaving the patient's skin (skin prep)	备皮	anesthesia	麻醉
postoperative care	手术后护理	applying elastic bandages	用弹性绷带
Emergency care (first aid)	急救护理	cardiopulmonary resuscitation	心肺循环复苏术
mouth-to-mouth (mouth-to-nose, mouth-to-stoma) resuscitation	口对口循环复苏术	emergency care for fainting (shock, stroke) victims	昏厥（休克、中风）患者急救
emergency care used to control hemorrhage	止血急救	postmortem care	死后护理
contagious diseases	接触性传染病	endemic diseases	地方病
epidemic diseases	流行病	functional diseases	机能病、官能病
infectious diseases	传染病	inherited diseases	遗传病
malignant diseases	恶性病	nutritional diseases	营养病
occupation diseases	职业病	organic diseases	器质性病
paroxysmal diseases	阵发性病	periodical diseases	周期病

primary (principal) diseases	原发（主导）病	secondary diseases	继发病
sexual (venereal, social) diseases	性病	terminal diseases	绝症
wasting diseases	消耗性疾病	chief complaint	主诉
clinical manifestation	临床表现	delivery history	分娩史
etiology	病因学	family history	家族史
history, medical history	病史	precipitating (induced)	诱因
marital status	婚姻状况	menstrual history	月经史
menarche	初潮	menopause	闭经
past history	既往史	pathogenesis	发病机制
personal history	个人史	symptoms	症状
cardinal symptom	主要症状	classical symptom	典型症状
concomitant symptom	伴发症状	constitutional (systemic) symptom	全身症状
indirect symptom	间接症状	induced symptom	诱发症状
local symptom	局部症状	mental symptom	精神症状
symptom-complex	征群	sign	体征
antecedent	前驱征	assident (accessory) sign	副征
commemorative	后遗症	sign of death	死征
diagnostic	诊断征	sign of disease	病征
subjective	自觉征，主观征	vein sign	静脉征
vital sign	生命体征	body length (height of the body)	身高
body weight	体重	barrel chest	桶状胸
cachexia	恶病质	compulsive position	被动体位
critical facies	病危面容	emaciation	消瘦
enophthalmos	眼球下陷	entropion	睑内翻
exophthalmos	眼球突出	flushed face	面色潮红
gain (loss) in weight	增加（减轻）体重	lock-jaw	牙关紧闭
lordosis	脊柱前凸	nasal ala flap	鼻翼扇动
nystagmus	眼震	obesity	肥胖
pallor	苍白	scoliosis	脊柱侧凸
agitation	焦急不安	debility, weakness	虚弱
diaphoresis	出汗，大量出汗	dizziness, vertigo	眩晕
lassitude, fatigue	无力，倦怠	malaise	不适
night sweat	盗汗	numbness	麻木
rigor, chill	寒冷，发冷	perspiration, sweating	出汗
pruritus, itching	痒，	somasthenia	躯体无力
tingling	麻刺感	abscess	脓肿
acidosis	酸中毒	adhesion	粘连
alkalosis	碱中毒	allergy	过敏

(续)

coagulation defect	凝血不良	congestion	充血
dehydration	脱水	distention	膨胀
edema	水肿	embolism	栓塞，栓塞形成
fluid and electrolyte imbalance	水电解质紊乱	gangrene	坏疽
hematoma	血肿	hemorrhage, bleeding	出血
infarction	梗死	infection	传染
inflammation	炎症	ketoacidosis	酮酸中毒
metastasis	转移	perforation	穿孔
necrosis	坏死	shock	休克
response	反应，应答	reaction	反应，感应
thrombosis	血栓形成	ulceration	溃疡
fever, pyrexia	发烧，发热	continuous fever	稽留热
intermittent fever	间歇热	low-grade fever	低热
remittent fever	弛张热	relapsing fever	回归热
pain	痛	burning pain	灼痛
chest (flank, ...) pain	胸（胁腹……）痛	cramp-like pain	痉挛性痛
dull, diffused pain	弥漫性钝痛	pleuritic pain	胸膜炎性痛
radiating pain (pain radiating to...)	放射性痛（放射到……疼痛）	angina	绞痛
cardiac angina	心绞痛	backache	背痛
colic	绞痛，急腹痛	earache	耳痛
headache	头痛	neuralgia	神经痛
migraine	偏头痛	rebound tenderness	反跳痛
somatalgia	躯体痛	sore throat	咽喉痛
stomachache	胃痛	toothache	牙痛
bloody sputum	带血的痰	cough	咳嗽
dry cough	干咳	expectoration	咳痰
expectoration of blood	咯血	hemoptysis	咯血
anoxia	缺氧	apnea	呼吸暂停，窒息
asthma	气喘，哮喘	hyperpnea hyperventilation	过度呼吸，换气过度
dyspnea	呼吸困难	hypoxia	低氧，缺氧
hypopnea	呼吸不全，呼吸浅表	respiratory arrest	呼吸停止
orthopnea	端坐呼吸	suffocation	窒息
fetid breath	口臭	tachypnea	呼吸急促
arrhythmia	心律失常，心律不齐	fruity breath	呼吸有水果味
cardiac arrest	心搏骤停	atelectasis	肺不张，肺膨胀不全
cyanosis	发绀，青紫	cardiac hypertrophy	心脏肥大
extrasystole	期外收缩	distension of jugular vein	颈静脉怒张
hemopleura	血胸	gallop rhythm	奔马律

(续)

hypovolemia	（循环）血容量减少	hepatojugular reflux	肝颈静脉回流
tachycardia	心动过速	palpitation	心悸
thrill	震颤	pneumothorax	气胸
dull sound	浊音	absent breath sounds	呼吸音消失
rale	啰音	hyperresonant	鼓音
wheeze	哮鸣音	rhonchus, rhonchi	鼾音，干啰音
anorexia, loss of appetite	食欲不振，厌食	occult blood	潜血
eructation	嗳气	dysphagia	吞咽困难
flatulence	气胀	belching	嗳气
gaseous distention	胃胀气	flatus	肠胃气，屁
hiccough, hiccup	打呃，呃逆	hematemesis	呕血
pyrosis	胃灼热	nausea	恶心
thirsty	口渴	regurgitation	反胃，回流
anal fissure, crack in the anal canal	肛裂	vomiting	呕吐
board-like rigidity of the abdomen	板状腹	ascites	腹水
esophageal varices	食管静脉曲张	decreased tactile fremitus	触觉性震颤减弱
hemorrhoid	痔	fistula	瘘，瘘管
hepatomegaly	肝脏肿大	hernia	疝
jaundice	黄疸	intussusception	肠套叠
peristalsis	蠕动	muscle guarding, defence of the abdominal wall	腹壁肌卫
mass peristalsis	总蠕动	loss of peristalsis	蠕动消失
prolapse	脱垂	retrograde (reversed) peristalsis	逆蠕动
rectal prolapse	直肠脱垂，脱肛	prolapse of anus	脱肛
calculus	结石，石	volvulus	肠扭转
vesical calculus	膀胱结石	biliary calculus	胆结石
defecation	排便	constipation	便秘
incontinence of feces	大便失禁	diarrhea	腹泻
fecal impaction	大便嵌塞	hematochezia	便血
bruise	挫伤，青肿	blotch	斑点
desquamation	脱皮，脱屑	acne	痤疮，粉刺
clay colored stools	陶土色便	painful straining with defecation	排便痛性牵动
fecal vomiting, stercoraceous vomiting	呕粪，吐粪	dark, granular/coffee ground emesis	咖啡样呕吐物
scanty and hard stools	便少而硬	foul fatty stools, steatorrhea	恶臭脂肪便，脂肪痢
anuria	无尿	tarry (black) stools	柏油样便
dysuria	排尿困难，尿痛	burning sensation of urination	排尿时的灼烧感

frequency of urination	尿频	enuresis, bed wetting	遗尿
micturation	排尿	uresis, urination, voiding	排尿
nocturia	夜尿	polyuria	多尿
oliguria	少尿	vesical tenesmus	排尿时里急后重
tenesmus	里急后重	urgency of urination	尿急
uremia coma	尿毒症昏迷	aciduria	酸尿
urinary incontinence	尿失禁	cylindruria	管型尿
chyluria	乳糜尿	hematuria	血尿
glycosuria	糖尿	pneumaturia	气尿
ketonuria	酮尿	pyuria	脓尿
proteinuria	蛋白尿	dysmenorrhea	痛经
amenorrhea	经闭，无月经	lochia	恶露
menorrhagia	月经过多	menstruation	月经
menorrhea	行经，月经过多	ecchymosis	瘀斑
uterine contraction	子宫收缩	nevus	痣
loss of skin turgor	失去皮肤充盈	petechia	瘀点，瘀斑
papule	丘疹	pustule	脓疱
pigmentation	色素沉着	red nodule	红结节
purpura	紫癜	scar	伤疤
roseola	玫瑰疹	spider angioma	蛛形痣
senile plaque	老人斑	urticaria	荨麻疹
subcutaneous nodule	皮下结节	vitiligo	白斑
vesicle	小水疱	blurred vision, visual disturbance	视力模糊
blindness	失明	lacrimation	流泪
impaired vision	视力下降	photophobia	畏光，羞明
papilledema	视神经盘水肿	deafness	聋
retinal detachment	视网膜脱离	tinnitus	耳鸣
hearing loss	听力丧失	impaired smelling	嗅觉障碍
epistaxis, nasal bleeding	鼻出血	nasal obstruction	鼻塞
nasal discharge	鼻涕	snore	打鼾
sneeze	喷嚏	hoarseness	嘶哑
aphonia, loss of voice	失音症	herpes labialis	唇疱疹，感冒疮
gum bleeding	齿龈出血	lead line of the gum	龈铅线
Koplik's spots	科普利克斑	strawberry tongue	草莓舌
salivation, drooling	流口水	atrophy	萎缩
tremulous tongue	舌震颤	deformity	畸形，变形
contracture	挛缩	fracture	骨折

(续)

dislocation	脱位	comminuted fracture	粉碎性骨折
closed (simple) fracture	无创骨折，单纯性骨折	knock-knee	膝外翻
compound fracture	哆开（开放性）骨折	prosthesis	假体
opisthotonos	角弓反张	tetany	（肌）强直，手足抽搐
spasm	痉挛	aphasia	失语
wrist drop	腕下垂	coma	昏迷
ataxia	共济失调	convulsion	抽搐，惊厥
consciousness	知觉，意识	delusion	妄想
delirium	谵妄	hallucination	幻觉
faint	昏厥	increased intracranial pressure	颅内压增高
hemiplegia	偏瘫	loss of orientation	定向丧失
insanity	精神错乱	memory defects, amnesia	记忆缺损，遗忘症
mania	躁狂	projectile vomiting	喷射性呕吐
paraplegia	截瘫，下身麻痹	somnolence, (lethargy)	昏睡，嗜睡
tetraplegia	四肢瘫痪	unconsciousness	失去知觉
yawning	打哈欠	crisis	危象
cerebral (febrile, hematic, hemolytic, hypertensive, thyrotoxic, ...) crisis	脑（热、血性、溶血、高血压、甲状腺中毒……）危象	failure	衰竭，故障
central (circulatory, cardiac, myocardiac, peripheral, congestive, renal, respiratory) failure	中枢（循环、心力、心肌、周围循环、充血性、肾、呼吸……）衰竭	diagnosis	诊断
auscultation	听诊	inspection	视诊
palpation	触诊	percussion	叩诊
laboratory examination	实验室检查	physical examination	体格检查
rectal (vaginal) touch	直肠（阴道）指诊	impression	印象
tentative diagnosis	暂定诊断	differential diagnosis	鉴别诊断
final diagnosis	最后诊断	prognosis	预后
prescription	处方	incubation (latent) period	潜伏期
prodromal stage	前驱期	incipient stage	初期
quiescent stage	静止期	alleviation	减轻，缓和
remission	缓解	attack	发作
convalescence (recovery) stage	恢复期	rehabilitation	康复
relapse	复发	sudden death	猝死
moribund	濒死的	course of the disease	病程

(续)

course of the treatment	疗程	indication	适应征，指征
complication	并发症	contraindication	禁忌征
side-effect	副作用	sequel (sequela), after effect	后遗症
radio-therapy	放射性疗法	supporting treatment	支持疗法
symptomatic treatment	对症疗法	cardiac massage	心脏按压
cardiac pacing	心脏起搏	electrotherapy	电疗法
electroshock treatment	电休克疗法	hemodialysis	血液透析
hyperbaric therapy	高压氧疗法	insulin-shock treatment	胰岛素休克疗法
light therapy	光疗法	therapeutic gymnastics	医疗体育
stupor	木僵，昏呆		

2.2.4 医院类型名称

general hospital	综合医院	children hospital	儿童医院
tumour hospital	肿瘤医院	chest hospital	胸科医院
field hospital	野战医院	isolation hospital	隔离医院
military hospital	陆军医院	municipal hospital	市立医院
maternity hospital	产科医院	mental hospital	精神医院
infectious hospital	传染医院	leprosy hospital	麻风医院
affiliated hospital	附属医院	training hospital	教学医院

2.3 普通英语词汇医学意义篇

词汇	普通词义	医学词义
(1)		
1. acquired	取得的，得到的	获得的，后天的
2. active	活跃的，积极的，灵敏的	活性的，速效的，放射性
3. acute	尖锐的，敏锐的，剧烈的	急性的
4. administration	管理，行政，执行	（药）给予，服法，用法
5. admit	让……进入，接纳，承认	让……住院
6. affect	影响，感动	（疾病）侵袭
7. agent	（发生作用的）动因	剂，因子
8. alienation	（情感上）疏远，离间；转让	精神错乱
9. angry	发怒的，（风雨）狂暴的	（患处）肿痛发炎的
10. attack	进攻，攻击，抨击	（疾病）侵袭，发作

（续）

词汇	普通词义	医学词义
(2)		
11. bedside	床边用的	临床的，护理的
12. benign	慈祥的，有益健康的	（瘤等）良性的
13. bulb	球茎，球状物	（解剖学中的）球
14. canal	运河，沟渠	管
15. carrier	搬运人，运送人	带菌者
16. cavity	洞，中空	腔，空洞
17. cell	小房间，单人牢房	细胞
18. chamber	房间，议院	腔，室
19. chest	箱子，柜子，金库	胸腔
20. clump	丛，簇，群，一团/块	细菌凝块
(3)		
21. colony	殖民地，一群	菌落
22. communicable	可传达（授）的	可传染的
23. complain	抱怨，诉苦，申诉	主诉
24. complement	补足物	（血清中的）补体，防御素
25. complication	复杂，混乱	合并征
26. congest	充满，拥挤	充血
27. consolidation	巩固，加强	坚实变化，实变
28. constitutional	宪法的，组成的	全身性的，体质的
29. contract	缔结，订（约）	得（病）
30. control	控制，支配，调节	（实验的）对照，对照物
(4)		
31. convulsion	震动，骚动	痉挛，抽搐
32. cortex	外皮	皮质
33. course	过程，道路，课程	病程，疗程
34. delivery	交货，交付，投递	分娩
35. depression	降低，沮丧，不景气	抑郁症，机能降低
36. discharge	卸（货），射出	让……出院；排出物
37. dislocate	使离开原来位置	使脱臼
38. disorder	混乱	（身心，机能）失调，轻病
39. disturbance	骚动，动乱	（身心等方面的）障碍，失调
40. dominant	支配的	显性的

(续)

词汇	普通词义	医学词义
(5)		
41. drainage	排水，下水道	导液法，引流（法）
42. dress	给……穿衣	敷裹（伤口）
43. effusion	流出，喷出	渗出（物）
44. elevation	高度，标高，高地	（皮肤上的）隆肿
45. embolism	（历法中的）加闰（日）	栓塞，栓子
46. enlarge	扩大，扩展，放大	肿大，肥大
47. entity	存在，实体	病（种）；本质
48. episode	一段情节，插曲	（一次）发作
49. erupt	爆发，迸出	（牙）冒出，（疹）发出
50. essential	本质的，必要的	特发的，原发的
(6)		
51. excision	删除	切除，切除术
52. extract	摘录，抽出物	提取物，浸膏
53. extremities	末端，极度	（人的）手、足
54. failure	失败，缺乏，衰退	衰竭
55. fatality	命运决定的事物，灾祸	死亡，致命性
56. filling	填补，充满	填补物
57. film	薄层，薄膜	胶片；（眼的）薄翳
58. focus (*pl.* foci)	焦点，（活动）中心	病灶
59. follow-up	补充报道	随访（诊断/治疗后，病人定期复查或与医生保持联系）
60. foreign	外国的，外地的	外来的，异质的
(7)		
61. frank	坦白的，直率的	症状明显的
62. fullness	充满，丰富	饭后饱胀感，饱闷
63. generalized	一般化了的	全身的
64. graft	嫁接，嫁接植物	移植，移植物
65. gross	总的，显著的	（不用显微镜）肉眼能看到的
66. growth	生长，生长物	肿瘤
67. history	历史	病史，病历
68. host	主人	宿主
69. immune	免除的	免疫的
70. inactivate	使不活动	灭活，使失去活性

(续)

词汇	普通词义	医学词义
(8)		
71. incidence	发生	发生率，发病率
72. incision	切入，切开	切口，切开
73. incubation	孵卵	潜伏
74. indicate	指示，表明	表示需要……作为治疗
75. infiltration	渗入	浸润
76. inflammation	点火，燃烧，激动	发炎
77. inherit	继承	遗传
78. insidious	阴险的，暗中为害的	（疾病）在不知不觉之间加剧的
79. inspection	检查，检验	望诊，视诊
80. insufficiency	不充分，不足	闭锁不全，机能不全
(9)		
81. insult	侮辱，凌辱	（对身体或其一部分）损害
82. intake	吸入，纳入	摄取，摄取量
83. involve	包缠，使卷入	累及，牵涉
84. irradiation	照耀，阐明，辐照	照射（法），扩散
85. irrigate	灌溉	冲洗（伤口等）
86. irritable	易激怒的	过敏性的，易激动的
87. joint	接合，接合处	关节
88. labo(u)r	劳动	分娩
89. laceration	撕裂	撕裂伤 [口]
90. lacrimal	泪的（$a.$）	泪腺（lacrimal gland）
(10)		
91. lobe	耳垂	（脑、肺、肝等的）叶
92. malignant	恶意的，邪恶的	恶性的
93. medium	中间，媒介物，工具	培养基
94. menstrual	每月一次的	月经的
95. migration	迁居，定期移居	移行，游走
96. moist	潮湿的，多雨的，含泪的	湿性的，有分泌物的
97. multiplication	增加，增多	繁殖
98. murmur	低沉连续的沙沙声，低语声	（心脏）杂音
99. naive	天真的，朴素的	首次用来进行实验的（鼠、兔等）
100. nonproductive	不能生产的	（咳嗽）干的

(续)

词汇	普通词义	医学词义
（11）		
101. onset	攻击，进攻，开始	发病，起病
102. open	开（着）的；开阔的	开放的，畅通的
103. oral	口述的，口头的	口的
104. origin	起源，出身，血统	起端
105. output	产量，产品	排泄物，排泄量
106. overflow	溢流，过剩	溢流口，溢流管，溢流受器
107. overgrowth	生长过度	增生，肥大
108. overhang	悬垂物，伸出量	悬突
109. pacemaker	定步速者，标兵	起搏器，起搏点
110. palpable	摸得出的，容易感觉到的	可触知的，触诊可按到的
（12）		
111. parasitism	寄生（现象、状态、习惯）	寄生物感染，寄生虫引起的疾病
112. pilot	引导的，导向的	（小规模）试验的，试点的
113. plaque	饰板，襟上饰物	斑，血小板
114. plate	盘	平皿，培养皿
115. premature	早熟的，过早发生的事物	早产婴儿
116. preparation	准备	制剂；（解剖或病理）标本
117. primary	初级的，原有的	原发的
118. purge	净化，清洗	泻药
119. regimen	政体，社会制度	摄生法
120. remission	宽恕，赦免	缓和，减轻
（13）		
121. removal	移动，迁居	切除，除掉
122. restorative	交还的	滋补的；兴奋剂
123. retention	保持，保留	停滞，潴留
124. rib	玩笑；（肉类）肋条，排骨	肋，肋骨
125. scan	细看，审视	扫描
126. secondary	第二位的，从属的	继发的
127. secretion	藏匿	分泌，分泌液
128. section	切断，段，节	切片
129. sedimentation	沉积（作用）	血沉（erythrocyte ~）
130. seizure	抓住，夺取	（疾病的）发作

（续）

词汇	普通词义	医学词义
（14）		
131. septic	引起腐烂的	脓毒性的，败血病的
132. sequel(=sequela)	继续而来的事，后果	后遗症，后发病
133. shock	冲击，震动，震惊，电击	休克，中风，心脏引起的昏迷
134. sigmoid	S形的，乙状形的	乙状结肠（的）
135. sign	符号，招牌，征兆	（病）症，（体）征
136. simple	简单的	单纯的
137. smear	污点，污迹，涂抹物	涂片
138. spatula	（涂敷等用的）抹刀，刮勺	压舌板，调药刀
139. sponge	海绵（用海绵揩拭）	纱布，棉球（用棉球擦洗）
140. spread	伸展，扩展	传播，蔓延
（15）		
141. starve	（使）饿死，以饥饿迫使	以节食治疗
142. stain	污点，瑕疵	着色（剂），染色（剂）
143. stone	石	结石，结石病
144. stool	凳子，厕所，马桶	粪
145. strain[1]	血缘，世系，种	菌株
146. strain[2]	拉紧	过劳，扭伤
147. strap	（用皮带）拴住	绑扎（伤口）（多用 strap up）
148. stricture	苛评，责难	狭窄
149. stroke	打，击，敲	中风，（疾病）突然发作
150. stunt	阻碍……的发展	阻碍……的生长（发育）
（16）		
151. subject	题目，学科；从属的	受治疗（实验）者，易患……的
152. subside	沉淀，（风、雨）平静下来	（肿、热度）减退
153. substrate	底层，地层	基质，底物
154. sufferer	受害者，受难者	患病者
155. surfeit	过度，过量	过食，过饮
156. swab	拖把	药签，拭子
157. sympathetic	同情的，和谐的	交感的，交感神经的
158. systemic	系统的	全身的
159. taint	玷污，败坏	污斑；遗传素质；使感染，沾染
160. take	取，拿	愈合，奏效

(续)

词汇	普通词义	医学词义
(17)		
161. tender	嫩的，脆弱的	一触即痛的
162. term	期限，学期	预产期，正常的分娩时刻
163. terminal	末端的	晚期的；致死的
164. test	测验，考验	分析，试验
165. theatre	剧院	手术室
166. tie	绳，带，领带	（手术时打的）结
167. tissue	薄绢，织物	组织
168. tract	一片（土地，森林）	道，系统，束
169. transfusion	移注，倾注，渗入	输血
170. transmit	传送，传达，传导	传播，传染
(18)		
181. valve	阀，活门	瓣，瓣膜
182. ventilator	通风装置，送风机	呼吸机
183. vessel	容器，器皿	脉管
184. victim	受害者	患者；残疾人
185. virtue	善，德，优点	功效，效能
186. virulence	毒力，恶毒	病毒性，致病力
187. viscid	胶粘的	黏稠的，半流体的
188. visit	访问	出诊，就诊
189. vital	生命的	有生命力的，充满活力的
190. vulnerability	易损性	易罹（疾病）性
(19)		
191. ward	保卫，监护	病房，病室
192. warn	警告	预先通知，警告
193. wash	洗	（用药）洗
194. wave	波浪	（心电图的）示波图，波
195. wheal	条痕，鞭痕	风块，荨麻疹团，水泡
196. whoop	高喊，呐喊	发喘息声，（百日咳似的）咳嗽
197. wind	风	肠胃中胀气
198. withdrawal	收回，撤退	断瘾；停止服药
199. work-up	印刷物表面的污迹，印痕	病情的检查
200. wrench	猛扭	扭伤

已知词	医学意义	同根词	医学意义
1. complication	并发症	complicate	并发……而使……（病）恶化
2. congest	充血	congestive	充血的
3. disturbance	障碍，失调	disturb	使失调，搅乱
4. dress	敷裹（伤口）	dressing	敷料
5. excision	切除，切除术	excise	切除
6. focus	病灶	focal	病灶的，病灶性的
7. immune	免疫的	autoimmunity	自体免疫
8. indicate	表明需要……作为治疗	indication	适应征
9. infiltration	浸润	infiltrate	浸润
10. tender	一触即痛的	tenderness	触痛

第六部分
词组搭配

全国医学博士英语
统考词汇巧战通关

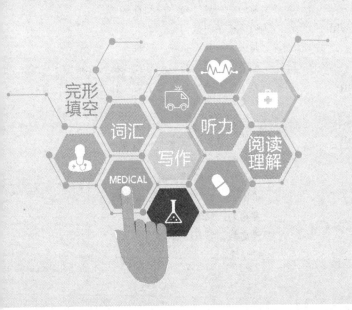

（按主词字母顺序排列）

abandon oneself to	沉溺于
with abandon	放任地，放纵地，纵情地
abide by	遵守，履行
to the best of one's ability	尽自己最大努力
keep abreast of	与……齐头并进，了解……的最新情况
be absent from...	缺席，不在
absence of mind	心不在焉
in the abstract	抽象地，在理论上
in abundance	充足，大量
be abundant in	富有，富于
by accident	偶然地，意外
of one's own accord	自愿地，主动地
with one accord	一致地
in accord with	与……一致，与……相符
out of one's accord with	同……不一致
in accordance with	与……一致，依照，根据
according to	据……所说，按……所载；根据，按照
on one's own account	为了某人的缘故，为了某人自己的利益；自行负责；依靠自己
on account	赊账
give sb. an account of	说明，解释（理由）
of no account	不重要的
on account of	为了……的缘故，因为，由于
on no account	决不，绝对不；不论什么原因
take account of	考虑到，顾及，体谅
take into account	考虑到，顾及，体谅
be accustomed to	习惯于

第六部分　词组搭配

be **acquainted** with	了解；熟悉
act as	扮演
act on	遵照……行动，奉行；作用于，影响
in the **act** of	在做……的过程中
add up	加起来；说得通
add up to	合计达，总括起来意味着
in **addition**	另外，加之
in **addition** to	除……之外（还）
adhere to	黏附；坚持，遵循
adjacent to	毗邻的，邻近的
in **advance**	在前面；预告，事先
have an **advantage** over	胜过
have the **advantage** of	胜过，处于有利条件
have the **advantage** of sb.	知道某人所不知道的事
take **advantage** of	利用，占……的便宜
again and **again**	再三地，反复不止地
in **agreement** with	同意，一致
in the **aggregate**	总共，总的来说
ahead of	比……提前，比……更早
in the **air**	流传中；不肯定，不具体
off the **air**	停播
on the **air**	广播
up in the **air**	悬而未决的
on the **alert**	警戒着，随时准备着，密切注意着
above **all**	首先，尤其是
after **all**	毕竟，终究，究竟
all but	几乎，差不多；除了……都
all in **all**	从各方面说，总的来说
all over	到处，遍及
at **all**	（用于否定句）丝毫，一点
for **all**	尽管，虽然
in **all**	总共，合计
allow of	容许，容许有……的可能
make **allowance(s)** for	考虑到，顾及；体谅，原谅

leave **alone**	不打扰，不惊动
let **alone**	不打扰，不惊动；更别提
along with	和……一道，和……一起
angle for	谋取，猎取
one **after another**	一个接一个，相继
one **another**	互相
answer for	对……负责任，保证，符合
in **answer** to	作为对……的回答
anything but	绝对不
for **anything**	（否定句中）无论如何
apart from	除……之外
to all **appearances**	就外表来看，根据观察推断
on **approval**	（商品）供试用的，包退包换的
apologize to sb. for sth.	为……向……道歉
appeal to sb. for sth.	为某事向某人呼吁
appeal to sb.	对某人有吸引力
apply to sb. for sth.	为……向……申请
apply to	与……有关；适用于
approve of	赞成
arise from	由……引起
arm in arm	臂挽臂
as for / to	至于，关于
as it is	实际上
as it were	可以说，宛如，好像
be **ashamed** of	以……为羞耻
aside from	除……之外
assert oneself	坚持自己的权利（或意见），显示自己的权威（或威力）
assure sb. of sth.	向……保证，使……确信
attach to	缚，系，结
make an **attempt** at doing sth. (to do sth.)	试图做……
attend to	注意，照顾；侍候，照料
attribute... to...	把……归因于，认为……是……的结果

avail oneself of	利用
on (the / an) average	按平均值,通常
be aware of	意识到,知道

back and forth	来回地,反复地
in back of	在……的后面/背后
be on one's back	卧病不起
at one's back	支持,维护
have sb. at one's back	有……支持,有……做后台
turn one's back on sb.	不理睬(某人),背弃某人,抛弃
back out	退出,撒手
back up	(使)倒退;支持
behind sb's back	背着某人,暗中
know…backwards	对……极其熟悉
go from bad to worse	每况愈下
in the balance	(生命等)在危急状态下,(命运等)未定
off balance	不平衡
behind bars	在狱中
bargain for / on	企图廉价获取;预料,指望
drive a hard bargain	杀价,迫使对方接受苛刻条件
barge in	闯入,干预
keep / hold sth. at bay	使无法近身
bear down on	施加压力,冲向
bear on / upon	对……有影响,和……有关
bear out	证实
bear up	撑持下去,振作起来
bear with	忍受,容忍
have a bearing on	对……有影响,与……有关
beat down	(太阳等)强烈地照射下来;打倒,平息
beat at	打赢

beat it	跑掉，走开，溜走
beat up	痛打，打（蛋），抬（价），搅拌
become of	使遭遇，发生
beg off	恳求免除（某种义务）
on / in **behalf** of	代表，为了
for the **benefit** of	为了……的利益（好处）
come into **being**	出现，形成
beyond **belief**	难以置信
beside oneself	极度兴奋，对自己的感情失去控制
at **best**	充其量，至多
get / have the **best** of	战胜
had **best**	应当，最好
make the **best** of	充分利用
better off	境况好的，生活优越的
get / have the **better** of	战胜，在……中占上风
in **between**	在中间，介乎两者之间
fill the **bill**	出类拔萃
kill two **birds** with one stone	一箭双雕，一举两得
by **birth**	生来，论出身，按照血统
do one's **bit**	做自己分内的事
in **black** and white	白纸黑字
be to **blame**	该受责备的，应承担责任的
blame sth. on sb.	把……推在某人身上
(at) full **blast**	大力地，全速地
blaze a trail	开拓道路，做先导
turn a **blind** eye (to)	（对……）视而不见
block off	封锁，封闭
block up	堵塞，垫高
in cold **blood**	残忍地
in (full) **blossom**	正开着花
blow up	爆炸；大怒；充气
come to **blows**	动手打起来，开始互殴
out of the **blue**	出乎意料地，突然地
across the **board**	包括一切地，全面地

above **board**	光明正大地，公开地
board up	用木板封闭（或覆盖）
on **board**	在船（车或飞机）上
boast of / about	吹嘘
in the same **boat**	处境相同，面临同样的危险
boil down to	意味着，归结为
a **bolt** from / out of the blue	晴天霹雳，意外事件
have a **bone** to pick with	与……争辩
make no **bones** about	对……毫不犹豫，对……直言不讳
book in	预订，办理登记手续
by the **book**	按规则，依照惯例
be **bound** up in	热衷于，忙于
be **bound** up with	与……有密切关系
know no **bounds**	不知限量，无限
pick sb.'s **brains**	（自己不下功夫）向……请教，占有别人的脑力劳动成果
rack sb.'s **brains**	绞尽脑汁，苦苦地动脑筋
branch out	扩充，扩大活动范围
break away	突然离开，强行逃脱
break down	损坏；（健康等）垮掉，崩溃
break in	非法闯入；打断，插嘴
break into	非法闯入，强行进入
break off	中断，突然停止
break out	爆发，突然出现；逃脱，逃走
break through	突围，冲破；取得突破性成就
break up	打碎，粉碎；散开，驱散；终止
make a clean **breast** of	彻底坦白，把……和盘托出
catch one's **breath**	喘息，气喘；呼吸；屏息
hold one's **breath**	屏息
out of **breath**	喘不过气来
take sb.'s **breath** away	使某人大吃一惊
in **brief**	简言之，简单地说
bring about	导致，引起
bring around / round	说服；使恢复知觉（或健康）

bring down	使落下，打倒；降低，减少
bring forth	产生，提出
bring forward	提前；提出，提议
bring off	使实现，做成
bring out	出版；使显出；激起，引起
bring through	使（病人）脱险，使安全度过
bring to	使恢复知觉
bring up	养育，教养；提出
on the **brink** of	濒临，处于……边缘
brush aside	不理，不顾
brush off	刷去，打发掉
brush up	重温，再练
buck up	使振奋，使打起精神
build in	使成为固定物，使成为组成部分
build on / upon	建立于，指望
build up	逐步建立；增强；集结
in **bulk**	大量，大批
bump into	偶然遇见，碰见
bundle up	把……捆扎（或包）起来；使穿得暖和
burn down	烧毁；火势减弱
burn out	烧光，烧毁……的内部；熄灭
burn up	烧掉，烧毁；烧起来
burst in on	突然出现（或到来）
burst into	闯入；突然……起来
burst out	大声喊叫，突然……起来
beat around / about the bush	转弯抹角，旁敲侧击
get down to **business**	认真着手办事
go out of **business**	歇业
have no **business** to do / doing sth.	无权做某事，没有理由做某事
in **business**	经商，经营
mind your own **business**	管好你自己的事，少管闲事
on **business**	因公，因事
mean **business**	是认真的
but for	要不是，倘没有

can not **but**	不得不；不禁要
last **but** one	倒数第二
on the **button**	击中下颌；准确地，准时地
buy off	出钱摆脱；向……行贿
buy out	买下……的全部股份
by and by	不久，迟早
by and large	大体上，总的来说
by the bye	顺便提一句

C

a piece of **cake**	容易的事
call back	回电话
call for	叫（某人）来；要求，需要
call in	叫……进来
call off	取消
call on / upon	访问，拜访；号召，要求
call up	打电话；召集；使人想起
be **capable** of	有……能力的；有……可能的
care for	照顾，照料；喜欢
take **care**	当心，注意
carry forward	结转
carry off	拿走，夺走
carry on	继续进行，坚持
carry out	实行，执行；完成，实现
carry over	（使）继续下去，将延后
carry through	实现，完成；使渡过难关
a **case** in point	有关的事例，例证
in any **case**	无论如何，不管怎样
in **case**	假使，以防万一
in **case** of	假如；防备

in no case	无论如何不，决不
cast about / around for	到处寻找，试图找到
cast aside	消除，废除，去掉
cast off	抛弃，丢弃
cast out	赶出，驱逐
catch at	试图抓住，拼命抓
catch on	流行起来；懂得，理解
catch out	发觉……有错误（或做坏事）
catch up with	赶上
be cautious of	谨防
center one's attention on	把某人的注意力集中在……上
be certain of	有把握，一定
for certain	肯定地，确切地
by chance	偶然，碰巧
by any chance	万一，也许
chance on / upon	偶然找到，偶然遇到
stand a chance of	有……的希望（可能）
take a chance	冒险，投机
chance of a lifetime	千载难逢的良机，一生中唯一的机会
for a change	换换环境（花样等）
in character	（与自身特性）相符
out of character	（与自身特性）不相符
in charge (of)	管理，负责
take charge	开始管理，接管
charge sb. with	控告某人犯有……
check in	（在旅馆、机场等）登记，报到
check out	结账离去，办妥手续离去
check up (on)	检查，核实
in check	受抑制的，受控制的
cheer on	为……鼓气，为……喝彩
cheer up	（使）高兴起来，（使）振作起来
chew over	深思，玩味
under no circumstances	无论如何不，决不
in the circumstances	在这种情况下，既然如此

under the **circumstances**	在这种情况下，因为这种情况
clamp down (on)	（对……）进行压制（或取缔）
clean out	把……打扫干净
clean up	把……收拾干净；清理，清除（犯罪现场等）
clear away	把……清除掉，收拾
clear off	离开，溜掉
clear out	清除，把……腾空；走开，赶出
clear up	清理；澄清，解决；（天）放晴
round the **clock**	日夜不停地
close by	在近旁，在旁边
close down	关闭，歇业
close in (on)	包围，围住
close up	堵住，关闭
come / draw to a **close**	渐近结束
in **collaboration** with	与……合作，与……勾结
come about	发生，产生
come across	偶然碰见，碰上
come along	出现，发生；进步，进展
come apart	破碎，崩溃
come around / round	苏醒，复原；顺便来访
come at	攻击，冲向；达到，了解
come between	分开，离间；妨碍（某人做某事）
come by	得到，获得；访问，看望
come down	（物价等）下跌，落魄，潦倒
come down to	可归结为
come in for	受到，遭到
come on	（表示鼓励、催促等）快，走吧；进步；发生
come out	出现，显露；出版，发表；结果是
come through	经历……仍活着，安然度过
come to	苏醒；总数为，结果是；涉及，谈到
come up	出现，发生；走上前来
come up against	突然（或意外）碰到（困难、反对等）
come up with	提出，想出；提供
commit oneself to	使自己承担

commit sb. to prison	把某人送进监狱
in **common**	共用的，共有的
be **common** to sb.	是与某人所共有的
keep **company** with	和……常来往
keep to one's own **company**	独自一人
beyond / without **compare**	无与伦比
by / in **comparison**	相比之下
in **comparison** with	与……比较
compensate for	补偿，赔偿，弥补
comply with	遵守，依从
be **composed** of	由……组成
as / so far as ... be **concerned**	就……而言
in **concert**	一起，一致
conceive of	想象，设想
be **concerned** with / about	与……有关
concern oneself about / with	关心
condemn sb. to	判决
on **condition** that	如果
out of **condition**	健康不佳
confide in	对……讲真心话，依赖
in **confidence**	私下地，秘密地
take into one's **confidence**	把……作为知己
confine… to…	把……限制在某范围内
confirm sb. in	使某人更坚定（信念）等
conform to	符合，遵照，遵守；服从
be **confronted** with	面对，面临
congratulate sb. on	祝贺
in **conjunction** with	与……共同，连同
in **connection** with	关于，与……有关
in (all / good) **conscience**	凭良心，公平地
be **conscious** of	觉察，知道
on one's **conscience**	引起某人的悔恨（或内疚）
consent to	同意
in **consequence**	因此，结果

in consequence of	由于，因为……的缘故
under consideration	在考虑中
in consideration of	考虑到，由于；作为对……的报酬
on no consideration	无论如何也不
take into consideration	考虑到，顾及
consist of	由……组成的
consist in	主要在于
be consistent with	与……一致
be consistent in	一贯的
consult sb. on / about sth.	向……征求……方面的意见，就……向……请教
be content with	满足于
be content to do sth.	愿意做某事
contrary to	与……相反
on the contrary	正相反
to the contrary	相反地
by / in contrast	对比之下
in contrast to / with	与……对比起来
contribute to	有助于
in control (of)	掌握着，控制着
out of control	失去控制
under control	处于控制之中
at one's convenience	在方便的时间或地点
be convenient to / for	对……方便
convince sb. of	使某人确信；劝说某人做某事
cool down / off	冷却，使冷静下来
cope with	应付，处理
to the core	彻底地，彻头彻尾地
around / round the corner	临近，在附近
turn the corner	出现转机
correspond to	对应于
correspond with	符合，一致
at all costs	不惜任何代价，无论如何
at the cost of	以……为代价
keep one's own counsel	将意见（或计划）保密

count against	（被）认为对……不利
count down	（发射火箭等）倒数数
count in	把……算入
count on / upon	依靠，指望
count up	算出……总数，共计
in the course of	在……期间，在……过程中
of course	当然，自然
a matter of course	理所当然的事
as a matter of course	当然地，自然地
cover up	掩盖，掩饰；盖住，裹住
take cover	隐蔽
under cover	秘密地，暗地里
crack down on / upon	对……采取严厉措施，镇压
crack up	（精神）崩溃
like crazy	疯狂地，拼命地
on credit	赊购
with credit	以优异成绩
to sb.'s credit	在（某人）名下，（某人）值得赞扬
to one's credit	使某人感到光荣
do sb. credit	使某人感到光荣
be critical of	爱挑毛病的，批评的
crop up	突然发生，突然出现
cross off / out	划掉，勾掉
cry out for	迫切需要
take one's cue from	学……的样，听……的劝告
cure sb. of	治好某人的疾病
curl up	卷起，撅起（嘴唇等）；使卷曲
cut across	抄近路穿过
cut back	急忙返回；削减，缩减
cut down	削减；砍倒，杀死
cut in	插嘴，打断；超车抢道
cut off	切断；使分离
cut out	切去，删去；戒除

a **danger** to	对……的危险
be in **danger** (of)	处于……危险中
be out of **danger**	脱离危险
dash off	迅速离去；迅速写（或画）
out of **date**	过时的
up to **date**	新式的，时兴的
date back to	可追溯到
date from	从某时期开始（有）
dawn on sb.	使开始明白
call it a **day**	今天到此为止
day and night	夜以继日
day in, day out	日复一日
to a / the **day**	恰好，一天不差
turn a **deaf** ear to	不愿听，充耳不闻
deal in	经营
deal with	处理，对付；论述，涉及
put to **death**	杀死，处死
to **death**	极，非常
in **debt**	欠债，负债
in sb.'s **debt**	欠某人的人情
decide on / upon	决定，选定
on the **decline**	在衰退中，在减少中
in **decline**	下降
deep down	实际上，在心底
in **defiance** of	违抗，无视
by **degrees**	渐渐地，逐渐地
to some **degree**	有点儿，稍微
take a **delight** in	以……为乐
to one's **delight**	令某人感到高兴
in **demand**	非常需要的，受欢迎的

demand sth. of sb.	向某人要求（非物质的东西）
demand sth. from sb.	向某人要求（物质的东西）
on **demand**	一经要求
deprive of	剥夺
derive...from	从……取得，由……来的
derive from	起源于
despair of	对……感到绝望
in **despair**	绝望
in **depth**	深入地，彻底地
out of one's **depth**	非……所能理解，为……所不及
go into **detail**(s)	详细叙述，逐一说明
in **detail**	详细地
deviate from...	偏离，不按……办
die **down**	变弱，逐渐消失
die out	逐渐消失，灭绝
on a **diet**	节食
differ from...in	与……的区别在于……
in **difficulties**	有困难，处境困难
make a **difference**	有影响，起重要作用
dig up	挖掘出，找出
dine out	外出进餐（尤指在餐馆）
dip into	随便翻阅，浏览；稍加研究
discharge sb. (from) ...	因……解雇，开除
in **disguise**	伪装，假扮
dish out	给予，分发
on **display**	陈列
at sb.'s **disposal**	任某人处理，供某人使用
dispose of	处理掉
in **dispute**	在争论中，未决的
in the **distance**	在远处
keep sb. at a **distance**	对某人冷淡，同某人疏远
be **distinct** from	与……截然不同
distinguish between	辨别

distinguish...from...	把……与……区别开
do away with	废除，去掉；杀掉，镇压
do for	毁坏，使完蛋
do up	系；修缮；打扮
have...to **do** with	与……有关系
do with	想要；对待；与……有关；以……对付过去
do without	没有……也行，用不着，将就
out of **doors**	在户外
beyond (any) **doubt**	无疑，确实
in **doubt**	不能肯定的，可怀疑的
no **doubt**	很可能，无疑是
without **doubt**	无可置疑地
down with	打倒，不要
drag on / out	（使）拖延
draw in	（天）渐黑，（白昼）渐短；到站
draw on	吸，抽（烟）；利用；接近
draw up	起草，拟订；（使）停住
dress up	穿上盛装；装饰，修饰
drink in	吸入，吸收；倾听，陶醉于
drive at	想说，打算
drop by / in	顺便（或偶然）拜访
drop out	退出，退学
drum up	竭力争取（支持），招揽（生意等）
dry out	（使）干透
dry up	（使）干透，（使）枯竭
due to	因为，由于
in **due** course	到时候，在适当的时候
off **duty**	下了班的，不在值班的
on **duty**	在上班的，在值班的
be in **duty** bound to	有义务
dwell on / upon	老是想着，详述

E

be **eager** for	想得到，盼望
by **ear**	凭记忆，不看乐谱
have an **ear** for	对……听觉灵敏，对……有鉴赏力
early on	在初期，早先
in **earnest**	认真地（的），坚定地（的）
on **earth**	究竟，到底
at **ease**	安逸，不拘束
ease off / up	减轻，减缓
with **ease**	容易，不费力
take it **easy**	不慌不忙；别紧张
economize on	节省
on **edge**	紧张不安，烦躁
bring / carry / put into **effect**	实行，实现，使生效
come / go into **effect**	开始实施，开始生效
be in **effect**	有效
in **effect**	实际上，实质上
take **effect**	生效，起作用
to the **effect** that	大意是，以便
or **else**	否则，要不然
end in	以……为结果
end up	结束，告终
no **end**	非常，极其
on **end**	连续地
enter into	参加，成为……的一个因素
enter on / upon	着手做，开始，占有
in **essence**	实质上，基本上
even as	正当，恰恰在……的时候
at all **events**	不管怎样，无论如何
in the **event**	结果，到头来
in the **event** that	万一，倘若

in the **event** of	万一，倘若
every now and then	时常，间或
every other	每隔……
in **evidence**	明显地，显眼地
make an **example** of	惩罚……以警戒他人
except for	除去；要不是
take **exception** to	反对，表示异议
with the **exception** of	除去……，除……以外
in **excess** of	超过
to **excess**	过度，过分，过量
exclusive of	除……外，不计算在内
in **excuse** of	作为……的借口
exert…on…	对……施加……
exert oneself	努力，尽力
make an **exhibition** of oneself	出洋相，当众出丑
in **existence**	存在，现有
come into **existence**	开始存在，成立
at the **expense** of	由……付费；以……为代价
explain away	为……辩解，把……解释过去
be **exposed** to	面临，遭受，暴露于
beyond **expression**	无法形容，难以表达
to a certain **extent**	在一定程度上
go to **extreme**	走极端
in the **extreme**	非常，极其
catch one's **eye**	被某人看到，引起某人的注意
close / shut one's **eyes** to	不理会，视而不见
in the **eyes** of	在某人看来，在某人眼里，在……的心目中
in one's **eye**	在某人看来，在某人眼里
look sb. in the **eye**	正视，打量某人
keep an **eye** on	照看，密切注意
see eye to **eye**	看法完全一致

F

face to face	面对面地
face up to	勇敢地对付（或接受）
in the face of	在……面前；尽管，不顾
on the face of it	表面看来，从表面判断
without fail	必定，一定，无疑，务必
in good faith	真诚地，善意地，老实地
keep faith with	对……守信用
lose faith in	对……失去信心
on faith	毫无怀疑地，依赖地，单凭信仰
fall back	后退，退却
fall back on	借助于，依靠
fall behind	落后
fall for	受……的骗；倾心，爱上
fall in with	同意，符合；与……交往
fall on / upon	袭击，攻击；由……承担
fall out	吵架，失和；脱落
fall short of	没达到，低于
fall through	落空，成为泡影
fall to	开始，着手
be familiar with	熟悉，了解
have a fancy for	（没有道理地）喜欢，想要
take a fancy to	喜欢上，爱上
by far	到目前为止，……得多
far and wide	到处，广泛地
far from	远远不，完全不
in so far as	到……程度，就……，至于
so far	迄今为止；到某种程度
in fashion	时兴，流行
after the fashion (of)	依照……
at fault	有责任，出毛病，感到困惑
find fault	抱怨，找茬

in **favor** of	支持，赞同
be in **favor** with	受宠，受偏爱
in one's **favor**	对……有利
be out of **favor** with	失宠，不受宠
for **fear** of	以防，由于怕
in **fear** of	担心
for **fear** that	生怕，以免
feed (sb.) on sth.	靠吃……，用……喂养
be **fed** up with	厌烦，腻了
feel like	想要，心想
on the **fence**	抱骑墙态度，保持中立
few and far between	稀疏的，稀少的，彼此距离很远
fit as a **fiddle**	非常健康
figure out	想出，理解，明白
on **file**	存档
fill in	填满，填写
fill in for	替代
fill out	填写；长胖，变丰满
find out	找出，查明，发现
keep one's **fingers** crossed	祈求成功
catch (on) **fire**	着火，开始燃烧
on **fire**	起火，着火
play with **fire**	玩火，轻举妄动
set **fire** to	使燃烧，点燃
set the world / **flames** on fire	有突出成就
first of all	首先
at **first** sight	乍一看，一见
for the **first** time	第一次
in the **first** place	首先，第一
fit into	刚好放入
fit in with	符合，适应
be **fit** for	适合
fix on	决定，确定
fix up	安排，安顿，照应

flatter oneself	自以为是,自鸣得意
in the flesh	本人,亲身,以肉体形式
focus on	集中在……上
as follows	如下
follow through	把……进行到底,完成
follow up	追究,追查;采取进一步的行动
be fond of	喜欢,喜爱
fool about / around	虚度光阴,闲荡
make a fool of	愚弄,使出丑
by force	靠武力,强行
force… on…	把……强加给……
first and foremost	首要的是,首先
and so forth	等等
be fortunate in	幸运,有好运气
for free	免费
set free	释放
be friends with	与……友好相处,跟……做朋友
make friends with	与……交朋友,和睦
in full	全部地,不省略地
for / in fun	取乐,闹着玩
make fun of	拿……开玩笑,取笑
make a fuss of / over	关怀备至,过分注意,大惊小怪
in future	今后,从今以后
in the future	在将来

G

gain on	赶上,逼近
gamble away	赌掉,输光
take a gamble	冒风险
give the game away	不慎泄露秘密,露出马脚
gear up	使准备好,使做好安排;使换快挡

in **general**	一般说来，大体上
get about	走动，（消息等）传开
get across	使被了解，将……讲清楚
get ahead	获得成功，取得进展
get along	前进，进展；过活，生活
get along with	与……相处融洽
get around / round	走动；克服，设法回避（问题等）
get around / round to	抽出时间来做（或考虑）
get at	够得着；意指；查明；指责
get away	离开；逃脱，走开
get away with	做了坏事而逃避责罚
get back	回到；取回，恢复
get back at	对……报复
get by	通过；过得去，（勉强）过活
get down	从……下来，写下；使沮丧
get down to	开始认真处理，着手做
get in	进入，抵达；收获
get in with	对……亲近
get into	对……发生兴趣；卷入；使进入
get off	从……下来；动身；结束工作；逃脱惩罚
get on	登上，骑上；进展，过活
get on to	靠近，接近；识破，明白过来
get on with	与……相处融洽；继续
get out	使离开，退出，泄露；生产，出版
get over	从……恢复过来；克服；讲清楚
get through	完成，度过；使通过考试，使获得通过，讲清楚；打通电话
get together	相聚，聚集
get up	起立；起床
give away	赠送，泄露
give back	归还
give in	认输，交上，呈上
give off	发出（光、声音等）；散发出（气味）
give out	分发；用完；发出（光、声音等）

give over to	留作,把……留作特定用途;沉溺于
give up	停止,放弃
give up oneself	自首
at a glance	一看就,即刻
at first glance	乍一看,一看就
be glued to	粘到……上,胶着在……上,盯住不放
go about	着手做,处理,忙于
go about with	常与……交往
go after	追赶,追求
go against	反对,违背;对……不利
go ahead	进行;开始
go along	进行,进展
go along with	赞同
go around / round	四处走动;流传;足够分配
go around / round with	常与……交往
go at	攻击,着手做,努力做
go back on	违背(诺言等)
go by	(时间)过去;遵守,依据
go down	下降;沉没,日落
go down with	生……病
go for	想要获得;袭击;喜爱;适用于
go in for	从事,爱好;参加
go into	进入,参加;开始从事;调查
go off	爆炸,开火;(电等)中断;不再喜欢
go on	继续;进行,发生;(时间)过去;灯亮
go out	外出;过时;退潮,熄灯;送出,公布
go over	仔细检查,查看;复习
go through	仔细检查,详细讨论;经历;获得通过
go through with	将……干到底
go under	失败,破产;沉没
go up	上升;正在建设中;烧毁,炸毁
go with	跟……匹配;与……相伴;附属于
go without	没有
as good as	和……几乎一样

do sb. **good**	对……有好处
for **good**	永久地
good and...	非常，完全地
in **good** time	早早地（做完、到达等）
make the **grade**	达到规定的目标、成功
take for **granted**	认为……是理所当然；因视为理所当然而对……不予重视
be **grateful** to sb. for sth.	因……感谢某人
come to **grief**	失败，遭受不幸
grin and bear it	无怨言地接受（或承受）
grind out	生拼硬凑地写出，用功做出
come / get to **grips** with	揪扭，认真处理
fall to the **ground**	（计划、希望等）失败，落空
gain **ground**	进展，占优势
get off the **ground**	开始，（使）取得进展
on (the) **ground**(s) of	根据……，以……为理由
grow on	越来越被……喜爱
grow out of	产生于；长大得……与不相称，因长大而不再做
grow up	长大，成熟；形成，发展
guard against	警惕，防止
off (one's) **guard**	没有提防地
on (one's) **guard**	站岗，值班；警惕，提防
be **guilty** of	犯有……罪或过失

break sb. of (a **habit**)	使某人改掉某习惯
get / fall into the **habit** of	养成了……的习惯
in the **habit** of	有……的习惯
get in sb.'s **hair**	惹恼某人
make sb.'s **hair** stand on end	使某人毛骨悚然
in **half**	成两半

go **halves**	均摊费用
come to a **halt**	停止；停住
at **hand**	近在手边，在附近
by **hand**	用手，用体力
change **hands**	转手，转换所有者
hand in glove (with)	狼狈为奸，密切合作
hand in hand	同时并进地，密切关联地
hand on	把……传下去
hand out	分发，散发
hand over	交出，移交
have one's **hand** full	忙得腾不出手来
in **hand**	在进行中，待办理；在控制中
in sb's **hand**	在某人掌握中，在某人控制中
join **hands**	联手，携手
lend sb. a **hand**	帮助某人，协助某人
live from **hand** to mouth	勉强度日，现挣现吃
on **hand**	在手边，在近处
out of **hand**	无法控制；脱手；告终；立即
take / have a **hand** in	参与，插手，干预
wash one's **hand** of	对……不再负责，洗手不干
hang about / around	闲荡，闲待着
hang on	坚持，抓紧；等待片刻，不挂断电话；有赖于
hang on to	保留（某物）；紧紧抓住
hang together	同心协力；一致，相符
hang up	挂断（电话）；悬挂，挂起
come to no **harm**	未受到伤害
in **harmony** (with)	与……协调一致，与……和睦相处
talk through one's **hat**	胡说八道，吹牛
have had it	受够了，累极了；完了，没有了
have it in for	想伺机惩罚（或伤害），厌恶
have on	穿着，戴着
above / over one's **head**	难以理解

come to a **head**	达到危急的关头
head for	向……方向前进
head over heels	头朝下；完全地，深深地
keep one's **head**	保持镇静
lose one's **head**	慌乱，仓皇失措
put one's **head** together	集思广益，共同策划
at **heart**	内心里，本质上
break sb.'s **heart**	使某人伤心
by **heart**	凭记性
from (the bottom of) one's **heart**	从心底
in one's **heart** of **hearts**	在内心深处；事实上
lose **heart**	失去勇气，丧失信心
set one's **heart** on	下决心做
take **heart**	鼓起勇气，振作起来
take to **heart**	对……想不开，为……伤心
to one's **heart's** content	尽情地
with all one's **heart**	全心全意地，真心实意
the **hell**	到底，究竟
like **hell**	拼命地，极猛地
can / could not **help**	禁不住，忍不住
help out	帮助解决难题（或摆脱困境）
here and now	此时此地
here and there	各处
neither **here** nor there	离题的，不重要的
over the **hill**	在走下坡路，在衰退
hinder…from	阻碍，使……不能做
hinge on / upon	依……而定，以……为转移
hit on / upon	忽然想起，无意中发现
catch / get / take **hold** of	抓住，得到
hold back	阻挡，抑制；踌躇，退缩；保守秘密等
hold down	阻止（物价等）上涨；压制；保持住
hold forth	滔滔不绝地讲，提供

hold off	推迟，拖延；阻止，抵挡住
hold on	等一会，（打电话时）不挂断；坚持住
hold on to	仅仅抓住，坚持
hold out	伸出；维持；坚持
hold over	延缓，推迟
hold up	支持，支撑；延迟；展示；抢劫
hold with	赞成，赞同
at home	在国内；舒适；精通，熟悉
bring home to	使清楚，使明白
be honest in	诚实
in honor of	为了向……表示敬意，为纪念
on / upon one's honor	以名誉保证
hook up	用钩钩起，连接；通电
hook up to	将（或与）……连接起来
off the hook	脱离困境
hope for	希望（某事发生），希望有
on the horizon	即将发生的
to one's horror	令某人感到恐惧的是
on the hour	在整点时刻
keep house	管理家务
on the house	由店家出钱，免费
how come	怎么会……

I

break the ice	打破僵局
on thin ice	如履薄冰，处境极其危险
be identical with	和……完全相同
be identified with	被视为与……等同
if only	要是……多好
be ignorant of	不知道
impose...on	把……强加给

impress...on	给……留下印象
make / leave an **impression** on	给……留下印象
under the **impression** that	有……的印象,认为
improve on / upon	改进,胜过
be **in** for	一定会遇到(麻烦等);参加(竞争等)
in that	因为,原因在于
every **inch**	完全,彻底
be **inclusive** of	把……包括在内
on the **increase**	正在增加,不断增长
be **independent** of	独立的,不受约束的
be **indicative** of	表明,说明
be **indifferent** to	对……漠不关心,冷淡,不在乎
be **inferior** to	比……差
inform sb. of sth.	通知,告诉
be **innocent** of	无罪的,无辜的
inquire after	问起,问候
inquire into	调查,探究
inside out	里面朝外,彻底地
insist on	坚持要
for **instance**	例如,比如
insure... against...	保险……以防……
in the **interest(s)** of	为了……的利益
in the **interim**	在其间
interfere in	干涉
interfere with	打搅,干扰
at **intervals**	每隔一段时间(或距离),不时
intervene in	干预
be **involved** in	卷入,参加
iron out	消除(困难等)
of **itself**	自发,自然,自行,自然而然地
by **itself**	自动地,独自地
in **itself**	本质上,就其本身而言

J

be **jealous** of	妒忌
on the **job**	在工作，上班
jog sb.'s memory	唤起某人的记忆
out of **joint**	脱臼，出了问题，处于混乱状态
get the **jump** on	抢在……前面行动，较……占优势
just about	差不多，几乎
bring sb. to **justice**	把……交付审判，使归案受审
do **justice** to	公平地对待，公正地审判

K

be **keen** on	喜爱，渴望
keep a close watch on	密切注视
keep at	继续做
keep back	阻止，抑制；隐瞒，保留
keep down	压制，镇压；使处于低水平，控制
keep from	阻止，抑制
keep off	使让开，使不会接近
keep on	继续进行，继续下去
keep to	遵守，信守；坚持
keep up	使继续下去，信守；坚持
keep up with	跟上
kick about / around	被闲置于；到处游荡；非正式讨论
kick off	开始，开球
kick up	引起混乱，激起混乱
in **kind**	以实物偿付，以同样的办法
kind of	有点儿，有几分
of a **kind**	同类的
knock about / around	到处游荡；粗暴地对待

knock down	击倒，撞昏；杀价，降价；拆除
knock off	下班；迅速而不费力气地完成；减价
knock out	（拳击中）击倒，打昏
knock over	弄翻，打倒；使不知所措；完成，干完
know better than	很懂得，明事理而不至于……
to one's **knowledge**	据……所知

L

lap up	欣然接受
at **large**	逍遥法外地；一般来说，普遍地；详尽地
by and **large**	大体上，总的说来
lash out (at)	猛烈抨击
at (long) **last**	终于
at the **latest**	最迟
later on	以后，后来
laugh at	因……而笑；嘲笑
lay aside	把搁置一边；留存，储存
lay down	放下，交出；规定，制定
lay off	暂时解雇，停止做
lay out	摆出，铺开；布置，设计
leaf through	匆匆翻阅，浏览
turn over a new **leaf**	翻开新的一页，改过自新
at **least**	至少
least of all	最不，尤其不
not in the **least**	丝毫不，一点不
to say the **least**	退一步说
leave alone	让……独自待着；不打扰
leave behind	忘了带；把……撇在后面；遗留
leave off	停止，中断
leave out	遗漏，省略；把……排除在外

take (one's) **leave** of	向……告辞
not have a **leg** to stand on	（论点等）站不住脚
at **leisure**	有空，闲暇时；从容不迫地
lend itself to	适合于，有助于
at **length**	详尽地；最终，终于
go to great **lengths**	竭尽全力
let alone	更别提；不打扰；不惊动
let down	使失望；放下，降低
let go (of)	松手，放开
let off	放过，宽恕；开枪，放炮或焰火等；排放
let out	放走，释放；发出，泄漏，放出
let up	减弱，放松，停止
to the **letter**	严格地
be **liable** to	易于……的，应受
be **liable** for	对……应负责任的
lie in	在于
bring to **life**	使复活，给……以活力
come to **life**	苏醒过来，开始有生气
for **life**	一生，终生
bring to **light**	揭露，将……曝光
come to **light**	显露，暴露
in (the) **light** of	鉴于，由于
light up	照亮，点燃；容光焕发
throw / cast **light** on / upon	使人了解，阐明
in **line**	成一直线，成一排
in **line** with	与……一致，与……符合
line up	使排成行，使排队
on the **line**	随时可支付的；危险的
out of **line**	不成一直线；不一致，出格
listen in	收听，监听，偷听
live off	依赖……生活
live on	靠……生活，以……为食物
live out	活过（某段时间）
live through	度过，经受住

live up to	遵守，实践；符合，不辜负
live with	与……在一起生活；忍受，忍耐
on **loan**	借贷
lock up	锁上，把……监禁起来
log in	进入计算机系统
log out	退出计算机系统
before **long**	不久以后
long for	渴望，希望得到
no **longer**	不再，已不
so **long**	再见
for **long**	很久，很长时间
in the **long** run	从长远来看；最后
look after	照料，照顾；注意，关心
look ahead	向前看，考虑未来
look at	朝……看；看待
look back	回头看
look back on	回顾，回忆
look down on / upon	看不起，轻视
look for	寻找，寻求；惹来，招来
look forward to	盼望，期待
look in	顺便访问，顺便看望
look into	调查，观察
look on	观看，旁观
look out (for)	注意，留神
look over	把……看一遍；查看，参观
look through	浏览；详尽核查
look to	照管，留心；指望，依靠
look up	好转；查找；看望，拜访
look up to	尊敬
at a **loss**	困惑，不知所措
cast / draw **lots**	抽签，抓阄
fall in **love** (with sb.)	爱上（某人）
in **luck**	运气好
out of **luck**	运气不好

in the **main**	大体上,基本上
be **made** up of	由……组成,由……构成
major in	主修(某课程)
make believe	假装,假扮
make for	走向;促成,有助于
make it	办成,做到;及时到达
make of	理解,推断
make off	匆忙离开;偷走,携……而逃
make out	辨认出;理解,了解;写出
make up	虚构;构成;化妆;补充;和解
make up for	补偿,弥补
many a	许多的(后接单数名词)
as a **matter** of fact	事实上,其实
for that **matter**	就此而言,而且
by all **means**	当然可以;不惜一切
by **means** of	用,依靠
by no **means**	决不,并没有
beyond **measure**	不可估量,极度,过分
meet with	会晤;偶然遇到;经历,遭遇
in **memory** of	纪念
mend one's ways	改过,改正错误
on the **mend**	好转,在康复中
mention sth. to sb.	向某人提起某事
not to **mention**	更不必说,不必提及
at the **mercy** of	任凭……摆布,完全受……支配
be in a **mess**	乱七八糟,处境困难
make a mess of	弄乱,打乱
mess about / around	瞎忙;闲荡;轻率地对待

mess up	把……弄乱 / 弄糟 / 弄脏
mess with	干预，介入
in the middle of	正忙于
in the midst of	在……之中，正当……的时候
bear / keep in mind	记住
bring / call to mind	使回想起
change one's mind	改变主意
have in mind	想到，考虑到
in one's mind's eye	在想象中
make up one's mind	下定决心，打定主意
never mind	不用担心；不要紧
to my mind	以我看，我认为
by mistake	错误地
mix up	混淆，弄混，弄乱
at the moment	此刻，目前
for the moment	暂时，目前
the moment that	一……就
gain / gather momentum	发展加快，势头增大
in the mood for	有情绪做，有心境做
mop up	擦去；扫荡，肃清；完成
what is more	更重要的，更有甚者，而且
at most	至多，不超过
make the most of	充分利用，尽量利用
get a move on	赶快，加紧
move in on	移近，向……逼近
move on	继续前进；走开，不要停留
move up	（使）升级，提升
on the move	在活动，在行进
be not much of	不是很好的
much as	虽然，尽管
a multitude / multitudes of	许多，大量

nail down	确定
in the **name** of	以……的名义
name after	用……名字命名
be **native** to	所产的
by **nature**	天生的，生来
in **nature**	本质上
of **necessity**	无法避免地，必定
in the **neighborhood** of	在……附近，大约
get on one's **nerve**	惹某人心烦
next to	紧靠……的旁边；几乎，近于
night and day	夜以继日
none but	除……之外，只有
none other than	不是别人，正是……
follow one's **nose**	笔直前进；凭直觉/本能行事
stick one's **nose** into	探问，探看；干预
compare **notes**	交换意见
take **note** of	注意，留神
for **nothing**	不花钱地；徒劳地
nothing but	只有，只不过
to say **nothing** of	更不用说
at short / a moment's **notice**	提前很短时间通知
do sth. at short **notice**	只给很少时间准备
until further **notice**	在另行通知前
take **notice** of	注意
(every) **now** and then / against	时而，偶尔
just **now**	现在；刚才，才不久
now (that)	既然，由于
get **nowhere**	使无进展，使不能成功
nowhere near	远远不，远不及

on / under **oath**	发誓
object to	反对
objection to	反对
on **occasion**(s)	有时，间或
occupy oneself with / in	忙于（某事）
it **occurs** to sb. that...	某人想到……
against all (the) **odds**	尽管有极大困难
at **odds** with	与……不和；与……不一致
odds and ends	零星杂物，琐碎物品
as **often** as not	往往，多半
every so **often**	有时，偶尔
more **often** than not	往往，多半
on and on	继续不断地，不停地
all at **once**	突然，忽然；同时，一起
at **once**	马上，立刻；同时，一起
once (and) for all	一劳永逸地，永远地
once in a while	偶尔，间或
(just) for **once**	就这一次
once more / again	再一次
once upon a time	从前
at **one** (with)	（与……）一致
one by one	一个一个地，一次地
(all) by **oneself**	独自（没有别人帮助）
only too	极，非常
in the **open**	在户外，在野外；公开地
open up	打开，开放；开发，开辟
operate on sb.	给某人做手术
bring / put into **operation**	实施，使生效，使运行
come / go into **operation**	施行，实行，生效
in **operation**	工作中；起作用，生效

be of the **opinion**	持有……的看法
be **opposed** to	反对
be **opposite** to	与……相反
in **order**	按顺序；整齐，处于良好状态
in short **order**	立即
on **order**	定购中，定制中
out of **order**	出故障的；不按次序；违反会议规程的
made to **order**	定做的（衣服）
out of the **ordinary**	不寻常的，非凡的
originate in / from	起源于，由……引起
on the **outskirts** (of)	在城郊
every **other**	每隔一个的
other than	不同于，非；除了
out of	由于；离开；缺乏；从……中
at / from the **outset**	开端，开始
at the **outside**	最多，充其量
outside of	在……外面；除……之外
all **over** again	再一次，重新
over and over (again)	一再地，再三地
over and above	除……之外（还），超过
owe...to...	把……归于……
owing to	由于，因为
hold one's **own**	坚守住；保持力量，不衰退
of one's **own**	某人自己的
on one's **own**	独自；独立地

P

keep **pace** (with)	（与……）并驾齐驱
set the **pace**	起带头作用
pack up	把……打包
go to great **pains**	下功夫，努力

take **pains**	努力，尽力，下苦功
palm off	用欺骗手段把……卖掉
on **paper**	以书面形式；在理论上
for one's **part**	就个人来说，至于本人
in **part**	部分地
on the **part** of	在……方面，就……而言
part with	放弃，出让
participate in	参加
be **particular** about	讲究，挑剔（吃、穿）
in **particular**	特别，尤其
pass away	去世
pass by	经过，从……旁边过
pass off (as)	充作，被看作，被当作
pass on	传授，传递
pass over	对……不加考虑
pass up	放过（机会），放弃
pat on the back	赞扬，鼓励
patch up	解决；修补，草草修理
pay back	偿还；回报，向……报复
pay off	还清；偿清工资解雇（某人）；取得成功
pay out	付钱，出钱
pay up	全部付清
at **peace**	处于和睦（或平静）状态
in **peace**	安静，平安
make **peace**	言和，和解
peel off	剥掉，脱去
be **peculiar** to	特有的，独具的
penalty for	对……的处罚/罚金
persist in	坚持，固执
in **person**	亲自，本人
pick at	吃一点点，无食欲地吃
pick on	找……岔子；挑选，选中
pick out	挑出；辨认出
pick up	拣起；用车接；获得；好转；继续

go to **pieces**	崩溃，垮掉
in **place**	在合适的位置
out of **place**	不在合适的位置；不适当的
take the **place** of	代替，取代
bring into **play**	使运转，启动
come into **play**	开始活动，投入使用
play at	玩，做游戏，假扮……玩
play back	放，播放
play down	降低……的重要性，贬低
play off... against...	使……相斗
play on	利用
play up	强调，突出
plug in	给……接通电源，连接
take the **plunge**	决定冒一次险，采取决定性步骤
in sb.'s **pocket**	在某人掌握之中，受制于某人
beside the **point**	离题的，不相关的
make a **point** of	特别注意，重视
on the **point** of	正要……之际/之时
point out	指出
to the **point**	切中要害，切题
come to the **point**	谈主要问题
there is no **point** in doing sth.	没必要做某事
be **popular** with / among	大众所喜爱的，拥戴
in the **position** of	处在……位置上
pour out	倾诉，倾吐
in **practice**	在实践中，实际上
out of **practice**	生疏的，荒废的
put in **practice**	实施，实行
bring / put... into **practice**	使……成为现实
prefer... to...	宁愿要，更喜欢
at **present**	现在，此刻
for the **present**	目前，暂时
preside over / at	主持（会议、业务等）

press on	加紧进行
presume on	（不正当地）利用；指望，过分依靠
prevail over	占优势，压倒，战胜
prevent... from	使……不，防止……做
be **previous** to	在……之前
at any **price**	不惜任何代价，无论如何
prick up one's ears	竖起耳朵注意听；立刻注意起来
take **pride** in	以……自豪
pride oneself on / upon	以……自豪
in **print**	以印刷的形式；已出版的，仍可买到的
out of **print**	已售完的，已绝版的
in **principle**	原则上
prior to	优先的，在前的
in **private**	在私下，秘密地
in all **probability**	十有八九，很可能
proceed from	由……出发，由……引起或产生
proceed with	继续进行
in **progress**	进行中
prohibit... from	禁止，阻止
in **proportion** to	与……成比例
protect... from...	阻止……不受，保护不受
be **proud** of	为……自豪
provide for	为……做准备
in **public**	公开地，当众
pull apart	把……拉开或拆开，被拉开或拆开
pull away	开走，（使）离开
pull down	拆毁
pull in	（车）停下/到站，（船）靠岸
pull off	（成功地）完成；扯下，脱去
pull out	拔出，抽出；驶出；（使）摆脱困境
pull over	驶到或驶向路边
pull through	渡过难关；恢复健康
pull together	齐心协力，团结起来

pull up	（使）停下
on **purpose**	故意
to the **purpose**	得要领的，中肯的
in hot **pursuit**	穷追不舍
push around	摆布，欺负
push on	匆忙向前，继续前进
put across / over	解释清楚，使被理解
put aside	储存，保留；暂不考虑
put away	放好，收好
put in	花费，付出；正式提出，申请
put off	推迟，拖延；阻止，劝阻
put on	穿上；上演；增加体重
put out	熄灭，关（灯）；出版；伸出；生产
put through	接通电话
put up	搭起；张贴；提高（价格等）
put up with	忍受，容忍
puzzle out	苦苦思索而弄清楚或解决

be **qualified** in	在某种科目或学科上合格
be **qualified** for	在某种职业上合格
in **quantity**	大量
beyond (all) **question**	毫无疑问
call in / into **question**	对……提出疑问/异议
in **question**	正在谈论的
out of the **question**	毫不可能的
without **question**	毫无疑问，毫无异议
jump the / a **queue**	不按次序排队，插队
on the **quiet**	秘密地，私下地

at **random**	随便地，任意地
range over	范围包括
the **rank** and file	普通士兵，普通成员
at any **rate**	无论如何，至少
at this **rate**	照这种情形，既然这样
had / would **rather** than	宁愿……而不愿……
rather than	与其……倒不如……，不是……而是……
in the **raw**	处在自然状态的；裸体的
beyond the **reach** of	无法达到，无法得到，无法理解
out of **reach** of	无法够到
within **reach** of / within one's **reach**	够得到，能拿到
react to	对……做出反应
react on / upon	对……产生影响
react against	做出反抗或反对
at the **ready**	准备立即行动
for **real**	严肃的，认真的；真正的，确实的
in **reality**	实际上，事实上
bring up the **rear**	处在最后的位置，垫后
beyond all **reason**	没有道理的
by **reasons** of	由于
it stands to **reason** that...	……理所当然
within **reason**	理智的，合理的
reckon with	估计；处理
on **record**	正式记录的，公开发表的
refer to... as...	把……称作 / 看作
with **reference** to	关于，就……而言
as **regards**	关于，至于
with / in **regard** to	关于，就……而论
give one's **regards** to sb.	向……问候
regardless of	不顾，不惜

in the region of	在……左右，接近
give (free) rein to	对……不加约束，放任
in relation to	有关，关于，涉及
relative to	有关，关于，涉及
be relevant to	与……有关的
to one's relief	令……感到放心的是
relieve... of...	解除，解脱；帮助拿；辞退
rely on	依靠，信赖
remark on / upon	对……发表评论
remedy for	对……治疗，补救，赔偿
remind sb. of	提醒某人，使某人想起
in good repair	处于良好状态
beyond reproach	不受责备的
resort to	诉诸……，求助于……
resort to force	诉诸武力
with respect to	关于，至于
in response to	作为对……的回应
rest on / upon	依靠，寄托
rest with	在……手中，是……的责任；由……决定；依靠
restrain... from	抑制……不……
restrict... to	把……限制于……
as a result	作为结果，因此
as a result of	作为……的结果，由于
result in	导致
with the result that	其结果是
in retrospect	回想起来，事后看来
in return (for)	作为报答（或回报、交换）
revolve around	以……为主要内容
get rid of	摆脱，除去，处理掉
ride out	安然度过，经受得住
by rights	按理说
in one's own right	凭本身的权利（或能力、资格等）
in the right	正确，有理

ring off	挂断电话
ring up	打电话给
run riot	胡作非为，撒野
give rise to	引起，导致，为……的原因
rise above	克服，不受……的影响
rise to	起而应付，证明能够应付
at risk	处境危险
at the risk of	冒着……的危险
run / take risk of	冒……的风险
on the road (to)	在去……的旅途中；在向……的转变中
root sth. out	根除，杜绝
rope in	用绳围圈起来，说服
go the round(s) (of)	传播，流行
round up	把……聚起来
in a row	一个接一个地，接连不断地
rub it in	反复提及令人不快的事
in ruins	成废墟，毁坏，毁灭
as a rule	通常，一般来说
rule out	把……排除在外，排除……的可能性
in the long run	从长远看，终究
in the short run	在不久的将来
on the run	忙碌，奔波；奔跑，逃跑
run across	撞见，碰见
run away with	战胜；偷走；与……私奔；轻易地赢得
run down	贬低；耗尽；减少，撞倒，查找出
run into	遭遇；撞在……上；偶然碰见；共计
run off	跑掉，逃跑；很快写出
run out	到期，期满
run out of	用完，耗尽
run over	在……上驶过；把……很快过一遍
run through	贯穿；匆匆阅读；排练
run to	跑向，达到，发展到；趋向
run up	积欠（账款、债务等）
run up against	遭遇，遇到

in **safety**	安全地
safe and sound	安然无恙
to be on the **safe** side	为了保险起见
sail through	顺利通过
set sail	起航
for the **sake** of	为了……起见
for **sale**	待售，供出售
on **sale**	出售；廉价销售
take with a **salt** / grain of salt	对……有保留，对……半信半疑
worth one's **salt**	胜任的，称职的，名副其实的
all the **same**	都一样；尽管如此，仍然
the **same** as	与……一致，与……相同的
be **satisfied** with	满意
save for	除……之外，除去
go without **saying**	不用说，不言而喻
I dare **say**	（我想）可能，（我想）是这样
to **say** nothing of	更不用说，何况
to **say** the least	至少可以说
on a **scale**	在……规模上
scale down	缩减
make oneself **scarce**	溜走，躲开
scarcely when	一……就……
behind the **scenes**	在幕后，不公开的
ahead of **schedule**	提前
be **scheduled** for	定在某时（进行）
on **schedule**	按时间表，及时，准时
on that **score**	在那一点上，就那一点来说
from **scratch**	从零开始，从头做起
up to **scratch**	合格，处于良好状态
put the **screw**(s) on	对……施加压力，强迫
screw up	拧紧；扭歪，把……弄糟

a **sea** of	大量,茫然一片
at **sea**	在海上;茫然,不知所措
in **search** of	寻找,寻求
in **season**	应时的,当令的,在旺季;及时的,适宜的
out of **season**	不当令的,不在旺季的
second to none	最好的
in **secret**	暗地里,秘密地
see about	办理,安排
see off	为……送行
see out	坚持到……的终点,完成
see through	看透,识破
see to	注意,照料
see (to it) that	一定注意到,务必使
seeing (that)	鉴于,由于
go / run to **seed**	花开结籽,衰老,走下坡路
seize on / upon	利用
seize up	(机器等)卡住,停顿
sell off	廉价出售(存货)
sell out	售完,脱销
sell up	卖掉(全部家产等)
send away	把……打发走
send for	派人去请,召唤;函购,函索
send in	递送,呈报,提交
send off	邮寄,发送
send out	发送;发出
be **senior** to	比……年长
in **sequence**	按顺序,按先后次序
come to one's **sense**	恢复理智,醒悟过来;苏醒过来
in a **sense**	从某种意义上说
make **sense**	讲得通,有意义,言之有理
talk **sense**	说话有理
set about	开始,着手
set against	使敌视;使抵消
set apart	使与众不同;留出,拨出

set aside	留出，拨出；把……置于一旁，不理会
set back	推迟，阻碍；使花费
set down	写下，记下
set forth	阐明，陈述
set in	开始（并将继续下去）
set off	出发，起程，激起，引起
set on	袭击；唆使
set out	动身；开始；摆放；阐明，陈述
set up	创立，建立；竖立；开业
settle down	定居；平静下来；定下心来
settle for	勉强认可
settle in / into	在新居安顿下来；适应
settle on / upon	选定，决定
settle up	付清，结清
sew up	缝合；确保……的成功
shade in / into	逐渐变成
shake down	敲诈，勒索；彻底搜查
shake off	抖落；摆脱
shake up	打击；使震惊
in (good) shape	处于（良好）状态
shape up	发展顺利，表现良好
take shape	成形，形成
share in / have a share in	分摊，分担
on the shelf	被搁置
be shocked at / by	对……感到震惊
in sb.'s shoes	处于……的地位（或境地）
cut short	中断，打断
fall short of	达不到，不符合
for short	缩写，简称
go / be short of	缺乏
in short	简而言之，总之
like a shot	立即，飞快地
shoulder to shoulder	肩并肩地，齐心协力地
shout down	用叫喊声淹没（或压倒）

shove off	动身，离开
show off	炫耀，卖弄
show up	暴露，显露；来到，露面
shrug off	对……满不在乎，对……不屑一顾
shut away	把……藏起来，隔离
shut down	（使）关闭，（使）停工
shut in	把……关在里面，禁闭
shut off	切断，关掉，使停止运转
at the side of	在……旁边，与……相比
on the side	作为兼职或副业；暗地里
side by side	肩并肩地，一起
at first sight	乍一看，初看起来
at / on sight	一见（就）
catch sight of	发现，突然看见
in sight	看得见；在望，在即
lose sight of	忘记，忽略
know sb. by sight	与……只是面熟
out of sight	看不见，在视野之外
sign away / over	签字放弃
sign for	签收
sign in	签到，登记
sign off	停止播送，结束
sign on / up	签约雇用 / 受雇
sign out	签名登记离开；登记携出（某物）
sink in	被理解，被理会
sit around	坐着没事干
sit back	在一旁闲着，袖手旁观
sit in on	列席会议，旁听
sit out / through	耐着性子看完（或听完），坐着熬到……结束
sit up	坐直；不睡，熬夜
size up	估计，判断
sketch out	简要地叙述
sleep off	以睡眠消除（疲劳等）
sleep through	未被吵醒

slow down / up	放慢，使减速
on the sly	秘密地，偷偷地
smell of	有……的气味
smooth over	缓和，减轻
snap out of	迅速从……中恢复过来
snap up	抢购；抢先弄到手
sniff out	发觉，发现
to be snowed under	忙得不可开交，被压倒
and so on / forth	等等
ever so	非常，极其
or something	诸如此类的什么
something of	在某种程度上，有点儿
would sooner	宁愿，宁可
of sorts / of a sort	马马虎虎的，较差的；各种各样的
out of sorts	身体不适，心情欠佳
sort of	有几分，有那么点儿
sort out	整理；弄清楚，解决
sound out	试探，探询
space out	把……间隔开
to spare	过剩，有余
speak for	代表……讲话，为……辩护；证明，表明
speak ill of	说……的坏话
speak out / up	大声地说，大胆地说
speed up	加快速度
spell out	详细地说明
spin out	拖长……时间；使（钱）尽可能多维持一些日子
spit sth. out	吐出
split up	断绝关系，离婚；划分
sponge on / off	依赖他人生活
on the spot	在场，到场；立即，当场
spread out	（人群等）散开；伸展，延伸
on the spur of the moment	一时冲动之下，当即
square off	把……做成方形；摆好（架势）
square up	付清，结账

stab in the back	背后中伤，背叛
at **stake**	在危急关头，在危险中
stamp out	踩灭，消灭
stand by	袖手旁观；坚持，遵守；支持，帮助；做好准备
stand down	退出，（从某职位上）退下
stand for	是……的缩写，代表；主张，支持；容忍，接受
stand in	代替，代表，做替身
stand out	清晰地显出，引人入胜；杰出，出色
stand up	站起来；（论点、论据等）站得住脚
stand up for	支持，维护，保卫
stand up to	勇敢地面对，抵抗；经得起，顶得住
take a **stand** against	采取某种立场反对
take a **stand** for	采取某种立场支持
start off	出发，动身；（使）开始从事
start on	开始进行，着手处理
start out	出发，动身；本来想要
start up	创办；开动，发动
to **start** with	首先，一开始
stay put	留在原地
in **step**	齐步，合拍，协调
out of **step**	不合拍，不协调
step aside / down	让位，辞职
step by step	逐步地
step in	介入，开始参与
step up	加快，加速；增加，逐步提高
stick around	等在旁边，留下等待
stick at	继续努力做，坚持干
stick by	忠于，对……真心；坚持，维护
stick sth. on	把……贴在……上
stick out	坚持到底；突出，显眼
stick out for	坚持要求
stick to	粘贴；紧跟，紧随；坚持，忠于，信守
stick together	团结一致，互相支持
stick up for	支持，为……辩护

stick with	紧随；继续从事
stir up	激起，挑起
out of stock	无现货的，脱销的
take stock of	对……估价，判断
stop by	顺便造访，串门
stop off / over	中途停留
in store	储藏着，准备着；必将到来，快要发生
set store by	重视，尊重
straight away / off	立即，马上
in strength	大量地
on the strength of	基于，根据
at a stretch	不停地，连续地
be strict with	对……严格要求
take in one's stride	轻而易举地应付，轻松地胜任
be / go on strike	罢工
strike off	删去，除名
strike out	独立闯新路，开辟
strike up	开始（谈话、相识等）
as such	就其本身而论
suck up	吸收
all of a sudden	突然，冷不防
in sum	总而言之
sum up	总结，概括
in summary	总的来说，概括起来
be superior to	优于……，比……好
for sure	确切地，肯定
make sure	查明，弄清楚；务必
sure enough	果然，毫无疑问
be taken by surprise	使吃惊，使感到意外；使措手不及
to one's surprise	使某人惊奇的是
suspect sb. of	疑心某人犯有……
be suspicious of	对……有疑心
swear by	极其信赖
swear in	使宣誓就职

swear off	保证戒掉,放弃
in full **swing**	正在全力进行中
switch off	(用开关)关掉
switch on	(用开关)开启

take aback	使吃惊,使困惑
take after	与……相像
take apart	拆除,拆开
be **taken** as	把……当作,认为
take away	减去
take back	收回(说错的话);使回忆起
take down	拆,拆卸;记下;写下
be **taken** for	把……认为是,把……看成
take in	接受,吸收;包括;领会,理解;欺骗
take off	脱下;起飞;匆匆离去
take on	开始雇用;呈现,具有;同……较量;承担,从事
take out	带……出去;除掉,毁掉
take out on	对……发泄
take over	接收,接管;承袭,借用
take the floor	起立发言
take to	开始喜欢;开始从事
take up	开始从事;把……继续下去;着手处理;占去
take up on	接受邀请或挑战
take up with	与……成朋友
talk back	回嘴,顶嘴
talk down to	以居高临下的口气说话
talk into	说服某人做某事
talk out of	说服某人放弃做某事
talk over	商议,商量,讨论

tangle with	与……争吵 / 或打架，与……有纠葛
be taken to task	指责，批评
taste of	有……味道
to (one's) taste	合……的口味，中意
in tears	流着泪，含着泪
tear at	撕，扯
tear away	使勉强离去
tear down	拆掉，拆除
tear into	攻击，抨击
tear up	撕毁
all told	总共，合计
tell apart	区分，辨别
tell... from	辨别，认出
tell off	责备；分派，指派，向……透露
lose one's temper	发脾气，发怒
be on good / bad terms with	关系好（不好）
in terms of	用……的话；按照
come to terms	妥协，和解
thanks to	由于，多亏
but then	但另一方面，然而
then and there / there and then	当场，当即
through thick and thin	不顾艰难险阻，在任何条件下
all things considered	从各方面考虑起来
for one thing	首先，一则
have a thing about	对……特别感兴趣或厌恶
make a thing of / out of	对……小题大做
think back to	回想，回忆
think better of	（经过考虑）对……改变主意（或看法）
think of	想出，提出；想起；考虑，关心
think of as	把……看作是，以为……是
think over	仔细考虑
think through	彻底地全面考虑
think up	想出，设计出
on second thoughts	再三考虑

at the **thought** of	一想到
on the **threshold** of	即将开始
be **through** with	做好，完成
through and through	完全，彻底
throw away	扔掉，抛弃；错过，浪费
throw in	外加，额外奉送
throw off	摆脱掉；轻易做出
throw out	扔掉；撵走
throw up	呕吐；产生（想法）
all **thumbs**	笨手笨脚
tick away / by	（时间一分一秒地）过去
tide over	使度过（困难时期）
tidy away	收起（某物），放好
tie down	限制，牵制
tie in with	与……一致，配合
tie up	拴住，捆牢；使（钱等）难以动用，阻碍
at full **tilt**	全速地，全力地
ahead of **time**	提前
all **the time**	一直，始终
at a **time**	每次，一次
at all **times**	随时，总是
at no **time**	从不，决不
at one **time**	曾经，一度
at the same **time**	同时；然而，不过
at **times**	有时，间或
behind the **times**	过时，落后
behind **time**	迟到，晚点
for the **time** being	眼下，暂时
from **time** to time	有时，不时
in no **time**	立即，马上
once upon a **time**	从前
take one's time	不着急，不慌忙
together with	同……一起，连同
by the same **token**	出于同样的原因，同样地

tone down	使缓和
on top	处于优势
on top of	除……之外
top up	装满，加满
in total	总共
in touch (with)	联系，接触
out of touch (with)	不联系，不接触
touch down	降落，着陆，底线得分
touch off	使爆炸，触发
touch on / upon	谈到，论及
touch up	润色，改进
in tow	被拖着，陪伴着
keep track of	与……保持联系
lose track of	失去与……的联系，不能跟上……的进展
track down	跟踪找到，追查到
trade in	以（旧物）贴换同类新物
trade on / upon	（为达到利己目的而）利用
trail along behind	没精打采地（跟在后面）走
by trial and error	反复试验，不断探索
a trifle	有点儿，稍微
trip up	把……绊倒；使犯错误
in trouble	陷入困境，倒霉
be true of	适合于
be true to	忠于
come true	实现，成为现实
trust... to	把……委托给
place / put / have trust in	依赖
in truth	的确，事实上
try on	试穿
try out	试验
tuck away	把……隐没在，把……藏起来；大吃
tuck in	痛快地吃；给……盖好被子；把……塞好
tuck up	给……盖好被子

tumble to	突然明白，领悟
in tune with	与……协调，与……一致
out of tune with	与……不协调，与……不一致；跑调
to the tune of	达……之多，共计
tune in	收听，收看
by turns	轮流地，交替地
in turn	依次地，轮流地；转而，反过来
take turns	依次，轮流
turn around / round	转变，使转好
turn away	回绝，把……打发走
turn back	使折回，使往回走
turn down	关小，调低；拒绝
turn in	交还，上交；上床睡觉
turn out	结果是；关掉；制造；驱逐
turn over	翻过来；仔细考虑；交，移交
turn to	求助于，查阅
turn up	开大；出现，来到
be typical of	是……的特点

up against	面临（问题、困难等）
up to	胜任……的；是……义不容辞的责任；取决于……的
in use	在使用着的，在用的
make use of	利用
out of use	不被使用，废弃
put to use	使用
use up	用完，用光
as usual	像平常一样，照例
do one's utmost	竭力，尽全力

in vain	徒然，白费力
be valid for	对……有效的
a variety of	种种，多种多样的
on the verge of	接近于，濒临于
in the vicinity of	在……附近，与……接近
in view of	鉴于，考虑到
in the view of	按……的意思
with a view of	为了，为的是
by virtue of	借助，由于

in the wake of	紧紧跟随；随着……而来
wake (up) to	认识到，意识到
walk away / off with	轻易获胜；顺手带走，偷走
walk out	（为表示抗议而）突然离去；罢工
walk out on	抛弃，舍弃，不履行
ward off	防止，避开
warm to	对……产生好感；对……变得感兴趣
warm up	使暖起来；使活跃起来；使热身
wash up	洗餐具；洗手洗脸；（浪头）将……冲上岸
waste away	日趋消瘦，日益衰弱
be on the watch for	不断监视看有没有……
be on the watch against	不断监视为了防范……
watch out (for)	密切注意，提防，留神
all the way	一直，完全
by the way	顺便地，附带地说说
give way	让路；让步，屈服；塌陷，倒塌
go out of one's way	特地，不怕麻烦地

in a **way**	在某种程度上，从某一点上
in no **way**	决不
in the / sb.'s **way**	挡某人的道，妨碍某人
make one's **way**	去，前往，行进
make **way**	让路，腾出地方或位置
no **way**	无论如何不，不可能
one **way** or another	以某种形式
out of the **way**	异常的，罕见的；偏远的
under **way**	在进行中
wear away	磨损，磨去；消磨，流逝
wear off	渐渐减少，逐渐消失
wear out	穿破，磨损，用坏；使疲乏
under the **weather**	不舒服，有病
carry **weight**	有分量，有影响
pull one's **weight**	干好本分工作
throw one's **weight** about / around	滥用权势，耀武扬威
just as **well**	没关系，无妨，不妨
may as **well**	还不如，不妨
all the **while**	始终
once in a **while**	偶尔
as a **whole**	作为一个整体，整个看来
on the **whole**	总的来说，大体上
go **wild**	狂怒，狂热
at **will**	任意，随意
with a will	有决心的
win over	说服，把……争取过来
in the **wind**	即将发生
wind up	上发条；结束，停止
in the **wings**	已准备就绪的，就在眼前的
wipe out	擦掉，擦净；彻底摧毁，消灭
at one's **wits'** end	智穷计尽
put in a (good) **word** for	为……说好话
in a **word**	总之
in other **words**	换言之

have a word with sb.	谈一谈
have words with sb.	争吵
have the last word	有决定权
keep one's word	遵守诺言
word for word	逐字地
work off	消除，去除
work at / on	从事，致力于
work out	算出；理解；想出；解决；产生结果
work up	激发，激起；制订出，精心制作
in the world	究竟，到底
what is worse	更糟的是
at (the) worst	在最糟的情况下
be worthy of	值得，够得上，配得上
write down	记下
write off	取消，注销，勾销
go wrong	出错，犯错误；发生故障

year after / by year	年年
yield to	对……屈服，投降，让步

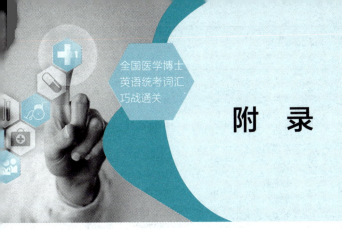

附 录

考博英语常见同义词一览表

a matter of speculation	supposition	phr.	推断	account	explain	v.	说明
a solicitation of	an invitation of	phr.	恳求；恳请	accumulate	collect	v.	积累；聚集
abandoned	left	a.	被遗弃的	accumulate	pile up	v.	积累；聚集
aberrant	abnormal	a.	脱离常轨的	accurate	correct	a.	正确的
abort	quit	v.	夭折；中止	accurately	correctly	ad.	正确地
abruptly	suddenly	ad.	突然地；意外地	acknowledge	recognize	v.	承认
absorb	appeal	v.	吸收；被……吸引	actually	in fact	ad.	事实上
absorb	learn（学习）	v.	吸收	added	extra	a.	附加的；额外的
absorb	take in	v.	吸收；被……吸引	adept	skilled	a.	熟练的
abstract	not concrete	a.	抽象的；非实际的	adherent	supporter	n.	拥护者
absurd	ridiculous	a.	荒谬的；可笑的	adjacent	nearby	a.	毗连的
abundance	large amount	n.	大量	adjacent	neighboring	a.	毗连的
abundance	great number	n.	大量	adjust	modify	v.	调整；改变……以适应
abundant	affluent	a.	丰富的；大量的	admit	let in	v.	准许进入

483

abundant	ample	a.	丰富的；大量的	agile	move and act quickly	a.	灵活的；敏捷的
abundant	numerous	a.	丰富的；大量的	air	feeling	n.	气氛
abundant	plentiful	a.	丰富的；大量的	alarm	sound	v.	警报
abundant	substantial	a.	丰富的；大量的	alarm	warning	n.	警告
abundantly	plentifully	ad.	丰富地；大量地	albeit	although	conj.	尽管；虽然
access	reach	v.	接近	albeit	even though	conj.	尽管；虽然
accessible	reachable	a.	可接近的	allow	enable	v.	允许
accessible	easy to reach	a.	易接近的	allude	suggest	v.	暗示
accidental	unexpected	a.	意外的；偶然的	allude to	refer to	phr.	提到
accommodate	provide for	v.	提供	ally with	link to	phr.	结盟
accomplished	achieved	a.	完成的	alter	change to	v.	改变
accomplished	skilled	a.	熟练的	amazing	remarkable	a.	令人惊讶的，非凡的
account	description	n.	说明	ambiguous	vague	a.	不明确的
adopt	enact	v.	采用	appreciable	noticeable	a.	相当可观的
advance	improvement	n.	发展；增长	approach	method	n.	方法
advent	arrival	n.	出现；到来	approach	move toward	v.	接近
advent	beginning	n.	出现；到来	approximately	roughly	ad.	大约
affair	matter	n.	事件；事情	architecture	structure	n.	构造
afford	provide	v.	提供；给予	archive	record	v.	存档
aggravate	increase	v.	加重；加剧	archive	stock	v.	存档
aggravate	annoy	v.	使恼火	archive	store	v.	存档
aggregate	overall	a.	聚集的；合计的	arduous	difficult	a.	艰巨的
aggregate	combined	a.	聚集的；合计的	arid	dry	a.	干旱的
agile	astute	a.	灵活的；敏捷的	arise	emerge	v.	出现
agile	clever	a.	灵活的；敏捷的	arrangement	configuration	n.	安排；布置
agile	quick and active	a.	灵活的；敏捷的	array	range	n.	一系列

ambivalent	mixed	a.	矛盾的	article	item	n.	物品
ample	plentiful	a.	充足的；丰富的	article	object	n.	物品
ample	spacious	a.	宽敞的	as a rule	in general	phr.	通常
anchor	hold in place	v.	使固定	assert	declare	v.	断言；宣称
ancient	old	a.	古老的	assertion	strong statement	n.	断言；主张
ancient	antique	a.	古老的	asset	advantage	n.	资产；有利条件
annihilate	destroy	v.	消灭	assimilate	combine	v.	同化
annihilate	completely remove	v.	消灭	assistance	help	n.	帮助；协助
annually	yearly	ad.	每年	assorted	various	a.	各式各样的
anomaly	irregularity	n.	异常的人或物	assume	believe	v.	假定；设想
antagonist	competitor	n.	对手；敌手	assume	suppose	v.	假定；设想
anticipate	expect	v.	预期	assume	take on	v.	承担
antiseptic	clean	a.	抗菌的	assumption	premise	n.	假设
antithesis	opposite	n.	对立面	astonishing	amazing	a.	惊人的
antler	horn	n.	鹿角	astute	clever	a.	敏锐的
anxiety	worry	n.	忧虑；担心	at random	without a definite pattern	phr.	随便地；任意地
apart from	exception	phr.	除了……之外	attachment to	preference for	phr.	依恋
apart from	except for	phr.	除了……之外	attain	achieve	v.	达到；获得
apparatus	equipment	n.	仪器；设备	attainment	achievement	n.	达到；获得
apparent	obvious	a.	显然的	attendant	accompanying	a.	伴随的
apparently	clearly	ad.	显然地	attest to	confirm	phr.	证实
appeal	attraction	n.	吸引力	attribute	accredit	v.	归于；认为
appealing	attractive	a.	有吸引力的	attribute	characteristic	n.	特点
appear	seem	v.	似乎	attribute to	credit with	phr.	归于；认为
appearance	rise	n.	出现	attribution	character	n.	属性
appearance	arrival	n.	出现	augment	increase	v.	增加；提高
appearance	showing up	n.	出现	available	obtainable	a.	可获得的
application	use	n.	应用	avenue	method	n.	途径；手段
avenue	means	n.	途径；手段	bulk	large part	n.	大部分
avid	enthusiastic	a.	热衷的	bulk	major part	n.	主体

barely	just	ad.	仅仅	bulk	large portion	n.	大部分
barge	boat	n.	泊船	bulk	great quantity	n.	大部分
barrier	obstacle	n.	障碍	burgeon	expand	v.	急速成长
barrier	impediment	n.	障碍	bustling	lively	a.	活跃的
battle	struggle	n.	搏斗；奋斗	camouflage	disguise	v.	伪装
incline	tend	v.	倾向	camouflage	hide	v.	伪装
be accustomed to	get used to	phr.	习惯	camouflage	decorate（装饰）	v.	伪装
be aware of	familiar with	phr.	了解	camouflage	blend with circumstances	v.	伪装
beforehand	foreordain	v.	预先	cardinal	fundamental	a.	基本的
be closer	be more like	phr.	非常相似	cargo	shipment	n.	船货；货物
be consistent with	be compatible with	phr.	一致的	celebrated	famous	a.	著名的
be entitled to	have the right	phr.	有……权利	central	essential	a.	主要的
beckon	invite	v.	召唤；引诱	certain	specified	a.	指定的
become extinct	die out	phr.	灭绝	chancy	risky	a.	冒险的
being	creature	n.	生命	channel	provide	v.	提供帮助
beneficial	advantageous	a.	有益的	channel	direct	v.	引导
blossom	flourish	v.	兴旺	channel	guide	v.	引导
blossom	thrive	v.	兴旺	chaotic	disorganized	a.	混乱的
boast	puff	v.	吹嘘	cherish	value	v.	珍爱
boast	exaggerate	v.	吹嘘	chief	major	a.	主要的
bombard	assail	v.	炮击；轰击	chisel	carve	v.	刻；凿
bombard	assault	v.	炮击；轰击	choose	opt	v.	选择
bombard	strike	v.	炮击；轰击	chronic	persistent	a.	长期的；不断的
boom	expansion	n.	激增；暴涨	chronic	confirmed	a.	长期的；不断的
boon	great benefit	n.	利益	chronic	habitual	a.	长期的；不断的
boost	raise	v.	增加；提高	chronic	inveterate	a.	长期的；不断的
boundary	periphery	n.	边界	chronically	constantly	ad.	长期地
branch	division	n.	分支	circuitous	indirect	a.	迂回的
breed	reproduce	v.	繁殖；饲养	circumstance	condition	n.	环境；情况

brilliant	bright	a.	光辉的；明亮的	cite	quote	v.	引用
brittle	breakable	a.	脆弱的	cite	refer to	v.	引用
brittle	fragile	a.	脆弱的	classic	typical	a.	典型的
broad appeal	wide popularity	phr.	广泛的吸引力	clear	visible	a.	容易看见的
broadly	generally	ad.	大体上	clear	apparent	a.	显然的
broadly	extensively	ad.	大体上	cling to	attach to	phr.	附着
bulk	majority	n.	大部分	close	careful	a.	严密的；周密的
clue	hint	n.	线索	consecutive	successive	a.	连续的
coating	cover	n.	覆盖层	consequence	result	n.	结果；重要性
coincide with	be as the sametime as	phr.	同时发生	consequence	importance	n.	结果；重要性
collaborate	cooperate	v.	合作	consequent	later	a.	随后的
collaboration	joint effect	n.	合作成果	consequent	resultant	a.	作为结果的
collect	gather	v.	收集	consequent	resulting	a.	作为结果的
collide	hit each other	v.	碰撞	consequential	significant	a.	重要的
collide with	run into	phr.	碰撞	consequently	therefore	ad.	因此
commemorate	celebrate	v.	庆祝；纪念	consequently	thus	ad.	因此
compact	concise	a.	紧密的；简明的	conserve	save	v.	保存
compact	compressed	a.	紧密的；简明的	consider	think as	v.	考虑；认为
comparable	equivalent	a.	可比较的	consider	view as	v.	考虑；认为
compel	push	v.	强迫	consider	think about	v.	考虑；认为
compelling	convincing	a.	令人信服的	considerable	substantial	a.	相当大的
compensate	reimburse	v.	赔偿；补偿	consist of	compose of	v.	由……组成
compensate for	balance	phr.	赔偿；补偿	consistent	regular	a.	一致的
complaint	protest	v.	抗议	consistently	regularly	ad.	一致地
complement	supplement	n.	补充物	conspicuous	notable	a.	明显的
complement	add to	v.	补充	constant	stable	a.	固定的；不变的
completely	totally	ad.	完全地	constantly	always	ad.	经常；不断地
complex	elaborate	a.	复杂的	constellation	collection	n.	一系列；一群
complex	system	n.	复合物；综合体	constellation	combination	n.	一系列；一群
complicated	complex	a.	复杂的	constitution	component	n.	构造

complicated	made things more difficult	a.	复杂的	constrain	restrict	v.	限制
component	constituent	a.	组成的	constraint	limit	n.	限制
composition	mixture	n.	合成物	constraint	restriction	n.	限制
comprehensive	understandable	a.	能理解的	consume	eat up	v.	消耗；吃；喝
comprehensive	complete	a.	全部的	consumed	used up	v.	消耗
comprise	form	v.	组成	contemplate	consider	v.	沉思
comprise	make up	v.	组成	contentious	disputed	a.	好争吵的
concern	interest	v.	感兴趣	continual	constant	a.	不间断的；连续的
conclusive	final	a.	最后的	continuous	uninterrupted	a.	连续的；持续的
conclusive	ultimate	a.	最后的	contrive	create	v.	发明
conducive	contributive	a.	有助于……的	contrive	invent	v.	发明
configuration	arrangement	n.	布局；结构	conventional	customary	a.	习惯的；惯例的
configuration	form	n.	布局；结构	conventional	traditional	a.	习惯的；惯例的
confine	limit	v.	限制	converging	concentrating	a.	收缩的；会聚的
confront	face	v.	面临	convert	transform	v.	使转变
congeal	solidify	v.	使凝结	convert into	change into	phr.	转变成
convict	condemn	v.	宣判	debate	argue	v.	辩论；争论
convict	sentence	v.	宣判	decimate	destroy	v.	大量毁灭
convict	doom（判决）	v.	宣判	decimation	destruction	n.	大量毁灭
conviction	belief	n.	相信；信念	degree	extent	n.	程度
conviction	strong belief	n.	坚定的信念	degree	measure	n.	程度
cope with	handle	phr.	应付；处理	delicate	dainty	a.	易碎的；精美的
cope with	deal with	phr.	应付；处理	delight	please	v.	使高兴
copious	plentiful	a.	丰富的；大量的	delight	pleasure	n.	高兴；愉快
core	center	n.	核心；要点	deluxe	lavish	a.	奢华的
correspondence	harmony	n.	一致	demand	need	v.	需要；需求
corroborate	confirm	v.	证实；确证	demise	extinction	n.	死亡
costly	expensive	a.	贵重的；昂贵的	demography	population	n.	人口统计

counsel	advise	v.	忠告	dense	crowded	a.	稠密的；密集的
counter	oppose	v.	反对	dense	thick	a.	稠密的；密集的
counter of	in the opposite of	phr.	相反的	depend	rely on	v.	依赖；依靠
counterpart	version（版本）	n.	复本；副本	dependable	reliable	a.	可信赖的
counterpart	similitude（类似物）	n.	复本；副本	depict	describe	v.	描述
counterpart	equivalent（同等物）	n.	复本；副本	depict	portray	v.	描写；描绘
countervail	compensate	v.	抵消；对抗	depletion	drain	n.	消耗；用尽
countervail	oppose	v.	抵消；对抗	deposit	accumulate	v.	沉积
couple	associate	v.	与……联系起来	deposit	lay down	v.	放下；放置
covered	included	a.	隐蔽的；有盖的	derive	arise	v.	源于；导出
crawl	move	v.	爬行；移动	design	create	v.	设计
create	invent	v.	创作；产生	designate	identify	v.	命名；指定
creative	inventive	a.	创造的	detractor	critic（批评者）	n.	诽谤者；恶意批评者
crest	peak	n.	顶峰	detrimental	harmful	a.	有害的；不利的
critical	crucial	a.	关键的	deviate	digress	v.	偏离
critical	essential	a.	关键的	deviation	departure	n.	背离
criticize	debate（争论；辩论）	v.	批评；责备	devise	create	v.	设计；发明
crucial	important	a.	重要的	devoid of	lack of	phr.	缺乏的
crucially	decisively	ad.	重要地	devoid of	without	prep.	缺乏的
crushed	ground	a.	碾碎了的	devoid of	scant of	phr.	缺乏的
cumbersome	awkward	a.	笨重的；麻烦的	devoted	dedicated	a.	虔诚的；专心致志的
cumbersome	clumsy	a.	笨重的；麻烦的	devoted to	concentrated on	phr.	虔诚的；专心致志的
cumbersome	unwieldy	a.	笨重的；麻烦的	dictate	determine	v.	口授；命令
curb	control	v.	控制；遏止	dictate	order	v.	命令

current	present	a.	现在的	differential	uneven	a.	差别的；独特的
dam	block	v.	筑坝；控制	diffuse	travel	v.	扩散；散布
dangle	hang	v.	悬挂；吊	diffuse	spread (out)	v.	扩散；散布
daring	bold	a.	大胆的	diligent	industrious	a.	勤奋的
diligently	industriously	ad.	勤奋地	divest	get rid of	v.	剥夺
dilute	reduce	v.	稀释；使薄弱	domestic	home	a.	家庭的；国内的
dim	decrease	v.	变暗淡	dormant	hibernated	a.	休眠的；不活动的
disassemble	break apart	v.	拆开	dormant	inactive	a.	休眠的；不活动的
disassemble	break up	v.	拆开	dramatically	greatly	ad.	戏剧性地
disband	dismiss	v.	解散；遣散	drastic	extreme	a.	激烈的；极端的
discard	throw away	v.	摒弃；丢弃	drastically	obviously	ad.	大大地；彻底地
discard	throw up	v.	摒弃；丢弃	drastically	Severely（严重地）	ad.	大大地；彻底地
discernible	noticeable	a.	可辨别的	dual	double	a.	双的；双重的
discernible	discriminating	a.	可辨别的	duplicate	copy	v.	复制
discharge	release	v.	释放	duplicate	repeat	n.	复本
disentangle	disband	v.	解开	durable	lasting	a.	经久的；持久的
disgust	distaste	v.	厌恶	earn	acquire	v.	赚得；赢得
disintegrate	break apart	v.	分解；碎裂	ease	facilitate（使容易）	v.	使减轻；使缓和
disintegrate	fall apart	v.	分解；碎裂	eccentric	erratic	a.	古怪的；反常的
disintegrate	tear apart	v.	分解；碎裂	eccentric	strange	a.	古怪的；反常的
dismantle	demolish	v.	拆开；拆除	efface	eliminate	v.	消去
disorder	anarchy	n.	混乱	elaborate	detailed	a.	精巧的；详尽的
dispensable	not necessary	a.	非必要的	elaborate	dainty	a.	精巧的；详尽的
dispersal	distribution	n.	散布；驱散	elapsed	passed	a.	过去的；经过的

displace	move out of position	v.	迫使（人）离开	element	weather condition	n.	（恶劣的）天气
disposition	temperament	n.	性格；性情	eliminate	remove	v.	排除；消除
dispute	contention	n.	争论；争执	elusive	difficult to catch	a.	难懂的；难捉摸的
dispute	argument	n.	争论；争执	emanate	emerge	v.	散发；产生
dissipate	disperse	v.	驱散	embark	on start	v.	从事；着手
dissipated	dispersed	a.	分散的	embed	insert	v.	插入；植入
dissuade	discourage	v.	劝阻	embed	implant	v.	插入；植入
distinct	clear and recognizable	a.	清楚的；明确的	embed	enclose	v.	插入；植入
distinction	difference	n.	差别	emergence	appearance	n.	出现
distinction	honor	n.	荣誉	emergency	crisis	n.	紧急情况
distinction	excellence	n.	优秀，卓越	emergent	developing	a.	新兴的
distinctive	characteristic	a.	有特色的	employ	use	v.	利用
distinguish	notice from the difference	v.	区别；识别	enable	allow	v.	使能够
distribute	spread	v.	分配；散布	enactment	establishment	n.	制定
distribution	dispersion	n.	散布	encapsulate	state briefly	v.	概述
distribution	geographic range	n.	分布区域	encourage	stimulate	v.	激励；刺激
disturb	upset	v.	打乱；扰乱	endangered	not abundant	a.	濒临绝种的
diverse	distinct	a.	不同的	endeavor	enterprise	n.	努力
diversification	emergence of many varieties	n.	多样化	endow	bestow	v.	捐赠
diversity	variety	n.	多样性	engulf	swallow	v.	吞没
divest	deprive	v.	剥夺	enhance	improve	v.	提高；增强
enhance	intensify	v.	提高；增强	excavate	dig out	v.	挖掘
enjoy	experience	v.	经历	excavation	dug-out	n.	挖掘
enlist	obtain	v.	谋取（支持、赞助等）	exceed	surpass	v.	超越；胜过
enormous	great	a.	巨大的	exceed	beyond above	v.	超越；胜过
enrich	enhance	v.	使富足	exceedingly	extremely	ad.	极其，非常
ensue	result	v.	因……产生	excess	go beyond	n.	超越；胜过
ensuing	subsequent	a.	接着发生的	exclusively	only	ad.	专门地；独占地
ensure	guarantee	v.	保证；担保	excrete	expel	v.	排泄；分泌
entail	involve	v.	牵涉	exercise	use	v.	运用

enthusiastic	eager	a.	热情的	exhausted	tired	a.	精疲力竭的
environment	setting	n.	环境	exhausted	used up	a.	耗尽的；用完的
ephemeral	short-lived	a.	短暂的	exhibit	demonstrate	v.	展示；陈列
ephemeral	transient	a.	短暂的	exhibit	display	v.	展示；陈列
episode	event	n.	事件	expand	stretch	v.	展开；增长
equilibrium	balance	n.	平衡	expand	increase	v.	展开；增长
era	period	n.	时代；年代	expanse	area	n.	一大片区域
eradicate	remove completely	v.	根除；消灭	expansive	large	a.	广阔的
erect	build	v.	建立	expediency	convenience	n.	方便；利己
erratic	unpredictable	a.	不稳定的；古怪的	expediency	advantage（优势；利益）	n.	方便；利己
erratic	irregular	a.	不稳定的；古怪的	expedient	fitting	a.	权宜的；方便的
escalate	extend	v.	逐步扩大	expend	use	v.	耗尽
essential	crucial	a.	极重要的	explicit	obvious	a.	明确的；清楚的
established	qualified	a.	已制定的	explicitly	clear	ad.	明确地
establishment	Formation（构成）	n.	建立；创立	exploit	utilize	v.	利用
estimate	projection	n.	估计	exploit	take advantage of	v.	利用
estimation	evaluation	n.	估计	exploit	make use of	v.	利用
euphoric	extremely happy	a.	心情愉快的	explore	investigate	v.	探测；探索
evaluate	judge	v.	评价	expose to	subject to（遭受）	phr.	使经历
eventual	later	a.	最后的	express	communicate	v.	表达
eventually	later	ad.	最后	extant	existing	a.	现存的；尚存的
eventually	ultimately	ad.	最后	extant	remaining	a.	现存的；尚存的
evidence	proof	n.	证据	extant	not extinct	a.	现存的；尚存的
evident	apparent	a.	明显的	extend	stretch	v.	延伸
evident	obvious	a.	明显的	extend	reach	v.	延伸
evoke	arouse	v.	唤起；引起	extol	praise	v.	赞美

evoke	draw	v.	唤起；引起	extraneous	inessential	a.	无关的；外来的
evoke	produce	v.	唤起；引起	extraneous	from outside	a.	无关的；外来的
evoke	promote	v.	唤起；引起	extraordinary	exceptional	a.	异常的
evoke	stimulate	v.	唤起；引起	exude	release	v.	渗出；发散
evoke	create in the mind	v.	唤起；引起	exude	give off	v.	渗出；发散
exaggerate	overstate	v.	夸张；夸大	fabricate	produce	v.	制造
far-reaching	extensive	a.	深远的；广泛的	fragmentation	break	n.	破裂
far-reaching	broad	a.	深远的；广泛的	fragmentize	break up	v.	使成碎片
fascinating	extremely attractive	a.	迷人的	frankly	openly	ad.	坦白地
fashion	make	v.	形成；造	frankly	sincerely	ad.	真诚地
fashion	way	n.	样子；方式	friction	conflict	n.	争执；不合
fashionable	popular	a.	流行的；时尚的	function	operation	n.	效用；作用
feasible	achievable	a.	可实行的	function	utility	n.	效用；作用
feasible	practical	a.	可实行的	fundamental	basic	a.	基础的
feast	eating	n.	盛宴	funds	money	n.	资金
ferry	transport	n.	渡轮	furthermore	in addition	ad.	此外
fertile	reproductive	a.	肥沃的；多产的	gap	opening	n.	缺口；裂口
fertile	productive	a.	肥沃的；多产的	gear	adjust	v.	使适合
figure out	map	phr.	计算出；解决（详细规划）	generate	produce	v.	产生
finding	discovery	n.	发现	genuinely	actually	ad.	真诚地
first andforemost	above all	phr.	首先；首要地	get accustomed to	become used to	phr.	习惯
flake	fragment	n.	小薄片	give rise to	produce	phr.	引起
flattery	praise	n.	恭维	given	particular	a.	规定的；特定的
flee	run away from	v.	逃走	govern	regulate	v.	统治；管理
flexible	adaptable	a.	易适应的	govern	control	v.	统治；管理

float	stay on the top	v.	漂浮	grasp	understand	v.	领会；理解
float upward	rise	phr.	浮起	groom	clean	v.	装扮；使整洁
flourish	prosper	v.	繁荣；兴旺	groom	make up	v.	装扮；使整洁
flourish	thrive	v.	繁荣；兴旺	groundless	unfounded	a.	无根据的
flourishing	prosperous	a.	繁荣的	grounds	reasons	n.	根据；理由
flow	movement	n.	流动	groundwork	base	n.	基础
fluctuate	change	v.	变动	groundwork	basis	n.	基础
fluctuation	variation	n.	变动；起伏	groundwork	foundation	n.	基础
focal point	centre area	phr.	焦点	grudging	unenthusiastic	a.	勉强的
follow	track	v.	跟随	guarantee	ensure	v.	保证；担保
for instance	for example	phr.	例如	hallmark	characteristic	n.	戳记，标志
forage	feed	n.	饲料	hamper	hinder	v.	妨碍；束缚
forage	search for food	v.	觅食	hamper	restrict	v.	妨碍；束缚
formidable	excessive	a.	巨大的	hamper	make difficulty	v.	妨碍；束缚
foster	encourage	v.	鼓励	handy	convenient	a.	便利的；灵活的
foster	urge	v.	培养；促进	haphazard	random	a.	随意的
foster	promote the development of	v.	培养；促进	harness	use	v.	利用
foul	pollute	v.	污染	harsh	drastic	a.	严厉的；严酷的
fragment	break up	v.	使成碎片	immensely	extremely	ad.	非常
hasty	hurried	a.	匆匆的；急忙	immigration	movement	n.	移居
haul	pull	v.	拉	immobile	fixed	a.	固定的；静止的
have nothing to do with	in no relation to	phr.	不相干	immobility	absence of motion	n.	固定；静止
havoc	destruction	n.	浩劫	immoral	indecent	a.	不道德的
hazard	danger	n.	危险	immoral	improper	a.	不道德的
heed	notice	v.	留心；注意	impermeable	impenetrable	a.	不能渗透的
heighten	increase	v.	增加；提高	impermeable	impervious	a.	不能渗透的
heir	inheritor	n.	继承人；后继者	impetus	stimulus	v.	刺激；促进
hence	therefore	ad.	因此	impetus	incentive	n.	刺激；促进
heritage	legacy	n.	遗产；传统	implausible	unbelievable	a.	难以置信的
heritage	tradition	n.	遗产；传统	implement	tool	n.	工具

heterogeneous	varied	a.	由不同种类组成的	imply	indicate	v.	意味
hide	conceal	v.	隐藏	imposing	impressive	a.	给人深刻印象的
hinder	interfere with	v.	妨碍	imprecise	inexact	a.	不精确的
hint	clue	n.	暗示；迹象	improbable	unlikely	a.	不大可能的
hint	implication	n.	暗示；迹象	in fact	actually	phr.	事实上
hint	indication	n.	暗示；迹象	in great demand	in popularity	phr.	普遍
hint	lead	n.	暗示；迹象	in respect to	in term of	phr.	就……而言
hire	employ	v.	雇用	hobby	pastime	n.	嗜好
hold	support	v.	支撑；保持	inadvertently	unintentionally	ad.	非故意地
hold	keep up	v.	支撑；保持	inadvertently	without knowing	ad.	非故意地
hollow	an empty space	n.	中空	inauspicious	unfavorable	a.	不吉利的
homogeneous	uniform	a.	同种的	incidentally	by the way	ad.	顺便一提
host	of great number	n.	大量	inclement	unfavorable	a.	（气候）严酷的
however	yet	conj.	然而	inconceivable	unimaginable	a.	难以置信的
hub	center	n.	中心	inconclusive	without result（毫无结果）	a.	不确定的
huge	large	a.	巨大的	incorporate	include	v.	包含
hurdle	fence	v.	用篱笆围	incorporate	merge	v.	吸收；并入
hypothetical	supposed	a.	假设的；假定的	incursion	invasion	n.	入侵
ice sheet	glacier（冰河）	n.	冰原	indicate	demonstrate	v.	指示；指出
identical	the same	a.	同样的	indigenous	native	a.	本土的；土生土长的
idiosyncrasy	peculiarity	n.	特性	indispensable	essential	a.	不可缺少的
ignite	set on fire	v.	点燃	indispensable	necessary	a.	不可缺少的
illusion	impression（印象）	n.	错觉；幻象	indispensable	needed	a.	不可缺少的
immediately	closest	ad.	接近；紧接着	indispensable	required	a.	不可缺少的
immense	great	a.	巨大的	indispensable	vital	a.	不可缺少的
immense	huge	a.	巨大的	indispensable	significant（重要的）	a.	必不可少的
immense	vast	a.	巨大的	induce	bring	v.	引起

induce	bring	v.	引起	induce	cause	v.	引起
ineffectively	without any result	ad.	无效地	inert	motionless	a.	迟缓的；惰性的
inert	motiveless	a.	迟缓的；惰性的	inevitable	unavoidable	a.	不可避免的
mundane	ordinary	a.	世俗的；平凡的	myriad	countless	a.	大量的；无数的
myriad	innumerable	a.	大量的；无数的	myriad	numerous	a.	大量的；无数的
narrow	limit	v.	使变窄	nature	character	n.	天性；本质
inaccessible	unreachable	a.	难接近的	nearly	almost	ad.	几乎；差不多
needless to say	obvious	phr.	不用说	nevertheless	however	ad.	然而；尽管
nevertheless	in spite of	ad.	然而；尽管	nocturnal	nighttime	a.	夜间的
notable	important	a.	显著的；重要的	notable	outstanding	a.	显著的；重要的
note	record	v.	记录	noticeable	obvious	a.	显而易见的
notwithstanding	despite	prep.	虽然；尽管	objective	purpose	n.	目标
oblige	force	v.	强迫	obscure	conceal	v.	使变暗；遮掩
obscure	hide	v.	使模糊	obscure	unclear	a.	模糊的
obscure	not clear	a.	模糊的	obsession	with fixation on	n.	痴迷；迷恋
obtain	acquire	v.	取得；获得	obvious	evident	a.	明显的
occasion	event	n.	重大活动	of legitimacy	lawful	phr.	合法的
of likelihood	probable	phr.	可能的	offset	compensate	v.	补偿；抵消
offset	balance	v.	补偿；抵消	offset	make up	v.	补偿；抵消
old male	aged male	phr.	老年男性	omit	exclude	v.	遗漏；删去
omit	neglect	v.	遗漏；删去	on the contrary	on the other hand	phr.	恰恰相反
on the contrary	whereas（然而；反之）	phr.	恰恰相反	on the whole	in general	phr.	大体上
ongoing	current	a.	进行的	onset	beginning	n.	开始
onset	start	n.	开始	opaque	impenetrable	a.	难理解的
optimal	most advantageous	a.	最佳的	option	choice	n.	选项；选择
orchestrate	stage-manage	v.	精心安排	orientation	perspective	n.	观点
orientation	introduction	n.	介绍	originally	at the first	ad.	起初
ornament	decorate	v.	装饰	ornamental	decorative	a.	装饰的
ornamentation	decoration	n.	装饰	outbreak	sudden increase	v.	爆发；突然发生

outcome	result	n.	结果	outermost	farthermost away	a.	最远的
overview	summary	n.	概要	overwhelming	powerful	a.	压倒性的
pacify	assuage	v.	使平静	paradox	contrary	n.	相反；矛盾
paradoxically	seemingly contradictory	ad.	似是而非地	parcel out	distribute	phr.	把……分成几份；分配
necessary	required	a.	必要的	pare	remove away	v.	修掉；削减
patch	spot	n.	斑点	patch	area	n.	小块土地
peak	maximum	n.	高峰（期）	peak	highest point	n.	高峰（期）
peak time	of the greatest period	phr.	高峰（期）	peculiar	strange	a.	奇怪的；独特的
penetrate	enter	v.	穿入；穿透	perceptible	appreciable	a.	可感知的
perceptible	noticeable	a.	可感知的	peril	danger	n.	危险
perilous	dangerous	a.	危险的	perilous	risky	a.	危险的
perilous	hazardous	a.	危险的	perilous	toxic	a.	危险的
periodically	regularly	ad.	周期性地	periodically	from time to time	ad.	周期性地
perishable	easy to spoil	a.	易腐坏的	permanent	lasting	a.	永恒的
permeate	penetrate	v.	渗透；弥漫	permit	allow	v.	允许
perpetual	constant	a.	永久的；连续的	persist	continue	v.	坚持；持续
persist	last	v.	坚持；持续	persistent	long lasting	a.	耐久的
personality	character	n.	个性；性格	pertinent	relevant	a.	相关的
pervasive	widespread	a.	普遍的	phenomena[pl.]	events	n.	现象
phenomenal	extraordinary	a.	异常的	phenomenon	occurrence	n.	现象
phenomenon	observable fact	n.	现象	piecing	joining	n.	接合
pigment	color	n.	色素	pigmentation	coloring		（生物的）天然颜色
pigmentation	dye	n.	染色	pinnacle	high point	n.	顶点；顶峰
pinpoint	precise	a.	精确的	pinpoint	describe precisely	v.	准确地解释或说明
pinpoint	identify	v.	准确地解释或说明	plausible	believable	a.	貌似有理的
plausible	paradoxical	a.	似是而非的	pledge	promise	n.	保证；誓言
plumage	feather	n.	羽毛	pocketbook	affordable	a.	负担得起的
popular	widespread	a.	流行的；广泛的	popular	appealing	a.	流行的；广泛的

pore	hole	n.	毛孔；细孔	pore	space（空间）	n.	毛孔；细孔
portion	part	n.	一部分	portion	constituent	n.	一部分
pose	place	v.	摆姿势；展现	pose	present	v.	摆姿势；展现
partly	in some degree	ad.	部分地	posit	propose	v.	断定；假定
posit	assume	v.	断定；假定	postulate	presume	v.	假定
postulate	hypotheses	v.	假定	potent	powerful	a.	有力的
potential	possible	a.	潜在的；可能的	practically	nearly	ad.	几乎；差不多
precarious	insecure	a.	不稳定的；危险的	precede	be beyond	v.	高于；超出
precede	come before	v.	在……之前	precious	valuable	a.	宝贵的
precipitate	bring about	v.	使……突然发生	precision	accuracy	n.	精确；正确
preclude	rule out	v.	排除；阻止	predicament	difficult situation	n.	尴尬的处境；困境
predicament	serious situation	n.	尴尬的处境；困境	prediction	prophecy	n.	预言
predominant	principal	a.	占优势的	predominant	most aggressive	a.	占优势的
predominant	very noticeable	a.	占优势的	predominantly	primitively	ad.	占优势地
predominately	mainly	ad.	主要地	preeminent	foremost	a.	卓越的；显著的
premise	assume	v.	假定	premise	assumption	n.	假定；前提
preoccupation with	concentration on	phr.	专注于	preordain	appoint	v.	预定；注定
preordain	foreordain	v.	预定；注定	preordain	ordain	v.	预定；注定
prerequisite	requirement	n.	必要条件	prerequisite	something required	n.	必要条件
prerequisite	something needed to happen	n.	必要条件	preserve	protect	v.	保存；保护
preserve	retain	v.	保存；保护	preserve	save	v.	保存；保护
presumable	probable	a.	可推测的；可能有的	prevailing	popular	a.	流行的
prevailing	dominant	a.	占优势的	prevalent	common	a.	普遍的；流行的
prevalent	prevailing	a.	普遍的；流行的	previous	past	a.	先前的；以往的
previously	before	ad.	以前；早先	primarily	mainly	ad.	主要地
primary	dominant	a.	主要的	primitive	early	a.	原始的

principal	essential	a.	主要的	principal	major	a.	主要的
principle	rule	n.	原则	principle	standard	n.	原则
posit	suggest	v.	断定；假定	prior	previous	a.	在先的；在前的
pristine	pure	a.	清新的；纯朴的	prized	valued	a.	有价值的
probe	explore	v.	探查；探测	process	purify（提纯；精炼）	v.	加工
procure	obtain	v.	获得；取得	procure	acquire	v.	获得；取得
profound	far-reaching	a.	深远的	programmed	determined	a.	计划……的
prohibitive	unaffordable	a.	抑止的	projection	estimate	n.	推测；估计
proliferation	increase	n.	增产；增加	prolifically	abundantly	ad.	多产地
prolong	extend	v.	延长	prominent	eminent	a.	显著的
prominent	outstanding	a.	卓越的；重要的	prominent	principal	a.	首要的；重要的
promote	encourage	v.	促进；增长	pronounced	clear	a.	明显的；显著的
pronounced	definite	a.	明显的；显著的	pronounced	notable	a.	明显的；显著的
propagate	multiply	v.	繁殖	propagate	reproduce	v.	繁殖
propel	push	v.	推进；激励	property	characteristic	n.	特性；属性
property	quality	n.	特性；属性	proponent	supporter	n.	拥护者
prosper	succeed	v.	成功；兴旺	prosperous	wealthy	a.	富有的；繁盛的
prototype	model	n.	原型	protrude	project	v.	伸出；凸出
protrude	extend	v.	伸出；凸出	protrude	stick out	v.	伸出；凸出
provoke	elicit	v.	激起；导致	prowess	expertise	n.	非凡的技能
prowess	ambition（雄心）	n.	英勇	proximity	closeness	n.	接近
proximity	nearness	n.	接近	proximity to quarters	close to residences	phr. n.	邻近；靠近 住处
pursue	chase	v.	追求；追赶	radical	extreme	a.	彻底的；极端的
radical	drastic	a.	彻底的；极端的	radically	completely	ad.	根本地
radical	fundamental	a.	根本的	ramification	branch	n.	分支；分派
raise to	come about	phr.	引起；使出现	range	vary	v.	变化；变动
ramification	consequence	n.	结果；衍生物	rate	classify	v.	评价；分等
rare	scarce	a.	稀有的；罕见的				

rather than	instead of	phr.	而不是	readily	easily	ad.	容易地
ready	receptive（能接纳的）	a.	甘心的；情愿的	realm	area	n.	领域
priority	preference	n.	优先	rebellion	revolt	n.	反抗；叛乱
receptacle	receiver	n.	容器	receptivity to	openness to	phr.	接受
recharge	refill	v.	再填充	recur	repeat	v.	反复出现
refine	improve	v.	精炼	refined	decent	a.	精致的
refined	with high quality	a.	精致的	refreshing	unusual	a.	别具一格的
refuse	garbage	n.	垃圾	regardless	without considering	ad.	无论如何
regulate	adjust	v.	调整；调节	regulate	control	v.	管理；控制
reinforce	strengthen	v.	加强	relative	comparative	a.	比较的
relatively	comparatively	ad.	相对地；对比地	relatively	correspondingly	ad.	相对地；对比地
relatively	oppositely	ad.	相对地；对比地	relevant	applicable	a.	有关的；恰当的
relic	remain	n.	遗物；遗迹	relic	remnant	n.	遗物；遗迹
reluctant	disinclined	a.	不情愿的	remarkable	notable	a.	非凡的；卓越的
remarkable	incredible	a.	非凡的；卓越的	remedy	cure	v.	治疗
remnant	remaining	a.	残留的	remnant	remains	n.	残余
remote	distant	a.	遥远的	remote	isolated（孤立的）	a.	遥远的
render	make	v.	使得	rendering	presentation	n.	演奏；表演
renowned	famous	a.	有名的	repercussion	effect	n.	回响；影响
replica	copy	n.	复制品	repudiate	reject	v.	否定；驳斥
reputation	fame	n.	名声	reserve	save	v.	保存；保留
resident	inhabitant	n.	居民	residual	remaining	a.	残留的
resilient	easy to recover	a.	迅速恢复的	resilient	quick to recover	a.	迅速恢复的
restricted	limited	a.	受限制的	retain	keep	v.	保持；保留
retreat	recede	v.	撤退	retrieve	bring back	v.	找回
reveal	manifest	v.	展现；揭露	reveal	show	v.	展现；揭露
reveal	make known	v.	展现；揭露	revenue	income	n.	税收
revival	restoration	n.	恢复；再生	revival	resuscitation	n.	恢复；再生
revolution	dramatic change	n.	彻底改革	revolutionize	change dramatically	v.	彻底改革

rigidly	strictly	ad.	严厉地	rigorous	demanding	a.	严厉的
rebound	recovery	n.	重新振作	rigorous	harsh	a.	严厉的
risk	danger	n.	危险	ritual	ceremonial	n.	仪式
rival	compete	v.	竞争；对抗	roam	wander	v.	漫游
robust	healthy	a.	强壮的；结实的	role	function	n.	作用
rotate	turn	v.	转动	roughly	approximately	ad.	大约
roundabout	circuitous	a.	迂回的	route	path	n.	路径；途径
routinely	commonly	ad.	常规地	rudiment	basic	n.	基础
rudimentary	basic	a.	根本的	rudimentary	primitive	a.	根本的
rupture	burst	v.	破裂	sacred	holy	a.	神圣的
sample	example	n.	样本；例子	satisfied	fulfilled	a.	令人满意的
save for	except for	prep.	除……之外	scale	magnitude	n.	大小；等级
scant	minimal	a.	少量的	scatter	distribute	v.	使分散
scatter	disperse	v.	使分散	scented	fragrant	a.	有气味的
scope	horizon	n.	范围；程度	scope	extent	n.	范围；程度
scorching	exceedingly hot	a.	酷热的	score	a large number of	n.	大量的；许多的
scorn	despise	v.	轻蔑；嘲笑	scrap	fragment	n.	碎片
screen	filter	v.	过滤	scrutinize	examine	v.	详细审查
scrutiny	examination	n.	详细审查	sculpt	shape	v.	雕刻；造型
secrete	produce	v.	分泌	sedentary	settled	a.	久坐的；固定的
seething	excited	a.	激昂的	seething	active	a.	激昂的
segment	portion	n.	部分；片断	seize	take	v.	抓住
seldom	rare	a.	很少的	separate	different	a.	个别的；不同的
serene	calm	a.	平静的	serene	silent	a.	平静的
set in motion	start	phr.	开动	set off	begin	phr.	出发；动身；引起
settle	inhabit	v.	定居；安顿	severe	harsh	a.	严厉的；严酷的
shallow	not deep	a.	浅的	shatter	destroy	v.	打碎
sheer	absolute	a.	完全的	shield	protect	v.	保护
shift	change	v.	转换；转移	shift	move	v.	转换；转移
shiver	tremor	v.	发抖；颤抖	showcase	display	v.	陈列
rise	emerge	v.	出现	shrink	contract	v.	缩水；收缩
significant	considerable	a.	重大的	significant	important	a.	重大的

significant	meaningful	a.	重大的	simulated	artificial	a.	假装的；仿造的
simultaneously	at the same time	ad.	同时地	singularly	particularly	ad.	非常；特别
sink	descend	v.	下沉；下陷	sink	drop to the bottom	v.	下沉；下陷
sink	pass out of sight	v.	下沉；下陷	site	locate	v.	选址；设置
size up	reckon up to	phr.	估计	skeptical	doubting	a.	怀疑的；多疑的
skeptical	suspected	a.	怀疑的；多疑的	slight	small	a.	轻微的；少量的
slightly	somewhat	ad.	稍微地	slope	incline	v.	倾斜
snap	break	v.	断裂	so far	until present	phr.	目前为止
so far	up to now	phr.	目前为止	so far	up to present	phr.	目前为止
soak	absorb	v.	吸收	sole	only	a.	单独的；唯一的
sole	unique	a.	单独的；唯一的	solicit	request	v.	恳求；请求
solitary	alone	a.	单独的；独自的	sophisticated	complex	a.	精致的；复杂的
sophisticated	elaborated	a.	精致的；复杂的	sophisticated	refined	a.	精致的；复杂的
sophistication	technology	n.	工艺	sort	kind	n.	品种；种类
sort	type	n.	品种；种类	sought-after	desired	a.	广受欢迎的
source	origin	n.	来源	span	period	n.	一段时间
spark	set off	v.	出发	sparse	not rich		稀少的；零星的
spawn	create	v.	产卵；产生	spawn	produce	v.	产卵；产生
speak of	indicate	phr.	提及	speciation	evolution（演化）	n.	物种形成
specific	particular	a.	特殊的；特定的	specify	state	v.	详细说明
spectacular	impressive	a.	引人入胜的	spectator	beholder	n.	目击者
spectator	viewer	n.	目击者	spectrum	range	n.	范围；系列
speed	increase the rate of	v.	加速	spell	period of time	n.	一段时间
sphere	area	n.	范围；领域	splendor	magnificence	n.	光彩；壮丽
split	divided		裂开的；分离的	spontaneous	impulsive	a.	自发的；非计划安排的

shy away from	avoid	phr.	回避；躲避	spontaneous	instinctive	a.	自发的；非计划安排的
sporadic	irregular	a.	偶尔发生的	sporadic	intermittent	a.	偶尔发生的
sporadically	occasionally	ad.	偶尔	spot	catch	v.	看见；发现
spot	see	v.	看见；发现	spot	identify	v.	看见；发现
spottily	occasionally	ad.	缺乏连续性	spread	distribute	v.	散布
spur	stimulate	v.	刺激	stabilize	hold in place	v.	使稳定
staggering	overwhelming	a.	巨大的	staple	important	a.	主要的
staunch	loyal	a.	坚定的；可靠的	staunch	strong	a.	坚定的；可靠的
steadfast	firm	a.	坚定的；固定的	stealthily	silently	ad.	悄悄地
stem	arise	v.	起源于	stimulate	cause	v.	刺激；促使
stimulate	prompt	v.	刺激；促使	stockpile	store up	v.	储备；贮存
strictly	only	ad.	仅仅	stride	step	n.	大步；阔步
strike	come into contract with	v.	撞击；冲击	striking	dramatic	a.	惊人的
string	series	n.	一系列	stringent	strict	a.	严厉的
strip	remove	v.	剥去	sturdy	strong	a.	结实的；强壮的
stylus	pen	n.	钢笔	subject to	vulnerable to	phr.	易受……影响的
subjected to	dominated by	phr.	控制	subsequent	ensuing	a.	后来的；随后的
subsequent	later	a.	后来的；随后的	subsidiary	less important	a.	次要的
substantial	sturdy	a.	坚固的	substantial	significant	a.	重大的；真实的
substantial	actual	a.	重大的；真实的	substantial	essential	a.	重大的；真实的
substantially	importantly	ad.	重大地	substantiate	confirm	v.	证明；证实
substitute	replace	v.	代替	substitute	replacement	n.	代替物
succession	series	n.	一系列	suitable	appropriate	a.	合适的
suited	appropriated	a.	合适的	sumptuous	luxurious	a.	奢侈的；豪华的
sunk down	to the bottom	phr.	下陷的	supplant	substitute	v.	代替；取代
supplant	replace	v.	代替	suppress	stop by force	v.	制止；镇压
surmise	assumption	n.	推测；猜测	surmise	guess	v.	推测；猜测
surmise	infer	v.	推测；猜测	surplus	excess	a.	过剩的

surplus	extra	a.	过剩的	surveillance	careful observation	n.	监视；检查
spontaneous	unplanned	a.	自发的；非计划安排的	susceptible to	prone to	phr.	易受……影响的
suspect	doubt	v.	猜想；疑有	suspend	hang	v.	悬挂
sustain	support	v.	支撑；支持	sustain	persist	v.	支持
sustenance	food	n.	生计；食物	sustenance	life	n.	生计；食物
sustenance	living	n.	生计；食物	swell	expand	v.	增大；肿胀
swell	enlargement	n.	增大；肿胀	swiftly	quickly	ad.	迅速地
symmetric	balance	a.	对称的；均衡的	synthesis	combination	n.	合成
tactual	textural	a.	触觉的	tailspin	total confusion	n.	混乱；失控
take	require	v.	需要	take place	occur	phr.	发生
tame	domesticate	v.	驯服；驯化	tangible	material	a.	有形的；实际的
tangible	physical	a.	有形的；实际的	tantalizing	anxious	a.	非常着急的
taper	diminish	v.	逐渐变小	task	work	n.	任务
technique	method	n.	手段；方法	teem with	be full of	phr.	充满；遍布
tempting	appealing	a.	吸引人的；诱人的	tend	care for	v.	趋于；照料
tendency	inclination	n.	倾向	tenet	belief	n.	原则；信条
tenet	principle	n.	原则；信条	tension	pressure	n.	紧张
terminal	final	a.	末端的；终点的	terrain	tract（大片土地）	n.	地形；地势
testify	give evidence	v.	作证	therefore	consequently	ad.	因此
therefore	in that purpose	ad.	因此	thoroughly	completely	ad.	完全地；彻底
threaten	endanger	v.	危及	threshold	limit	n.	界限；起始点
through	by	prep.	通过	thus	consequently	ad.	因此
tie	connection	n.	连接；关系	tie	relation	n.	连接；关系
timid	fearful	a.	胆怯的	toil	work	v.	辛勤劳动
tolerate	endure	v.	忍受	toxic	poisonous	a.	有毒的
track	follow	v.	跟踪；追踪	track	observe（观察；观测）	v.	跟踪；追踪
tracts (of land)	area	n.	大片土地	transfer	move	v.	转移；转变
transform	deform	v.	转变	transformation	conversion	n.	转化；转换
suspect	believe	v.	猜想；疑有	transformation	change	n.	转化；转换
transformation	shuffle	n.	转化；转换	transforming	changing	n.	转化；转换

transitory	ephemeral	a.	短暂的	transitory	short-lived	a.	短暂的
transitory	temporary	a.	短暂的	transitory	transient	a.	短暂的
trappings	decorations	n.	装饰	trauma	damage	n.	损伤；精神创伤
traverse	cross	v.	横过；穿过	trend	movement	n.	趋势；走向
trend	tendency	n.	趋势；走向	tricky	difficult	a.	狡猾的；棘手的
trigger	start	v.	触发；引发	trigger	initiate	v.	触发；引发
truism	it was evidence that	n.	不言而喻的道理	turbulent	agitated	a.	激动的
turn	change to	v.	使变成	typical	ordinary	a.	平常的
ubiquitous	common	a.	到处存在的	ultimately	eventually	ad.	最终
ultimately	finally	ad.	最终	unadorned	not decorative	a.	未装饰的
unanimity	total agreement	n.	一致同意	undergo	experience	v.	经历；经受
underlying	inner	a.	潜在的；隐含的	underpinning	foundation	n.	基础；支柱；支撑
underpinning	support	n.	基础；支柱；支撑	underrate	underestimate	v.	低估；看轻
underrate	undervalue	v.	低估；看轻	underscore	stress	v.	强调
undertake	attempt（努力；尝试）	v.	承担；担任	undertaking	enterprise	n.	事业；企业
uneasy	unstable	a.	不稳定的	uniform	without variation	a.	统一的；一致的
uniformly	evenly	ad.	一致地	uniformly	consistently	ad.	一致地
unintendedly	occasionally（偶然地）	ad.	非计划中的	unique	distinct	a.	特有的
unique	sole(唯一的)	a.	特有的	unique to	only found in	phr.	特有的
universally	without exception	ad.	在各种情况下	unleash	release	v.	释放
unprecedented	initial	a.	空前的	unprecedented	new	a.	空前的
unprecedented	novel	a.	空前的	unprecedented	unique	a.	空前的
unqualified	complete	a.	不合格的；无条件的	unreceptive	unresponsive	a.	接受能力差的
transformation	rotation	n.	转化；转换	unresolved	undecided	a.	未解决的
unsophisticated	simple	a.	简单的	unsuitable	inappropriate	a.	不适合的
unsurpassed	superior	a.	非常卓越的	unwieldy	cumbersome	a.	笨重的

urbane	cultivated	a.	文雅的	utilitarian	practical	a.	实用的
utilitarian	functional	a.	实用的	utterly	completely	ad.	完全
vagary	uncertainty	n.	难以预测的变化	vaguely	slightly	ad.	模糊的
vanish	disappear	v.	消失	variability	tendency to change	n.	可变性；反复不定
variation	difference	n.	变更；变化	varied	different	a.	不相同的
vast	immense	a.	巨大的	vast	extended	a.	辽阔的
vast	extensive	a.	辽阔的	vast	large number	a.	大量的
vastly	greatly	ad.	巨大地	vehicle	way	n.	手段；工具
vehicle	means	n.	手段；工具	vehicle	method	n.	手段；工具
versatile	adaptable	a.	多才多艺的	via	by means of	prep.	经过；凭借
via	by the way of	prep.	经过；凭借	vial	bottle	n.	小瓶
vibrant	vivid	a.	生气勃勃的	vigor	energy	a.	生气勃勃的
vigorous	strong	a.	精力旺盛的	vigorous	energetic	a.	精力旺盛的
virtually	nearly	ad.	差不多	virtually	almost	ad.	差不多
virtually	actually	ad.	事实上地	virtually	in fact	ad.	事实上地
visual barrier	obstacle toview	phr.	视觉阻碍	vital	essential	a.	极重要的
vivid	bright	a.	鲜明的	volume	quantity	n.	数额
vulnerable	susceptible	a.	易受伤害的	vulnerable	weak	a.	易受伤害的
vulnerable	open to attack	a.	易受伤害的	vulnerable	open to break	a.	易受伤害的
wanting	inadequate	a.	不够好的	warrant	justify	v.	使正当
warrant	authorize	v.	授权	wary	cautious	a.	小心的；谨慎的
way	station	n.	（长途旅行的）小站	whatever	in any case	ad.	不管怎样
whereas	however	conj.	然而	whereby	in which	conj.	凭借；如何
while	although	conj.	虽然	wholly	completely	ad.	完全地；全部
wield	exert	v.	行使	with respect of	in terms of	phr.	关于
within	inside	ad.	在里面	withstand	resist	v.	承受；经得住
withstand	tolerate	v.	承受；经住	witness	observe	v.	目击
yearly	annual	a.	一年的	yearning	longing	a.	思念的；渴望的
yet	however	conj.	然而	yield	produce	v.	产生；提供
yield	provide	v.	产生；提供	zenith	peak	n.	顶点
unrestricted	unlimited	a.	没有限制的				

高频词复习检测表

以下词汇按组规划，旨在为不同情况的考生提供一个更便捷高效的复习通道。这部分内容为高频词汇的精练版，既可以作为单词表检测自己的学习效果，同时也能作为复习工具按照规划内容按组复习。复习时看到英文能迅速反应出其英文意思即可，无须记住拼写。

第一组

pace 步伐	persist 坚持	pose 姿势	prime 首要的	property 财产
panic 恐慌	personnel 人事的	positive 正面的，积极的	primitive 原始的	proportion 比例
partial 部分的	perspective 角度	possess 拥有（动词）	principal 校长	protest 抗议
participate 参与	pessimistic 悲观的	possession 拥有，财物	principle 原则	provided 假如
particularly 尤其	phase 阶段	postpone 延迟	prior 在……前面	provision 提供，供应
partner 伙伴	phenomenon 现象	potential 潜在的	privilege 优势	provoke 激发
passion 激情	philosophy 哲学	practical 实际的	procedure 程序	psychological 心理的
passive 被动的	physical 物理的，身体的	pray 祷告	proceed 前进	publication 出版
peculiar 特殊的	physician 内科医生	precious 珍贵的	process 进程	publicity 公开，宣传
peer 同辈	physicist 物理学家	precise 精确的	procession 过程	publish 出版
penalty 惩罚	pill 药片	predict 预测	produce 产生	punch 打孔
penetrate 穿透	plot 情节	prejudice 偏见	profession 职业	punctual 按时的
pension 养老金	poisonous 有毒的	prescribe 诊断	profit 利润	purchase 购买
perceive 观察	polish 擦光	presence 出席，存在	progressive 进步的	purpose 目的
perception 观察	poll 民意调查	preserve 保留	prominent 突出的	pursue 追求
performance 表演，业绩	pollute 污染	pretend 假装	promote 提倡	puzzle 谜
permanent 永久的	portable 可携带的	prevail 显示	prompt 迅速的	
permission 允许	portion 部分	previous 以前的	proof 证据	

第二组

radical 激进的	relieve 解放	resume 简历
ratio 比率	religious 宗教的	retail 重播
rational 理性的	reluctant 不情愿的	retain 滞留
raw 生的，未加工的	remain 保留	reveal 显示，表明
readily 有备地	remark 评论	revenue 岁入，税收
rebel 反叛	remarkable 显著的	revise 修改
recall 回忆，叙述	remedy 药方	reward 奖励，报酬
receipt 收据	remind 提醒	ridiculous 荒谬的
reception 接收，接待	remote 偏僻的，遥远的	rival 敌人
recession 退化	removal 挪移	rotate 旋转
reckon 思考	render 考虑	routine 路线
recognition 认出	repetition 重复	rumor 谣言
recommend 推荐（动词）	represent 代表	rural 郊区的
recommendation 推荐（名词）	representative 代表	restrain 限制，抑制（动词）
recovery 复苏	reputation 规范，规则	restraint 限制，抑制（名词）
recreation 娱乐	request 要求	restrict 限制
recruit 招收	rescue 挽救	relevant 相关
reference 参考	resemble 反映	reliable 可靠的
refine 精炼	reservation 保留	relief 解放
reflect 反映	resident 居民	responsible 负责任的
reform 改革	resign 辞职	restless 无休止的，不停歇的
refresh 新鲜	resist 抵制	restore 保留
refugee 避难	resort 求助，采用，度假胜地	reinforce 加强
refusal 拒绝	respectively 各自，分别地	reject 反对
register 登记	respond 反馈	release 解放，发行
regulate 规范	responsibility 责任	

508

第三组

sacrifice 牺牲；祭品	spark 火花	surrender 投降
sake 目的；理由	specialist 专家	surround 周围
sample 样品，样本	species 种	survey 调查
sanction 批准；[常用复] 制裁	specific 具体的	survive 幸免于
scandal 丑闻	specify 规定	suspect 怀疑
scarce 不足的；稀少的	spectacular 壮观的	suspend 吊起；暂停
scare 害怕	speculate 思索；投机	suspicion 怀疑
scatter 分散	sphere 球	sustain 支撑
scenery 风景	spill 使溢出	swallow 吞
schedule 日程，时间表	spoil 溺爱	sway 摇晃
scope 范围；眼界	sponsor 发起人；发起	swear 起誓
section 部分；部门	squeeze 压榨	swift 疾速的
sector 部分；断片	stable 稳定的	swing 挥舞
secure 安全可靠的；牢固的	stain 玷污	switch 开关；改变
security 安全	statistic 统计	symbol 符号
seek 寻找	status 状态	sympathetic 同情的
segment 部分	steady 稳定的	sympathize 同情
sensible 明智的；明显的	steer 驾驶	sympathy 同情
sensitive 有感觉的；敏感的	stiff 硬的，挺的	symptom 症状
sequence 顺序	stimulate 刺激，激发	systematic 系统的
shallow 浅的	stock 股票	superior 较高的；上级
shelter 隐蔽处	strain 种，族	surgery 外科
shield 盾牌；屏	stroke 打击；中风	surplus 剩余
shift 替换；转移	structure 结构	sour 酸的
shrink 收缩	stuff 物品	source 来源
significant 有意义的	subject to 使……服从	span 跨度
sincere 真诚的	submit 提交	suicide 自杀
slice 片	subsequent 以后的	summit 顶点
slight 轻微的	substance 物质	superficial 表面的
smash 摔碎	substantial 实质的	somewhat 稍微
solar 太阳的	substitute 代替	sore 疼痛的
sole 仅有的；鞋底	succeed 成功	sorrow 悲痛
solve 解决	succession 连续	

第四组

calculate 计算	classical 古典的	competent 有能力的,胜任的	conquest 征服	contradiction 矛盾
cancel 取消	classification 分类	competition 竞争	conscience 良心	contrary 相反的
candidate 候选人	classify 分类	competitive 竞争的	conscious 有意识到	contrast 对比
capture 捕获	client 沉默	complain 抱怨	consequence 结果	contribute 贡献
casual 偶然的	clue 线索	complete 完成	consequently 从而	controversy 辩论
category 种类	code 代码	complex 复杂的	conservative 保守的	convenience 方便
cautious 谨慎的	collapse 倒塌	complicated 复杂的	considerable 相当大的	convenient 方便的
cease 停止	collision 碰撞	component 成分	considerate 考虑周全的	convention 大会
certify 证明	column 圆柱,专栏	compose 组成	consist 由……组成	conversion 转变
chain 链(条)	combat 战斗	comprehensive 全面的	consistent 一致的	convey 表达
challenge 挑战	comedy 戏剧	comprise 包含	constant 一致的,不变的	conviction 深信
charity 慈善	comfort 安慰,舒适	concentrate 集中	constitute 制定	convince 使确信
chase 追赶	command 命令	concept 概念	construct 建构	crazy 疯狂的
chief 小偷	comment 评论	concrete 具体的	consult 咨询	create 创作
chill 寒意,寒冷的	commission 委任,佣金	condemn 谴责,判刑	consume 消费	credit 信任
choke 窒息,阻塞	commit(犯)错误	conference 会议	contact 接触	critical 重要的,危急的
chop 砍	community 团体,社会	confident 自信的	contain 包含	crucial 至关紧要的
circulate 循环	companion 同伴	confine 限制	contemporary 当代的	crush 粉碎
circumstance 情况	comparable 可比较的	confirm 确定	content 内容	cue 暗示
civil 市民的	comparative 比较的	conflict 冲突	contest 竞争	cultivate 培养
clarify 澄清	compass 罗盘,圆规	confront 使面临	context 上下文	curiosity 好奇心
clash 冲击	compel 强迫	confuse 搞乱	continue 继续	current 目前的
classic 杰作,一流的	compete 比赛	conquer 征服	contract 合同	curse 诅咒

第五组

abandon 放弃	alert 警惕	arrest 逮捕
aboard 在船（飞机、车）上	allowance 津贴	artificial 人工的
absent 缺少	ally 结盟	aspect 方面
absolute 绝对的	alter 改变	assemble 集合
absorb 吸收	alternative 选择性的	assess 估定
abuse 滥用	amateur 业余爱好者	asset 资产
academy 研究院，学会	amaze 使吃惊	assign 分配
accent 口音	ambition 雄心	assist 帮助
access 接近	ambulance 救护车	associate 交往
accommodate 供应，供给	amuse 使发笑	association 协会
accomplish 完成	analysis 分析	assume 假定
accordingly 于是	ancestor 祖先	assumption 假定
account 账户	ancient 古代的	assure 保证
accumulate 积累	anniversary 周年纪念	astonish 使吃惊
accurate 精确的	annoy 使烦恼	atmosphere 气氛
accuse 控告	annual 每年都	attach 附上
accustomed 通常的	anticipate 期望	attack 攻击
acknowledge 承认	anxiety 焦虑	attain 获得
acquaintance 相识，熟人	anyhow 无论如何	attempt 尝试
acquire 获得	anyway 无论如何	attend 参加
acquisition 获得	apparent 显然的	attitude 态度
adapt 使适应	appeal 吸引	attract 吸引
addition 加	appliance 用具	attraction 吸引
adequate 足够的	application 应用	attractive 吸引人的
adjust 调整	apply 申请	attribute 属性
admire 羡慕	appoint 指定	audience 观众
advocate 支持	appointment 约会	authority 权威
affect 影响	approach 方法	automatic 自动的
affection 影响	appropriate 适当的	available 可用的
afford 提供	approve 赞成	average 平均的
agency 代理处	approximate 大约	avoid 避免
agenda 日程	architect 建筑师	award 奖
agent 代理人	arise 出现，发生	aware 意识到的
aggressive 好斗的	arouse 引起	awful 可怕的
alarm 警报		awkward 笨拙的

第六组

badly 严重地	data 数据	detect 侦查	effect 效果	evaluate 评价
bankrupt 使破产	dawn 黎明	determination 决定	effective 有效的	eventually 最终
banner 旗帜，标语	deadline 最终期限	devise 设计	efficiency 效率	evidence 证据
bare 赤裸的，空的	deal 交易	devote 投入于	efficient 有效率的	evident 明显的
bargain 议价	debate 争论	dimension 尺度	elaborate 精心制作的	evolution 进化
barrier 障碍	debt 债务	diplomatic 外交的	elegant 文雅的	evolve（使）发展
bearing 轴承	deceive 欺骗	directly 径直地	elementary 初步的	exaggerate 夸张
behalf 代表	decent 正派的	discipline 纪律	eliminate 出去	exceed 超越
behave 举动	declaration 宣布	discuss 讨论	embarrass 使困窘	exchange 交换
belong 属于	decline 下降	disguise 假装	embrace 拥抱	exclaim 惊叫
beloved 心爱的	decorate 装饰	dismiss 解散	emerge 出现	exclude 排出
bend 弯曲的	defeat 打败	display 陈列	emergency 紧急事件	exclusive 排外的
beneficial 有利的	defect 缺点	disposal 处理	emit 发出	execute 执行
blame 责怪	defend 防御	dispute 争论	emotion 情绪	exhaust 用尽
bleed 流血	definitely 明确地	distinct 清楚的	emphasis 强调	exhibit 展示
blend 混合	delegate 代表	distinguish 区别	employ 雇佣	existence 存在
bloom 花开	delete 删除	distress 悲痛	enclose 装入	exit 出口
boast 夸大	deliberate 故意的	disturb 打扰	encounter 遇到	expand 扩展
boil 沸腾	delicate 精巧的	diverse 不同的	endure 忍受	expectation 期望
bold 大胆的	delight 高兴	divorce 离婚	enforce 强迫	expense 花销
bomb 炸弹	deliver 递送	document 文档	engage 从事	expert 专家
boom 繁荣	democracy 民主	domestic 国内的	enhance 提高	exploit 开拓
boost 推进	demonstrate 示范	dominant 支配的	enormous 巨大的	explore 探测
border 边界	deny 否认	dominate 支配	ensure 保证	explosion 爆炸
bore 令人厌烦的人	deposit 存放	donation 捐款	entertain 娱乐	export 出口
boring 令人厌烦的	depress 使沮丧	draft 草稿	entitle 给……授权	expose 使暴露
bounce 弹起	depression 沮丧	drag 拖	envy 嫉妒	exposure 暴露
bound 跳跃	derive 起源	drain 消耗，排水	episode 插曲	extend 扩充
boundary 边界	descend 下降	dramatic 戏剧性的	equation 等式	extent 广度，范围
bow 弓	deserve 值得	drift 漂流	equip 设备	extraordinary 非凡的
broadcast 广播	despair 失望	drip 水滴	equivalent 相等的	extreme 极端的
broom 扫帚	desperate 不顾一切的	durable 持久的	erect 直立的	
budget 预算	despite 尽管	dynamic 动态的	essential 基本的	
burden 负担	destruction 毁灭	ease 安心，悠闲	establishment 确立	
burst 爆炸	detail 细节	economical 节约的	estimate 估计	

第七组

facility 设施	frequency 频率	harness 马具	infect 传染	interval 间隔
factor 因素	frustrate 挫败	harsh 粗糙的	infer 推断	interview 面试
faculty 全体教员	fulfill 完成	haste 匆忙	inferior 下等的	intimate 亲密的
fade 减弱下去	function 功能	hatred 憎恨	infinite 无限的	invade 侵略
faint 晕倒	fund 资金	hazard 冒险	inflation 通货膨胀	invasion 入侵
faith 信任	fundamental 基础的	heading 标题	influence 影响	invest 投资
faithful 信任的	furnish 供应	headline 大字标题	influential 有影响的	investigate 调查
fantastic 幻想的	gain 获得	heal 治愈	inform 通知	invitation 邀请
fascinating 迷人的	gap 裂开，隔阂	hedge 树篱	ingredient 成分	involve 卷入
fasten 扎牢	gaze 凝视	heel 脚后跟	inhabitant 居民	isolate 孤立
fatal 致命的	gene 基因	hesitate 犹豫	inherit 继承	issue 发行
fatigue 疲劳	generate 产生	highlight 突出	initial 初步的	jealous 妒忌的
faulty 有过失的	generous 大方的	hostile 敌对的	initiative 主动	joint 连接
favorable 讨人喜欢的	genuine 真正的	humble 卑下的	injure 受伤	journal 杂志
favorite 喜爱的	germ 细菌	identical 同一的	innocent 无辜的	junior 年少的
feasible 可行的	gesture 手势	identify 识别	insert 插入	justice 正义
feature 特征	glance 扫视	identity 同一性，身份	insight 见识	justify 证明……正义的
feedback 反馈	glimpse 一瞥	ignore 忽略	inspect 检查	keen 热心的，渴望的
fertile 肥沃的	glow 发光	illustrate 阐释	inspire 鼓励	label 标签
fiction 虚构	govern 统治	image 形象	install 安装	lag 落后
fierce 凶猛的	grab 抢夺	imagination 想象	instance 实例	landscape 风景
figure 轮廓	gradual 逐渐的	imagine 想象	instant 立即	launch 下水
file 文件	graduate 毕业	imitate 模仿	instinct 本能	laundry 洗衣店
finance 财务	grant 同意	immense 无边的	institute 学院	leak 泄漏
flame 火焰	grasp 抓住	impact 影响	instruction 指示	lease 租借
flash 动画	grateful 感激的	implement 执行	insult 侮辱	legislation 立法
flexible 灵活的	gratitude 感激	implication 暗示	insure 确保	leisure 空闲
flourish 繁荣	greedy 贪婪的	imply 暗示	integrate 整合	lest 以免
fluent 流利的	grind 磨碎	impose 强加，征税	intellect 智力	liable 有义务的
focus 焦点	grip 紧握	impress 印，留下印象	intelligence 聪明	license 许可证
fond 喜爱的	gross 总的	improve 提高	intend 想要	limitation 限制
forbid 禁止	guarantee 保证	in (en) quire 询问	intense 强烈的	literary 文学的
forget 忘记	guidance 指导	incident 事件	intensity 强烈	loan 贷款
forgive 原谅	guideline 方针	incline 使倾向于	intention 意图	local 当地的

format 格式	guilty 有罪的	indicate 表明	interaction 交互作用	logic 逻辑
formula 公式	halt 停止	indifferent 无所谓的	interfere 干涉	lower 降下
fragment 部分	handle 处理	indispensable 不可缺少的	interior 内部的	loyal 忠实的
frame 框架	handy 便利的	individual 个人的	interpret 解释，口译	luxury 奢侈
freight 货运	harmony 和谐	inevitable 不可避免的	interrupt 打断	

第八组

machinery 机器	myth 神话	outcome 结果	transform 转换	vanish 消失
magnificent 华丽的	namely 即	outlet 出口	translation 翻译	variable 可变的
maintain 维持	nationality 国籍	outline 轮廓	transmission 传播	variety 多样性
manual 手册	neglect 忽略	outlook 前景	transmit 传播	vary 改变
manufacture 制造	negotiate 谈判	output 输出	transparent 透明的	vast 巨大的
margin 页边的空白	nest 巢	outstanding 突出的	transport 运输	vehicle 交通工具
marvelous 非凡的	neutral 中立的	qualification 资格	trash 垃圾	version 版本
massive 大量的	nevertheless 然而	qualify 具有资格	treatment 对待	via 通过
mature 成熟	normal 正常的	quality 质量	treaty 条约	victim 受害人
maximum 最大的	noticeable 引人注意的	quantity 数量	tremble 颤抖	vigorous 精力旺盛的
mechanic 机械的	notify 通知	quotation 引用	tremendous 巨大的	violate 违犯
mechanism 机制	notion 概念	tackle 处理	trend 趋势	violence 暴力
media 媒体	novel 小说	tag 标签	trim 修整	virtual 实质的
medium 媒体，中间的	numerous 大量的	talent 天才	triumph 胜利	virtue 美德
membership 成员资格	objection 异议	tame 驯服	troop 部队	virus 病毒
mend 改进	objective 目标	target 目标	tropical 热带的	visible 可见的
mental 神经的	obligation 义务	technique 技术	twin 双胞胎	visual 视觉的
mention 提及	oblige 强迫	tedious 单调的	twist 扭曲	vivid 生动的
mercy 仁慈	observe 观察	temper 脾气	typical 典型的	volume 卷，量
mere 仅仅的	obstacle 障碍	temporary 临时的	ultimate 最终的	voluntary 自愿的
merit 有点	obtain 获得	temptation 诱惑	uncover 揭开	volunteer 志愿者
mess 混乱	obvious 明显的	tend 趋向	undergo 经历	vote 投票
mild 温和的	occasion 场合	tendency 趋向	unique 独一的	wage 工资
minority 少数	occasional 偶尔的	tender 温柔的	unity 团体	wander 徘徊
miracle 奇迹	occupation 职务	tense 紧张的	universal 普遍的	weed 野草

mirror 镜子	occupy 占领	terminal 终点	upright 垂直的	welfare 福利
miserable 痛苦的	occur 发生	terror 恐怖	upset 不安的	whereas 然而
mislead 误导	occurrence 发生	textile 纺织品	up-to-date 最新的	wipe 擦
mission 使命	odd 奇怪的	theme 主题	urban 城市的	withdraw 撤销
mobile 移动的, 手机	offend 冒犯	theoretical 理论的	urge 促进	withstand 抵挡
mode 模式	offensive 进攻性的	therapy 治疗	urgent 紧急的	witness 证据
moderate 适中的	omit 忽略	thirst 渴	utilize 利用	worship 崇拜
modest 谦逊的	operate 操作	thrive 繁荣	utter 发出声音	worth 价值
modify 修改	opportunity 机会	tissue （动物的）组织	vacant 空的	worthwhile 值得做的
motion 运动	opposite 相反地	toast 吐司	vacuum 真空的	worthy 值得的
motivate 激发	optical 光的	tolerate 忍受	vague 模糊的	wound 创伤
motive 动机	optimistic 乐观的	tough 强硬的	vain 徒然的	wreck 残骸
mount 爬上	option 选项	trace 痕迹	valid 有效的	yield 产出
multiple 多重的	organ 机构	tragedy 灾难	valuable 有价值的	zeal 热情
mutual 相互的	origin 起源	transfer 迁移	value 价值